This book is to be returned on
or before the date stamped below

UNIVERSITY OF PLYMOUTH

PLYMOUTH LIBRARY

Tel: (01752) 232323
This book is subject to recall if required by another reader
Books may be renewed by phone
CHARGES WILL BE MADE FOR OVERDUE BOOKS

NAILS:
Therapy ▪ Diagnosis ▪ Surgery

NAILS:
Therapy ▪ Diagnosis ▪ Surgery

SECOND EDITION

Richard K. Scher, MD
Professor of Dermatology
College of Physicians and Surgeons
Columbia University
New York, New York

C. Ralph Daniel III, MD
Clinical Professor of Medicine (Dermatology)
University of Mississippi Medical Center
Jackson, Mississippi

W.B. SAUNDERS COMPANY
A Division of Harcourt Brace & Company
Philadelphia ▪ London ▪ Toronto ▪ Montreal ▪ Sydney ▪ Tokyo

W.B. SAUNDERS COMPANY
A Division of Harcourt Brace & Company

The Curtis Center
Independence Square West
Philadelphia, PA 19106

Library of Congress Cataloging-in-Publication Data

Nails: therapy, diagnosis, surgery / [edited by] Richard K. Scher, C. Ralph Daniel.—2nd ed.

p.   cm.

Includes bibliographical references and index.

ISBN 0–7216–7026–1

1. Nails (Anatomy)—Diseases.   2. Nails (Anatomy)—Surgery.
  I. Scher, Richard K.   II. Daniel, C. Ralph.
  [DNLM: 1. Nail Diseases. 2. Nails—surgery.   WR 475 N156 1997]

RL 165.D56 1997   616.5'47—dc21

DNLM/DLC   96–36756

Nails: Therapy, Diagnosis, Surgery   ISBN 0–7216–7026–1

The senior author (RKS) wishes to dedicate this edition to those other new additions (grandchildren) who were not present when the 1990 book was produced. They are Jacob Samuel Ohlbaum, Jessica Marie Alexander, and Jonah Kyle Scher-Zagier.

CRD again wishes to thank Melissa, his wife, and Carl and Jon, his sons, for allowing him to spend the time on this endeavor.

Contributors

Edward Akelman, M.D.
Associate Professor,
Brown University School of Medicine,
Providence, Rhode Island; Surgeon-in-Charge,
Hand, Upper Extremity, and Microvascular
Surgery, Rhode Island Hospital, Providence,
Rhode Island
Advanced Surgery

Pamela J. Besuk, M.D.
Attending Physician, Southside Hospital,
Bayshore, New York and Good Samaritan
Hospital, West Islip, New York
Dermatologic Diseases of the Nail Unit

Mary Ellen Brademas, M.D.
Assistant Clinical Professor of Dermatology,
New York University, New York, New York;
Director of Sexually Transmitted Diseases
Clinic, Bellevue Medical Center and Chief of
Dermatology, St. Vincent's Hospital,
New York, New York
Embryology

Maria A. Charif, M.D.
Assistant Professor of Dermatology, Case
Western Reserve University School of
Medicine, Cleveland, Ohio
Onychomycosis

Robert A. Christman, D.P.M.
Assistant Professor and Director of Radiology,
Department of Medicine, Pennsylvania
College of Podiatric Medicine,
Philadelphia, Pennsylvania
*Subungual Exostosis and Nail Disease
and Radiologic Aspects*

Philip R. Cohen, M.D.
Assistant Professor, Department of
Dermatology, University of Texas–Houston
Medical School, Houston, Texas; Assistant
Professor, Department of Medical Specialties,
Dermatology Section, University of Texas
M.D. Anderson Cancer Center,
Houston, Texas
The Nail in Older Individuals

John Thorne Crissey, M.D.
Clinical Professor of Medicine (Dermatology),
University of Southern California School of
Medicine, Los Angeles, California; Senior
Attending Physician, Los Angeles County,
University of Southern California Medical
Center, Los Angeles, California
Historic Aspects of Nail Disease

C. Ralph Daniel III, M.D.
Clinical Professor of Medicine (Dermatology),
University of Mississippi Medical Center,
Jackson, Mississippi
*An Approach to Initial Examination of the Nail;
Onychomycosis; Nonfungal Infections and
Paronychia; Pigmentation Abnormalities; Nails
in Systemic Disease; Nail Changes Secondary
to Systemic Drugs and Ingestants; Glossary;
Appendix 1; Appendix 2*

Melissa P. Daniel, M.C.S.
Assistant Professor, University of Mississippi
Medical Center, School of Health Related
Professions, Jackson, Mississippi
Nonfungal Infections and Paronychia

James Q. Del Rosso, D.O.
Director of Clinical Dermatology, Mohs
Micrographic Surgery Laboratory Director,
Mohave Skin and Cancer Clinic, Laughlin,
Nevada; Clinical Dermatologist, Las Vegas
Skin and Cancer Clinics, Las Vegas, Nevada
Dermatologic Diseases of the Nail Unit

Madelein Duvic, M.D.
Professor of Dermatology and Internal
Medicine, University of Texas Medical School,
Houston, Texas; Chief, Section of
Dermatology, M. D. Anderson Cancer Center,
Houston, Texas
*The Possibility of HIV Transmission by Manicure;
Appendix 5*

Boni Elizabeth Elewski, M.D.
Associate Professor of Dermatology, Case
Western Reserve University School of
Medicine, Cleveland, Ohio
Onychomycosis

Patricia G. Engasser, M.D.
Clinical Professor of Dermatology, Stanford
University School of Medicine, Stanford,
California and University of California,
San Francisco, California; Attending Staff,
Kaiser Hospital, Redwood City, California
Nail Cosmetics

Philip Fleckman, M.D.
Associate Professor of Medicine
(Dermatology), University of Washington
School of Medicine, Seattle, Washington
Basic Science of the Nail Unit

Richard C. Gibbs, M.D.
Clinical Professor of Dermatology,
New York University Medical Center,
New York, New York; Attending in
Dermatology, University Hospital, New York,
New York
Pedal Biomechanics and Toenail Disease

Aldo González-Serva
Department of Dermatology, Boston University
School of Medicine, Boston,
Massachusetts; Attending, Veterans Adminis-
tration Hospital and Carney Hospital, Boston,
Massachusetts
Structure and Function

Aditya K. Gupta, M.D.
Assistant Professor, Division of Dermatology,
Department of Medicine, University of
Toronto, Toronto, Canada
Nonfungal Infections and Paronychia

Leanor D. Haley, Ph.D.
Deceased May 18, 1996
Appendices

James H. Herndon, M.D., M.B.A.
David Silver Professor and Chairman,
Department of Orthopaedic Surgery,
University of Pittsburgh Medical Center,
Pittsburgh, Pennsylvania; Associate Senior
Vice Chancellor for the Health Sciences
and Vice President, Medical Services,
University of Pittsburgh Medical Center,
Pittsburgh, Pennsylvania
Advanced Surgery

Suthep Jerasutus, M.D.
Consultant to Department of Dermatology,
Ramathibody Hospital, Mahidol University,
Bangkok, Thailand; Director of
Suphannahong Dermatology Clinic, Bangkok,
Thailand
Histology and Histopathology

Warren S. Joseph, D.P.M.
Associate Professor of Medicine and Chief,
Infectious Diseases, Pennsylvania College
of Podiatric Medicine, Philadelphia,
Pennsylvania
Pediatric Approach to Onychomycosis

David G. Kern, M.D., M.O.H.
Associate Professor of Medicine and Director,
Program in Occupational Medicine, Brown
University School of Medicine, Providence,
Rhode Island; Director, Division of General
Internal Medicine, Memorial Hospital
of Rhode Island, Pawtucket, Rhode Island
Occupational Disease

Noreen Lemak, M.D.
Research Associate, Department of
Dermatology, The University of Texas
Medical School, Houston, Texas
*The Possibility of HIV Transmission by Manicure;
Appendix 5*

Harvey Lemont, D.P.M.
Director, Foot Dermatology Clinic, Foot
and Ankle Institute, Pennsylvania College of
Podiatric Medicine, Philadelphia,
Pennsylvania; Director, Laboratory
of Podiatric Pathology, Philadelphia,
Pennsylvania
*Subungual Exostosis and Nail Disease
and Radiologic Aspects*

Steven R. Myers, M.D.
Orthopedic Surgeon, Colorado Springs
Orthopedic Group, Colorado Springs,
Colorado
Advanced Surgery

Lawrence A. Norton, M.D.
Clinical Professor Emeritus of Dermatology,
Boston University School of Medicine,
Boston, Massachusetts
Tumors

Lawrence Charles Parish, M.D.
Clinical Professor of Dermatology and
Cutaneous Biology and Director, Jefferson
Center for International Dermatology,
Jefferson Medical College of Thomas Jefferson
University, Philadelphia, Pennsylvania
Historic Aspects of Nail Disease

Anthony R. Ricci
Miriam Hospital, Providence, Rhode Island
Dermatologic Diseases of the Nail Unit

Stuart J. Salasche, M.D.
Clinical Associate Professor of Dermatology,
University of Arizona, Tucson, Arizona
Surgery

W. Mitchell Sams, Jr., M.D.
Professor and Chairman, Department
of Dermatology, University of Alabama
at Birmingham, Birmingham, Alabama
Nails in Systemic Disease

Richard K. Scher, M.D.
Professor of Dermatology, College
of Physicians and Surgeons, Columbia
University, New York, New York
*The Nail in Older Individuals; Dermatologic
Diseases of the Nail Unit; Nails in Systemic
Disease; Nail Changes Secondary to Systemic
Drugs and Ingestants*

Robert A. Silverman, M.D.
Associate Clinical Professor, Department of
Pediatrics, Georgetown University,
Washington, D.C.; Assistant Clinical
Professor, Department of Dermatology, Case
Western Reserve, Cleveland, Ohio; Director,
Pediatric Dermatology, Georgetown
University Children's Medical Center,
Washington, D.C.
Pediatric Disease

Justin Wernick, D.P.M.
Professor, Department of Orthopedics,
New York College of Podiatric Medicine,
New York, New York
Pedal Biomechanics and Toenail Disease

Preface

It is indeed a privilege to be able to write the second edition of a practical, easy-to-use textbook on nails that is easy to carry and not overweight. This book, like its predecessor, should be useful to virtually all health care providers because it stresses treatment after accurate diagnosis is made. The content elaborates in great detail how to identify nail disease so that subsequent therapy will be effective. The book goes significantly further than providing medical treatment protocols in its extensive development of nail surgical techniques from the simple everyday procedures to the more complex, so that both the generalist, whatever his or her field—and the trained surgeon—will find significant value in it.

The chapter on onychomycosis has been vastly expanded and rewritten in view of the breakthrough developments that have occurred since 1990. Thus a broad and complete discussion of all the new antifungal medications used for treatment of nail mycoses is presented in an easily applicable manner for everyday office implementation. A new chapter for podiatrists has been added and earlier podiatric chapters have been updated and expanded so that the podiatrist, who cares for a major segment of the onychodystrophies, will find this an invaluable text. Readers will also benefit from an important and unique chapter devoted to geriatric nail problems. This discussion should prove invaluable considering the huge increase in this segment of the population. The nail salon advice material is particularly appropriate considering that annually several billion dollars are spent on nail cosmetics in the United States alone. Another noteworthy portion of the book is devoted to nail disorders in the HIV-positive patient, a topic not elaborated on significantly elsewhere. All the remaining chapters have been revised and made current to keep pace with the rapidly progressive field of onychology.

The editors are grateful to all those health care practitioners who have made this book the most successful one ever devoted to nail disorders. This text has found worldwide distribution in large numbers, including translations into several languages. The authors are most appreciative of this. We look forward to this second edition as a bridge to the twenty-first century. All the authors have worked together to produce an integrated work that is not fragmented or overloaded with scores of unnecessary references.

RICHARD K. SCHER
C. RALPH DANIEL III

Contents

xiii

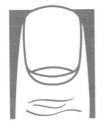 # The Normal Nail

CHAPTER 1

Historic Aspects of Nail Disease

John Thorne Crissey and Lawrence Charles Parish

Nails fit awkwardly into the dermatologic scheme of things. They are altered by internal disturbances and by skin diseases as well. They are subject to the effects of environment and the whims and cosmetic manipulations of their owners and have, in addition, a set of diseases all their own. In dealing with nails, authors of dermatologic texts for 200 years have had to compromise with the tenets of orderliness and sound organizational procedures to distribute information concerning nails here and there in the body of their works, wherever it seemed appropriate. Yet they have still found it necessary to create large, elastic catchall categories in which to stow whatever is left. These problems are brought into particularly sharp focus when one attempts, as we have here, to track the development of our knowledge of nail structure, function, and disease. The accumulation of facts was painfully slow. It followed no discernible pattern and was recorded in the literature of a variety of disciplines that communicated poorly with one another.

Nails also present clinical problems. They are capable of no more than a narrowly limited number of morphologic responses to a very large number of pathologic stimuli, and nail dystrophies, therefore, tax the diagnostic abilities of even the most experienced clinicians. Moreover, the nail complex, unlike the skin, does not readily lend itself to biopsy. Pa-

tient resistance and the ever present risk of producing permanent damage with biopsy procedures involving the nail more often than not deprived dermatologists of their favorite diagnostic aid. Anatomic and physiologic difficulties also confront the examiner. In accordance with medical wisdom, the intelligent management of nail disease requires a thorough understanding of normal structure, growth, and function. Authors face a maximum challenge to their ingenuity and literary skills to lay these matters out for their readers in a manner that is both interesting and easily understood. This challenge has not been successfully met in the past. An examination of the older dermatologic texts that were issued in paper covers and later bound in cloth often shows the sections on nail anatomy and physiology have been left uncut and never read. Nor do we see many finger marks, or underlining, or dog-ears on the analogous pages of similar sections in more modern works.

If it is difficult to splice together a coherent and useful picture of the nail and its diseases even equipped as we now are with all the advantages, techniques, and accumulated knowledge—imagine the obstacles faced by interested physicians in the days before the simple fact was known that tissue is made up of cells. This extract from an 1827 paper by London's renowned surgeon-anatomist Sir Astley Patson Cooper illustrates the sort of thinking that went into the precellular approach[1]:

Opposite the hollow at the root of the nail is placed a highly vascular and villous surface, which I call the ungual gland, and the portion of the nail over this surface is thinner than the rest. Beyond this secreting surface appear a number of laminae, like the underpart of the mushroom, which are parallel with those placed in the inner part of the nail, and which pass in the direction of the axis of the finger. The parts of the nail usually cut project beyond these laminae.

The ungual gland is a very vascular surface, and its use is to secrete the nail, which proceeds from it between the laminae placed before it, so that the nail grows from its root, as may be easily seen by cutting a notch there, which grows gradually out in about three months, advancing until it reaches the extremity of the nail.

The first investigator to consider nail structure in any detail after the acceptance of the cellular theories of Schwann was Rudolph Albert von Kölliker, of Würzburg, whose *Manual of Human Histology* (1852) ranks as one of the most important works in 19th-century medicine. The 15-page description of the nail complex, which appears in the first edition of Kölliker's manual, is rich in detail and reads very smoothly even now.[2]

The transfer of cellular anatomic concepts to the study of nail diseases was accomplished in the same era by Gustav Simon, of Berlin, whose *Hautkrankheiten Durch Anatomische Untersuchungen Erlaütert,* published in 1848, was the earliest textbook devoted entirely to dermatohistopathology.[3] Virchow's 1854 essay on the subject was also a contribution of considerable importance.[4]

Studies on nail growth rates were mentioned as early as 1684, in the work of the remarkable British investigator Robert Boyle, whose *Experiments and Considerations About the Porosity of Bodies* also marked the beginning of investigations into the transfer of substances across the natural barrier of the skin.[5] Actual data on nail growth appeared first in 1741 in Albrecht Haller's addition to Boerhave's *Predilectiones Academicae.* He estimated, from the movement of gold salt stains on nails, that transit from cuticle to free edge took place in 3 months. Nail growth and its corollaries have long intrigued individuals in a broad spectrum of disciplines—for example, in the biologic sciences, anthropology, and sociology. The subject also has been of interest to Asian princesses, Siamese actresses, Brazilian zither virtuosos, the compilers of the *Guinness Book of World Records,* and certainly Herr Otto Kellner, whose

25-year collection of his own nail clippings (Fig. 1–1) was considered impressive enough to be placed on display in the Royal Anatomical Museum in Berlin. However, in the more prosaic world of science, the measurement and study of nail growth were placed on a modern footing in 1850 in the assiduous and detailed research carried out by Arnold Berthold of Göttingen.[6]

In the early years of the 19th century, tissues belonging to "horny substance" class were regarded as among the simplest in the animal organism and considered merely as different forms of the same matrix, which, in the 1854 words of C. G. Lehmann, one of the era's leading authorities on chemistry, "certain chemists were ready enough to discover and to designate by the name Keratin." "The zealous labours of recent histologists," he added, "have, however, shown us that even these ap-

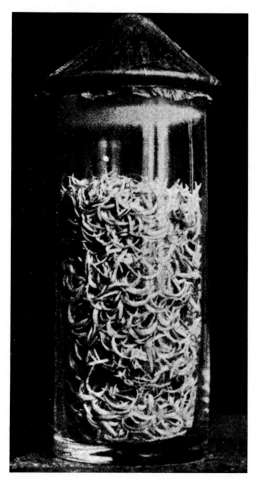

Figure 1–1. Herr Otto Kellner's personal nail clippings, collected over a 25-year period and placed on display in the Royal Anatomical Museum in Berlin. Total weight, 51.5 g.

parently homogeneous tissues have a complicated and, in many respects, a variable structure."[7] He was referring of course to the work of Kölliker, Simon, and Virchow.

The first biochemical study of nails with any claim to modernity is to be found in the 1837 inaugural dissertation of Theodore Theophil Matecki of Breslau, *De ungue humano*.[8] Destined later to become one of Poland's most prominent citizens, Matecki in this early work outlined the results of distillation, alcohol extraction, and residual ash experiments along with investigations into acid and base solubilities and the like. However, real progress along these lines was not possible until the publication in 1838 of the classic papers on the nature of protein by Gerardus Mulder,[9] an associate at the time of the renowned Julius Liebig of Giessen, who trained most of the important biochemists of the era. In 1840, Johann Joseph Scherer, another associate of Liebig, followed the lead of Mulder and calculated for the first time the C, H, N, L, and S percentages for nails, hair, horn, and feathers.[10] By the end of the 19th century, individual amino acid constituents of various proteins were routinely being reported, and K.A.H. Mörner of the Caroline Institute in Stockholm, whose enormous paper on sulfur-protein combinations (1902) is now considered a classic, noted the surprisingly high content of sulfur in hair, mostly in the form of cystine.[11] In 1907, Hans Buchtala of Graz used Mörner's techniques to demonstrate that such was also the case for nails.[12] It is one of history's many little quirks that cystine, the first of the amino acids to be discovered (1810), was the last to be identified in horny tissues.[13] Extraction methods used throughout the 19th century unfortunately ensured denaturation of cystine before it could be detected. From this point on, the elucidation of the nature of nail protein merges with the study of molecular structure of keratin in general, our knowledge of which owes so much to experiments on wool fibers conducted in the 1930s by W.T. Astbury, H.J. Woods, and J.B. Speakman, all of whom worked at the University of Leeds in England.[14]

Paul Unna and L. Golodetz published the first detailed analysis of the fatty substances associated with the nail matrix (1909),[15] although the presence of fat had been duly noted in the 1837 thesis of Matecki.

That disturbances in the nails can be secondary to larger problems in the organism is an ancient idea. Indeed, the earliest reference of any sort to nails in the medical literature is a one-liner included in the *Prognostics* of Hippocrates as one of the symptoms of empyema: "The nails of the hand are bent"—which is to say, curved over the tips of the fingers. The association with clubbing to complete the picture of the "Hippocratic fingers" is later described from time to time in a large number of pulmonary diseases.

The Parisian Dr. Joseph Honoré Simon Beau described his famous transverse line in 1846 as a part of an in-depth study of nail growth in general.[16] His suspicions that the temporary interference in keratin formation represented by the lines could follow innumerable disturbances in the body economy have been confirmed many times over in the perpetual rediscovery of his sign, which, because it is so easily demonstrated, continues to interest clinicians to a degree beyond its practical worth.

The association of nail changes with specific skin diseases is a 19th-century phenomenon made possible by the successful separation of these clinical entities one from another by Robert Willan in England and by his energetic disciples in France. Willan himself was the first to describe the nail changes in psoriasis. In his chef d'oeuvre *On Cutaneous Diseases* (1808), he set up a special category, Psoriasis unguium, to accommodate the condition[17]:

> The Psoriasis unguium sometimes occurs alone, but it is usually connected with scaly patches on the arms, hands, etc. In some cases, the nails from the middle appear brown or yellowish; they bend upwards and are ragged at the ends and rough on the surface. In other cases they are thickened, deeply indented, and bent downwards over the ends of the fingers.

The association of nail dystrophy with eczematous eruptions is first described in the 1835 treatise of Pierre Rayer (Fig. 1–2). The clinical *verismo* that characterizes all of the work of this Parisian master is evident again in his account of the condition as it occurred in an 80-year-old man under his care[18]:

> For the last 12 years he has been subject to eczema, at one time in the squamous, at another in the humid state, between the buttocks and about the margin of the anus. Two years ago an aggregation of the same kind made its appearance about the nails of the toes, and subsequently about those of the fingers. The nails of the toes are particularly remarkable for their deformity; they are of a greenish-yellow color, and are detached from their matrices, being raised upon a mass of solid matter of the same color, and of a faint and sickly smell, three or four lines in thickness, which even extends beyond their ends and edges. The nails are painful when cut, the action of the knife or scis-

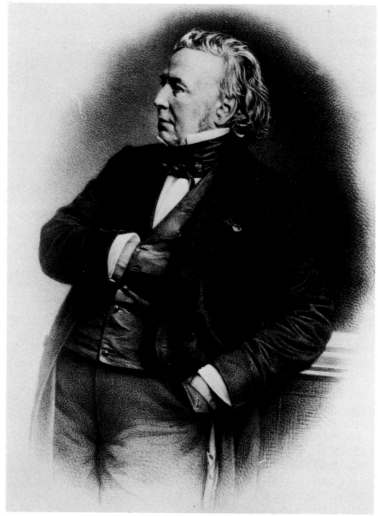

Figure 1–2. Pierre François Olive Rayer (1793–1867). Rayer was the leading authority on nail diseases (among many other things) in the early decades of the 19th century.

sors jarring the roots. A yellowish liquid matter occasionally exudes from under the lateral parts of the nails, which are then more than usually painful.

The Rayer treatise is by far the best source of information on nails and nail diseases in the early part of the 19th century. It is in fact the first publication in which these structures were considered in any detail at all and also the first to feature illustrations of nail problems. Indeed, Plate XXI (Fig. 1–3) in the atlas that accompanied the magnificent second edition of the treatise no doubt set some sort of record in the annals of medical illustration.[19] Onychomycosis, onychogryphosis, acute paronychia, traumatic onychia, subungual wart, and congenital deformities of the nail all make their initial appearance there in picture form—along with the first illustrations of verruca vulgaris, verruca filiformis, black hairy tongue, and alopecia of the beard. Nail changes associated with eczema, psoriasis, tuberculosis, and syphilis are also illustrated, again for the first time, in other plates. Paul Gerson Unna regarded the Rayer treatise as one of the finest works ever written on skin diseases, and certainly we concur with his opinion.

Pityriasis rubra pilaris can also affect the nails. The original descriptions of the disease appear in the works of Rayer[20] and Alphonse Devergie,[21] but the disease was distinguished from psoriasis and lichen planus only after an incredible amount of clinical bickering in print. The matter was settled late in the 19th century when case presentations at various international dermatologic meetings demonstrated the disease to be a clinically distinct entity. The

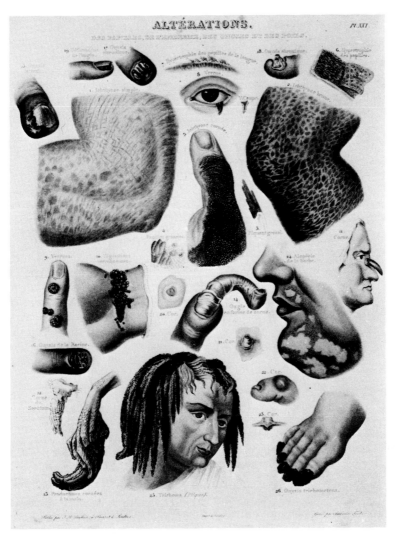

Figure 1–3. Plate XXI from Rayer's *Traité Théorique et Pratique des Maladies de la Peau* (1835). Rayer's treatise was the first in which nail diseases were considered in any detail. A number of nail problems were illustrated in Plate XXI for the very first time.

nail changes were first noted by Jonathan Hutchinson in 1878 in a review paper on nail problems that was much admired at the time[22]:

> *Pityriasis rubra [pilaris] is a rare and very peculiar malady. We know nothing of its causes, and most of which we know of its course can be summed up in the following statements: In certain adult persons a state of persistent congestion of the whole integument with exfoliation of epidermis may occur, the patient becoming everywhere of vivid red colour, and the epidermis peeling off in large flakes. Where the skin is thick, as in the palms and soles, the epidermis may accumulate in layers like the leaves in a book, sometimes making up a thickness of half an inch, or even more. The disease is chronic, prone to relapse, and often attended by great debility. For our present purpose we are concerned with this malady only because in it there is usually much disease of the nails. The changes consist in opacity of the nail, with deposit of epidermis between it and its bed. When the skin disease subsides, the nails participate in the benefit. In these cases the nails are implicated as parts of the general integument, the whole skin being affected. It is, however, remarkable that they should suffer so severely. I have rarely seen nails so much thickened and deformed as in some of these cases.*

The earliest pictures of pityriasis rubra pilaris, including the nail changes (Fig. 1–4), were also prepared under the direction of Hutchinson for the New Sydenham Society Atlas (1860–1875).

We note in passing that Hutchinson was fascinated by nail diseases throughout his life, as he was by all disturbances in the integument and its accessory structures, and he was always on the lookout for new ways of looking

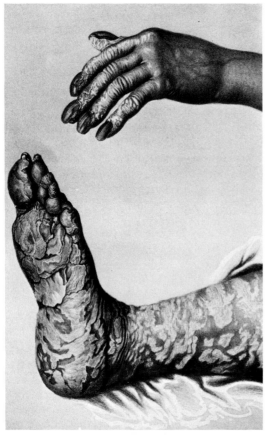

Figure 1–4. Pityriasis rubra pilaris. Section of a lithograph prepared under the direction of Jonathan Hutchinson for the *New Sydenham Society Atlas* (1860–1884).

at dermatologic problems. "It is convenient," he wrote, "to think of a nail as a gigantic flattened hair, the walls of the follicle of which are flattened on one side."[22] This idea helped explain to the clinicians of the time the simultaneous involvement of hair and nails in so many conditions and even now remains valid, if one takes into account the obvious difference that hair growth is cyclic, whereas nails grow continuously.

Lichen planus affects the nails in some 5 to 10 per cent of cases, and yet the nail changes were not noticed until 1901, four decades after Erasmus Wilson's original description of the disease itself. The association was made by the remarkable William Dubreuilh of Bordeaux, clinician extraordinaire and restless experimenter, who could also claim among his many accomplishments the first description of plantar warts. The heart of his "lichen plan des ongles" report reads like this[23]:

> The nails are profoundly altered. They show very fine longitudinal striations. These striations are per-

fectly parallel and occupy the entire length of the nail; they are at least a third of a millimeter in width, are deep and contiguous, and at some points are clearly formed by longitudinal splitting in narrow elevated grooves. The nail appears uneven, as though roughened by a rasp or coarse grit. In short, the appearance corresponds exactly to the changes I have previously described under the name onychorrhexis. The general shape of the nails is preserved; they do not appear to be reduced in thickness, but according to the patient, they are fragile and often break; they are adherent to the bed, which is normal, and the external surface alone is altered. However, both little fingers show a cornified pad under the free edge of the nail, brownish in color, and attributable to hyperkeratosis of the bed.

Syphilis of the nails received a great deal of attention in the dermatologic and venereologic literature of the 18th and 19th centuries. The first description of any length is to be found in John Hunter's *Treatise on Venereal Diseases* (1786), the same great compendium in which the hunterian chancre description appears, along with the account of the author's celebrated and unlucky self-inoculation experiment. Hunter described the nail changes as follows[24]:

> The disease on its first appearance often attacks that part of the fingers upon which the nail is formed, making that surface red which is seen shining through the nail, and if allowed to continue, a separation of the nail takes place, similar to the cuticle in the before described symptoms; but here there cannot be that regular succession of nails as there is of cuticle.

That simple account gave way to more and more elaborate descriptions as the disease became the subject of intense investigation in the middle and later decades of the 19th century. By 1879, for example, the handsome and eminently successful New York venereologist Freeman J. Bumstead, America's first authentic genitourinary expert, was able in his textbook to spin out several thousand words on the subject.[25] It had become clear by this time that nail involvement was more likely to be associated with relapsing or late syphilis than with the early stages, as well as with the congenital form of the disease. Until the 20th century, syphilis of the nails was often called onychia maligna. The name, which finally succumbed to its obvious disadvantages, was coined by James Wardrop of London in a famous and much quoted review of the diseases of fingers and toes published in 1814.[26] It is a measure of the distance we have come that today's busy dermatologists or even venereologists might spend a lifetime without ever seeing such a case.

The earliest references to diseases originating in the nail complex itself are also ancient. Celsus (53 B.C.–A.D. 7) considered both acute paronychia and the swollen flap of skin, with or without granulation tissue, that often extends over the nail plate in these cases.[27] He recommended surgical intervention when conservative methods failed. No doubt his clinical material included ingrown toenails, although he did not mention that condition specifically. Paulus Aeginita, a seventh-century Greek physician, dealt with similar problems.[28] He also made recommendations for the treatment of subungual hemorrhages and furnished several prescriptions containing sulfur, arsenic, and cantharides for the removal of diseased nails, especially those that were "leprous," whatever that may have meant.

Chiropodists would have us believe that Lewis Durlacher of London was the first to delineate accurately the lowly ingrown toenail and the troubles that surround it.[29] Durlacher, who was by far the best-known practitioner of his profession in England in the middle decades of the 19th century, was the first to emphasize or perhaps even to mention that incorrect cutting of the nail was usually the cause of the problem. However, in every other aspect of precedence, he was far down on the list. Paulus Aeginita gave an easily recognizable description of the condition,[28] as did most of the ancients. Indeed, along with paronychia, the ubiquitous ingrown toenail must have been a common cause of limping about in the caves of the Cro-Magnons and Neanderthals, contributing in a small way to the natural surliness of the species.

In 1726, Daniel Turner described ingrown nails in his remarkable treatise on skin diseases,[30] but it was not until the beginning of the 19th century that the condition was considered in any detail. Diseases sometimes become fashionable subjects for medical writing for mysterious reasons that have little to do with new discoveries or with perceived alterations in the course or demography of the conditions, and such would appear to be the case with unguis incarnatus at that time. Baron Dupuytren, then the leading surgeon, supplied the most influential of the many accounts available. He managed the condition as follows[31]:

I pass one blade of a pair of straight, strong, sharp scissors rapidly under the middle of the nail almost to its base, and divide it at a single stroke into two nearly equal halves. With a pair of pliers I then grasp the half that lies over the ulceration and pull it off by

turning it back upon itself. If the other side is also diseased, I remove it in the same way. In those cases in which the fungoid tissue adjacent to the wound is considerably elevated I apply the hot cautery to destroy it and to ensure, in so far as possible, a cure for the disease.

Dupuytren claimed that the procedure was not particularly painful, but Pierre Prosper Baumès, the notable dermatologist from Lyons, was more honest about it when he admitted that even the most stoic of his patients "suffered horribly" and cried out in agony when the operation began.[32] It is of course possible that in those days before the advent of anesthesia, the pain of so trivial an operation failed to impress a general surgeon like the baron, who had to inflict great suffering every working day of his life.

The original description of subungual malignant melanoma is attributed to Dubourg, who called the lesion "melanic subungual cancer" and described it as a large, black, spherical tumor more than 4 inches in diameter, with a knobby surface, growing steadily for 3 years at the site of a preexisting thin, black line beneath the nail. The line had persisted unchanged for 27 years.[33] The tumor "creaked" when cut across with the knife, a sign considered indicative of cancer at the time. Melanotic whitlow was redescribed, and named, by Jonathan Hutchinson in 1857.[34] Three decades and a half a dozen disastrous cases later (1886), he warned his colleagues that these lesions were extraordinarily dangerous, always malignant, and in need of prompt, effective intervention.[35]

Descriptions of mycotic infections of the nail, identifiable as such, appear first in the 1829 treatise on scalp ringworm by the Parisian empiric Mahon the younger.[36] Mahon was the most prominent member of a family that contracted to take care of favus and allied scalp conditions at l'Hôpital St. Louis in Paris in the early and middle decades of the 19th century. The family, no member of which was a physician, used "secret" remedies in their scalp treatment station, mostly depilatories consisting of sulfur and sodium carbonate. In his treatise, Mahon extolled the virtues of his secret pomades and advertised his skills in an unconscionable manner. Despite its commercial approach, the book contained much of value—for example, the earliest description of "gray patch," or microsporum tinea capitis, which was new to Europe at the time. Mahon also used his treatise as a forum from which to attack some of the dangerous and brutal methods then used for the treatment of favus, and his efforts led to much-needed therapeutic reforms. In this remarkable work the first description of favus of the nails appears[36]:

> The nails of the toes and fingers showed to the highest degree those changes attributable to the favic influence; they were very thick and split into layers at the tips, as it were, reminding the observer of the statue of Daphne changing into the laurel tree, in which the transformation of human into ligneous material is depicted—although there is, to be sure, a considerable distance between the graceful aspect of that artistic production and the appearance of this unfortunate individual who was reduced to that deplorable state which some would leave to nature alone to cure.
>
> The alterations in the nails caused by favus would appear to result from a disturbance and an increase in the corneous secretion of which they are composed, because they increase in thickness and grow outward to an unusual degree. The regularity and polish of the normal state gives way to a longitudinal rugosity; they become frayed at the ends; they do not fall off, but become more sensitive than normal; they take on the yellow color characteristic of favus.

The metaphor was labored—Daphne changed into a laurel tree to escape from the amorous advances of Apollo—but the clinical description, the first of onychomycosis, was perfectly satisfactory. In a later section, Mahon noted similar nail changes in a case of gray patch ringworm but observed that the yellow color was lacking.

Credit for the discovery of the dermatophyte itself in nail substance belongs to George Meissner (the discoverer of the corpuscles that go by his name), who in 1853 observed hyphae in a potassium hydroxide preparation of a "thick finger nail, bent clawlike," taken from an 80-year-old man.[37] The term *onychomycosis* appears to have been coined by Virchow 3 years later in 1856.[38]

Candida albicans infection of nails was first reported by Dübendorfer in 1904.[39]

Finally, for those who wish to pursue the subject further, we offer a helpful suggestion. As Rayer was the most knowledgeable authority on nails in the early decades of the 19th century, so Julius Heller (1864–1931) of Berlin was the Herr Nägel, the "Mr. Nails," at the beginning of the 20th century. His *Krankheiten der Nägel*[40] (Fig. 1–5), a 300-page *Meisterstück*, appeared in print in 1900. Thoroughly Teutonic in its treatment, organization, and detail, this work contains many original observations and references to almost everything worth knowing about nails in the literature of the time. Heller's lifelong preoccupation with nails culminated in an exhaustive essay on the subject in the Jadassohn *Handbuch* of 1927. Serious reviews of the older literature should begin with these two works.

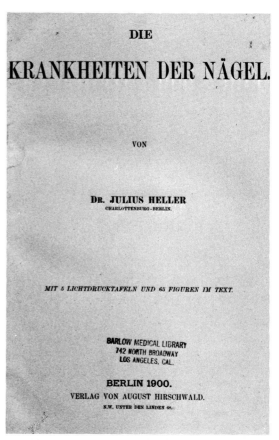

Figure 1–5. Title page of Heller's *Krankheiten der Nägel (Diseases of the Nails)*, 1900. Julius Heller (1864–1931) was the "Mr. Nails" of the medical world in the early decades of the 20th century. The exhaustive treatment of the subject in his treatise far exceeded anything that had gone before.

References

1. Cooper A: Diseases of the nails. Lond Med Phys J 57:289, 1827.
2. Kölliker RA: Manual of Human Histology. Sydenham Society, London, 1853, pp 153–168.
3. Simon G: Hautkrankheiten durch anatomische Untersuchungen erläutert. G. Reimer, Berlin, 1848, pp 366–375.
4. Virchow R: Zur normalen und pathologischen Anatomie der Nägel. Verhandl Med Phys Gesellschft Würzburg 5(B):83, 1854.
5. Boyle R: Experiments and Considerations About the Porosity of Bodies. Samuel Smith, London, 1684.
6. Berthold A: Beobactungen über das quantative Verhältniss der Nägel—und Haarbildung beim Menschen. Müller's Arch, 1850.
7. Lehmann CG: Physiological Chemistry. Cavendish Society, London, 1854, p 53.

8. Matecki TT: De ungue humano. Inaugural dissertation, Wratislaviae, 1837.

9. Mulder GJ: Guzammensetzung von Fibrin, Albumin, Leimzucker, Leucin, usw. Ann Pharm 28:73, 1838.

10. Scherer JJ: Animal Chemistry of Organic Chemistry. Taylor and Walton, London, 1842.

11. Mörner KAH: Zur Kentniss der Bindung des Schwefels in den Proteinstoffen. Hoppe-Seyler's Z Physiol Chem 34:207, 1902.

12. Buchtala H: Ueber das Mengenverhältnis des Cystins in Hornsubstanzen. Hoppe-Seyler's Z Physiol Chem 52:474, 1907.

13. Vickery HB, Schmidt CL: History of the discovery of the amino acids. Chem Rev 9:169, 1931.

14. Fraser RDB, Gillespie JM: Wool structure and biosynthesis. Nature 261:650, 1976.

15. Unna PG, Golodetz L: Die Hautfette. Biochem Z 20:469, 1909.

16. Beau JHS: Note sur certains charactères de séméologie rétrospective présentés par les ongles. Arch Gén Méd (4s) 11:447, 1846.

17. Willan R: On Cutaneous Diseases, Vol VI. J Johnson, London, 1808, p 169.

18. Rayer P: Theoretical and Practical Treatise on the Diseases of the Skin. Carey and Hart, Philadelphia, 1845, p 383.

19. Rayer P: Traité des Maladies de la Peau, Atlas. JB Baillière, Paris, 1835.

20. Rayer P: Traité des Maladies de la Peau, Vol 2. JB Baillière, Paris, 1835, p 158.

21. Devergie A: Pityriasis Pilaris. Traité Pratique des Maladies de la Peau, ed 2. Libraire de Victor Masson, Paris, 1857, pp 454–455.

22. Hutchinson J: On the nails and the diseases to which they are liable. Medical Times Gazette, April 20, 1878, pp 423–426.

23. Dubreuilh W: Lichen plan des ongles. Ann Dermatol Syphilig 2:606, 1901.

24. Hunter J: Treatise on the Venereal Disease. 13 Castle St, London, 1786, p 321.

25. Bumstead FJ, Taylor RW: Pathology and Treatment of Venereal Diseases, ed 4. Henry C Lea, Philadelphia, 1879, pp 578–582.

26. Wardrop J: An account of some diseases of the toes and fingers, with observations on their treatment. Med Clin Trans 5:129, 1814.

27. Celsus: Of Medicine, in eight books [lib VI, chap XIX]. H Renshaw etc., London, 1838, pp 335–336.

28. Paulus Aeginita: The Seven Books of Paulus Aeginita, Vol 6, pp 679–683, Vol 2 pp 414–416. Sydenham Society, London, 1844.

29. Dagnall JC: Durlacher and "the nail growing into the flesh." Br Chirop J 27:263, 1962.

30. Turner D: De Morbis Cutaneis, ed 3. R and J Bonwicke etc, London, 1726, pp 267–273.

31. Dupuytren G: Leçons Orales de Clinique Chirurgicale de Dupuytren, Vol 4. Paris, 1834, p 392.

32. Baumès PP: Nouvelle Dermatologie, Vol 2. JB Baillière, Paris, 1842, pp 381–387.

33. Dubourg NI: Cancer mélané du petit doigt de la main droite. J Hébdom Méd 7:73, 1830.

34. Hutchinson J: Melanotic whitlow. Trans Pathol Soc 8:404, 1857.

35. Hutchinson J: Melanosis often not black; melanotic whitlow. BMJ 1:491, 1886.

36. Mahon M Jr: Recherches sur la Siège et la Nature des Teignes. JB Baillière, Paris, 1829, pp 59–61, 139.

37. Meissner G: Pilzbildung in den Nägeln. Arch Phys Heilkünde 12:193, 1853.

38. Virchow R: Beitrage zur Lehre von den beim Menschen vorkommenden pflan zlichen Parasiten. Virchows Arch 9:557, 1856.

39. Dübendorfer E: Ein Fall von Onchomycosis blasomycetica. Dermatol Zentralbl 7:290, 1904.

40. Heller J: Krankheiten der Nägel. August Hirschwald, Berlin, 1900.

CHAPTER 2

Structure and Function

Aldo González-Serva

The human nail, the horny covering of the upper surface of the tip of each finger and toe, is a set of complex structures that can most accurately be called the nail unit.

The visible nail plate is the ultimate product of the continuous pathway of maturation that occurs in this very active, specialized keratinizing unit. It is mainly through observations of this plate that patient and clinician become aware of the presence of disease in the unit as a whole.[15,17–20] However, it is important to understand the functional and structural organization of the deeper, concealed components of the system, which account for the external findings clinically seen in the nails. This chapter deals with those components that are responsible for development of a normal nail plate. For the most part, morphologic components are discussed, but physiologic aspects of nail growth are also included.

FUNCTIONS OF THE NAIL

The nail has evolved phylogenetically with the development of manual dexterity. From the claw of lower mammals, birds, reptiles, and other phyla, both hoof and nail have evolved divergently in higher species.[21]

The hooves of bovines and other quad rupeds are suited to the lifestyles of these ani-

mals, which graze and run. The nails of primates and humans developed with the ability of these animals to grasp and manipulate objects. These manual abilities could not have evolved without the support of the nails. Indeed, the nail plates act as buttresses that appose the fingertips,[17] increasing the discriminatory ability of the acral pulp and skin whenever an object is felt or grasped between two fingers: A half or a full pincer is provided by rigid peripheral nail plates. Such a pincer grip is even more efficient than the blunt support that would be provided solely by a pair of phalangeal bones.

The intensified sensory discrimination provided by the nail-enhanced pincer grip also permits additional dexterity when handling minute objects because it improves the capability for fine digital movements.

The nails fulfill the more general and indispensable function of protecting the terminal phalanx and fingertip from traumatic impact.

In primates and humans, the nails serve also as scratching organs[22] and are used more frequently for grooming and alleviation of itching than for offense or defense against sexual rivals and predators.

In humans, the nails may serve an aesthetic and cosmetic purpose through a variety of manipulations and modifications. Even social status can be silently communicated by the

12

condition of the nails. Chinese noblemen grew long nails to demonstrate their avoidance of any type of manual work. Table 2–1 is a summary of the functions of the nail unit.

COMPONENTS OF THE NAIL UNIT

The nail unit consists of six main components,[17,19,20] which form, ensheathe, support, anchor, and frame the nail plate:

1. The generating portion, which is represented by the nail matrix.

2. The product portion, or nail plate.

3. The ensheathing portion, or cuticular system, which dorsally comprises the obvious and visible "cuticle," or eponychium, and more deeply and proximally the less obvious but indispensable true cuticle. These cuticles are derived from the marginal dorsal part and from the ventral part of the proximal nail fold, respectively. The cuticular system beneath the nail plate is represented by the hyponychium and, more deeply and proximally, by the solehorn and the bed horny layer.[23] These latter keratinous products derive from the hyponychial epithelium and from the bed epithelium (the solehorn from the "fertile" distal part and the bed horny layer from the proximal bed epithelium), respectively.

Table 2–1. **FUNCTIONS OF THE NAIL UNIT**

Protection of the phalanges and fingertips
Enhancement of fine touch and fine digital movements
Scratching and grooming
Aesthetic and cosmetic organ

4. The supporting portion, which consists of nail bed mesenchyme ("dermis") and of phalangeal bone.[13,24]

5. The anchoring portion, represented by the specialized mesenchyme, which is most likely ligamentary and which exists proximally between the phalanx and the matrix and distally between the phalanx and the lateral and distal grooves.

6. The framing portion, which is composed of the nail folds ("nail walls")—specifically, the dorsal part of the proximal nail fold, the lateral folds, and the distal fold.

Spatial Disposition of Components of the Nail

On external observation from above and from the side, the visible parts of the nail unit are as follows (Fig. 2–1):

Dorsal aspect of the proximal nail fold
Lateral nail folds
Obvious "cuticle" (eponychium)

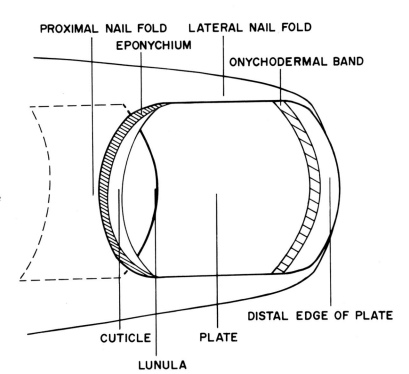

Figure 2–1. Dorsal view of the nail unit.

Subtle true cuticle (nail vest)
Plate
Distal matrix (lunula)
Onychodermal band
Distal free edge of the plate

On gross and microscopic observation of the nail unit along a sagittal section (longitudinally) through the main axis of the finger, the parts to be observed, in addition to those just mentioned, are as follows (Fig. 2–2A):

Ventral aspect of the proximal nail fold
Occult portion of the true cuticle
Remaining proximal matrix
Bed (epithelium and horny layer)
Distal, highly keratinizing (fertile) bed epithelium and horn (solehorn)
Hyponychium (angle, epithelium, and horn)

Distal groove
Distal nail fold
Nail field mesenchyme ("dermis" and ligaments)
Phalanx

Modes of Keratinization of the Epithelial Components of the Nail

Among the epithelia composing the generating, ensheathing, and framing portions of the nail unit, various modes of differentiation are manifested by the production of histologically distinct, specific types of keratin. These keratinizing modes are as follows:

1. Onychokeratinization, which occurs in the matrix epithelium. The product is the hard keratin of the plate.

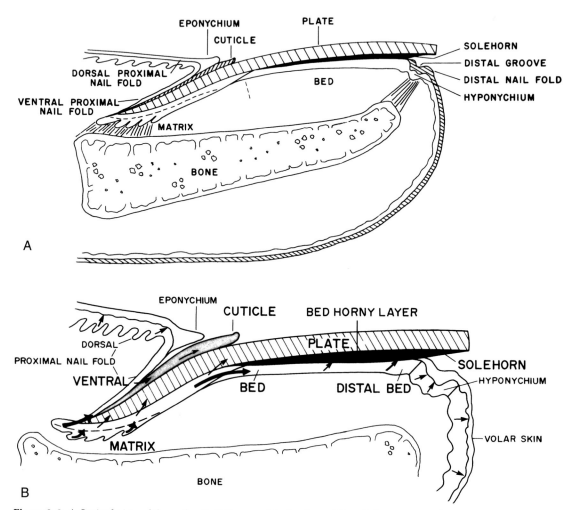

Figure 2–2. A, Sagittal view of the nail unit. B, Proposed derivations of the adult structures of the nail unit. The thick arrows indicate epithelial derivatives of the matrix; the thin arrows, the cornified products therefrom (the proportions of cuticle, bed horny layer, and solehorn—onycholemmal components—have been exaggerated in regard to the true plate for diagrammatic purposes).

2. Onycholemmal keratinization, which occurs in the epithelium of the ventral portion of the proximal nail fold and in the bed epithelium, particularly in the distal bed epithelium. The products are the thin layers of semihard keratins of the true cuticle and of the bed horny layer and the thicker solehorn, respectively.[16]

3. Epidermoid keratinization, which occurs in the epithelium of the dorsal portion of the proximal nail fold, the lateral folds, and the hyponychium. The products are the soft keratins (orthokeratin) of the overt "cuticle" (eponychium), of the hyponychial horn, and of the cornified layer of volar skin.

Onychokeratinization and onycholemmal keratinization are intrinsic and specific to the nail unit. Epidermoid keratinization is similar to the compact orthokeratinization of volar skin.

The epithelia undergoing these types of keratinization display very specific traits:

1. The onychokeratinizing epithelium of the matrix shows a prominent keratogenous zone that is not preceded by a granular layer.

2. The onycholemmal keratinizing epithelia of the ventral proximal nail fold and bed are somewhat different: the former has a granular layer, and the latter is agranular. Both types of epithelium, however, appear barely to be proliferating, lack regular rete ridges, and are devoid of the keratogenous zone that is observed on the epithelium of the matrix.

3. The epidermoid keratinizing epithelia of the dorsal proximal nail fold, lateral folds, distal fold, and hyponychium resemble true epidermis and, in contrast to the onychokeratinizing and onycholemmal keratinizing epithelia, display prominent granular layers (keratohyalin) beneath variably thick and compact orthokeratin. These products are not as firmly compressed as those of the nail plate and cuticular system, however.

Thus, as shown in Table 2–2, the generating portion of the nail unit onychokeratinizes, some of the ensheathing portion or cuticular system onycholemmokeratinizes, and the framing and a fraction of the ensheathing portions orthokeratinize. Perhaps the lack of a distinction between these keratinizing modes has been the source of the disagreements about one versus three layers in the nail plate and about the intermediate matrix versus the intermediate-dorsal-ventral matrices as the site of origin of the nail plate.[5,25]

Development of the Components of the Nail Unit

Embryology

Detailed studies of the embryology of the nail unit have been conducted by Zaias[26] and by Hashimoto and colleagues.[27]

The chronology of events may be described as follows. Development starts in the ninth week of embryogenesis with the differentiation of a nail field composed of a histologically distinguishable epithelium, with a thickness of from one to several cells, delineated by the circumferential grooves (the proximal, distal, and lateral grooves). An underemphasized fact about the formation of these grooves is that their induction is probably mediated by a denser underlying mesenchyme, which would be responsible for the retraction of the margins of the nail field. The proximal groove will eventuate between the 11th and 12th weeks as a proliferative wedge of cells that constitutes the matrix primordium. At approximately the same time, a distal ridge is formed cephalad to the distal groove, and the inner area of the nail field orthokeratinizes, beginning from the ridge backward in a proximal or cephalad direction. By the 13th week, the matrix primordium has given rise to the developing matrix, already visible externally as a lunula, while an incipient plate starts to appear proxi-

Table 2–2. **MODES OF KERATINIZATION OF THE NAIL UNIT**

Mode	Component	Product
Onychokeratinization	Matrix	Plate
Onycholemmal keratinization	Ventral proximal nail fold	Dorsal cuticle
	Bed epithelium (proximal and distal)	Bed horny layer, solehorn, and ventral cuticle
Epidermoid keratinization	Marginal proximal nail fold	Eponychium
	Hyponychium	Hyponychial horn
	Paronychial skin	Volar horn

mally. At about the same time, the neighboring mesenchymal structures (cartilage and bone) and epithelial structures (epidermal rete and sweat glands) are being formed.

By the 20th week of fetal life, when the matrix is mature and exhibits an adult type of onychokeratinization and the plate is being completed, the bed epithelium has already begun to lose its granular layer in a receding, caudad fashion that coincides with the forward movement of a more developed plate. When this plate reaches the distal ridge, this ridge may become important as the ramp for launching the free edge of the nail and as the site of insertion of the plate into the nail field. This insertion is most probably mediated by the onycholemmal keratin of the distal bed (solehorn).

The development of the toenails lags 4 weeks behind that of the fingernails, maintaining the cephalic-caudal trend of maturation of the integument of the embryo and fetus.

Table 2–3 and Figure 2–2B show a proposed pathway for the derivation of the adult structures of the nail unit based on the events just described.

Regeneration of the Plate

Although the adult nail plate is not shed physiologically as hair shafts are, its regenera-

tion after avulsion somewhat replicates the embryologic steps of nail formation, in a manner that is equivalent to the way in which the hair cycle recapitulates the embryology of hair.

When avulsion occurs, the detached plate carries with it the keratogenous zone of the matrix and the bed epithelium and leaves behind a naked basal matrix and an exposed bed mesenchyme.[28] The bare surfaces are immediately covered by a crust. Epithelial repair beneath the crust is provided by epidermis that migrates from the lateral folds and hyponychium. This reparative epidermis is hyperplastic and hyperkeratotic and contains a granular layer of keratohyalin, as is typical of regenerative epidermis elsewhere in the body.

As the new plate is formed and advances forward, an epithelium with a different appearance gradually progresses caudally and takes the place of the reparative epithelium. This new epithelium is thinner and devoid of a granular layer and is the normal, permanent bed epithelium.

As mentioned, during embryonic development the early bed epithelium is also epidermoid (and has been referred to as the forenail or false nail); hence, it is a bearer of granular and cornified layers. This early-appearing epithelium is initially found distally, but it then proceeds in a cephalad direction to involve the

Table 2–3. **DERIVATION OF STRUCTURES OF THE NAIL FIELD DURING DEVELOPMENT IN UTERO**

Early (9th Week)	Middle (11th–13th Weeks)	Late (and Adult) (18th–20th Weeks On)
Proximal groove	Matrix primordium	Dorsal proximal nail fold (and eponychium)
		Ventral proximal nail fold (and cuticle)
		Matrix
		Plate
		Late bed epithelium
Inner field	Early bed epithelium (fore- or false nail)	None
Distal groove	Distal ridge	Distal bed (and solehorn) –proximal hyponychium juncture
		Hyponychium (and horn)
		Distal groove and distal nail fold
Lateral grooves		Lateral grooves and lateral nail folds

nail field between the distal ridge and the developing matrix. When the matrix matures and a plate is formed and impelled forward, this early or provisional epithelium recedes caudally and is replaced by a late or definitive bed epithelium without a granular layer or any obvious epidermoid keratinization.

Both after avulsion and in utero, the transformation from early provisional epithelia to late definitive epithelia may indicate one of two possibilities:

1. The two types of epithelium may be the same, the late epithelium being produced by the differentiation or maturation in situ of the temporary epidermis. However, such differentiation or maturation is unlikely in view of the gradual, migratory character of the events just described, as well as in view of the improbability that epidermis redifferentiates into a more specialized type of epithelium (onycholemmal bed epithelium).

2. Most probably, the two types of epithelium are different, the late definitive epithelium being produced by the replacement, through displacement, of the temporary epithelium by a permanent epithelium derived from the matrix.

This definitive epithelium produced de novo would, in either case, advance synchronously with the emerging plate, because both plate and bed epithelium are products of the matrix. Furthermore, it is reasonable to assume that the processes of regeneration and the primary generation of the first fetal plate are remarkably similar in terms of their histologically recognizable differentiation (Fig. 2–3).

Metaplastic Epidermidization of the Nail Bed

Abnormal regeneration of the bed epithelium is a probable source of those traits that are common to different inflammatory diseases of the nail bed.

Diseases of the nail that involve the matrix may damage it reversibly (e.g., psoriasis) or irreversibly (e.g., lichen planus) and may result in an abnormal or absent plate.[8]

These and many other diseases may also, or primarily, affect the bed (e.g., onychomycosis). Because the bed does not form the plate, the plate will be present but may be altered in its shape, position, or adhesiveness.

Among the diseases that affect the bed are those that are autochthonous to the zone and those that may also appear on the skin (e.g.,

psoriasis, lichen planus, superficial mycosis). The histologic examination of involved tissue, when the disease is able to afflict both the nail bed and skin, usually reveals different microscopic features in the two locations.[29] In addition to changes like those of skin are superimposed manifestations in the nail bed. Surprisingly, these additional features are shared by unrelated diseases—namely, psoriasis, lichen planus, and onychomycosis—which are histologically distinct when observed in the skin. These alterations include increased hyperplasia or unexpected exudative phenomena, which do not occur when the same diseases are entirely cutaneous.

Some of the features that accompany disease processes in the nail bed include a more intense and usually papillated or often digitated hyperplasia, prominent hypergranulosis, and marked hyperkeratosis. The exudative phenomena include spongiosis, sometimes even with the presence of globules of serum and scaly crust, and, more frequently, evidence of hemorrhage.

These shared characteristics of disease processes may depend more on a common response of the bed epithelium to injury than on the nature of the disease itself. The histologic basis for this common response could be epidermidization of the bed epithelium. A previ-

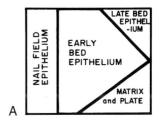

EMBRYONIC DEVELOPMENT

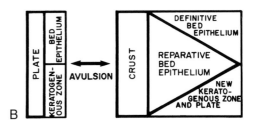

POST-AVULSION DEVELOPMENT

Figure 2–3. Schematic representation of the development of the nail: (A) Embryonic development. (B) Postavulsion development.

ously onycholemmal epithelium may, at the microscopic level, be transformed to an epithelium that resembles epidermis and even to an epidermis that has diverted the usual production of onycholemmal keratin to the production of a greater proportion of ortho- or parakeratin. This excessive accumulation of epidermoid cornified layer, abnormal for the site, will lodge between the nail plate and bed and, in addition to modifying the normal character of the plate, will obstruct the shedding of newer keratin.

Under these circumstances, the metaplastic epidermis reacts to mechanical (pressure) trauma in the same way as the normal epidermis would react—namely, with exudation, hyperkeratosis, and hyperplasia, phenomena not unlike those of lichen simplex chronicus or of secondary lichenification superimposed on previous diseases.

This sequence of events may be why extraneous histologic features shared by many unrelated diseases of the nail bed combine with the specific features of any given disease. The disparate combination of histologic data so obtained from a biopsy of nail bed, then, makes interpretation very difficult and occasionally impossible.

Comparisons and Homologies Between Components of the Nail Unit and Those of the Hair Unit

When homologies have been sought between the nail unit and the hair unit (Table 2–4), it has usually been assumed that the nail can be compared with only one half of the hair follicle.[20,23] This assumption has ignored some of the dorsal structures of the nail. These structures, although admittedly less conspicuous, smaller, and less developed than the ventral structures, nonetheless demonstrate some similarities with the other half of the hair follicle.

Table 2–4. **PUBLISHED SYSTEMS OF HOMOLOGIES BETWEEN NAIL AND HAIR UNITS**

Hair	Nail	
	Achten, 1968[53]	*Zaias, 1980*[20]
Matrix	Matrix	Matrix
Shaft	Plate	Plate
Inner root sheath	Lower nail plate	Bed epithelium and horn
Outer root sheath	Nail bed	Hyponychium

These dorsal structures give bilaterality to the nail unit; however, in contrast to the hair follicle, which is almost bilaterally symmetric, the bilaterality of the nail is rather asymmetric.

1. If the plate (hair shaft equivalent) is considered as the midplane of bilaterality, the thinnest proximal plate is surrounded dorsally by a short, inconspicuous, dorsal matrix and ventrally by a longer, obvious, ventral matrix. This composite region probably represents the level of maximal unilaterality or asymmetry that can be found in the nail unit, if it is compared with the hair matrix.

2. Beyond this composite region, the plate is surrounded dorsally and ventrally by epithelial products of the matrix—namely, the epithelium of the ventral proximal nail fold and the bed epithelium. In turn, these epithelia produce cuticular keratin (cuticle and bed horny layer), which is not necessarily identical to the true cuticle of the hair shaft but instead approximates the inner and outer root sheaths of the hair follicle.

In both nails and hair, these epithelia, and particularly their products, will resolve and disintegrate after fulfilling their ensheathing functions. A noticeable feature of the asymmetry between the dorsal and ventral halves of the nail unit at this point is the highly developed cuticular product present at the end of the bed epithelium: the solehorn. This onycholemmal keratin does not have a dorsal equivalent that can easily be discerned. The probable role of the solehorn (incorrectly termed the ventral nail) as a fastener, in addition to its role as an ensheather of the plate, may explain the absence of a dorsal equivalent at the ventral proximal nail fold, a structure that is a less important provider of support to the nail plate. It is possible, then, that both the ventral proximal nail fold and the poorly keratinizing bed epithelia are homologous to the inner root sheath of the hair follicle, whereas the solehorn keratin and epithelium may be the unilateral equivalent of the outer root sheath, at the level of the isthmus of the hair follicle.

3. Farther ventrally, the underside of the free edge of the plate will face the hyponychium and the distal groove, as the emerging hair shaft faces the infundibulum of the hair unit. Dorsally, likewise, the infundibular equivalent could be represented by the somewhat steep margin of the dorsal proximal fold and its conspicuous product, the eponychium.

Table 2–5. **PROPOSED SYSTEM OF HOMOLOGIES WITHIN NAIL AND BETWEEN NAIL AND HAIR UNITS**

Nail		Hair
	Dorsal	*Ventral*
Short matrix (non-plate forming)	Long matrix (plate forming)	Matrix
Ventral proximal fold (cuticle)	Proximal bed epithelium (thin bed horny layer)	Inner root sheath
?	Distal bed epithelium (thick solehorn)	Outer root sheath (isthmus)
Margin of proximal fold (eponychium)	Hyponychium (hyponychial horn)	Infundibulum
Digital proximal fold	Distal fold Lateral folds	Follicular ostium and peri-follicular skin
Mesenchyme of ventral proximal fold	Mesenchyme of matrix and bed	Fibrous root sheath

4. Most distally, the typical volar skin at the proximal dorsal fold, the lateral folds, and the distal fold could constitute an equivalent to the skin that surrounds the ostium of the hair follicle, in a manner suggestive of the outskirts of a very wide, albeit flattened, nail ostium.

5. Finally, the specialized mesenchyme of the nail unit shares characteristics of a fibrous sheath, similar to that of the fibrous root sheath of the hair follicle. This similarity, perhaps, provides the reason why a disease of the interface—particularly a lichenoid disease that destroys the basement membrane zone, such as lichen planus—is scarring (and sterilizing) in both the hair follicle and the nail unit, whereas such a disease process is reversible when it occurs elsewhere in the skin.

A summary of this interpretation is given in Table 2–5.

COLOR OF THE NAIL

The nail plate and the anatomic structures around and beneath it exhibit colors that are influenced by the histologic components, singly or in combination, described previously.

Consideration is given to the colors of the cuticular and ensheathing system, the underplate structures, and the nail plate.

Cuticle

The term *cuticle* has been applied by some authors only to the webbed, thick rim of keratinous material that borders the free margin of the proximal nail fold and that is in close proximity to the site of emergence of the nail plate. This easily visible component results

from the orthokeratinization of the dorsal portion of the proximal nail fold and, to a lesser degree, of the lateral folds. These epithelia resemble the more proximal dorsal skin of the digit, except that they are thinner and less papillated, do not carry fingerprints, and have no hairs and few sweat glands. Nonetheless, their product, a somewhat flaky deposit of compact orthokeratin that resembles orthokeratin in other locations, is white and should more accurately be termed eponychium.

A less well understood and less conspicuous portion of the dorsal cuticular system is the thinner, predominantly colorless, true cuticle.[26]

This cuticular material derives from the ventral portion of the proximal nail fold. This epithelium is even thinner than that of the dorsal proximal nail fold and lacks rete ridges, dermal papillae, melanocytes, and adnexae. Because the resulting true cuticle, or "nail vest," resembles very compact orthokeratin but adheres intimately to the underlying plate, it might be better described as a probable variant of onycholemmal keratin. This membranous keratin is largely transparent, except at the site where it starts to detach and to disintegrate, somewhere beyond the eponychium. Here the true cuticle can be identified as a delicate and barely perceptible whitish line that is parallel to both the eponychium and the proximal nail fold.

Hyponychium

The term *hyponychium* includes the space, the epithelium, and the keratinous products of an area bordered by the line of dissociation of the plate and the nail bed and by the distal groove and fold. The white appearance of its cornified products is, as in the eponychium, the result of the compact disposition of the often retained orthokeratin that has been produced by its epidermis-like epithelium. This epithelium, except for the absence of fingerprints and adnexae and of a denser "dermis," resembles modified volar skin.

Another keratinous product whose existence is more difficult to demonstrate is the exteriorized subungual solehorn, which is intimately attached to the undersurface of the free edge of the plate. This membranous ventral cuticle is a very compact, thin, and adherent layer of onycholemmal keratin and is probably transparent and colorless. This ventral cuticle is the outward extension of the solehorn that lies between the plate and the distal bed epithelium. Some authors have described it as a part of the hyponychium.[20]

Lunula

The lunula[1] is the visible portion of the nail matrix. It is grayish white because of the prominent and special nature of the keratinization of its epithelium. The lunula or visible matrix, like the occult matrix, contains a keratogenous zone that at the microscopic level consists of a relatively abrupt and well-circumscribed, multilayered band of heavily keratinized cells with incipient (pyknotic) nuclear debris above the layer of basal cells. This keratogenous zone, resembling parakeratin, is the basis for the onychokeratinization that leads to the formation of the nail plate by the matrix.

The cells of the keratogenous zone contain abundant eosinophilic cytoplasm and progressively fragmented nuclei (as the cells move upward). Fragmentation continues until the cells are predominantly anucleated, eosinophilic, and arranged in the very compact sheets of the nail plate. As in the case of parakeratotic horn at other locations (e.g., in the abnormal scales of eczematous dermatitides or psoriasis), the parakeratotic keratogenous zone scatters light in such a manner that it appears white.

Most of the color of the lunula is derived from the keratogenous zone because, after forcible avulsion of the plate, a lunular ghost remains attached to the nail plate,[19,30] a probable indication of the tenaciously adherent character of the keratogenous zone to its product, the plate. However, there may also be a minor contribution from the basal epithelium of the matrix (which, however, is very thin distally) or from the submatrical mesenchyme.

An additional factor enhancing the visibility of the whitish keratogenous zone of the lunula may be the thinness of the nail plate over the entire area of the matrix.

Nail Bed

The nail bed is confined between the distal edge of the lunula and the onychodermal band. It is composed of epithelium that is flat topped and longitudinally ridged, and the parallel alignment of these ridges is very regular. The epithelium consists of barely proliferating, stratified cells that exhibit no mitoses and keratinize very gradually throughout most of the extension of the bed. A layer of basaloid cells, more prominent in the immediate vicinity of the lunula and more likely still representing a portion of the matrix, is followed distally by an indistinctly stratified layer of predominantly squamoid cells with an inconspicuous upper layer of horny cells.

The nail bed is pink but not uniformly colored.[31] The more intense pink hue is noted within two arciform bands, anterior and posterior, circumscribed sharply by the lunula proximally and by the onychodermal band distally. The opposing margins, which face each other at the midportion of the bed, are not sharply defined. The middle bed is of a paler, less pronounced pink. After application of pressure to the pulp, this middle bed turns pinker while the distal bed that precedes the onychodermal band becomes whiter. This response to pressure, in the presence of the only gradually thickening nail plate and of a relatively uniform bed epithelium, supports the role of the bed vasculature as the main source of the pink color of the bed.

The systematized regional variations in the pink color of the nail bed could depend on gradients of anatomic or functional vascularization of the bed mesenchyme, perhaps with vascularization being richer toward the lunula and onychodermal band and poorer under the midbed.

Another color that may be noted on or often over the nail beds of black[32] or Asian individuals is the color of melanin in the bed epithelium, plate, and corresponding onychotomal matrix. This pigment can be observed as a diffuse or streaked gray-black discoloration of these structures. Sparse melanocytes, more numerous in blacks and Asians, may be seen within the epithelium of the matrix and, less often, within the bed epithelium.[33,34] The production of melanin by these melanocytes does not necessarily signify the presence of a melanocytic nevus or a melanoma in the matrix but more often the existence of melanocytes in a hyperactive state,[35] perhaps similar to that of a freckle.

The occasional splinter hemorrhage seen in otherwise healthy individuals as a longitudinal reddish-brown or brown streak corresponds to the deposit and mobilization of extravasated erythrocytes after spontaneous bleeding. These are contained in the horny layer of the bed epithelium and extruded between the solehorn-derived ventral cuticle and the plate.[36]

Onychodermal Band

The onychodermal band is the external expression of the solehorn, that distal part of the bed that precedes both the launching of the free distal edge of the plate and the hyponychial epithelium. It consists, grossly, of a glassy-gray arciform band,[37] which most probably is seated on the proximal slope of the attenuated distal ridge of the adult.

Microscopically, it corresponds to that distal portion of the bed epithelium that, in contrast to the poorly keratinizing proximal and middle portions, produces a heavier load of cuticular keratin, which may even be contained in occasional microcystic pegs[38] that resemble miniature trichilemmal or pilar cysts. This onycholemmal keratin seals off what would otherwise be a space between the plate and the bed epithelium, playing a role in the ensheathing and fastening of that plate and also in determining the site of its detachment.

Plate

The nail plate, the final product of the nail unit, is a hard, relatively inflexible multilayered sheet of cornified cells that covers from one seventh (on the little finger) to one half (on the big toe) of the dorsal surface of every digit.[17] Histologically, the nail plate is formed by eosinophobic, strongly acid-fast (basic fuchsin positive) cells, the onychocytes, derived from the cells of the keratogenous zone of the matrix. The product of these cells is onychokeratin, the result of the most specific of the maturational pathways of the nail unit.

The onychocytes are, for the most part, anucleated and are smaller on the surface than on the bottom of the plate.[39] Occasional islands of retained parakeratotic cells, similar to those from the underlying keratogenous zone, can be seen in otherwise healthy individuals at a considerable upward or forward distance from the onychotomal matrix. This phenomenon is the source of the so-called leukonychial spots. Their white color responds to the same factor as that which renders the lunula white, namely parakeratosis.

The plate has two distinct colors depending on its location. The plate over the nail bed is transparent and colorless, whereas the portion of the plate forming the free edge is yellowish white.

Although the plate is thinner at the site of its inception and grows thicker distally as the distal matrix contributes to it, the histologic appearance of the plate at these extremes is quite similar. Therefore, the most probable factor determining the absence or the presence of color in the plate is the nature of the interfaces at the ventral (or lower) side of the plate. Although the interface of the attached portion is between an adherent keratinous plate and an airtight bed epithelium (a solid–solid interface), the interface of the detached edge is with the air present in the hyponychial angle (a solid–gas interface). The light refracted at these different interfaces will be refracted unequally. The refraction will be minimized in the solid–solid interface, and the plate will appear transparent and translucent, allowing for clear visualization of the nail bed.

The increased refraction at the solid–gas interface will make the plate appear as an opaque structure, however, despite its intrinsic ability to be transparent. This phenomenon is like that occurring when the top of an aquarium, the bottom of a swimming pool, or a preparation under a high-power microscope objective is observed without the benefit of the solid–liquid interface provided by a glass wall, a swimming mask, or immersion oil. An approximately similar situation occurs in the cornea. Transparent and colorless under normal circumstances, the cornea may become opaque or cloudy if the anterior epithelium, which provides the necessary solid–solid interface to the very dense and avascular lamina propria, becomes edematous, abraded, or lost.

Refraction at the interfaces probably explains the paradox observed in an avulsed plate, in which the areas originally transparent

Table 2–6. **FACTORS CONTRIBUTING TO NAIL COLOR**

Structure	Color	Factor

Cuticles
  True dorsal
  Subungual solehorn of free edge
    of plate (ventral cuticle)
	Transparent	Membranous compact (cuticular)
		  onycholemmal keratin

Eponychium and hyponychium	Opaque white	Flaky compact (volar) orthokeratin
Lunula	Matte grayish white	Thick keratogenous zone of matrix
Bed	Pink	Bed capillary network

	Diffuse or streaked gray-
	  black pigmentation
		Melanocytes in matrix (or less likely
		  in bed epithelium)
		Melanin in plate

Onychodermal band	Glassy gray	Bed–hyponychium–plate juncture (solehorn)
Plate (over bed)	Transparent, colorless	Adherent keratin plate (solid–solid interface)
Plate (on distal free edge)	Yellowish white or white	Nonadherent keratin plate (solid–gas interface) Hyponychium

become opaque while the site of the lunula ghost, where the keratogenous zone is still contributing a solid–solid interface, can easily be transilluminated.[30]

In addition to the phenomenon just discussed, another factor that may influence the distinct color of the distal edge of the plate may be the presence of the often-retained cornified products of the hyponychium, which could contribute further refraction and also some of their own color.

The cuticular keratin of the solehorn-derived ventral cuticle, which is attached to the lower aspect of the free edge, is less likely to contribute significantly to the color of the free plate because it is membranous, thin, and adherent and is possibly as transparent as the true cuticle present above the proximal plate.

A summary of the factors that influence the color of the nail is given in Table 2–6.

CONFIGURATION OF THE NAIL PLATE

The parameters that define the delicately balanced configuration of the nail plate are as follows:

1. Shape
2. Convexity
3. Outline of the distal edge
4. Thickness
5. Horizontality of the silhouette (flat emergence)

The first four parameters account for the morphology of the plate, the fifth for the position of the plate.

Shape

The predominant orientation of the longer axis of the plate will define whether the plate is closer to rectangular in shape (fingernails) or quadrangular (toenails). As shown in Figure 2–4, this characteristic is influenced by

1. The breadth of the matrix, which will determine a relatively narrow or a relatively broad plate.
2. The length of the bed, which will determine if the plate will be relatively long or relatively short. In turn, this length depends on the position of the onychodermal band (solehorn), which is the real boundary of the nail bed and precedes the airborne plate.

This position of the onychodermal band in adults probably derives from the embryonic distal ridge, which, although attenuated under the pressure of the plate, still seems to be the seat of the distal bed epithelium on its proximal slope and of the hyponychial epithelium on its distal slope.

Beyond the onychodermal band, the length of the plate is a matter of personal or environmental rather than natural design.

Because the matrix, the bed, and the positioning of the onychodermal band must ultimately accommodate to the breadth and

Plate I

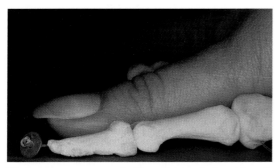

The bone as mattress and pillow of the nail plate. There is an intimate relation between the shape of the nail and the subjacent bone. The bony prominences at the beginning and end of the nail field are the sites wherein the ligaments that keep the field constant and relatively immutable are inserted.

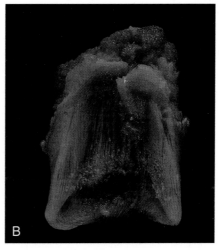

Anatomy of the nail. *B,* Ventral portion of the same plate as in *A:* The longitudinally oriented mushroom-like striations of the rear of the plate reflect the corrugated interaction of the plate and attached bed epithelium with the nail mesenchyme.

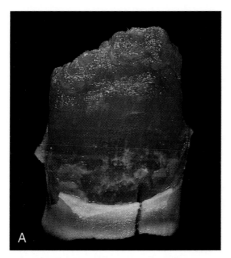

Anatomy of the nail. *A,* Dorsum of dislodged nail: There are degenerative (senile) changes of the plate. The true cuticle appears as a sepal near the proximal border of the nail, which it covers dorsally.

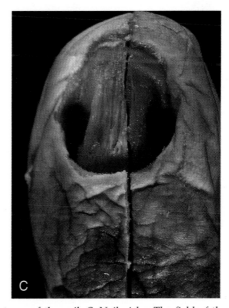

Anatomy of the nail. *C,* Nail niche: The field of the dislodged nail shows the close attachment and embracing of the plate (now absent) to the subjacent bony structures. Distally, the arciform bony tuberosity is seen as an area on which the similarly shaped onychodermal band sits.

Plate II

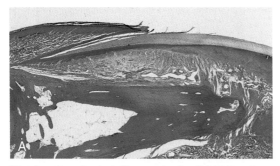

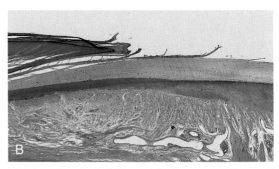

Histology (monkey). *A*, The proximal nail fold lies above the junction of the lunula and the bed. The eponychium, or "false cuticle," is in the spur of epithelium of the proximal nail fold, whereas the true cuticle appears as the detached membrane just beyond it.

Histology (monkey). *B*, The matrix shows several layers of cells, the basal one of which is mammillated. The bed epithelium is uniform and poorly stratified or cellular and appears distal to the matrix that it follows as a derivative.

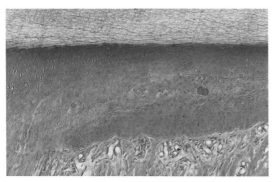

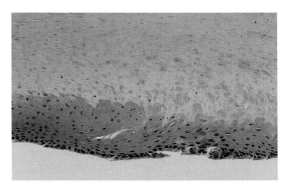

Nail bed. Fully active squamoid epithelium (but not true epidermis) attached to the nail plate. There is no contribution of new plate at this level.

Nail bed epithelium. Onycholemmal keratinization, resembling that of the outer root sheath of the hair at the level of the isthmus, is noted in the nail bed.

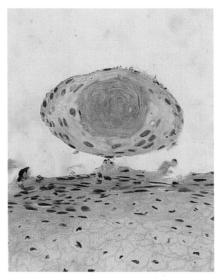

Onycholemmal peg. An outgrowth of onycholemmal epithelium of the bed configures a microcyst, which is a relatively common finding in nail biopsies and almost certainly reflects the forward movement of the bed epithelium.

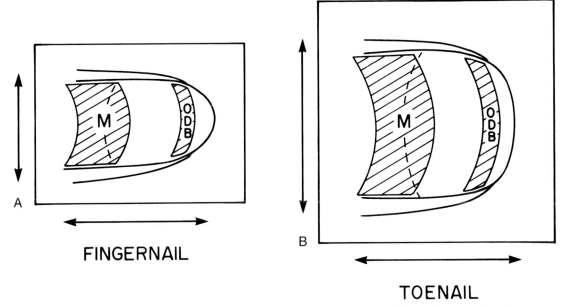

Figure 2–4. Shape of the nail plate. *A,* Fingernail. *B,* toenail. (M, matrix; ODB, onychodermal band.)

length of the underlying bone, the role of the phalanx in shaping the plate should not be underestimated.

Convexity

The anterior and posterior slopes of the surface of the nail plate, as well as the transverse curvature of the plate, define the convexity that causes the nail to assume the shape of a crystal of a watch or half a thimble. This convexity derives from

1. The degree of arching of the matrix (Fig. 2–5), which is responsible for the more or less pronounced arching of the transverse axis of the plate.
2. The bifrontal sloping of the bed (Fig. 2–6), which determines the degree of curvilinearity of the longitudinal axis of the plate.

Just as the underlying bone ultimately influences the shape of the plate, the convexity ("height") of the nail plate is related to the accommodation of matrix and bed to the subjacent bone-related mesenchyme and to the phalanx. The somewhat convex plates of fingernails are probably a response to the more elongated and flat-topped morphology of the finger phalanges, and the more curved plates over the toes reflect the shorter and plumper bones in these digits.[7]

Outline of the Distal Edge

To the extent that the length of the free edge of the plate is environmental and variable, so the outline of the distal plate is also environmental and variable. Generally, however, the distal edge often follows a parallel or parabolic course at a variable distance from the true and constant landmark, which is the onychodermal band (Fig. 2–7). Because of its stability, the contour of the onychodermal band is the important parameter to consider. This contour reflects the arciform distal contour of the lunula and is usually remarkably parallel to it, expressing an almost exact correspondence to every variation found among the lunulae of the same individual. This correspondence of outlines between the onychodermal band and distal margin of the lunula suggests that, among meridians of maturation in the bed epithelium and plate, the speed of movement is constant. Therefore, the peripheral portions of the plate–bed subunit will arrive "late" at the onychodermal band not because they departed later from the site of origin but because they departed at the same time from different positions in the more backward peripheral (lateral) portions of the lunula and occult matrix. In sum, at the site of the onychodermal band, a cross-section of every meridian of the plate is probably formed by onychokeratin sheets that have equivalent ages at any given depth.

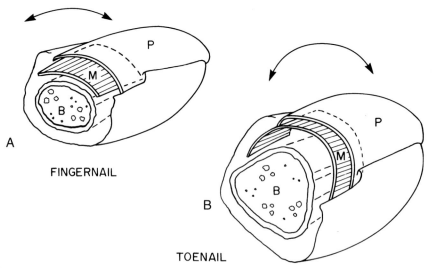

Figure 2–5. Transverse convexity of the nail plate and arching of the matrix. *A,* Fingernail. *B,* Toenail. (M, matrix; P, plate; B, bone.)

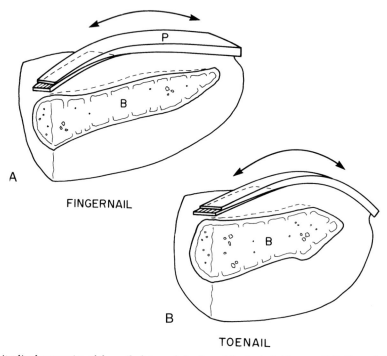

Figure 2–6. Longitudinal convexity of the nail plate and sloping of the bed. *A,* Fingernail. *B,* Toenail. (B, bed; P, plate.)

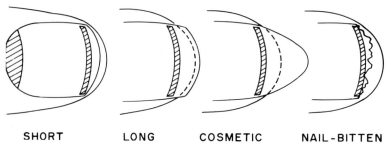

SHORT   LONG   COSMETIC   NAIL-BITTEN

Figure 2–7. Outline of the onychodermal band: relationship to the outline of the lunula. The same nail may have differently outlined distal edges; the onychodermal band is constant.

Thickness

It is known that the plate is thinner proximally and thicker distally. Both differential and average thicknesses depend on

1. The length of the matrix because the matrix is the only structure responsible for the formation of true plate (the plate without the onycholemmal components of true cuticle and solehorn). The superficial portion of the plate will derive from the proximal matrix, the deeper portion from the distal matrix.[40]

2. The gradient of speed of forward movement between the superficial and the deep levels of the plate, result from a fast-moving surface and a more slowly moving bottom. These speeds in turn derive from a more actively proliferating proximal matrix and a less actively proliferating distal matrix.

Histologically, some indication of the proliferative gradients of the matrix is given by the thicker, denser, and more rete-bearing proximal matrical epithelium and by the presence of small onychocytes in the superficial (proximally derived) sheets, in contrast with larger and broader onychocytes in the deep (distally derived) sheets of the plate.[39,41]

When time-lapse autoradiography has been used in dynamic studies,[40,42] both these heterogeneously proliferating segments of the matrix and the different speeds with which the layers of the plate move forward can be definitively visualized. The different speeds can be observed, when tritiated glycine has been used, as successive same-instant planes of onychokeratinization that travel forward with a progressively slanting deflection (from parallel above the matrix to oblique above the bed), derived from a faster production of material by the proximal matrix and a slower production of material by the distal matrix.

This deflection in each particular same-instant plane of onychokeratinization can be quantified with respect to its degree of inclination toward an imaginary horizontal line (A in Fig. 2–8). Each of the angles of deflection represents a particular gradient of speed among all the layers that comprise the plate at a given moment.

The vertex of the angle advances and the size of the angle increases as the plate moves forward. The vertex of this movable angle is formed by the distal inferior end of the same-instant plane and is originally located at the anterior border of the lunula. The position of the vertex subsequently changes as it moves along the lowermost sheet of onychokeratin,

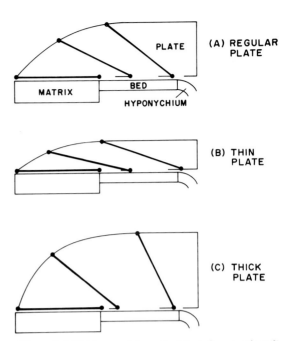

Figure 2–8. Thickness of the nail plate: influence of gradients of speeds of superficial and deep sheets as shown by slowly or rapidly deflecting same-instant onychokeratinization planes.

which is derived from the most distal point of the matrix.

The proximal superior end is originally situated at the most proximal point of the matrix and subsequently in the uppermost sheet of plate keratin derived therefrom. The distal inferior end eventually reaches the distal edge of the plate and arrives much earlier than the proximal superior end of the corresponding same-instant plane of onychokeratinization. This earlier arrival, in spite of the slower speed, is the result of the shorter distance to be covered by this distal portion of the same-instant plane of onychokeratinization.

Within the confines of the nail field, the angles of deflection range from near 0° to less than 45°. If, hypothetically, the angle were to reach 90° (with the same-instant plane being perpendicular to the upper and lower surfaces of the plate) within the extent of a nail field, the plate would at this point be approximately as thick as the matrix is long.

As in a wave in the sea, if the speed of the upper stream of water is too high and in particular disproportion to the speed of the lower stream, the crest of the wave is high and stormy. If both speeds are approximately equal, the crest will be lower and quiet. Similarly, if the angles of deflection of the nail plate increase quickly if there is a large gradient of speed between plates on the upper and lower

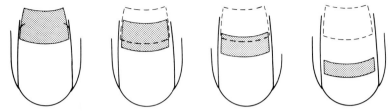

Figure 2–9. The probable course of one same-instant plane of onychokeratinization: representation of idealized results of time-lapsed autoradiography. Open area, matrix; dotted area, same-instant plane.

levels, the nail will attain a sizable thickness more rapidly (C in Fig. 2–8). Likewise, if the angles in the same nail remain small for some distance within the plate (low gradient of speeds), the slow deflection will induce a thinner plate (B in Fig. 2–8) that can only reach its full potential thickness after some time (perhaps never if the nail is clipped).

In this manner, given a constant length of the matrix, functional differences between portions of the matrix can modify the thickness of a given plate.

This hypothesis regarding the deflection angle also helps to explain why physiologic variations in healthy individuals, senility,[43] or matrical diseases[29] produce variations in thickness of the nail plate in the presence of a matrix of invariable length. This hypothesis also disqualifies studies of plate growth that are exclusively concerned with linear and not also with volumetric parameters, including thickness. A model of the hypothetical advancement and deflection of a single onychokeratinization plane is shown in Figure 2–9.

FLAT Silhouette of the Plate

Despite the presence of the angle formed by the proximal nail fold and the emerging plate (Lovibond's angle),[44] the overall silhouette of the plate is relatively flat if it is considered that the levels of the margin of the proximal nail fold and the onychodermal band are approximately similar and that the upper and lower surfaces of the plate are largely parallel despite the variable thickness of the plate.

The reasons for this ultimately flat silhouette of the plate are complex and interrelated and involve the special arrangement of the matrix, the dynamics of the matrix, the differentiation and growth of the plate, the shaping effects of neighboring soft and hard structures, the adhesiveness and fastening pro-

vided by the nail coverings, and the anchoring exerted by the special mesenchyme that supports the nail unit.

Intrinsic Arrangement of Matrical Epithelium

The vertical axes of the rete and of the basal cells of the epithelium of the matrix are not perpendicular to the line formed by the uppermost layer of basal cells.[27] The vertical axes are oriented outward and forward rather than upward (i.e., they are slanted in a caudad direction) (Fig. 2–10). This histologic factor alone greatly influences the oblique and centrifugal direction of growth of the cells that form the diagonally oriented keratogenous zone and early plate, the latter of which is the superficial portion of the definitive plate.

Dynamics of Differentiation of the Matrix and Growth of the Plate

As discussed, the direction of growth in the nail is predominantly centrifugal along the entire extension of the plate. Some centripetal tendency, however, is present in the distal segment of the plate, expressed perhaps in the anterior slope of some more convex nails, which not only reflect an accommodation of the bed to the mesenchyme and to the bone but also an

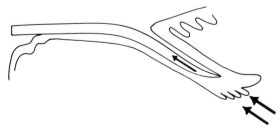

Figure 2–10. Horizontal slope of the nail plate: slanted orientation of the epithelial rete of the matrix inducing an early diagonal plate.

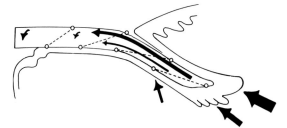

Figure 2–11. Horizontal slope of the nail plate: dominant superficial vectors in the plate (as an effect of dissimilar proliferative rates of matrix—graded thick (arrows) determine the centripetal (rotational) trend of growth of plate in its mid- and distal course.

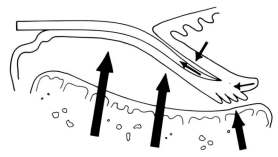

Figure 2–12. Horizontal slope of the nail plate: external molding resulting from forces exerted by proximal nail fold and bone.

intrinsically curved vector within the plates. These directions are an expression of the growth pressures exerted by portions of the plate that move with different speeds as they grow.

The various speeds of the different levels of the nail plate are correlated with the different proliferative rates found in the corresponding parts of the matrix: highest in the proximal, lower in the distal, and lowest in the middle matrix.[20] As in the regulation of the thickness of the plate, a more active, faster-growing proximal matrix will produce superficial sheets that move more quickly and probably mature and harden more quickly or even in a manner different from those sheets derived from the more slowly proliferating anterior matrix.[23,45] The higher speed with which these superficial layers move, even though they remain inseparably adhered to the deeper layers, probably imposes a rotational effect on the whole plate (Fig. 2–11). According to the impetus supplied by these upper layers, a relative elevation or depression of the main vector of the plate will be obtained. This change in the main vector is probably why extremely long human nails, as well as claws (in animals with a dominant proximal matrix), tend to run a curvilinear or even spiral course that is initially centrifugal and subsequently markedly centripetal.

External Molding

The growth pressures from the matrix, transmitted heterogeneously to the plate, are channeled by the confines provided dorsally by the nail folds[47,48] and ventrally by the underlying phalangeal bone (Fig. 2–12).

Because a relatively normal plate can grow in the absence of folds,[6,48] the most important factor is probably the molding provided by the bone.

As if it were a pillow for the nail, the proximal or epiphyseal portion of the phalanx generates an anatomic slant in the most proximal matrix, giving the nail root a downward tilt at its inception. Although the tilt of the matrical epithelium is widely represented in numerous photographs throughout the literature, its significance has probably been underestimated. When this tilt is added to the intrinsic obliqueness of the matrical rete and basal cells, the position of the nail-generating component is anatomically prone to produce a plate with a relatively flat spread, notwithstanding the dominant upward and outward inclination of its proximal portion.

Likewise, as if they were a mattress for the nail, the middle and distal portions of the phalanx contribute further, as a base, to the tendency toward almost horizontal growth of the remaining plate.

It is clear that the role of the phalanx in determining the shape, convexity, and spread of the nail field, as well as the silhouette of the plate, should be taken as crucial rather than accessory. The nail is the shield or protective cover of those bones, and because the protection of the distal digits is one of the primary functions of nails, it is logical that the configuration of the plate conforms to that of the protected object.

Adhesion to the Nail Bed

The bed epithelium provides the plate with the means to adhere to the nail bed and also with a mechanism that facilitates its mobility, ensuring that the plate will maintain its original direction of growth and its flatness.

The bed epithelium adheres so tenaciously to the plate that even after avulsion of the latter, the epithelium sticks to it and not to the "dermis."[19] Moreover, the bed epithelium travels at the same speed as the nail plate, as has been shown by the kinetics of migration of ^{3}H-thymidine–labeled matrically derived keratinocytes to progressively advancing locations within the space occupied by the bed epithelium.[40,42] The horny layer, formed by the bed epithelium, appears to have special adhesive properties. The stronger attachment of the bed epithelium to the plate than to the mesenchyme may be dependent on the onycholemmal quality of the keratin produced. The bed horny layer, although inconspicuous proximally, is thick and prominent distally where the bed epithelium differentiates into a solehorn-producing epithelium. The adhesiveness provided by these two horns and, most particularly, by the solehorn, which act as a soldering plane and band for the plate, respectively, is an important factor in guiding the nail plate into the flat position that it adopts over the nail bed (Fig. 2–13).

Furthermore, the anatomic disposition of bed epithelium and bed "dermis" probably functions to allow the smooth and efficient channeling of the plate–bed epithelium subunit over the bed mesenchyme rather than to allow the plate to glide over a stable, immovable bed epithelium (Fig. 2–14). The peculiar arrangement of the ridges in the bed epithelium may serve to enhance the synchronous movement of the subunit composed of the intimately attached and inseparable plate and bed epithelium. The bed epithelium, albeit flat topped, has an undulated bottom (on cross-section) composed of longitudinal ridges that are parallel to each other and to the longitudinal axis of the plate and that interdigitate with corresponding corrugations in the bed mesenchyme (dermis). These complementary anatomic dispositions would, then, be the microscopic basis for the channeling effect that permits the normal flat ride of the plate in its mid and late course. The integrity of the bed mesenchyme rather than that of the bed epithelium, which can regenerate more easily, is then essential for an integral, normal distal plate. A severed bed epithelium (e.g., after partial avulsion) does not have independent motion,[49] perhaps as a result of the loss of forward traction provided by the preceding flowing epithelium or even by the plate.

The movement in unison of the plate–bed epithelium subunit probably indicates that the bed epithelium has a proximal site of origin and a distal end.

The bed epithelium is completely derived from the matrix epithelium and is not a self-

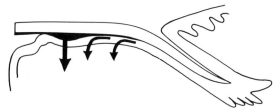

Figure 2–13. Horizontal slope of the nail plate: tenacious adhesion of plate to bed epithelium, provided by the bed horny layer and, particularly, by the solehorn.

generating and independent structure. This relationship is supported by the following histologic observations. The basal cell layer of the bed epithelium is more prominent in the proximity of the lunula (distal matrix). In addition, this basal cell layer is wedged beneath the inferior angle formed by the recession of the spurlike end of the keratogenous layer of the matrix, not unlike the wedging of the locally thinned inner and outer root sheaths around the matrix of the hair bulb. Whether this portion of the nail is named the germinative layer of the bed epithelium or whether it should be recognized as part of the matrix is probably irrelevant to the physiologic interdependence, rather than independence, of bed and matrix. Furthermore, the main layer of the bed epithelium is composed of indifferent-looking cells without mitoses, without conspicuous nuclei, and without other signs of very active proliferation in situ. These cells are indicative of a passive, almost terminal epithelium. Finally, the high rate of uptake of ^{3}H-thymidine that occurs simultaneously in the classic matrix and in the germinative layer of the bed epithelium (in contrast to the practically absent uptake of the bed epithelium ahead of it) and the slow, forward migration of marked bed cells, which coincides with the advance of the plate,[20,42] support the hypothesis discussed previously.

The bed epithelium disappears or resolves through complete horny maturation at the distal zone of the bed, where it meets the hyponychial epithelium. At this point, the epithelium is thicker, there is a heavier accumulation of onycholemmal keratin, and the keratin–epithelium junction is wrinkled, very much like the wrinkling observed in tricholemmal keratinization.[38,50] This distal "fertile" zone of the bed epithelium is the solehorn[23] or "ventral nail,"[51] which extends outward as the solehorn cuticle, which in turn is located beneath the free edge of the plate. This interpretation may explain the fate of the bed epithelium at that critical junction of the plate, bed, and hy-

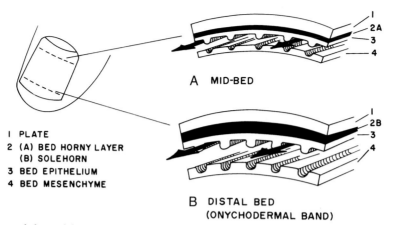

Figure 2–14. Horizontal slope of the nail plate: channeling effect of sliding plate–bed epithelium subunit over corrugated mesenchyme.

ponychium: complete resolution, extrusion, and sloughing off as a half-ensheathing product rather than as a portion of the true plate.

The functions of the bed epithelium—both the channeling throughout its length and the adhesion throughout its length, but predominantly distally—will give the plate both the movable support and the soldering to a base that it requires to sustain its normal configuration and position.

Mesenchymal Anchoring

The dense sclerotic mesenchyme underneath the nail unit exerts a stabilizing effect on the configuration of the plate by holding all overlying structures together and close to the bone.

In contrast to the dermis-like mesenchyme of the nail folds, the matrical and bed mesenchyme is composed mainly of fibroconnective and vascular tissue that is not organized in classic papillary or reticular patterns. This mesenchyme lacks adnexa and is seated on periosteum and tendons rather than on a subcutaneous layer.[11,52] In fact, the matrical and bed mesenchyme have almost a ligamentary or even tendon-like character. This subungual mesenchyme (Fig. 2–15) can be tentatively divided into three portions when observed sagittally: the matricophalangeal (posterior) ligament, the bed dermis, and the hyponychial-phalangeal (anterior) ligament. The bulkier portion is the bed dermis, whereas the proximal and distal portions are narrow and connect the proximal and distal segments of the phalangeal bone to the matrix and distal groove, respectively. Ligaments to the lateral grooves probably complete a ligamental oval around the nail field.

The bed dermis does not resemble dermis anywhere else in the skin, and if an analogy needs to be drawn, a comparison with the reticular dermis would barely be applicable. Rather, this mesenchyme approaches the histologic appearance of an exaggerated fibrous sheath, not unlike that of hair and of the hair follicle.

Nonetheless, the bed mesenchyme shares with the cutaneous dermis the ability to form a papilla equivalent—namely, the longitudinal corrugations that mirror the reciprocal ridges of the bed epithelium. This bed mesenchyme is richly innervated and vascularized[9,10,12] by means of numerous neural receptors (Vater-Pacini and Meissner's corpuscles), a profuse capillary network that courses throughout the upper corrugations, and a prominent lymphatic system. In addition, the prevalent glomus bodies, those peculiar neural and myoepithelial arteriovenous fistulas that regulate distal microcirculation under different thermal conditions, are also present.

Because this specialized mesenchyme is ultimately responsible for keeping the constant

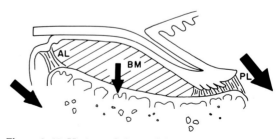

Figure 2–15. Horizontal slope of the nail plate: organization of the mesenchyme of the nail field allowing anchoring of proximal and distal nail grooves and support of the nail bed. (AL, anterior ligament; BM, bed mesenchyme; PL, posterior ligament.)

Table 2–7. **CONFIGURATION OF THE NAIL PLATE**

Dimension	Factor(s)
	Morphology of Plate
Shape (rectangular vs. quadrangular)	Breadth of matrix
	Length of bed (secondary to position of onychodermal band)
Convexity	
Transverse	Arching of matrix
Longitudinal	Sloping of bed
Outline of onychodermal band ± distal edge	Semilunar contour of lunula
Thickness of plate	Length of matrix
	Translational angles of same-instant onychokeratin planes (secondary to speeds gradient between superficial and deep portions of the plate)
	Position of Plate
Horizontality of plate silhouette (flat emergence)	Slanted matrix papillae
	Centrifugal and centripetal direction of plate growth (secondary to the fast surface and slow bottom of the plate)
	External molding by
	Nail folds (minor)
	Phalanx (major): bone as nail pillow proximally, and as nail mattress distally
	Channeling effect of tenaciously adherent (to plate) bed epithelium sliding over bed mesenchyme
	Mesenchymal anchoring provided by nail "dermis" and ligaments: matricophalangeal, proximally (proximal groove), phalangeal-hyponychial groove, distally (distal groove), and lateral ligaments

positional relationships and the critical distances between matrix, bed, hyponychium, and bone, any disturbance of it by osseous, soft tissue, or periosteal diseases will result in a distorted or misdirected plate.[14]

Table 2–7 summarizes the factors that are most probably involved in the normal configuration, both morphologic and positional, of the nail plate.

In conclusion, this chapter has attempted to combine common histologic observations, recent dynamic studies, and analogies with the hair unit in an effort to understand the structures and mechanisms that eventuate in a normal nail plate.

References

1. Cohen PR: The lunula. J Am Acad Dermatol 34:943, 1996.
2. Ditre CM, Howe NR: Surgical anatomy of the nail unit. J Dermatol Surg Oncol 18:665, 1992.
3. Dykyj D: Anatomy of the nail. Clin Podiatr Med Surg 6:215, 1989.
4. Goldminz D, Bennett RG: Mohs micrographic surgery of the nail unit. J Dermatol Surg Oncol 18:721, 1992.
5. Johnson M, Shuster S: Continuous formation of nail along the bed. Br J Dermatol 128:277, 1993.
6. Kato N: Vertically growing ectopic nail. J Cutan Pathol 19:445, 1992.
7. Parrinello JF, Japour CJ, et al: Incurvated nail. Does the phalanx determine nail plate shape? J Am Podiatr Med Assoc 85:696, 1995.
8. Sinclair RD, Wojnarowska F, et al: The basement membrane zone of the nail. Br J Dermatol 131:499, 1994.
9. Smith DO, Oura C, et al: Artery anatomy and tortuosity in the distal finger. J Hand Surg [Am] 16:297, 1991.
10. Smith DO, Oura C, et al: The distal venous anatomy of the finger. J Hand Surg [Am] 16:303, 1991.
11. Soon PS, Arnold MA, et al: Paraterminal ligaments of the distal phalanx. Acta Anat (Basel) 142:339, 1991.
12. Wolfram-Gabel R, Sick H: Vascular networks of the periphery of the fingernail. J Hand Surg [Br] 20:488, 1995.
13. Zook EG: Anatomy and physiology of the perionychium. Hand Clin 6:1, 1990.
14. Zook EG, Russell RC: Reconstruction of a functional and esthetic nail. Hand Clin 6:59, 1990.
15. González-Serva A: Anatomía macro- y microscópica de la uña. (Macro- and microscopic anatomy of the nail.) Camacho Martínez F (ed): Monografías de Dermatología (Spain) IV (5):256, 1991.
16. González-Serva A: Onycholemmal keratinization: Ensheathing and fastening of the nail plate (Abstract). J Invest Dermatol 98:582, 1992.
17. Dawber RPR, Baran R: Structure, embryology, comparative anatomy and physiology of the nail. *In* Baran R, Dawber R (eds): Diseases of the Nails and Their Management. Blackwell Scientific Publications, Oxford, 1984.
18. Norton LA: Nail disorders. A review. J Am Acad Dermatol 2:451, 1980.
19. Samman PD: Anatomy and physiology. *In* Samman PD, Fenton DA (eds): The Nails in Disease, ed 4. Year Book, Chicago, 1986.

20. Zaias N: The Nail in Health and Disease. Spectrum Publications, New York, 1980.
21. Chapman RE: Hair, wool, quill, nail, claw, hoof, and horn: *In* Bereiter-Hahn J, Matoltsy AG, Richards KS (eds): Biology of the Integument. Vol 2. Vertebrates. Springer-Verlag, New York, 1986.
22. Barron JN: The structure and function of the skin of the hand. Hand 2:93, 1970.
23. Achten G: L'ongle normal et pathologique. Dermatologica 126:229, 1963.
24. Zook EG, Van Beek AL, Russell RC, et al: Anatomy and physiology of the perionychium: A review of the literature and anatomic study. J Hand Surg 5:528, 1980.
25. Lewis BL: Microscopic studies of fetal and mature nail and surrounding soft tissue. Arch Dermatol Syphilol 70:732, 1954.
26. Zaias N: Embryology of the human nail. Arch Dermatol 87:37, 1963.
27. Hashimoto K, Gross BG, Nelson R, et al: The ultrastructure of the skin of human embryos. III. The formation of the nail on 16–18 weeks old embryos. J Invest Dermatol 47:205, 1966.
28. Zaias N: The regeneration of the primate nail: Studies of the squirrel monkey, Saimiri. J Invest Dermatol 44:107, 1965.
29. Jerasutus S: Histology and embryology of the nail unit. Histopathology of nail diseases. *In* Scher RK, Daniel CR III (eds): Nail Therapy. WB Saunders, Philadelphia, 1990.
30. Terry R: Red half-moons in cardiac failure. Lancet 2:842, 1954.
31. Terry R: White nails in hepatic cirrhosis. Lancet 1:757, 1954.
32. Monash S: Normal pigmentation in the nails of the Negro. Arch Dermatol Syphilol 25:876, 1932.
33. Higashi N: Melanocytes of nail matrix and nail pigmentation. Arch Dermatol 97:570, 1968.
34. Higashi N, Saito T: Horizontal distribution of the DOPA-positive melanocytes in the nail matrix. J Invest Dermatol 53:163, 1969.
35. Leyden JJ, Spott DA, Goldschmidt H: Diffuse and banded melanin pigmentation in nails. Arch Dermatol 105:548, 1972.
36. Stone OJ, Mullins JF: The distal course of nail matrix hemorrhage. Arch Dermatol 88:186, 1963.
37. Terry RB: The onychodermal band in health and disease. Lancet 1:179, 1955.
38. Lewin K: The normal finger nail. Br J Dermatol 77:421, 1965.
39. Branca A: Notes sur la structure de l'ongle. Ann Dermatol Syphiligr 1:353, 1910.
40. Zaias N, Alvarez J: The formation of the primate nail plate. An autoradiographic study in squirrel monkey. J Invest Dermatol 51:120, 1968.
41. Germann H, Barran W, Plewig G: Morphology of corneocytes from human nail plates. J Invest Dermatol 74:115, 1980.
42. Norton LA: Incorporation of thymidine-methyl-H^3 and glycine-2-H^3 in the nail matrix and bed of humans. J Invest Dermatol 56:61, 1971.
43. Lewis BL, Montgomery H: The senile nail. J Invest Dermatol 24:11, 1955.
44. Lovibond JL: Diagnosis of clubbed fingers. Lancet 1:363, 1938.
45. Jarrett A, Spearman RIC: The histochemistry of the human nail. Arch Dermatol 94:652, 1966.
46. Kligman AM: Why do nails grow out instead of up? Arch Dermatol 84:313, 1961.
47. Kligman AM: Nail growth direction revisited (response). J Am Acad Dermatol 4:82, 1981.
48. Baran R: Nail growth direction revisited. J Am Acad Dermatol 4:78, 1981.
49. Zaias N: The movement of the nail bed. J Invest Dermatol 48:402, 1967.
50. Pinkus H, Iwasaki T, Mishima Y: Outer root sheath keratinization in anagen and catagen of the mammalian hair follicle. A seventh distinct type of keratinization in the hair follicle: Trichilemmal keratinization. J Anat 133:19, 1981.
51. Samman PD: The ventral nail. Arch Dermatol 84:1030, 1961.
52. Zook EG: Injuries of the fingernail. *In* Green DP (ed): Operative Hand Surgery. Vol 1. Churchill Livingstone, New York, 1982.
53. Achten G: Normale histologie und histochemie des nagels: *In* Gans O, Steigleder GK (eds): Normale und Pathologische Anatomie der Haut, Vol I/1. Springer-Verlag, New York, 1968.

CHAPTER 3

Embryology

Mary Ellen Brademas

Less is known about the embryology of the nail than about any other cutaneous appendage,[1] perhaps because of the difficulty in obtaining adequate material for study. Until 1954, dermatologists considered the nail plate a uniform sheet of cells originating solely from the ventral nail matrix. In that year, Lewis[2] concluded, on the basis of histochemical findings, that the nail plate consisted of three layers, each of separate and distinct origin. Zaias, however, in two studies of the embryology of the human nail, arrived at different conclusions. Zaias found the nail plate to be a unit structure derived entirely from the ventral nail matrix. Achten[3], on the other hand, concluded that the nail plate consisted of three layers, the first two originating from the ventral and dorsal matrices and the third from the nail bed. Results of elegant investigations by Hashimoto and his colleagues using electron microscopic techniques supported Achten's findings.[3,4]

COMPOSITION OF THE NAIL PLATE

In its broadest sense, epidermal keratinization involves the transformation of committed basal and spinous layer cells through the stage of the granular cell and into the flattened squamae of the stratum corneum.[5] The process involves synthesis of one or more polypeptides that subsequently become stabilized by the formation of cystine bridges.[6] The polypeptides polymerize into helical filiments with an alpha-type x-ray diffraction pattern. Each filament is a repeating unit composed of three elongated, aligned polypeptide chains containing regions of coiled alpha-helix interspersed with regions of nonhelix.[7] Filaggrin, a basic protein contained in keratohyalin granules in the granular cell layer, causes keratin filaments to become densely packed in the terminally differentiating cornified cells.[8] The nail plate keratinizes without the formation of keratohyalin granules.[9]

Elaborated by specialized epidermal cells, the nail plate is hardened epidermal tissue composed of multiple layers of horny cells firmly cemented together and filled with keratin.[10] The keratin proteins belong to a family of neutral buffer-insoluble polypeptides with a molecular weight of 40,000 to 70,000 and are characteristic of epithelial tissue.[11]

Mammalian hard keratin—for example, hair, nails, and hooves—contains a complex mixture of proteins showing considerable variation in their proportions among different species, between different individuals of the same species, between different body locations in an individual, between in vivo epidermis versus cultured cells, between normal ver-

32

sus pathologic skin, and in the epidermal cell (keratinocyte) itself as it undergoes differentiation from the basal cell to the flattened cell of the stratum corneum.[12–15]

Comparative studies show that despite different morphologic characteristics, hair and nails are differentiated along similar lines. Human hair and nails contain the same proteins, although, in addition to the acidic sulfur–rich hard keratins seen in both, nails contain 10 to 20 per cent more basic soft proteins.[16,17]

GENETICS

The development of the vertebrate limb requires, the coordinated action of multiple signals to achieve proper arrangement of adult tissues. The spatial organization of differentiating cells and tissues and ultimately of the body as a whole is called pattern formation.[18] Patterning of the digits is dependent on a group of cells located at the base of the limbs on their posterior border known as the zone of polarizing activity (ZPA). At early stages of development, there appears a characteristic accumulation within the limb mesoderm of a still unidentified morphogen (a substance involved in the formation and differentiation of tissues) diffusing from the ZPA.[19] This substance, together with several recently identified morphogens, plays a central role in patterning of the limb buds. These morphogens include retinoic acid and homeobox genes (*HOX* genes).[18] *HOX* genes are "master" genes that regulate the expression of other genes by producing transcriptional factors (small proteins that activate genes by binding to their promotor regions). Molecular studies of the chick wing have yielded the exciting finding that, during normal development, at least four different *HOX* genes are activated at different times and in a craniocaudad sequence. Cells in the limb bud possess receptors for retinoic acid. Evidence suggests that when retinoic acid occupies these receptor sites it activates specific *HOX* genes, which causes the cell to differentiate.[21]

HISTOGENESIS

The limb buds begin to appear toward the end of the fourth week as slight elevations of the ventrolateral body wall. The leg buds develop slightly after the arm buds, and, throughout fetal development, toenail development lags behind fingernail development by about 4 weeks.[9] The tissues of the limb buds are derived from two main sources: the somatic mesoderm of the lateral plate and the ectoderm.[22]

The nails are derived from the epidermis, which is first segregated from the ectoderm during the process of neurulation. Nail development represents specialized differentiation of epidermal cells and, therefore, is histogenesis rather than organogenesis.[23]

At the fifth gestational week, the human fetus has no fingers or toes, only limb buds. The most distal extensions of these are mitten-like structures, the future hands and feet (Fig. 3–1). The sectioned arm bud (Fig. 3–2) at this stage reveals a seeming disarray of mesenchymal tissue separate from the ectoderm. Interestingly, the mesenchymal cells, although appearing to be loosely arranged, exhibit specialized contact where their processes are apposed.[24]

With the evolution of two layers of surface cells, the periderm and the germinative layer become defined. Results of studies show the dynamic layer of periderm cells to be involved with interface transport. The periderm overlies the developing keratinocytes, which appear to produce keratin during the 11th week; keratin accumulates at the tip of the digit as globular blebs.[25] Production of keratin will persist, undergoing gradual degradation until epidermal cornification is complete at about the 23rd week.[26] At this stage of development, no distinct basal cell layer is present, and a basement membrane cannot be recognized.

Figure 3–3 shows a longitudinal section of the human toe at 8 weeks. Although incomplete, bone formation is clearly discernible, and loose collections of blood cells appear in the mesenchymal tissues, which are separated from the orderly basal cell layer by a clear

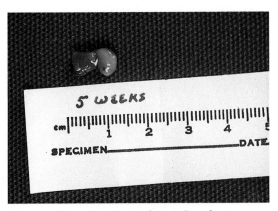

Figure 3–1. Human fetus at 5 weeks.

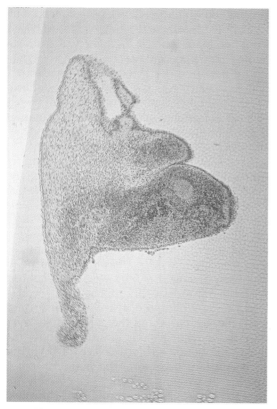

Figure 3–2. Longitudinal section of arm bud.

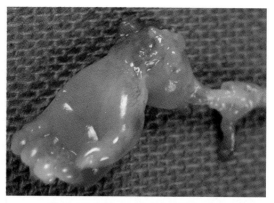

Figure 3–4. Human hand at 10 weeks.

zone. Merkel cells are detected in the nail anlage as early as the ninth week. They increase, particularly in the epithelium of the proximal nail fold and dorsal and ventral sides of the apex region, until the 22nd week, when they recede. Merkel cells in the adult nail matrix are very rare.[27]

At 10 weeks, the human hand is 8 mm long and outwardly, except for the absence of nails (Fig. 3–4), is an exact miniature of the hand at term. Histologically (Fig. 3–5), the cells have

begun to flatten over the dorsal aspect of the distal phalanx, the site of the future nail bed, called the primary nail field. At the proximal end of this flattened area, the cells appear crowded together. This crowding phenomenon of epidermal cells presages incipient nail formation and has been observed to coincide with the earliest stages of hair shaft formation in embryonic skin (Fig. 3–6).[26] No periderm is included in the matrix.[28]

Vessel formation can be observed at the 12th week, and a true invagination of epidermal cells has begun on the dorsal surface proximal to the developing nail bed (Fig. 3–7). This invagination, termed the *matrix primordium*, will continue to grow ventrally and proximally until it reaches a distance of 1 mm from the bony phalanx in the full-term finger.[9] The matrix primordium becomes the proximal nail groove.

At 14 weeks, extension of the matrix primordium can be seen (Fig. 3–8). The future nail—its dorsal layer and midlayer elaborated by the centrodistally oriented cells of the dorsal, apical, and ventral matrices (the ventral surface of the nail plate is made by the nail

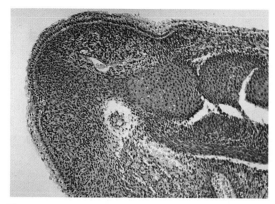

Figure 3–3. Longitudinal section of human toe at 8 weeks.

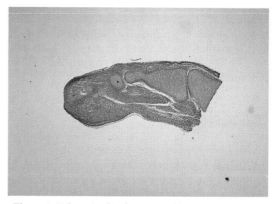

Figure 3–5. Longitudinal section of finger at 10 weeks.

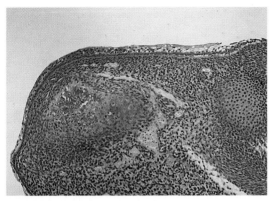

Figure 3–6. Higher magnification of finger at 10 weeks.

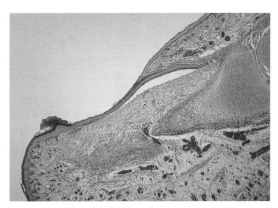

Figure 3–8. Longitudinal section of finger at 14 weeks.

bed)—will occupy the space separating the ventral surface of the proximal nail fold and the nail matrix, which forms the floor of the proximal nail groove and which is seen as the lunula when it extends beyond the edge of the proximal nail fold.[29] Actual keratinization occurs at approximately one fourth of the distance between the apex of the proximal nail fold and the cuticle. This area has been designated by Hashimoto and his colleagues as the vertical level of keratinization of the nail. The process of keratinization occurs even as the matrix primordium undergoes invagination.[4]

The linear extension of eosinophilic material from the tip of the proximal nail fold is the cuticle. It is thought to be a persisting remnant of the periderm. The accumulated mass of eosinophilic material on the most distal aspect of the nail represents the distal ridge. The ridge will be sheared off by the nail plate as the plate passes over it and will persist as a small rise of epidermis called the hyponychium.[13] Rudimentary epidermal rete ridges extend ventrally beyond the hyponychium. At this stage, both the nail bed and the invaginated nail fold develop a granular layer with

typical keratohyalin granules (Fig. 3–9). These disappear when the hard nail plate is formed. The ventral part of the root, which later forms the intermediate matrix, never develops a granular layer. Electron microscopy reveals peculiar dense cytoplasmic bodies associated with ribosomes appearing in cells about to undergo keratinization, but the significance of these bodies is unknown.[23]

At 17 weeks, the nail plate emerges.[30] Vessels and rete are well formed (Fig. 3–10). The discrete islands of basophilic cells within the mesenchyme are eccrine glands. Bridging the area between these islands and the epidermis are even smaller collections of basophilic cells, the future eccrine ducts. Formation of the matrix primordium is complete. The granular layer of the nail bed epithelium will recede in a distal direction concomitantly with the distal movement of the formed nail plate. The nail plate eventually grows out over the nail bed and projects distally as a free edge while its lateral borders are enveloped in the lateral nail folds.[9]

The nail plate is visible to the unaided eye at the tips of the digits by the 26th week.[31] The

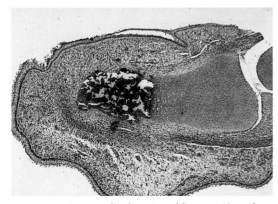

Figure 3–7. Longitudinal section of finger at 12 weeks.

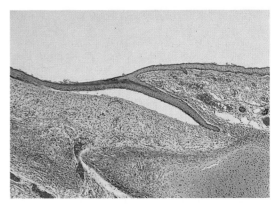

Figure 3–9. Higher magnification of finger at 14 weeks.

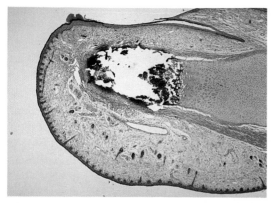

Figure 3–10. Longitudinal section of finger at 17 weeks.

free edge of the nail plate extends beyond the hyponychium by the 32nd week.

Acknowledgment

I thank A. Bernard Ackerman, MD, for the photomicrographs used in this chapter and John Brademas, MD, for his editorial assistance.

References

1. Montagna W, Parakkal PE: The Structure and Function of Skin, ed 3. Academic Press, New York, 1974, p 272.
2. Lewis BL: Microscopic studies of fetal and mature nail and surrounding soft tissue. Arch Dermatol Syphilol 70:732–744, 1954.
3. Achten G: L'ongle normal of pathologique. Dermatologica 126:229–245, 1963.
4. Hashimoto K, Gross BG, Nelson R, et al: Ultrastructure of the skin of human embryos: The formation of the nail in 16–18 week old embryos. J Invest Dermatol 47:205, 1966.
5. Breathnach AS: Aspects of epidermal ultrastructure. J Invest Dermatol 66:622, 1975.
6. Mercer EH: Keratin and Keratinization. An Essay in Molecular Biology. Pergamon Press, New York, 1961, p 21.
7. Freedberg IM: Epidermal protein synthesis and its control. In Goldsmith LA (ed): Biochemistry and Physiology of the Skin. Oxford University Press, New York, 1983, pp 282–291.
8. Manabe M, Sanchez M, Sun T-T, Dale BA: Interaction of filaggrin with keratin filaments during advanced stages of normal human epidermis differentiation in Ichthyosis vulgaris. Differentiation 48:43, 1991.
9. Zaias N: The Nail in Health and Disease. Spectrum Publications, New York, 1980.
10. Hashimoto K: Ultrastructure of the human toenail.
11. Baden HP: The keratinocyte has become the subject of intense investigation. J Invest Dermatol 84:305, 1984.
12. Gillespie JM, Marshall RC: Proteins of the hard keratins of echidna, hedgehog, rabbit, ox and man. Aust Biol Sci 30:401, 1977.
13. Steinert PM, Peck GL, Idler WW: Structural changes of human epidermal keratin in disorders of keratinization. In Bernstein IA, Seiji M (eds): Biochemistry of Normal and Abnormal Epidermal Differentiation. Tokyo University Press, Tokyo, 1980, pp 391–406.
14. Ball RD, Walker GK, Bernstein IA: Histadine-rich proteins as molecular markers of epidermal differentiation. J Biol Chem 253:5861, 1978.
15. Baden HP, Goldsmith LA, Fleming B: A comparative study of the physiochemical properties of human keratinized tissues. Acta Biochem Biophys 322:269, 1973.
16. Marshall RG: Genetic variation in the proteins of the human nail. J Invest Dermatol 785:264, 1980.
17. Lynch MH, O'Guin M, Hardy C, et al. Acidic, basic hair/nail (hard) keratins: Their colocalization in the upper cortical and cuticle cells of the human hair follicle and their relationship to "soft" keratins. J Cell Biol 103:2593, 1986.
18. Larsen WJ: Human Embryology. Churchill Livingstone, New York, 1993, p 300.
19. Sadler TW: Langman's Medical Embryology. Baltimore, MD, Williams & Wilkins, 1995, p 155.
20. Macias D, Ganan Y, Hurle JM: Modification of the phalangeal pattern of the digits in the chick embryo leg bud by local microinjection of RA, staurosporin and TGF betas. Anat Embryol 188:201, 1993.
21. Yokouchi Y, Ohsugi K, Sasaki H, Kuroiwa A: Chicken homeobox gene Msx-1 structure, expression in the limb buds and effect of retinoic acid. Development 113:431, 1991.
22. Moore K: The Developing Human, ed 4. WB Saunders, Philadelphia, 1988.
23. Balinski BI: An Introduction to Embryology, ed 5. WB Saunders, Philadelphia, 1981.
24. Breathnach AS: The Herman Beerman lecture: Embryology of human skin, a review of ultrastructure studies. J Invest Dermatol 57:133, 1971.
25. Mazzarello V, Dessi CA: Ontogenesis of the human fetal nails. I. Observations using the scanning electron microscope. Bollettino-Societa Italiana Biologia Sperimentale. 66:441, 1994.
26. Holbrook KA, Odland GF: The fine structure of the developing epidermis: Light, scanning and transmission electron microscopy of the periderm. J Invest Dermatol 65:16, 1975.
27. Moll I, Moll R: Merkel cells in ontogenesis of human nails. Arch Dermatol Res 285:366, 1993.
28. Steinert PM, Cantier JS: Epidermal keratin. In Goldsmith LA (ed): Biochemistry and Physiology of the Skin. Oxford University Press, New York, 1983, pp 135–169.
29. Fleckman P: Anatomy and physiology of the nail. Dermatol Clin 3:373, 1985.
30. Baran P, Dawber RPR: Diseases of the Nails and their Management. Cambridge, MA, Blackwell Scientific, 1994, p 3.
31. Jarrett A: The Physiology and Pathophysiology of the Skin, vol 5. Academic Press, New York, 1978.

Cell migration, keratinization and formation of the intercellular cement. Arch Dermatol Res 240:1, 1971.

CHAPTER 4

Basic Science of the Nail Unit

Philip Fleckman

Published interest in the nails arose in the 19th century.[1–3] This chapter provides a review of the embryology, anatomy and cell biology, physiology, biochemistry, biophysics, and pharmacology of the nail unit. When appropriate, clinical correlations with basic science are discussed. The term *nail unit*, defined by Zaias as the four structures that together form what is commonly called the nail,[4] is used throughout this review. The terms *nail plate* and *nail* are used interchangeably.

In a book devoted to the treatment of nail disorders, it is appropriate to focus what is known about the basic science of nails by asking the following questions:

1. What explains the optical properties of the nail? Why is the lunula white?
2. What seals the proximal nail fold to the nail plate, and how is this affected by pathologic processes that produce chronic paronychia?
3. What holds the nail down, and how is this affected by pathologic processes that produce onycholysis?
4. What is the source of pigment in the nail unit? How can this information be used to understand and treat leukonychia and abnormalities of nail pigmentation?
5. What factors control the rate of nail growth? Can these factors explain pathologic

processes such as the decreased rate of growth in the yellow nail syndrome and increased rate of growth in psoriasis?
6. What holds the nail together? Why is the nail hard? What causes brittle, thin, or split nails?
7. What controls the penetration of substances into the nail? How can effective topical therapies be designed for the treatment of nail bed and nail matrix diseases?

EMBRYOLOGY

The embryology of the nail unit was investigated as early as the late 19th century (reviewed in Lewis[5] and Zaias[6]). Lewis,[5] Zaias,[6] Hashimoto and colleagues,[7] and Holbrook[8] studied the embryology of the human nail. Their work has been reviewed.[9,10]

Fingers are first recognized in the sixth week in utero; toes are recognized the following week. By the eighth week, digits are separated, but the earliest visible external changes defining the nail unit are appreciated only in the 10th week. A smooth, shiny, quadrangular surface, the primary nail field is at this time delineated on the dorsum of the distal digit by shallow grooves. The distal groove—the most distal of these shallow grooves—delineates the distal edge of the primary nail field. By the

11th week, well-formed fingers with joints are seen. At the tip of the finger in the distal part of the primary nail field just proximal to the distal groove, the distal ridge appears as an area of thickened epidermis. This distal ridge is the first area in the embryo to become keratinized. The distal ridge becomes the hyponychium, the area first invaded by dermatophytes in distal subungual onychomycosis.[11] At the same time, an area in the proximal primary nail field, the matrix primordium, grows into the substance of the distal phalanx. The matrix primordium grows proximally and ventrally, isolating a wedge of dermis dorsally that becomes the proximal nail fold. Beginning at its distal end and proceeding proximally, the matrix primordium differentiates into the matrix. By the 14th week, a recognizable nail plate can be seen emerging from beneath the proximal nail fold. The entire nail bed is covered by a stratum corneum. By the 16th week, the nail plate covers one half of the nail bed. The plate initially forms via keratohyalin granules. Only later, after the nail plate has grown over the matrix, does the nail plate form via the parakeratotic process seen in the adult. By the 17th week, the nail plate covers almost the entire nail bed. From this time on, changes in the nail unit are mainly those of growth. As the nail plate grows over the distal ridge, the distal ridge progressively flattens, forming the hyponychium.

ANATOMY AND CELL BIOLOGY

The topography of the nail unit was described by Zaias (Fig. 4–1).[6] The nail unit consists of the proximal nail fold, the matrix, the nail bed, and the hyponychium (Figs. 4–2 to 4–4). These structures together form the nail plate, the flat, rectangular, convex, translucent, hard structure sitting on top of the digits and extending past their free edge.

The nail plate consists of close-packed, adherent, interdigitating cells that lack nuclei or organelles. Cells in the plate are very flat, lying with the smallest diameter perpendicular to the plane of the nail plate surface. There is a progression from the top (dorsal surface) of the plate, where cell borders are straight, to the middle of the plate, where cell borders are much more "meandering."[12] Many intercellular links are present, including tight, intermediate, and desmosomal junctions.[13] The cells at the surface of the nail plate overlap, slanting from "proximal-dorsal to distal-volar."[14] Scan-

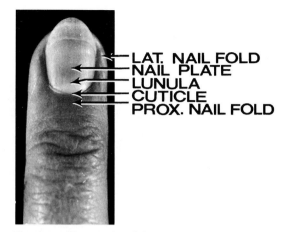

Figure 4–1. Topography of the nail unit. The surface landmarks of the nail unit viewed from the top (courtesy of Karen Holbrook, PhD).

ning electron microscopy reveals that the dorsal surface of the nail plate is smooth but the palmar surface is irregular.[15] The nail plate is approximately 0.5 mm thick in women and 0.6 mm thick in men.[16] In normal nails, distal plate thickness can be ranked as thumb > index > middle > ring > little finger.[17] On the basis of radioautographic data, the length of the matrix determines the thickness of the nail plate.[4] The progressive increase in nail plate thickness with age may be due to the increasing size of the cells in the plate.[16] This view is supported by cytologic study of the cells of the dorsal nail plate, which shows that the area of the cells correlates with growth rate, increasing with decreasing growth rate and with the age of the patient.[18]

The nail plate is formed by a progressive broadening and flattening of cells in the matrix as they mature to form nail plate cells, with fragmentation and lysis of nuclei and retention of nuclear membranes in nail plate cells.[5,6] There is an increase in intermediate (tono)filaments, with clumping, lateral accretion, and the eventual formation of the keratin pattern (a morphologic pattern seen with the electron microscope in stratum corneum)[19] as basal cells differentiate and rise to form nail plate cells. Lamellar granules are observed extruding contents into the extracellular space, and marginal band formation is seen. With the exception of second-trimester embryonic nail formation, the matrix cells form nail plate by a process in which no keratohyalin granules are produced. No keratohyalin granules are seen.[20,21] Frequent gap junctions are observed near the area where lamellar granules are dis-

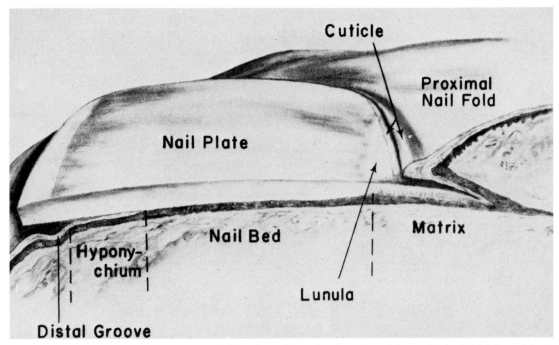

Figure 4–2. Diagram of a sagittal section through the nail unit. The nail unit consists of the proximal nail fold, the matrix, the nail bed, and the hyponychium. Together, these structures form and support the nail plate. From Zaias N: The embryology of the human nail. Arch Dermatol 87:39, 1963. Copyright 1963, American Medical Association. Used with permission.

charging their contents, and it has been suggested that a substance with the size of lanthanum complex might be able to pass through the nail plate via such intercellular channels. Perhaps such channels explain why the nail plate is more permeable to polar solvents than is skin.[22]

If the nail plate is removed, three potential spaces become apparent: the proximal nail groove (see Fig. 4–3) and the two lateral nail grooves. Folds of skin, the proximal and lateral nail folds, overlap the nail plate to form these grooves. The proximal nail fold (PNF) (see Figs. 4–1 to 4–4) is an invaginating, wedge-shaped fold of skin on the dorsum of the distal digit. The nail plate arises from under this fold. The dorsum of the PNF consists of a continuation of the epidermis and dermis of the dorsal digit with sweat glands but no follicles or sebaceous glands. At the distal tip of the PNF, the skin reflects proximally and ventrally, traveling about 5 to 8 mm toward the distal interphalangeal joint. The skin of the ventral surface of the PNF is quite thin, has no appendages, and is closely applied to the dorsal surface of the nail plate. The epithelium of the ventral surface of the PNF has also been called the eponychium.[23] The stratum corneum of the tip and the ventral surface of

the PNF grow out a short way on the dorsal surface of the nail plate as the cuticle (see Figs. 4–1 to 4–4) before being shed. The cuticle seals the PNF to the dorsal surface of the nail plate. Disruption of this seal results in production of a real space from the potential space between the ventral surface of the PNF and the dorsal surface of the nail plate and may result in chronic paronychia.

The ventral surface of the PNF forms the roof of the proximal nail groove; the nail matrix (see Figs. 4–2 and 4–3) forms its floor; the nail plate lies between the two. In fact, the matrix begins just before the roof of the proximal nail groove makes its distal bend toward the tip of the digit. The matrix is a thick epithelium and has no granular layer. Because of this, the transition from the ventral surface of the PNF to matrix is easily appreciated. Nail matrix cells have been cultured and shown to express both epithelial ("soft") and "hard" keratins (see discussion of biochemistry).[24,25] The basal surface of the matrix cells interdigitates in finger-like projections.[20] Despite this interdigitation, one can undermine and move the matrix surgically with ease.

The matrix of Caucasians contains sparse, poorly developed melanocytes.[26] Melanocytes are more numerous in distal than in proximal

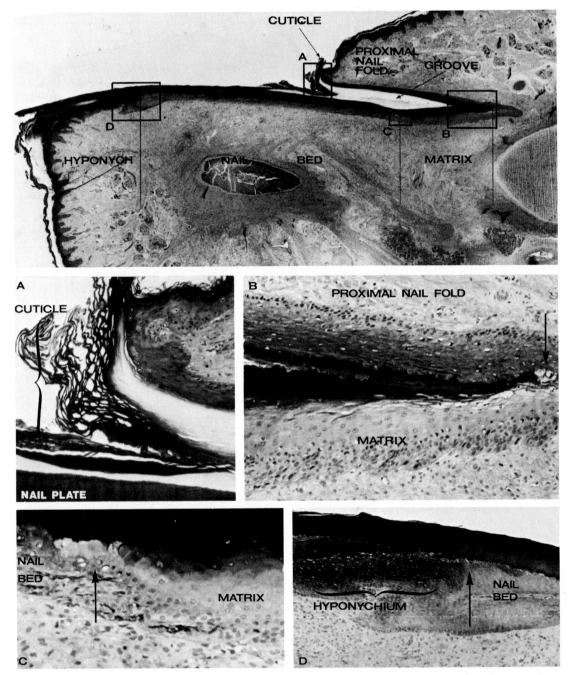

Figure 4–3. Photomicrograph of a sagittal section through the nail unit. *A–D,* Enlargements taken from the upper figure from the indicated areas. The proximal nail fold is artifactually separated from the nail plate, revealing the upper half of the proximal nail groove (groove). In the upper figure, vertical lines indicate the junction between the matrix, nail bed, and hyponychium (hyponych). In this nail unit, no lunula would be seen, as the matrix–nail bed junction is beneath the proximal nail fold (Richardson stain, original magnification × 18). *A,* The distal tip of the proximal nail fold. Note the cuticle growing out on the nail plate (Top plate 13×18 *A–D,* × 600; *B,* The proximal margin of the proximal nail groove. Arrow indicates the transition in the roof (ventral surface) of the proximal nail fold from normal epithelium to nail matrix, with loss of keratohyalin granules. *C,* The junction of the matrix with the nail bed. Note the thinness of the epithelium of the nail bed with the matrix. Neither epithelium contains keratohyalin granules. *D,* The junction of the nail bed and the hyponychium. Note the abrupt appearance of keratohyalin granules and a normal, keratinized (orthokeratotic) stratum corneum (arrow) (*A–D,* Richardson stain, original magnification × 600) (courtesy of Karen A. Holbrook, PhD).

whites, the number of melanocytes and the intensity of the dopa reaction in those melanocytes are much greater in distal than in proximal (Japanese) matrix. Investigators have speculated that the proximal–distal difference is because those melanocytes in the proximal matrix are protected by the PNF from stimulation by ultraviolet light and other exogenous agents.[28] The location of melanocytes in the matrix is directly related to the location of pigmented bands, most of which originate in the distal matrix and do not involve the proximal matrix.[29] Langerhans' cells have also been identified in matrix,[26] and Merkel cells have been found in the matrix and nail bed epithelium.[30]

When the matrix extends beyond the edge of the PNF, it is seen as the lunula (see Figs. 4–1, 4–2, and 4–4). The lunula is the white, half-moon–shaped area seen on some but not all nails. The shape of the lunula determines the shape of the nail plate.[31] Several hypotheses have been proposed to explain why the lunula is white. Burrows suggested that the matrix was not firmly adherent to the underlying connective tissue, became separated, and produced a reflecting surface that appeared white.[32] Lewin[33] stated that the flat, shiny surface (in contrast to the rougher, distal part of the nail), the opacity of the proximal nail plate, the relative avascularity of the subepidermal layer, and the loose texture of the dermal collagen contributed to the color of the lunula. Zaias commented that the nail plate is thinner over the lunula than over the nail bed and that the area of the lunula corresponds with that of the keratogenous zone, the zone of cytoplasmic condensation in the matrix just before cells form the nail plate.[4] Samman and Fenton pointed out that the lunula remains apparent in both the nail plate and the underlying nail bed after nail avulsion and stated that the color is likely due to a combination of incomplete keratinization in the nail plate and loose connective tissue in the underlying dermis.[34] This hypothesis is supported by high-resolution magnetic resonance imaging, which reveals a well-defined area beneath the nail matrix that histologically is composed of loose connective tissue.[35] The area is supplied by large regular meshes of vascular networks.[36] Zaias suggested that the color is the same as that seen in leukonychia, in which nucleated cells are often found in the nail plate.[4,37]

The nail bed begins where the lunula or distal matrix ends (see Figs. 4–2 to 4–4). Like the lunula, the nail bed has no granular layer,

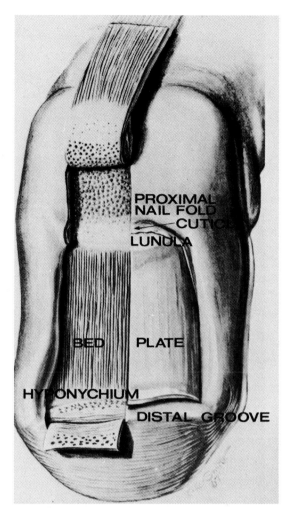

Figure 4–4. Diagram of the nail unit with the proximal nail fold, matrix, nail bed, and hyponychium reflected. The epidermis of the proximal nail fold, matrix, and nail bed is reflected back, and the epidermis of the hyponychium is reflected forward to expose the underlying dermal papillae. Note the parallel, tongue-in-groove spatial arrangement of the epidermal rete and dermal papillae of the nail bed compared with the conventional rete of the papillary dermis seen in the matrix and hyponychium. From Zaias N, Ackerman AB: The nail in Darier-White disease. Arch Dermatol 107:193, 1973. Copyright 1973, American Medical Association. Used with permission.

matrix; the cells are located both in the basal layer and suprabasally, as single cells and in small clusters of three to four cells.[27] The distal matrix of people of color is thought to contain more melanocytes than are seen in whites; this is in contrast to interfollicular skin, in which pigment formation is increased but the number of melanocytes is the same. For example, the distal matrix of Japanese individuals contains several hundred well-developed melanocytes per square millimeter.[28] As with but unlike the lunula, the nail bed is an extremely thin epithelium. Thus, the end of the matrix and beginning of the nail bed are easily appreciated histologically (see Figs. 4–2 and 4–3). The nail bed has a unique, longitudinal, tongue-in-groove spatial arrangement of papillary dermal papillae and epidermal rete ridges (see Fig. 4–4). In transverse section, this arrangement is appreciated as a serrated interdigitation of papillae and rete (Fig. 4–5). When spirally coiled vessels in the hyponychium rupture,[38] the blood extravasates into these longitudinal grooves to form splinter hemorrhages. If one avulses the plate and studies the undersurface by scanning electron microscopy, one sees grooves.[39] Rand and Baden speculated that the nail plate adheres to the nail bed by way of these grooves.[40] It is unclear whether the ridges seen belong to the nail bed epithelium that remains attached to the nail plate after avulsion[41] or are actually etched into the undersurface of the plate, although they are not seen at the free edge of the plate and avulsed epidermis was not removed from the undersurface of the nail plate before it was studied by scanning electron microscopy (Montagna W: Personal communication, June 10 1988). A combination of the deep interdigitation of the nail bed epithelium with underlying papillary dermis and the thin epithelium of the nail bed probably makes moving the nail bed difficult surgically.

The nail bed ends beneath the nail plate at the beginning of the hyponychium (see Figs. 4–2 to 4–4). The hyponychium marks the beginning of normal volar epidermis. As with the dorsal skin of the PNF, a granular layer and eccrine glands are present, and this epithelium undergoes normal keratinization. The hyponychium is the first site of keratinization in the nail unit[5,6] and of all epidermis in the embryo.[8] The hyponychium is said to make waterproof the area where the nail plate lifts off the nail bed.[14] The hyponychium is the initial site of invasion by dermatophytes in the most common type of onychomycosis: distal subungual onychomycosis.[11]

Beneath the distal nail plate, just proximal to the white line that marks the separation of the nail plate from the hyponychium, lies the onychodermal band.[42] This narrow band, normally from 0.5 to 1.5 mm wide, was described by Terry[42] as paler than the pink nail bed, with a slightly amber tinge and a translucent quality. However, Stewart and Raffle commented that "many normal onychodermal bands are actually a *deeper* pink" than the adjacent distal

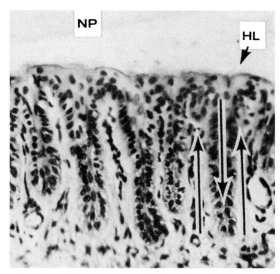

Figure 4–5. Photomicrograph of a coronal (transverse) section through the midline of the nail bed. Note the serrated, interdigitating nail bed epidermal rete ridges (arrow down) and dermal papillae (arrows up). (NP, nail plate; HL, horny layer of the nail plate.) (Hematoxylin and eosin, original magnification × 450.) From Zaias N: Psoriasis of the nail. Arch Dermatol 99:569, 1969. Copyright 1969, American Medical Association. Used with permission.

nail bed[43]; I agree. The band may be pigmented in black skin. Terry speculated that this area had a blood supply different from the remainder of the nail bed; this is supported by the work of Martin and Platts.[38] The area of the onychodermal band can become prominent in chronic renal failure, cirrhosis, and other chronic disease.[42,44–46] Sonnex and coworkers[47] described the onychocorneal band, which they pointed out was originally described by Pinkus.[1] This is a thin, tranverse white line, 0.1 to 1 mm wide, that transects the accentuated pink band at the distal edge of the nail bed that is the onychodermal band. The authors described this as the point of attachment of the epidermis of the skin of the fingertip to the undersurface of the nail plate and proposed that the area was necessary for "maintaining the integrity of nail attachment." They stated that this was the site of resistance to a probe passed proximally from beneath the undersurface of the free edge of the nail plate, although Terry stated that the site of resistance was at the proximal edge of the onychodermal band. How can all this be interpreted? The onychodermal band and the onychocorneal band are easily observed when one extends the finger. The point of attachment of the undersurface of the nail plate to the volar epidermis of the fingertip is obviously vital in sealing the nail plate to the nail bed and preventing onycholysis. If the observations of Sonnex and colleagues withstand the scrutiny of others, the onychocorneal band marks this site.

The most distal boundary of the nail unit is marked by the distal groove (see Figs. 4–2 and 4–4). This indentation of the volar epidermal skin marks the distal site of demarcation of the primary nail field, the earliest external change in the embryonic development of the nail.[6]

The basement membrane zone of the nail unit resembles that of interfollicular epidermis and expresses target antigens in an identical manner.[48]

The distal phalanx lies immediately below the structures of the nail unit. An extensor tendon runs over the ventral surface of the distal interphalangeal joint and attaches to the distal phalanx, proximal to the reflection of the proximal nail groove. Lateral ligaments extend from the ungual processes of the distal phalanx to the lateral ligaments of the distal interphalangeal joint (Fig. 4–6). The importance of the phalanx in normal development of the nail unit has been emphasized by Kelikian and others.[49,50] Because the dermis is quite thin and there is no subcutis in this area, pressure from tumors lying in the nail unit may erode the bone; likewise, bony tumors of the distal phalanx often manifest as nail abnormalities. Even simple surgical procedures in the nail unit, such as punch biopsy, extend to the periosteum; therefore, careful attention to sterile technique is indicated.

BLOOD AND NERVE SUPPLY OF THE NAIL UNIT

The blood supply of the nail unit derives from the lateral digital arteries [51–53] (see Fig. 4–6). These arteries give off medium-sized branches that cross over the dorsal surface of the distal interphalangeal joint to supply a superficial arcade, which supplies the PNF and matrix. The lateral digital arteries then enter the distal digit adjacent to the volar surface of the bone and give off branches to the bone and the superficial arcade.[5,53] The digital arteries then course dorsally around the "waist" of the distal phalanx in the confined space between the bone and the lateral ligament and perforate the septum of the pulp space. Here they divide to form proximal and distal arcades, which supply the matrix and nail bed. Thus, the matrix has two sources of blood supply: the superficial and the proximal arcades.[51,53] This is beneficial when disease (e.g., scleroderma) affects the vessels in the pulp.

The digital arterial system manifests two characteristic anatomic features: arched anastomotic arteries in the deep dermis and more superficial terminal arteries that branch to supply the rete.[52] The arteries possess inner

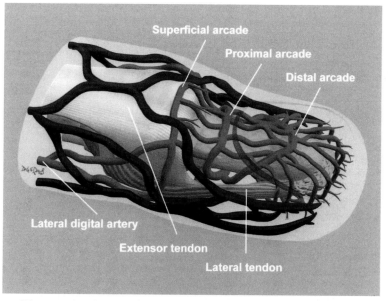

Figure 4–6. Diagram of the arterial and venous blood supply and tendons of the nail unit. Drawing by Dale Davis, MT, ASCP, based on references 5, 36, 38, 51–53 and the representations of Andrew Morgan, MD. Used with permission.

longitudinal and outer circular coats of smooth muscle but no internal elastic lamina. The vasculature of the nail bed is unique in that it must supply a vascular structure between two hard surfaces: the nail plate and the bone. Venous drainage combines proximally, forming two veins, one on each side of the plate in the PNF.[52]

Below the hyponychium, where the longitudinal rete ridges are replaced by conventional papillary dermis, long, thin-walled, spirally wound, looped vessels of wide caliber are found.[38] These vessels rupture, filling the longitudinal troughs formed by the rete and papillae in the nail bed with blood to form splinter hemorrhages. Large arteriovenous (AV) anastomoses are found at the level of the anastomotic arteries and the deep venous circulation in all areas of the nail unit except the PNF. These AV anastomoses vary morphologically, from simple, unmodified anastomoses to a complex association of vessels.[52] The simple structures probably function as AV shunts. The more complex structures are confined to the nail bed and volar areas; their function is speculative. It is unclear whether the occurrence of glomus tumors is restricted to either structure. The innervation of the nail unit roughly parallels the blood supply.

NAIL PLATE GROWTH

The rate of nail growth has been studied extensively.[54,55] A consensus about these numbers has evolved despite failure to assess variation within or between patients, inconsistent statistical analysis, and the use of many different techniques.[56] Normal fingernail growth varies from less than 1.8 to more than 4.5 mm per month and varies markedly between individuals but is more constant among members of the same family.[16] The average growth rate of 0.1 mm/day (3 mm/month)[4] is invaluable for determining the approximate time of trauma to a nail and for predicting future events. For example, a nail that has a rim of polish 3 mm distal to the PNF was last painted about 1 month previously. It takes a normal fingernail about 2 months to grow the 5 to 8 mm out from under the PNF. A normal fingernail, therefore, grows out completely in about 6 months. Toenails grow at half to one third the rate of fingernails, so a normal toenail takes 12 to 18 months to grow out.[34] Approximately 3 g of fingernail plate is produced annually.[57]

Nails grow faster when regenerating after avulsion.[4] In any individual, nail growth is proportional to the length of the finger.[58,59] Nail growth is faster in the dominant hand and faster in males than in females.[16] Nail growth is faster than normal during pregnancy,[60] in nail biters,[59] in warm climates,[59,61] and in persons with psoriasis[58] and onycholysis (psoriatic and idiopathic).[63] The rate of nail growth peaks between the ages of 10 and 14 years and begins an inexorable decrease with age after the second decade of life.[16,54,58,64] The rate of nail growth is less than normal in persons who are immobilized or paralyzed[65]; those with decreased circulation,[55] malnutrition,[66] or the yellow nail syndrome[67]; at night[68]; during lactation[55]; in acute infection[54,69]; and during therapy with antimitotic drugs.[58]

The question of where the nail plate is formed is disputed.[4,34,70,71] Unna[3] and Pinkus[1] believed that the nail plate was formed by the matrix. On the basis of staining of the nail plate with a silver protein stain and on morphology of keratinizing cells, Lewis concluded that the nail plate was the product of three different matrices.[5] He postulated the dorsal matrix in the roof of the PNF, which made the dorsal part of the nail plate; the conventional matrix, which made the intermediate nail; and the ventral matrix on the nail bed, which made the ventral part of the nail plate. The ventral and dorsal parts of the nail were produced by an "inflation–deflation cycle," whereas the intermediate nail was made by "gradient parakeratosis." The dorsal nail was thin compared with the intermediate nail, whereas the ventral nail varied from absent to one third the thickness of the intermediate nail. Lewis' hypothesis was supported by differential staining of the nail plate,[72] by Zeiss-Nomarski differential interference contrast microscopy,[20] by ultrastructural observation of keratohyalin granules in embryonic nail,[20] and by physical properties of dissected nail clippings.[12] Johnson and colleagues suggested that approximately 20% of normal nail plate is contributed by the nail bed.[73,74] On the other hand, Zaias and Alvarez used radioautography to show that the nail plate was formed exclusively by the matrix in squirrel monkey.[75] They showed that the most proximal part of the matrix makes the dorsal nail plate, whereas the distal matrix makes the distal nail plate. This work was criticized by Hashimoto.[20] These criticisms were answered when Norton confirmed Zaias' work by following the incorporation of

3H-labeled glycine and thymidine in human toenails.[71] Samman reported other evidence supporting the exclusive formation of the nail plate by the matrix[53]; Caputo and Dadati[13] and Forslind[12] reported that ultrastructurally the nail plate was a homogeneous structure with no evidence of formation from three different matrices; Forslind and colleagues[76,77] and Robson and Brooks[78] used electron probe microanalysis (analytic electron microscopy) to show that there was no difference between dorsal and intermediate nail plate in dry mass, sulfur content, calcium, or potassium levels; and Hashimoto[20] reported that all parts of the adult nail plate keratinized similarly. Monoclonal antibody staining of nail-associated keratin proteins also supports exclusive formation of the nail plate by the (conventional) matrix[24,79] (see discussion of biochemistry). To add one final bit of confusion, Samman suggested that although under normal conditions the nail plate is made exclusively by the matrix, in certain pathologic conditions the nail bed adds a ventral nail to the undersurface of the nail plate.[53,80]

Why has there been so much effort to complicate the matrix, and where *is* the nail plate formed? Lewis seized on his histochemical findings to explain the nail plate dystrophy observed in paronychia (ventral matrix inflammation) and in diseases of the nail bed (e.g., psoriasis and distal subungual onychomycosis). Samman could not confirm the dorsal nail findings but supported the idea of a ventral nail in disease. The data of Zaias and Norton are irrefutable; the nail plate is formed predominantly by the matrix under normal conditions, with a possible small contribution of cells to the undersurface of the nail plate by the nail bed. Rather than postulate a dorsal matrix, dorsal nail plate dystrophy produced by PNF disease (e.g., paronychia) is best explained by an effect of inflammation on the underlying proximal matrix, which produces the dorsal surface of the nail plate.[75] Whether a ventral nail exists under pathologic conditions remains to be proved.

Why do nails grow out instead of up? Kligman postulated that the cul-de-sac of the proximal nail groove forced the cells of the matrix to grow out.[81] He showed that nail matrix transplanted to the forearm produced a vertical cylinder of hard keratin that had histologic characteristics of nail. Hashimoto stated that the long axis of the matrix cells in embryonic nail was directed upward and distally.[7] Baran disputed Kligman's findings on the basis of observations of surgically excised proximal nail folds and the lack of bone under the forearm graft.[82] Kikuchi and colleagues' examination of a congenital ectopic nail supports Kligman's hypothesis.[83] Dawber and Baran summarized the literature and concluded that all hypotheses are partially correct.[56] One can only agree with Kligman in his assessment of the problem: "the subject of nail growth . . . is worthy of further consideration."[84]

The manner in which the nail plate grows out and the relationship between the nail plate and the nail bed in nail growth are issues directly related to the clinical problems of onycholysis and nail growth. Pinkus was quoted by Silver and Chiego in discussing the observation that splinter hemorrhage, which occurs between the plate and bed, grows forward with the plate.[85] If the plate merely moved over the bed, the extravasated blood would not move; therefore, the upper part of the bed must move out with the plate. Krantz removed the distal two thirds of one side of the plate, marked the underlying nail bed, and observed these marks moving forward.[86] From this he concluded that there is no "gliding" of the nail plate over the bed; rather, the two grow forward together. Kligman removed a transverse strip of nail plate distal to the lunula so that there was a strip of plate on the distal nail bed not connected to the more proximal plate.[87] He observed the distal strip of plate move forward and shed before the gap was closed and concluded that "the hyponychium is dragging the nail plate." Zaias observed that the crust produced after nail avulsion was pushed off by regrowing nail instead of growing forward with the nail bed.[41] Zaias repeated the experiment of Kligman but did not find that the distal strip of nail plate moved forward.[88] He suggested that Kligman's observations were based on the result of trauma. He also repeated the experiment of Krantz, with the exception of removing the entire side of a nail plate instead of the distal two thirds of one side. Zaias observed that although the proximal nail bed marks moved out as Krantz reported, the distal marks did not. He concluded that the proximal nail bed moves out either by "pressures by the advancing [regrowing] plate" or because of trauma, but that the distal nail bed and hyponychium do not move. Norton's findings support the movement of cells from the distal matrix to the proximal nail bed.[71] More recently, Zaias reported data clarifying the mechanism of nail plate growth and its relationship to the nail bed.[4] From the data he concluded that "basal cells labeled at the nail bed origin [proximal nail bed] move distally and differentiate to the [under-] surface [of the plate] along the entire length of the nail bed. The growth rate or movement of the matrix and nail bed cells is identical."

What attaches the nail plate to the nail unit? The nail bed contributes significantly to the attachment of the nail plate to its underlying structures. When one avulses a nail plate, most of the resistance is encountered in the nail bed (personal observation, supported by Samman and Fenton[34]). Zaias and others observed that most of the epithelium of the nail bed remains attached to the undersurface of the avulsed plate.[41] Zaias commented that although the nail bed contributes nothing to the mass of the plate, it does contribute a few cells to the undersurface of the plate.[4] The hyponychium contributes cells to the undersurface of the free edge of the nail plate.[14,87] A combination of the small contribution of cells by the nail bed to the undersurface of the plate and the interdigitating, tongue-in-groove spatial arrangement of the nail bed rete and dermal papillae probably holds the plate to the bed.[40] The area is sealed distally by the hyponychium-onychocorneal band. One question remains, however: if the nail bed contributes directly to the undersurface of the nail plate and the nail plate is firmly attached to the nail bed, how does the plate move out? Does the plate slide over the bed? To quote Hashimoto, "It is difficult to conceive that the nail bed provides just a sliding floor for the nail plate produced more proximally."[20] How does the unique spatial arrangement of the nail bed rete and dermal papillae contribute to the attachment and movement of the nail plate? Does the nail bed grow out with the plate, or is there some other mechanism of attachment and release akin to the making and breaking of desmosomal contacts between keratinocytes as the cells differentiate and rise in the epidermis? The answers to these questions remain to be clarified.

BIOCHEMISTRY OF THE NAIL UNIT

What is the nail plate composed of? Many investigators have studied the composition of the nail plate with the idea that nail plate, as an epithelial product, will reflect body mineral metabolism. A second assumption is that the slow growth of nail plate will temper transient factors that may perturb serum mineral levels

and confuse understanding of overall mineral metabolism. Their findings are summarized in Table 4–1 and highlighted in the following text.

Components of the nail plate can be divided into two groups: inorganic and organic. Inorganic elements can be divided into trace metals and electrolytes (circulating ions in the plasma and other body fluids). Serious technical difficulties arise in measuring inorganic elements in nail plates. External (environmental) contamination and the accuracy of the technique used probably account for both the wide range of values reported by individual investigators and the differences reported between investigators. Variability between investigators may be compounded by different washing procedures aimed at removing environmental contaminants but resulting in differential extraction of the elements from the nail plate being studied.[89] Large variations among patients,[90] twofold variation between fingers of the same individual,[91] 25 per cent variation between sections of one nail plate, and great variations between successive segments of the same nail over time[92] have been reported in the measurement of one element. Unfortunately, despite such large variation in measured results, statistical evaluation of data is often not reported. Therefore, the significance of the reported observations can be questioned. Some methods (e.g., emission spectroscopy and spark source mass spectrometry) are useful for the detection of several metals on small samples of one specimen (including toxic metals such as arsenic) but are too insensitive to detect small variations occurring in metabolic disease. More sensitive techniques, such as chemical methods, flame photometry, and atomic absorption spectroscopy, are better suited for smaller changes.[90,91,93]

In spite of technical difficulties in measurement of inorganic elements in nail plates, many interesting observations have been reported: calcium and zinc are higher and magnesium is lower in nail plates from males than from females,[93] magnesium and sodium are higher in the nails of children than in the nails of adults,[86,92] and copper is increased in the nail plates of patients with Wilson's disease.[94] Iron has been reported to be decreased in the nail plates of adolescents and either decreased[95] or unchanged[96] in patients with iron deficiency anemia. Magnesium was increased in the nails of two patients undergoing chronic dialysis,[91] and sodium and calcium are higher and magnesium is lower in nail plates of children with kwashiorkor than in normal children.[78,97] The concentration of sodium is increased in nail plates from patients with cystic fibrosis and may be useful in the diagnosis of the disease when sweat test results are inconclusive and in patients living in remote areas.[98,99] The level of arsenic in the nail plate increases within hours of exposure and can be useful for demonstrating acute and chronic arsenic intoxication.[100,101]

Organic elements are less difficult to quantify. Although carbon is technically the only organic element, sulfur and nitrogen are included because in the nail plate they are found almost exclusively in amino acids.[102] Nitrogen content of nails is reduced in neonates,[103] slightly higher in white than in black adolescents, but unaffected by nutritional status.[104] In the nail plate, sulfur is found almost exclusively in the amino acid cystine.[102] Hess detected lower concentrations of cystine in nails from patients with arthritis.[105] Klauder and Brown showed that the sulfur content of nails was reduced in a number of cutaneous and systemic diseases, but they concluded that determination of the concentration of sulfur in diseased nails or in nails of patients with systemic disease was of no value.[102] Reduced nail plate cystine has been reported in uranium mine workers.[106] Cystine content does not

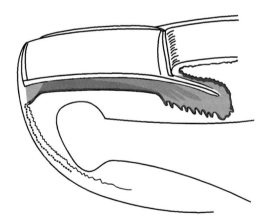

Figure 4–7. Pattern of keratin expression in the nail unit. Red, keratins 5 and 14 expressed in the basal layer; green, keratins 1 and 10 expressed in the suprabasal layers of the proximal nail fold, the matrix, and the volar epidermis of the finger tip; purple, hard keratins (including Ha1) expressed sporadically in the upper parts of the suprabasal layers of the nail matrix; blue, keratins 6, 16, and 17 expressed in the suprabasal layers of the nail bed epithelium. The thickness of the nail bed epithelium is artifactually thickened to demonstrate the limited expression of keratins 6, 16, and 17. Drawing is based on data from references 24 and 79.

vary as a function of ethnic group, differing dietary habits, or pregnancy[107] but may be reduced in nails when koilonychia is present.[108]

Nail plates, like hair and epidermis, contain a group of tough, fibrous proteins called keratins (from the Greek word for "horn").[109] Early studies of wool revealed two components—fibrous proteins (keratins) and less-structured globular matrix proteins—that surround the fibrous proteins. Compared with the fibrous proteins, matrix proteins contain high levels of the sulfur-containing amino acid cystine. Wool chemists speculated that the matrix proteins hold the fibrous proteins together, with the disulfide bonds of cystine acting as a glue. The proteins of nail are similar to those of wool and can be divided into fibrous and globular (nonfibrous) proteins on the basis of solubility, amino acid composition, electrophoretic mobility, and x-ray diffraction pattern.[110] Compared with stratum corneum of epidermis, the proteins of nail plate are quite different. Not only is the pattern of the keratin expression distinct,[110–113] but also no high-sulfur matrix component has been found in stratum corneum.

The fibrous proteins, the keratins, belong to the group of intermediate filament proteins that contribute to the cytoskeleton of the cell (reviewed in Fuchs[114]). More than 30 keratin proteins have been described. Keratins can be divided into two groups of acidic and neutral-basic proteins; they are expressed as a pair, one from each group. The keratin pairs expressed vary with both the tissue and the stage of differentiation (e.g., the pair expressed in suprabasal epidermis is different from that expressed in suprabasal esophagus or from that expressed in the basal layer of epidermis). A number of "hard" keratins have been identified in hair and nails.[113] The nail unit expresses both hard keratins and keratins seen in other epithelia[24,79,113] (Fig. 4–7). Mutations in epidermal keratins have been demonstrated in individuals with pachyonychia congenita.[115,116]

Baden and colleagues studied the proteins of normal nail plates and showed a genetic variant in the (low-sulfur) keratins.[117] The variant appeared in approximately 5 per cent of the population studied and appeared to be inherited as an autosomal dominant trait. This likely reflects keratin polymorphisms.[118] Gillespie and Marshall confirmed the presence of high- and low-sulfur-containing proteins in nail plate and showed that among species there were considerable differences among the fi-

Table 4-1. SUMMARY OF FINDING ON NAIL COMPOSITION

	N	Ca	Mg	Na	K	Fe	Cu	Zn	Au	Mn	P	S[a]	Cys[a]
Baden et al[110] (4)[b,c]												3.2%[o] 5.5%[n] 20.3%[n]	10.6%[n] α-helix "matrix" 12.0%
Block[151,f(?),c]	14.9%[d]											3.8%	
Cotzias et al[152] (3)[b,e]										0.2–0.8			
Djaldetti et al[96] (17)[h]		18.74 ±2.68%				0.80 ±0.84%	0.78 ±0.52%	1.26 ±0.80%				78.24 ±3.08%	
Forslind[12.77,f]		1060[g] [720–1880]										3–6%[h]	
Goldblum et al[90] (18b,i) (90)[b,i]		940–5900	23–110			18–65	9.4–81	116–3080		<1	82–278		137 × 10³
Grozdanovic et al[36a] (40)[c,f]													
Harrison et al[91,93] Female (7)[b,g]		821 [701–982]	111 [68–152]			38 [14–90]	44 [28–53]	222 [130–360]					
Male (10)[b,g]		904 [687–1270]	106 [68–140]			41 [28–109]	62 [45–102]	178 [135–391]					
Both (17)[b,j]		[450–1600]	[11–380]			[16–200]	[17–64]	[62–360]					
Hein et al[104,b,d] White (49) Black (127)	141 × 10³ 137 × 10³												
Hess[105,f(?),e] Normal Arthritic								821 [701–902]					12.0%[o] 9.8%[o]
Jacobs et al[95] (50 adults)[b,c]						129–227							
Jalili et al[108,c,f,o] Normal (29) Koilonychia (6) Anemia (17)													8.12 ± 1.17% 2.54 ± 0.83% 6.32 ± 1.4%
Kanabrocki et al[92,e,k] Adults (13) Children (6)				900 ± 538 2370 ± 1836			51 ± 23 86 ± 45		0.5 ± 0.6 0.4 ± 0.6	0.9 ± 0.3 1.9 ± 1.4			
Kile[128] (5)[b,c]		725									310		
Klauder & Brown[102] (11)[f(?),c]												3.2%[o]	12.0%[o]
Kopito et al[99f,l,n] Children with CF (149)				3220 ± 1220	1680 ± 1060								

48

Study								
Healthy children (44)				1060 ± 550	700 ± 390			
Parents of CF (87)				800 ± 600	550 ± 740			
Healthy adults (32)				670 ± 480	430 ± 430			
Sibs of CF (64)				1450 ± 740	1020 ± 630			
Leonard et al[97] (25)[f(?)]		3070 ±2010[m]	2480 ±1660[m]	3010 ±970[l]	2400 ±1150[l]			
Lockard et al[103] Adult (24)[f,d]		146 ± 6 × 10³						
Neonates (67)		131 ± 14 × 10³						
Normal (40)		136 ± 14 × 10³						
Ill (27)		123 ± 17 × 10³						
Martin[94,b,c] Normal male (6)							14.8 ± 3.8	
Normal female (7)							10.6 ± 2.8	
Wilson's disease male (2)							21.1, 32.2	
Wilson's disease female (1)							11.4	
Pascher[153,b,c]								9.4%
Petuschkov et al[79] (3)[f(?)]				[240−3900]		—	[1200 − 2700][0.006 − 0.085]	
Pruzanski et al[107] Males (67)[c,f(?)]								88 ± 9 × 10³
Females (52)[c,f(?)]								89 ± 13 × 10³
Sobdewski et al[155] Healthy adult (40)[b,g]						12.5[6−26]		
Iron deficient (5)						1.6[4−3]		
Iron deficient, under treatment (4)						10[8−16]		
Cadaver (15)						8.9[<1−21]		
Vellar[57] (10)[f(?)]	148 ± 1 × 10³[d]	368 ± 53[g]	83 ± 9[g]	440 ± 92[g]	357 ± 72[g]	27 ± 4[c]	73 ± 8[g]	—[g]
Way (discussed in Kile[128])	14.7-17.6%[o]						2.47-3.12%	

—, failed to detect; blank, not determined; CF, cystic fibrosis.

Numbers in parentheses indicate number of patients studied. Numbers in brackets indicate range. Numbers following ± indicate standard deviation.

[a]Cystine contains 26.7% sulfur. [b]Dry weight. [c]Chemical. [d]Kjeldahl. [e]Neutron activation. [f]Wet weight. [g]Atomic absorption. [h]Figures for quantitative x-ray microradiography reported as percentage of the total weight of the elements examined. [i]Spectrography. [j]Spark source mass spectrometry. [k]Air dried. [l]Flame photometry. [m]Fluorometric; [n]Residues/100 residues; [o]g/100 g.

brous proteins but that the electrophoretic pattern of the high-sulfur matrix proteins was preserved.[119] Marshall defined the keratin and matrix proteins of nail using two-dimensional electrophoresis and showed that there are genetic variants not only in the keratin proteins but also in the matrix proteins.[120] When the variant keratin proteins are present, the variant matrix proteins are also found; however, the variant matrix proteins can be found in the absence of the variant keratins. No differences in the physical properties of the nail plates have been associated with the variant proteins.

The cornified cellular envelope is a chemically resistant structure found in the stratum corneum of the epidermis[121] and in the nail plate.[21] A cornified cellular envelope-enriched fraction of protein from nail plates has been prepared and shown to contain relatively high levels of proline.[122]

BIOPHYSICAL PROPERTIES OF THE NAIL PLATE

X-ray diffraction studies of the nail plate have shown that the fibrous proteins (the keratins) are oriented in the plane of the plate, perpendicular to the axis (longitudinal) of growth.[123–126] There is no specific axis of fiber orientation in newly formed plate other than in the plane of the plate; as the plate grows out, fibers develop an overall directional orientation parallel to the free edge of the plate.[124]

Nail plates of normal thickness transmit approximately 30 per cent of grenz rays and 85 per cent of x rays.[127] Transmission of grenz rays is directly correlated with the thickness of the nail plate. Attempts to treat the nail bed through thick nails with grenz ray are futile; superficial x rays should be used.

The water content of nails varies from 10 to 30 per cent[110,128] and is directly related to relative humidity.[110] At high humidity, much less water is held by the nail plate than by the stratum corneum.[110] The rate of water diffusion through a nail plate is approximately 10 times greater than through abdominal skin.[110,129,130] Therefore, considering that stratum corneum thickness is about 1/100 that of the nail plate, the diffusion constant of water through nail is several hundred times that through most skin. Although in stratum corneum the water-holding capacity is decreased and the diffusion of water through skin is increased by extraction of lipids, water-holding capacity and diffusion

of water through nail plate are unaffected by lipid extraction.[124] The loss of water through the nail plate can be stopped by applying a layer of petroleum jelly or nail polish on the plate.[131,132]

HARD NAILS, BRITTLE NAILS

Although technically this topic should be included in the section on biophysical properties, so much attention has been devoted to the subject that it deserves a place of its own. Why is the nail plate hard, or what makes nails brittle? To discuss this, one must first define hard and brittle. Most definitions of brittleness include longitudinal or horizontal cracking or splitting of the free end of the nail plate into laminae.[128,133,134] Hard nails have been defined as "'normal' nails, where this does not happen."[128] Others have attempted to define hardness and brittleness by more easily evaluated clinical parameters, such as photographs[133] and scanning electron microscopy,[135] or by more easily quantified physical parameters, such as Knoop hardness number, which measures indentation under a fixed weight[136–138]; flexural characteristics[139–141]; modulus of elasticity, which quantifies the relationship between force-area and deformation produced[110,124,126]; and tensile strength, tearing resistance, and impact absorption.[140]

Silver and Chiego reviewed the association of brittle nails with systemic and cutaneous disease.[85] Their investigations included many exogenous factors, among them occupation, trauma, avitaminosis, iron metabolism, the coefficient of nail plate expansion, unsaturated fats, the pH of the skin, and solvents.

Forslind attributed nail plate hardness to physical properties, including the double curvature (longitudinal and transverse) of the nail plate, the very flat adhesive pattern of cells in the plate, and the orientation of the fibers in the plane of the plate perpendicular to the direction of growth.[12] Baden suggested that the mechanical properties of the nail plate might be due in part to cell wall attachments.[124]

Cystine is decreased in brittle nails.[102,105] The high cystine content of nail matrix protein has been discussed previously. In sheep, as the consumption of sulfur is reduced, the amount of matrix protein in wool decreases; however, once the intake of sulfur is reduced below a critical level, the growth of wool decreases progressively, suggesting that the glue function of the high-sulfur matrix protein is necessary for the synthesis of the appendageal product.[109] The solubility of matrix protein is such that it would be extracted by alkaline solutions that increase lamellar splitting.[34,128,142] This suggests that extraction of matrix protein may be responsible for splitting in this problem.

No association of calcium with brittle nails has been documented.[128] Calcium is increased in the nails of individuals with kwashiorkor.[78] Such nails have a higher Knoop hardness number than normal nails.[137] The increase in hardness has been attributed to the increase in calcium, but the arguments are not supported by analytic electron microscopic studies.[77] X-ray diffraction studies contain no suggestion of a separate phase (e.g., a calcium mineral, such as in bone) in nail plate.[12] Heterotopic calcification of the nail plate can occur after injury.[143] The preoccupation with calcium in relationship to nail hardness "probably stems from the hardness of bones and teeth, where large quantities of calcium are present. Thus the idea may have evolved that the more calcium in the system, the harder the nails."[128]

The importance of water in nail hardness, brittleness, and flexibility has been emphasized repeatedly.[12,128,144] In homemakers, brittle nails are an occupational hazard.[85] Solvents probably exert adverse effects on nail plates not through lipid extraction[124] but through dehydration[85] and may be overrated in causing adverse effects. The modulus of elasticity,[124,126] flexibility,[141] and the number of times a nail plate can be flexed before breaking[139] all increase when the nail plate is hydrated. Changes seen by scanning electron microscopy similar to those seen in onychoschizia have been produced by repeated wetting and drying and by exposure of nail clippings to detergent and water.[144]

Thus, the hardness of nails is determined by several factors: the physical properties of the nail plate, the matrix proteins that may glue the fibrous protein together, and the hydration of the nail plate. The function of the cornified cellular envelope and the role, if any, of intercellular cement substance[145] in nail hardness remain to be determined.

PHARMACOLOGY OF THE NAIL UNIT

As with water diffusion out of the nail plate, nail plate permeability to water is greater than that of the stratum corneum.[22] n-Alkanols have been used as model compounds with varying polarity. Unlike stratum corneum, the permeability coefficient of nail to n-alkanols decreases as the compound becomes increasingly hydrophobic. If the alkanol permeabilities could be extrapolated to other low-molecular-weight organics, "then very polar compounds might be surprisingly easily delivered through the nail plate to underlying tissues."[146]

Pharmacodynamic studies of systemic drugs have shown rapid delivery of drug to the entire nail plate.[147–150] Studies of drugs topically applied to the dorsal nail plate surface have demonstrated penetration to the ventral surface.[62] These observations suggest fertile avenues for topical drug treatment of subungual diseases such as psoriasis of the nail bed and distal subungual onychomycosis.

Acknowledgments

I thank Ms. Judy Carpenter and Ms. Betsy Williams for secretarial assistance and Kris Carroll for assistance with Figure 4–7. Dale Davis created Figure 4–6 on the basis of the work of Andrew Morgan, MD. Irene Leigh, MD, graciously shared prepublication material for Figure 4–7.

References

1. Pinkus F: Der Nagel. In Jadassohn J (ed): Handbuch der Haut und Geschlechtskrankeiten, Springer-Verlag, New York, 1927, pp 266–289.
2. Rainey G: On the structure and formation of the nails of the fingers and toes. Trans Microscop Soc London 2:105, 1849.
3. Unna PG: Entwichtlungsgeschichte und Anatomy. In Ziemessen (ed): Handbuch der Speciellen Patholgie und Therapie, vol 14. Leipzig, F.C.W. Vogel, 1883, pp 38–51.
4. Zaias N: The nail in health and disease, ed 2. Appleton & Lange, Norwalk, CT, 1990, pp 1–255.
5. Lewis BL: Microscopic studies of fetal and mature nail and surrounding soft tissue. AMA Arch Dermatol Syphilis 70:732, 1954.
6. Zaias N: Embryology of the human nail. Arch Dermatol 87:77, 1963.
7. Hashimoto K, Gross BG, Nelson R, Lever WF: The ultrastructure of the skin of human embryos: III. The formation of the nail in 16–18 weeks old embryos. J Invest Dermatol 47:205, 1966.
8. Holbrook KA: Human epidermal embryogenesis. Int J Dermatol 18:329, 1979.
9. Holbrook KA: Structural abnormalities of the epidermally derived appendages in skin from patients with ectodermal dysplasia: Insight into developmental errors. Recent advances in ectodermal dysplasias. In Salinas CF, Opitz JM, Paul NW (eds): Birth Defects:

Original Article Series, vol 24. Alan R. Liss, New York, 1988, pp 15–44.

10. Holbrook KA: Structure and function of developing skin. *In* Goldsmith LA (ed): Physiology, Biochemistry, and Molecular Biology of the Skin, ed 2. Oxford University Press, New York, 1991, pp 63–110.

11. Zaias N: Onychomycosis. Arch Dermatol 105:263, 1972.

12. Forslind B: Biophysical studies of the normal nail. Acta Dermatovener 50:161, 1970.

13. Caputo R, Dadati E: Preliminary observations about the ultrastructure of the human nail plate treated with thioglycolic acid. Arch Klin Exp Dermatol 231:344, 1968.

14. Runne U, Orfanos CE: The human nail. Curr Probl Dermatol 9:102, 1981.

15. Forslind B, Thyresson N: On the structure of the normal nail: A scanning electron microscopic study. Arch Derm Forsch 251:199, 1975.

16. Hamilton JB, Terada H, Mestler GE: Studies of growth throughout the lifespan in Japanese: Growth and size of nails and their relationship to age, heredity and other factors. J Gerontol 10:401, 1955.

17. Finlay AY, Moseley H, Duggan TC: Ultrasound transmission time: An in vivo guide to nail thickness. Br J Dermatol 117:765, 1987.

18. Germann H, Barran W, Plewig G: Morphology of corneocytes from human nail plates. J Invest Dermatol 74:115, 1980.

19. Brody I: The keratinization of epidermal cells of normal guinea pig skin as revealed by electron microscopy. J Ultrastruct Res 2:482, 1959.

20. Hashimoto K: Ultrastructure of the human toenail. Cell migration, keratinization, and formation of the intercellular cement. Arch Derm Forsch 240:1, 1971.

21. Hashimoto K: Ultrastructure of the human toenail: II. Keratinization and formation of the marginal band. J Ultrastruct Res 36:391, 1971.

22. Walters KA, Flynn GL, Marvel JR: Physicochemical characterization of the human nail: I. Pressure sealed apparatus for measuring nail plate permeabilities. J Invest Dermatol 76:76, 1981.

23. LeGros Clark WE: Nails. *In* Press C (ed): Tissues of the Body, ed 5. Clarendon Press, Oxford, England, 1965, pp 315–319.

24. Kitahara T, Ogawa H: Cultured nail keratinocytes express hard keratins characteristic of nail and hair in vivo. Arch Dermatol Res 284:253, 1992.

25. Picardo M, Tosti A, Marchese C, et al: Characterization of cultured nail matrix cells. J Am Acad Dermatol 30:434, 1994.

26. Hashimoto K: Ultrastructure of the human toenail: I. Proximal nail matrix. J Invest Dermatol 56:235, 1971.

27. Tosti A, Cameli N, Piraccinin BM, et al: Characterization of nail matrix melanocytes with anti-PEP1, anti-PEP8, TMH-1, and HMB-45 antibodies. J Am Acad Dermatol 31:193, 1994.

28. Higashi N, Saito T: Horizontal distribution of the dopa-positive melanocytes in the nail matrix. J Invest Dermatol 53:163, 1969.

29. Higashi N: Melanocytes of nail matrix and nail pigmentation. Arch Dermatol 97:570, 1968.

30. Hashimoto K: The ultrastructure of the skin of human embryos. X. Merkel tactile cells in the finger and nail. J Anat 111:99, 1972.

31. LeGros Clark WE: The problem of the claw in primates. Proc Zool Soc 1:1, 1936.

32. Burrows MT: The significance of the lunula of the nail. Johns Hopkins Hosp Rep 18:357, 1919.

33. Lewin K: The normal finger nail. Br J Dermatol 77:421, 1965.

34. Samman PD, Fenton DA: The Nails in Disease, ed 4. William Heinemann, London, 1986.

35. Drape JL, Wolfram-Gabel R, Idy-Peretti I, et al: The lunula: A magnetic resonance imaging approach to the subnail matrix area. J Invest Dermatol 106:1081, 1996.

36. Wolfram-Gabel R, Sick H: Vascular networks of the periphery of the fingernail. J Hand Surg 20B:488, 1995.

37. Mitchell JC: A clinical study of leukonychia. Br J Dermatol 65:121, 1953.

38. Martin BF, Platts MM: A histological study of the nail region in normal human subjects and in those showing splinter hemorrhages of the nail. J Anat 93:323, 1959.

39. Montagna W, Parakkal PF: The Structure and Function of Skin, ed 3. Academic Press, New York, 1974, p 275.

40. Rand R, Baden HP: Pathophysiology of nails—Onychopathophysiology. *In* Soter NA, Baden HP (eds): Pathophysiology of Dermatologic Diseases. McGraw-Hill, New York, 1984, p 209.

41. Zaias N: The regeneration of the primate nail studies of the squirrel monkey, Saimiri. J Invest Dermatol 44:107, 1965.

42. Terry RB: The onychodermal band in health and disease. Lancet I:179, 1955.

43. Stewart WK, Raffle EJ: Brown nail-bed arcs and chronic renal disease. BMJ 1:784, 1972.

44. Holzberg M, Walker HK: Terry's nails revisited: Revised definition and new correlations. Lancet I:896, 1984.

45. Lindsay PG: The half-and-half nail. Arch Intern Med 119:583, 1967.

46. Raffle EJ: Terry's nails. Lancet I:1131, 1984.

47. Sonnex TS, Griffiths WAD, Nicol WJ: The nature and significance of the transverse white band of human nails. Semin Dermatol 10:12, 1991.

48. Sinclair RD, Wojnarowska F, Leigh IM, Dawber RPR: The basement membrane zone of the nail. Br J Dermatol 131:499, 1994.

49. Baran R, Juhlin L: Bone dependent nail formation. Br J Dermatol 114:371, 1986.

50. Kelikian H: Congenital Deformities of the Hand. WB Saunders, Philadelphia, 1974, p 201.

51. Flint MH: Some observations on the vascular supply of the nail bed and terminal segments of the finger. Br J Plast Surg 8:186, 1955.

52. Hale AR, Burch GE: The arteriovenous anastomoses and blood vessels of the human finger. Medicine 39:191, 1960.

53. Samman PD: The human toenail: Its genesis and blood supply. Br J Dermatol 71:296, 1959.

54. Bean WB: Nail growth: A twenty-year study. Arch Intern Med 111:476, 1953.

55. Bean WB: Nail growth: 30 years of observation. Arch Intern Med 134:497, 1974.

56. Dawber R, Baran R: Nail growth. Cutis 39:99, 1987.

57. Vellar OD: Composition of human nail substance. Am J Clin Nutr 23:1272, 1970.

58. Dawber R: Fingernail growth in normal and psoriatic subjects. Br J Dermatol 82:454, 1970.

59. LeGros Clark WE, Buxton LHD: Studies in nail growth. Br J Dermatol 50:221, 1938.

60. Halban J, Spitzer MZ: Uber das gesteigerte wachstum der nagel in der schwangerschaft. Monatsschrift fur Geburtshulfe und Gynakologie 82:25, 1929.

61. Geoghegan B, Roberts DF, Sampford MR: Possible climatic effect on nail growth. J Appl Physiol 13:135, 1958.
62. Ceschin-Roques CG, Hanel H, Pruja-Bougaret SM, et al: Ciclopirox nail lacquer 8%: In vivo penetration into and through nails and in vitro effect on pig skin. Skin Pharmacol 4:89, 1991.
63. Dawber RPR, Samman PD, Bottoms E: Fingernail growth in idiopathic and psoriatic onycholysis. Br J Dermatol 85:558, 1971.
64. Orentreich N, Markofsky J, Vogelman JH: The effect of aging on the rate of linear nail growth. J Invest Dermatol 73:126, 1979.
65. Head H, Sherren J: The consequence of injury to the peripheral nerves in man. Brain 28:263, 1908.
66. Gilchrist ML, Buxton LHD: The relation of fingernail growth to nutritional status. J Anat 73:575, 1939.
67. Samman PD, White WF: The "yellow nail" syndrome. Br J Dermatol 76:153, 1964.
68. Basler VA: Wachstumsvorgange am Vollentwickelten Organismus (Growth processes in fully developed organisms). Med Klin 33:1664, 1937.
69. Sibinga MS: Observations on growth of fingernails in health and disease. Pediatrics 24:225, 1959.
70. Baran R, Dawber RPR: Diseases of the Nails and their Management, ed 2. Oxford, England, Blackwell Scientific, 1994, pp 21–24.
71. Norton LA: Incorporation of thymidine-methyl-H3 and glycine-2-H3 in the nail matrix and bed of humans. J Invest Dermatol 56:61, 1971.
72. Jarrett A, Spearman RIC: The histochemistry of the human nail. Arch Dermatol 94:652, 1966.
73. Johnson M, Comaish JS, Shuster S: Nail is produced by the normal nail bed: A controversy. Br J Dermatol 125:27, 1991.
74. Johnson M, Shuster S: Continuous formation of nail along the bed. Br J Dermatol 128:277, 1993.
75. Zaias N, Alvarez J: The formation of the primate nail plate: An autoradiographic study in squirrel monkey. J Invest Dermatol 51:120, 1968.
76. Forslind B, Lindstrom B, Philipson B: Quantitative microradiography of normal human nail. Acta Dermatovener 51:89, 1971.
77. Forslind B, Wroblewski R, Afzelius BA: Calcium and sulfur location in human nail. J Invest Dermatol 67:273, 1976.
78. Robson JRK, Brooks GJ: The distribution of calcium in fingernails from healthy and malnourished children. Clin Chim Acta 55:255, 1974.
79. Leigh I, et al: Expression of "hard" keratins in the nail unit. In press.
80. Samman PD: The ventral nail. Arch Dermatol 84:192, 1961.
81. Kligman AM: Why do nails grow out instead of up? Arch Dermatol 84:181, 1961.
82. Baran R: Nail growth direction revisited. J Am Acad Dermatol 4:78, 1981.
83. Kikuchi I, Ogata K, Idemori M: Vertically growing ectopic nail. J Am Acad Dermatol 10:114, 1984.
84. Kligman AM: Response. J Am Acad Dermatol 4:82, 1981.
85. Silver H, Chiego B: Nails and nail changes: II. Modern concepts of anatomy and biochemistry of the nails. J Invest Dermatol 3:133, 1940.
86. Krantz W: Beitrag zur Anatomie des Nagels. Dermatol Zeitschrift 64:239, 1932.
87. Kligman AM: Nails. In Pillsbury DM, Shelley WB, Kligman AM (eds): Dermatology, WB Saunders, Philadelphia, 1956, pp 32–39.
88. Zaias N: The movement of the nail bed. J Invest Dermatol 48:402, 1967.
89. Bank HL, Robson J, Bigelow JB, et al: Preparation of fingernails for trace element analysis. Clin Chim Acta 116:179, 1981.
90. Goldblum RW, Derby S, Lerner AB: The metal content of skin, nails and hair. J Invest Dermatol 20:13, 1953.
91. Harrison WW, Clemena GG: Survey analysis of trace elements in human fingernails by spark source mass spectrometry. Clin Chim Acta 36:485, 1972.
92. Kanabrocki E, Case LF, Graham LA, et al: Neutron-activation studies of trace elements in human fingernail. J Nucl Med 9:478, 1968.
93. Harrison WW, Tyree AB: The determination of trace elements in human fingernails by atomic absorption spectroscopy. Clin Chim Acta 31:63, 1971.
94. Martin GM: Copper content of hair and nails of normal individuals and of patients with hepatolenticular degeneration. Nature 202:903, 1964.
95. Jacobs A, Jenkins DJ: The iron content of finger nails. Br J Dermatol 72:145, 1970.
96. Djaldetti M, Fishman P, Hart J: The iron content of finger-nails in iron deficient patients. Clin Sci 72:669, 1987.
97. Leonard PJ, Morris WP, Brown R: Sodium, potassium, calcium and magnesium contents in nails of children with kwashiorkor. Biochem J 110:22P, 1968.
98. Bock H, Koch E, Stephan U, et al: Investigations on electrolyte concentrations in the nails of cystic fibrosis patients and controls. Mod Probl Pediatr 10:279, 1967.
99. Kopito L, Mahmoodian A, Townley RRW, et al: Studies in cystic fibrosis. N Engl J Med 272:504, 1965.
100. Lander H, Hodge PR, Crisp CS: Arsenic in the hair and nails. J Forensic Med 12:52, 1965.
101. Shapiro HA: Arsenic content of human hair and nails: Its interpretation. J Forensic Med 14:65, 1967.
102. Klauder JV, Brown H: Sulphur content of hair and of nails in abnormal states: II. Nails. Arch Dermatol Syphilis 31:26, 1935.
103. Lockard D, Pass R, Cassady G: Fingernail nitrogen content in neonates. Pediatrics 49:618, 1972.
104. Hein K, Cohen MI, McNamara H: Racial differences in nitrogen content of nails among adolescents. Am J Clin Nutr 30:496, 1977.
105. Hess WC: Variations in amino acid content of finger nails of normal and arthritic individuals. J Biol Chem 109:xliii, 1935.
106. Grozdanovic J, Ulbert K: Oscillopolarographic determination of cysteic acid level in the fingernails followed chronic irradiation in humans. Strahlentherapie 139:735, 1970.
107. Pruzanski W, Arnon R: Determination of cystine and other amino acids in the fingernails of members of various ethnic groups in Israel. Israel J Med Sci 2:465, 1966.
108. Jalili MA, Al-Kassab S: Koilonychia and cystine content of nails. Lancet III:108, 1959.
109. Fraser RDB: Keratins. Sci Am 221:86, 1969.
110. Baden HP, Goldsmith LA, Fleming B: A comparative study of the physicochemical properties of human keratinized tissues. Biochim Biophys Acta 322:269, 1973.
111. Baden HP, Kubilus J: A comparative study of the immunologic properties of hoof and nail fibrous proteins. J Invest Dermatol 83:327, 1984.
112. Heid HW, Werner E, Franke WW: The complement of native α-keratin peptides of hair-forming cells: A

subset of eight polypeptides that differ from epithelial cytokeratins. Differentiation 32:101, 1986.

113. Lynch MH, O'Guinn WM, Hardy C, et al: Acidic and basic hair/nail ("hard") keratins: Their colocalization in upper cortical and cuticle cells of the human hair follicle and their relationship to "soft" keratins. J Cell Biol 103:2593, 1986.

114. Fuchs E: Keratins: Mechanical integrators in the epidermis and hair and their role in disease. Prog Dermatol 30:1, 1996.

115. Bowden PE, Haley JL, Kansky A, et al: Mutation of a type II keratin gene (K6a) in pachyonychia congenita. Nat Genet 10:363, 1995.

116. McLean WH, Rugg EL, Lunny DP, et al: Keratin 16 and keratin 17 mutations cause pachyonychia congenita. Nat Genet 9:273, 1995.

117. Baden HP, Lee LD, Kubilus J: A genetic electrophoretic variant of human hair α polypeptides. Am J Hum Genet 27:472, 1975.

118. Mischke D, Wild G: Polymorphic keratins in human epidermis. J Invest Dermatol 88:191, 1987.

119. Gillespie JM, Marshall RC: Proteins of the hard keratins of echidna, hedgehog, rabbit, ox and man. Aust J Biol Sci 30:401, 1977.

120. Marshall RC: Genetic variation in the proteins of human nail. J Invest Dermatol 75:264, 1980.

121. Reichert U, Michel S, Schmidt R: The cornified envelope: A key structure of terminally differentiating keratinocytes. In Darmon M, Blumenberg M (eds): Molecular Biology of the Skin: The Keratinocyte. Academic Press, San Diego, 1993, pp 107–150.

122. Shono S, Toda K: The structure proteins of the human nail. Curr Prob Dermatol 11:317, 1983.

123. Astbury WT, Sisson WA: X-ray studies of the structure of hair, wool, and related fibres. Proc R Soc Lond 150:533, 1935.

124. Baden HP: The physical properties of nail. J Invest Dermatol 55:115, 1970.

125. Derksen JD, Heringa GC, Weidinger A: On keratin and cornification. Acta Neerlandica Morph 1:31, 1937.

126. Forslind B, Nordstrom G, Toijer D, Eriksson K: The rigidity of human fingernails: A biophysical investigation on influencing physical parameters. Acta Dermatovener 60:217, 1980.

127. Gammeltoft M, Wulf HC: Transmission of 12 kv grenz rays and 29 kv x-rays through normal and diseased nails. Acta Dermatovener 60:431, 1980.

128. Kile RL: Some mineral constituents of fingernails. AMA Arch Dermatol Syphilis 70:75, 1954.

129. Burch GE, Winsor T: Diffusion of water through dead plantar palmar and torsal human skin and through toe nails. Arch Dermatol Syphilis 53:39, 1946.

130. Spruit D: Measurement of water vapor loss through human nail in vivo. J Invest Dermatol 56:359, 1971.

131. Jacobi O: Die Nagel des lebenden Menschen und die perspiratio insensibilis. Arch Klin Exp Dermatol 214:559, 1962.

132. Spruit D: Effect of nail polish on the hydration of the fingernail. Am Cosmet Perfum 87:57, 1972.

133. Rosenberg SW, Oster K: Gelatin in the treatment of brittle nails. Conn St Med J 19:171, 1955.

134. Tyson TL: Preliminary and short reports: The effect of gelatin on fragile finger nails. J Invest Dermatol 14:323, 1950.

135. Shelley WB, Shelley ED: Onychoschizia: Scanning electron microscopy. J Am Acad Dermatol 10:623, 1984.

136. Michaelson JB, Huntsman DJ: New aspects of the effects of gelatin on fingernails. J Soc Cosmet Chem 14:443, 1963.

137. Robson JRK: Hardness of finger nails in well-nourished and malnourished populations. Br J Nutr 32:389, 1974.

138. Robson JRK, El-Tahawi HD: Hardness of human nail as an index of nutritional status: A preliminary communication. Br J Nutr 26:233, 1971.

139. Finlay AY, Frost P, Keith AD, Snipes W: An assessment of factors influencing flexibility of human fingernails. Br J Dermatol 103:357, 1980.

140. Maloney MJ, Paquette EG, Shansky A: The physical properties of fingernails: 1. Apparatus for physical measurements. J Soc Cosmet Chem 28:415, 1977.

141. Young RW, Newman SB, Capott RJ: Strength of fingernails. J Invest Dermatol 44:358, 1965.

142. Dixon S: Nail-splitting: A survey. Nursing Times 63:1760, 1967.

143. Blakey PR, Earland C, Stell JGP, Swift D: Heterotopic calcification of human nail and hair. Nature 207:190, 1965.

144. Wallis MS, Bowen WR, Guin JD: Pathogenesis of onychoschizia (lamellar dystrophy). J Am Acad Dermatol 24:44, 1991.

145. Rosenberg S, Oster KA, Kallos A, Burroughs W: Further studies in the use of gelatin in the treatment of brittle nails. AMA Arch Dermatol 76:330, 1957.

146. Walters KA, Flynn GL, Marvel JR: Physicochemical characterization of the human nail: Permeation pattern for water and the homologous alcohols and differences with respect to the stratum corneum. J Pharm Pharmacol 35:28, 1983.

147. Cauwenbergh G, Degreef H, Heykants J, et al: Pharmacokinetic profile of orally administered itraconazole in human skin. J Am Acad Dermatol 18:263, 1988.

148. Faergemann J, Zehender H, Denouel J, Millerioux L: Levels of terbinafine in plasma, stratum corneum, dermis-epidermis (without stratum corneum), sebum, hair, and nails during and after 250 mg terbinafine orally once per day for four weeks. Acta Derm Venereol (Stockh) 73:305, 1993.

149. Finlay AY: Pharmacokinetics of terbinafine in the nail. Br J Dermatol 126 (Suppl 39):28, 1992.

150. Matthieu L, De Doncker P, Cauwenbergh G, et al: Itraconazole penetrates the nail via the nail matrix and the nail bed—An investigation in onychomycosis. Clin Exp Dermatol 16:374, 1991.

151. Block RJ: The composition of keratins. The amino acid composition of hair, wool, horn, and other eukeratins. J Biol Chem 128:181, 1939.

152. Cotzias GC, Papavasiliou PS, Miller ST: Manganese in melanin. Nature 201:1228, 1964.

153. Pascher G: Bestandteile der menschlichen hornschicht. Arch Klin Exp Dermatol 218:111, 1964.

154. Petushkov AA, Linekin DM, Balcius JF, Brownell GL: High-resolution gamma ray spectrometry in the determination of trace elements in human fingernails. J Nucl Med 10:730, 1969.

155. Sobolewski S, Lawrence ACK, Bagshaw P: Human nails and body iron. J Clin Pathol 31:1068, 1978.

CHAPTER 5

Histology and Histopathology

Suthep Jerasutus

A variety of skin diseases may involve the nails or the area around nails in the absence of cutaneous lesions. Nail biopsy is one investigation that not only provides etiologic, diagnostic, and prognostic information but also aids in improving the understanding of the pathogenesis of the nail diseases.

The knowledge of the histopathology of nail disease is much more limited than that of skin disease not only because of its small number of biopsy specimens but also because of its distinct anatomic structures, which are more complex than those of the skin. Thus, close communication between the clinician and the pathologist is required regarding orientation and handling of the specimen for proper interpretation. The main problem with a small specimen, as is usually obtained from a nail unit biopsy, is the same as for a skin biopsy: proper orientation may be lost. Therefore, the clinician must mark the specimen and request the pathologist to cut it in a particular orientation; orientation may be important in histologic diagnosis.

Understanding pathologic processes in the nail, as in any organ, requires a thorough grounding in normal structure and function.

HISTOLOGY OF THE NAIL UNIT

The nail unit consists of the nail plate and the four epithelial structures around and be-

neath it. These epithelial structures—beginning proximally, the proximal nail fold, nail matrix, nail bed, and hyponychium—can be seen on longitudinal section. The proximal nail fold consists of both dorsal and ventral surface epithelia (Fig. 5–1). The dorsal surface is a continuation of the dorsal skin of the digit, containing sweat glands but no pilosebaceous units. The epidermis includes all four layers found in normal skin with its undulating rete ridge–dermal papilla pattern (Fig. 5–2). The ventral surface epithelium is also cornified and includes all four layers of the normal epidermis; however, it is quite thin and has neither a rete ridge–dermal papilla pattern nor epidermal appendages. The epithelium of the ventral surface of the proximal nail fold has also been called the "eponychium." The cornified layer at the ventral surface and at the tip of the proximal nail fold grows over the dorsal surface of the nail plate to constitute the cuticle (Fig. 5–3).

The nail matrix, the germinative epithelium, has no granular cell layer and consists mostly of matrix cells. The matrix epithelium is thick and has broad, club-shaped rete ridges that point downward and proximally (Figs. 5–4 and 5–5). The proximal margin of the nail matrix is the ventral surface of the proximal nail fold, and the distal margin is the nail bed. Melanocytes are present in the normal nail matrix and nail bed; however, they differ from

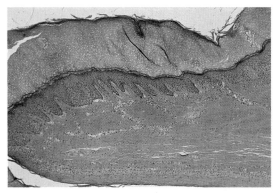

Figure 5–1. The proximal nail fold consists of two surfaces of epidermis: dorsal and ventral.

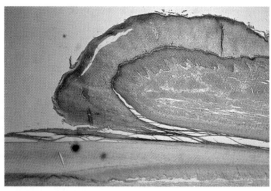

Figure 5–3. The ventral surface of the proximal nail fold cornifies by forming the cuticle, which extends over the dorsal surface of the nail plate.

those elsewhere in the skin. They are poorly developed and fewer in number, whereas the proximal matrix contains a lower density of melanocytes than the distal matrix.[1,2] The difference in number of melanocytes exists probably because those melanocytes are protected from ultraviolet stimulation by the proximal nail fold. The nail plate contains melanin by melanosome transfer from these melanocytes to the differentiating matrix cells.[1,3] Nail pigment is quite common in blacks and quite rare in whites. Langerhans' cells and rare Merkel cells have also been identified in the matrix.[1] The lunula—the white, halfmoon area—corresponds with the keratogenous zone, which consists of epithelial cells with flattened nuclei and eosinophilic cytoplasm[4] (see Fig. 5–5). These keratogenous zone cells lose their nuclei and form the nail plate cells, or onychocytes.

The nail plate consists of closely packed cornified cells arranged in lamellae that stain

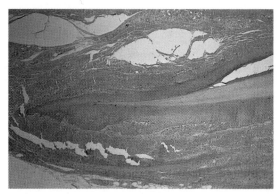

Figure 5–4. Junction between the nail matrix and the ventral proximal nail fold. The latter shows flat epithelium with a granular layer.

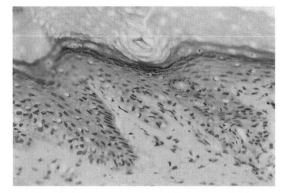

Figure 5–2. The dorsal surface of the proximal nail fold. Four layers can be recognized: (1) basal, (2) spinous, (3) granular, and (4) cornified. Note the presence of an intraepidermal eccrine duct.

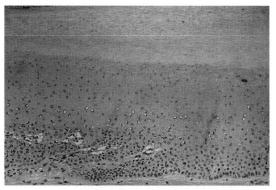

Figure 5–5. Nail matrix consists of a thick epithelium with no granular layer. Note the keratogenous zone, lined by keratinocytes with dark, small nuclei and eosinophilic cytoplasm, between the nail matrix and the nail plate.

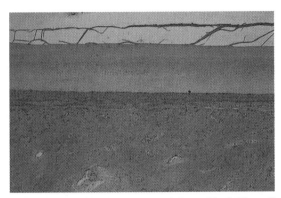

Figure 5–6. Longitudinal section of the nail bed. The nail bed epithelium is relatively thin, lies beneath the nail plate, and weakly stains with eosin.

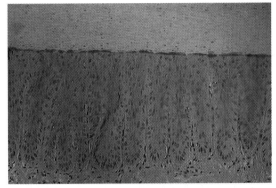

Figure 5–9. Transverse section of the nail bed. Note the serrated interdigitating nail bed epithelium and dermal papillae.

weakly with eosin and strongly with acid-fast stains (Figs. 5–6 and 5–7). The dorsal surface of the nail plate is smooth, but the ventral surface is irregular, as demonstrated by electron microscopy.[5] The nail plate is approximately 0.5 mm thick; the nail plate over the lunula is thinner than that over the nail bed.[6]

The nail bed epithelium lies beneath the nail plate and is bordered proximally by the nail matrix and distally by the hyponychium. The epithelium of the nail bed has no granular cell layer, relatively thin epithelium, in sagittal section, and few parakeratotic cells (Figs. 5–6 and 5–8). The parakeratotic cells of the nail bed tightly adhere to the undersurface of the nail plate and move forward as the nail plate grows toward the distal groove. The nail bed, in transverse sections, is firmly attached to the underlying dermis by long, narrow epithelial rete ridges that are interlocked with dermal papilla, forming regular longitudinal folds along the nail bed (Fig. 5–9).

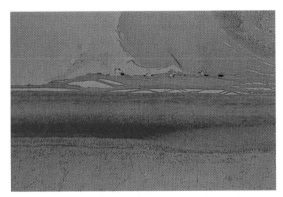

Figure 5–7. The nail plate is strongly positive with acid-fast stains.

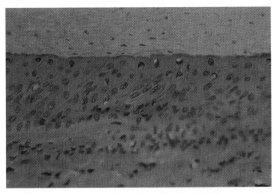

Figure 5–8. Higher power magnification of the nail bed showing a thin layer of parakeratotic cells and no granular layer.

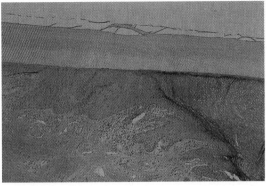

Figure 5–10. Hyponychium. It is composed of all four layers of the epidermis, with a thick, compact, cornified layer as volar skin.

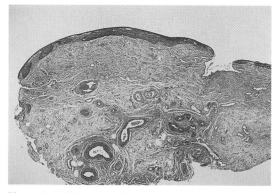

Figure 5–11. Dermis of the nail unit, a region characterized by prominent blood vessels and neural structures devoid of epithelial adnexa.

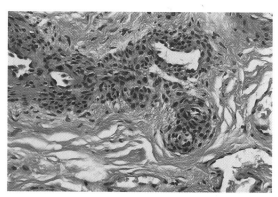

Figure 5–13. Glomus cells surrounding arterioles and venules of special shunts; known as glomus bodies.

The hyponychium is a narrow zone of epidermis beneath the free edge of the nail plate and between the nail bed and distal nail groove. The hyponychium cornifies like volar skin (i.e., it produces a granular cell layer and a thick, compact cornified layer) (Fig. 5–10).

The dermis of the nail unit is highly vascular and is supplied by digital arteries. In addition, there are numerous glomus bodies, which function as special arteriovenous shunts to regulate the temperature of the digits (Figs. 5–11 to 5–13). Nerve endings and nerve trunks are also numerous, with special nerve structures such as Meissner's corpuscles and Vater-Pacini corpuscles. There are no adnexal epithelial structures in the ventral surface of the proximal nail fold, nail matrix, nail bed, and hyponychium. The dermis of the nail

unit lies directly on the phalanx without subcutaneous fat tissue. The upper reticular dermis is composed of thick collagen bundles primarily arranged parallel to the skin surface, whereas in the lower reticular dermis the collagen fibers are thin and loosely arranged. Proportionally, there are more plump fibroblasts and ground substance in the lower reticular dermis. Infrequently, lipocytes can be found within the deep dermis.

EMBRYOLOGY: HISTOLOGIC ASPECTS

At the gestational age of 7 to 8 weeks, the epidermis of the digits consists of a single layer of epithelium, whereas the dermis is composed of abundant undifferentiated mesenchymal cells (Fig. 5–14). Numerous mitotic figures are present in both the epithelial and mesenchymal components. Fetal cartilage is also present at this stage (Fig. 5–15).

The nail unit first appears at about 9 weeks gestation. The invagination of the surface epithelium forms the proximal, lateral, and distal grooves. The area outlined by these grooves is termed the *nail field* (Fig. 5–16A). The surface epithelium of the nail field is more developed than the surrounding epithelium and consists of multiple epithelial cell layers, including a granular cell layer (Fig. 5–16B). Along the proximal groove, there is a wedge of epithelial cells, the matrix primordium, growing downward proximally to form the precursor of the nail matrix and the ventral surface of the proximal nail fold. Endochondral ossification and cartilage are present at this stage (Fig. 5–17).

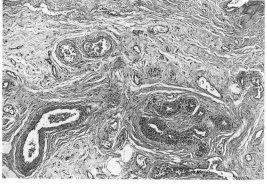

Figure 5–12. The lower dermis, which is composed of thin, loosly arranged collagen fibers in contrast to superficial dermis. Note the abundant blood vessels and glomus bodies.

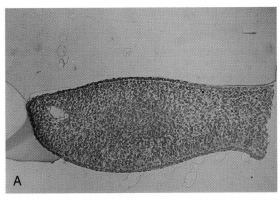
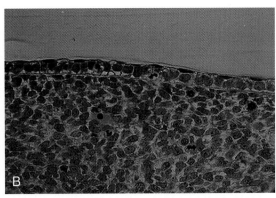

Figure 5–14. *A* and *B*, Longitudinal section of finger at 7 weeks gestation consisting of a single layer of epithelium and dermis with abundant undifferentiated mesenchymal cells.

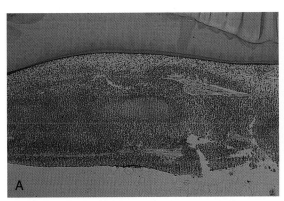
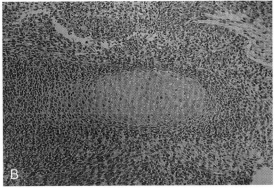

Figure 5–15. *A* and *B*, Longitudinal section of finger at 8 weeks gestation. In this stage, formation of fetal cartilage appears in the mesenchymal tissues.

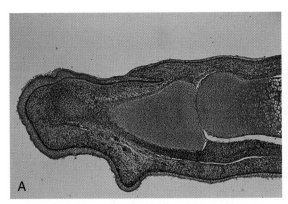
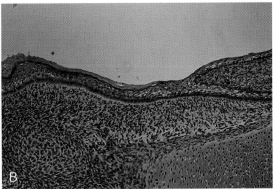

Figure 5–16. *A* and *B*, Longitudinal section of finger at 9 weeks gestation. Note the matrix primordium, which grows downward proximally at the nail field.

At 15 weeks gestation, the matrix primordium differentiates and separates into two components. The upper component forms the ventral surface of the proximal nail fold, whereas the lower component forms the nail matrix. The rete ridges and eccrine sweat primordia are also developed in the dermis of volar epithelium at this stage (Fig. 5–18).

When the fetus reaches 20 weeks of gestational age, the nail unit is virtually complete. The nail matrix produces mature onychocytes, which can be demonstrated with

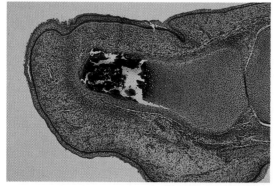

Figure 5–17. Cartilage and endochondral ossification in the dermis at 10 weeks gestation.

Table 5–1. **MANIFESTATIONS OF PSORIASIS IN THE NAILS AND SKIN**

Nail Psoriasis	Skin Psoriasis
Mild to moderate hyperkeratosis	Marked hyperkeratosis
Hypergranulosis not unusual	Hypergranulosis unusual
Serum globules in corni-fied layer usual	Serum globules in corni-fied layer unusual
Hemorrhage in the corni-fied layer usual	Hemorrhage in the corni-fied layer unusual
Papillomatous epidermal hyperplasia common (transverse section)	Papillomatous epidermal hyperplasia uncommon
Spongiosis common	Spongiosis uncommon

sulfhydryl stains. The nail plate grows along the surface of the nail bed from the proximal nail fold toward the distal groove, whereas its lateral surfaces are bordered by the lateral nail folds. The nail unit of the toes develops in the same manner as the nail unit of the fingers, but the development occurs more slowly.

HISTOPATHOLOGY OF NAIL DISEASES

A number of diseases affect the skin and nail unit. Some of them may occur only as changes in the nails; therefore, a nail biopsy is often required for diagnosis. The histologic changes in the nail unit are usually similar to those in the skin, but some findings are rather specific to the nail.

Psoriasis

Nail involvement in psoriasis is quite common, varying from 10 to 50 per cent of cases.[7–9] Psoriasis involving only the nail unit is not uncommon. However, it is slightly more difficult to diagnose clinically on the basis of the nail changes alone. The histologic study may, therefore, be necessary to confirm the clinical diagnosis.

Nail psoriasis has the same pathogenesis as skin psoriasis, but the clinical manifestations are quite different from the skin lesions, namely pitting and other nail plate abnormalities, discoloration of the nail bed, subungual hyperkeratosis, onycholysis, and splinter hemorrhages (Table 5–1).

Psoriasis can involve any part of the nail unit and cause a variety of clinical and pathologic manifestations. The majority of changes can be observed in and under the nail plates.

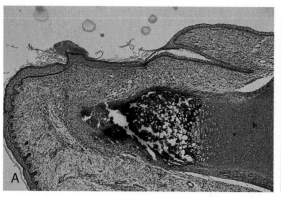
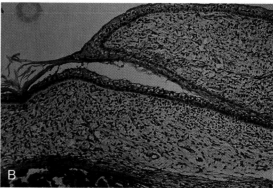

Figure 5–18. *A* and *B,* Longitudinal section of finger at 15 weeks gestation. Formation of nail matrix and ventral portion of the proximal nail fold occurs by separation of the matrix primordium.

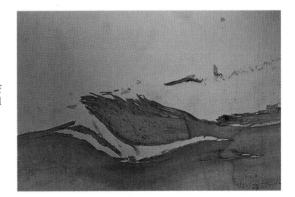

Figure 5–19. Pitting nail, evolving lesion. Small clusters of parakeratotic cells are shed from the surface of the nail plate. This lesion has evolved into pitting nail.

Psoriatic involvement of the proximal nail matrix causes pitting and a rough-surfaced nail plate. The histology of nail pitting reveals foci of parakeratotic cells in the upper portion of the nail plate. When the parakeratotic cells fall off, they produce pits on the dorsal nail plates (Fig. 5–19). Psoriatic involvement of the middle and distal nail matrix produces a smooth-surfaced leukonychia that histologically reveals foci of parakeratotic cells in the deeper portion of the nail plates. It may also produce focal onycholysis.

Psoriasis of the nail bed results in a discoloration of the nail bed, subungual hyperkeratosis, onycholysis, and splinter hemorrhages. The nail biopsy in psoriasis is usually taken from the nail bed and nail plate. Psoriasis of the nail bed and skin has many histologic features in common, among them neutrophils in the epidermis, psoriasiform hyperplasia, and a superficial infiltrate of lymphocytes and neutrophils around widely dilated capillaries and venules (Figs. 5–20 and 5–21). However,

some features of psoriasis of the nail bed differ from those of psoriasis of the skin (see Table 5–1). Nail bed psoriasis shows more spongiosis and hyperplasia in the epidermis and more serum accumulation in the cornified layer than does skin psoriasis. The prominent granular cell layer, a feature not usually seen in normal nail bed or skin psoriasis, is usually present in nail psoriasis (Figs. 5–22 to 5–29).

In late lesions of psoriatic nails, there is an absence of neutrophils in the cornified layer. However, these lesions can be diagnosed as psoriasis because of the psoriasiform hyperplasia with thin, elongated rete ridges, thin suprapapillary plates, and dilated, tortuous capillaries in the papillary dermis. Lichen simplex chronicus is often superimposed on old lesions of psoriatic nails, especially when there is partial or complete absence of the nail plate secondary to persistent rubbing and picking of the nail bed and hyponychium. These lesions are also characterized

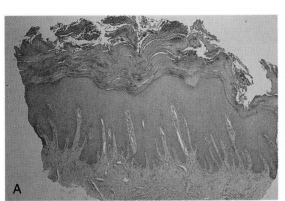

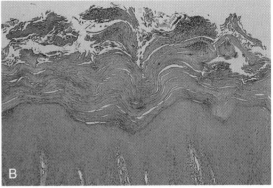

Figure 5–20. *A* and *B,* Nail psoriasis. The diagnostic features are focal parakeratosis admixed with neutrophils, psoriasiform epidermal hyperplasia, superficial perivascular lymphocytic infiltrate, and dilated tortuous capillaries in the papillary dermis.

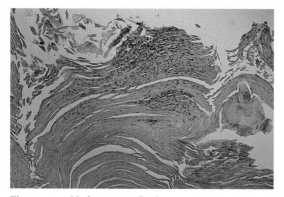

Figure 5–21. Nail psoriasis (high-power magnification of Figure 5–20). Tiers of neutrophils within mounds of parakeratosis are diagnostic of active lesions.

by compact orthokeratosis, hypergranulosis, and coarse collagen in vertical streaks in a thickened papillary dermis (Figs. 5–30 and 5–31).

Onycholysis results from psoriatic involvement of the nail bed and hyponychium. Histologic study of the nail plate of onycholytic nails shows mounds of parakeratosis containing neutrophils in the subungual cornified layer, and the separation is actually between the layer of neutrophils containing the parakeratotic horn of the nail bed and hyponychium, not between the nail bed and nail plate (Figs. 5–32 and 5–33).

Reiter's syndrome and psoriasis have the same histologic changes.

Lichen Planus

Nail involvement occurs in approximately 10 per cent of lichen planus cases and may occur without skin or mucous membrane in-

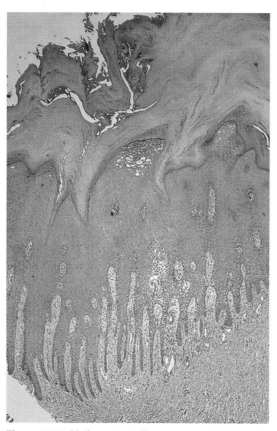

Figure 5–22. Nail psoriasis (low-power magnification). One observes hyperkeratosis, spongiosis, acanthosis, and papillomatosis.

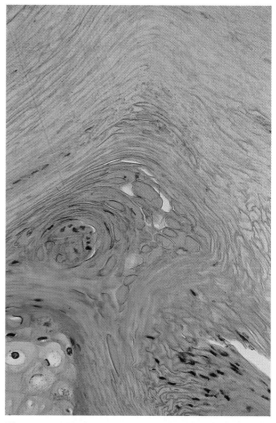

Figure 5–23. Nail psoriasis (high-power magnification of Figure 5–22). Scaly crusts lie in the thickened cornified layer.

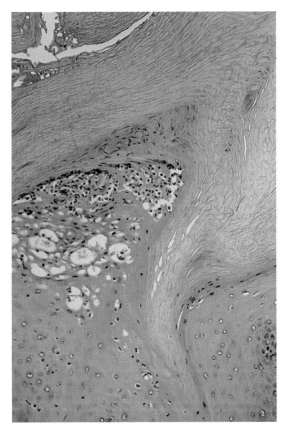

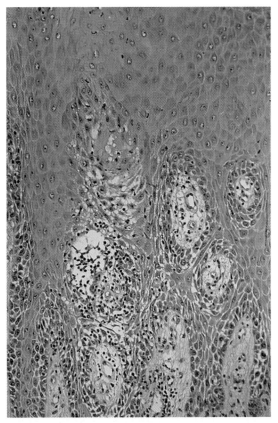

Figure 5–24. Nail psoriasis (high-power magnification of Figure 5–22). Neutrophils within epidermis in spongiform are important diagnostic features of acute stage. Note a small area of hemorrhage in the thickened, cornified layer.

Figure 5–25. Nail psoriasis. Spongiosis and spongiotic vesicles within epidermis are common features in nail psoriasis.

volvement.[10] The nail changes in lichen planus are not pathognomonic for the disease. Severe involvement of the nail unit can produce permanent damage; therefore, early nail biopsy is necessary to make a specific diagnosis and institute appropriate therapy to prevent sequelae.

Lichen planus of the nail unit has many features in common with that of the skin, among them hyperkeratosis, hypergranulosis, irregular epidermal hyperplasia, necrotic keratinocytes (Civatte bodies—round, homogeneous eosinophilic bodies resulting from necrotic keratinocytes), vacuolar alteration, dense lichenoid lymphohistiocytic infiltrate with melanophages in the upper dermis that obscures the dermal–epidermal interface, and coarse collagen bundles in a thickened papillary dermis (Figs. 5–34 and 5–35). In contrast, lichen planus of the nail unit has certain histologic features that differentiate it from lichen

Table 5–2. HISTOLOGIC FEATURES OF LICHEN PLANUS IN NAILS AND SKIN

Nail Lichen Planus	Skin Lichen Planus
Marked compact orthokeratosis and focal parakeratosis	Slight to moderate compact orthokeratosis
Scaly crust in cornified layer common	Scaly crust in cornified layer uncommon
Diffuse hypergranulosis	Wedge-shaped hypergranulosis
Marked fibrosis in the papillary and reticular dermis	Slight fibrosis in the papillary dermis
May resolve with scar	Usually resolves without scar

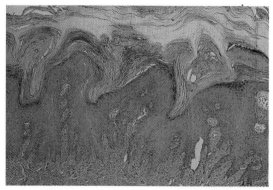

Figure 5–26. Nail psoriasis. Foci of parakeratosis, acanthosis, papillomatosis, and dilated tortuous capillaries are features of chronic lesion.

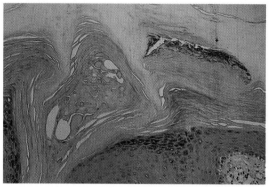

Figure 5–27. Nail psoriasis (high-power magnification of Figure 5–26). Neutrophils within mounds of parakeratosis, scaly crusts, and hypergranulosis are common features in nail psoriasis.

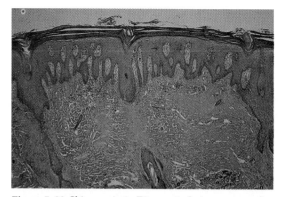

Figure 5–28. Skin psoriasis. Diagnostic features are confluent parakeratosis, hypogranulosis, psoriasiform epidermal hyperplasia, dilated tortuous capillaries, and perivascular lymphocytic infiltrate.

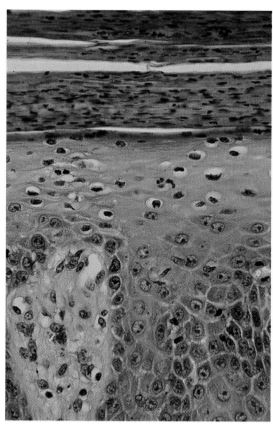

Figure 5–29. Skin psoriasis (high-power magnification of Figure 5–28). Note the neutrophils within confluent parakeratosis and epidermis with absence of granular layer.

planus of the skin (Table 5–2). The compact hyperkeratosis of the cornified layer in nail lichen planus is usually associated with focal parakeratosis or scaly-crust, but the same is not true of skin lichen planus. Hypergranulosis of skin lichen planus is situated focally in an otherwise normal granular cell layer, whereas that of nail lichen planus tends to be diffuse (Figs. 5–34 to 5–41). In addition, in the late lesion of nail lichen planus, fibrosis occurs more prominently in the upper dermis, and may result in permanent atrophy and scarring (Figs. 5–43 to 5–47). In contrast, in skin lichen planus, postinflammatory pigmentary alteration and slight fibrosis result (Fig. 5–42).

Onychomycosis

The nail changes in onychomycosis sometimes cannot be distinguished clinically or histologically from other nail diseases; therefore,

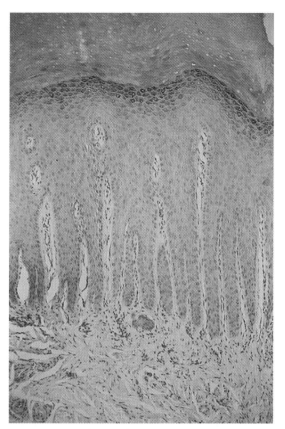

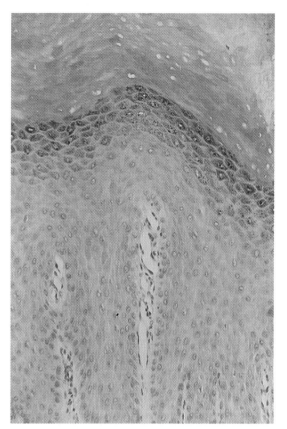

Figure 5–30. Nail psoriasis; chronic, persistent lesion. It shows compact hyperkeratosis, hypergranulosis, psoriasiform epidermal hyperplasia with thin, elongated rete ridges and dilated tortuous capillaries.

Figure 5–31. Nail psoriasis (high-power magnification of Figure 5–30). Note the compact orthokeratosis, hypergranulosis, thin suprapapillary plates and dilated tortuous capillaries, and absence of neutrophils within epidermis.

potassium hydroxide (KOH) preparation and fungus culture are often used to confirm the clinical diagnosis. Scrapings of the nail specimen are usually too superficial because the spores and hyphae of fungi are characteristically located in the cornified layer of the nail bed or the deep portion of the nail plate, resulting in negative cultures and KOH preparations (Fig. 5–48A and B). Norton found 50 per cent of infected nails to have negative results on KOH preparation and fungus culture.[11] Hence, nail biopsy is warranted to demonstrate fungi in such culture-negative cases. Furthermore, a biopsy can also be helpful in the decision as to whether a nondermatophytic fungi cultured from an abnormal nail is a pathogen or merely a contaminant.

The histologic diagnosis of onychomycosis is based on the clinical types of distal and proximal subungual onychomycosis, necessitating the presence of spores and hyphae in the cornified layer of the nail bed, the deep

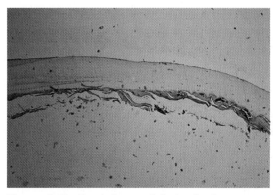

Figure 5–32. Psoriatic onycholysis. It demonstrates mounds of parakeratosis in the undersurface of the nail plate.

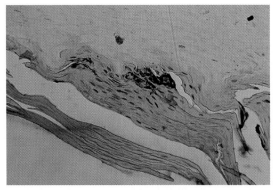

Figure 5–33. Psoriatic onycholysis (high-power magnification of Figure 5–32) demonstrates neutrophils within mounds of parakeratosis. Separation occurs between cells in the parakeratotic nail bed.

portion of the nail plate, or the hyponychium for accurate diagnosis. In the absence of fungal elements, the diagnosis of psoriasis must be considered.

Dermatophytosis and subungual onychomycosis have many histologic features in common, namely hyperkeratosis containing neutrophils, spongiosis, epidermal hyperplasia, and a lymphocytic infiltrate with occasional neutrophils in the papillary dermis (Figs. 5–49 to 5–55). However, some features of subungual onychomycosis differ from those of dermatophytosis. In contrast to dermatophytosis, onychomycosis tends to have marked hyperkeratosis often associated with plasma in scaly crust and small collections of blood clots (Table 5–3).

The nondermatophytic fungi are often causative agents of distal subungual ony-

Text continued on page 71

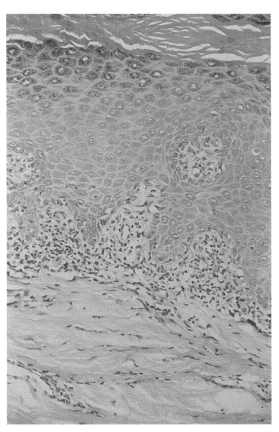

Figure 5–35. Nail lichen planus (high-power magnification of Figure 5–34). Several features are evident: compact orthokeratosis; diffuse hypergranulosis; irregular epidermal hyperplasia, with jagged sawtooth appearance of the rete; vacuolar alteration; and lichenoid infiltrate of lymphocytes.

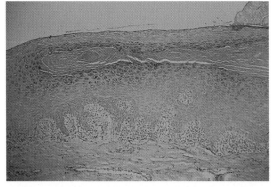

Figure 5–34. Nail lichen planus. Diagnostic features seen in this photomicrograph include orthokeratosis, hypergranulosis, epidermal hyperplasia, and lichenoid infiltrate of lymphocytes that obscure the dermoepidermal junction.

Table 5–3. **SUBUNGUAL ONYCHOMYCOSIS VERSUS DERMATOPHYTOSIS**

Onychomycosis	Dermatophytosis
Marked hyperkeratosis	Slight to moderate hyperkeratosis
Hyphae present in compact horn	Hyphae present between basketweave horn and compact horn or between orthokeratosis and parakeratosis (sandwich sign)
Scaly crust common	Scaly crust uncommon
Papillomatous epidermal hyperplasia common (transverse section)	Papillomatous epidermal hyperplasia uncommon
Extravasated erythrocytes usually in cornified layer	Extravasated erythrocytes usually in papillary dermis

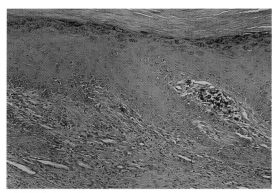

Figure 5–36. Nail lichen planus, old lesion. This lesion is differentiated from the early ones by less lichenoid infiltrate of lymphocytes with numerous melanophages in the thickened papillary dermis in addition to hyperkeratosis and hypergranulosis.

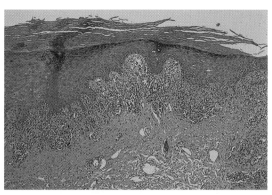

Figure 5–39. Skin lichen planus. Diagnostic features are orthokeratosis, focal hypergranulosis, irregular epidermal hyperplasia, and lichenoid infiltrate of lymphocytes that obscure the dermoepidermal junction.

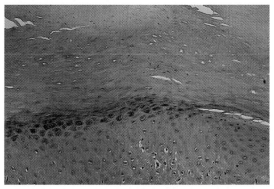

Figure 5–37. Nail lichen planus (high-power magnification Figure 5–41). Note the presence of focal parakeratosis in the thickened, cornified layer and diffuse hypergranulosis.

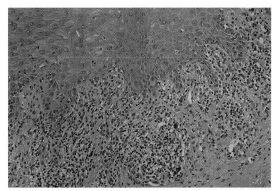

Figure 5–40. Skin lichen planus (high-power magnification of Figure 5–39). Irregular epidermal hyperplasia with jagged sawtooth appearance of the rete, lichenoid infiltrate of lymphocytes, and melanophages are evident.

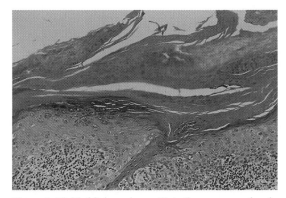

Figure 5–38. Nail lichen planus. Note the presence of scaly crusts in the cornified layer.

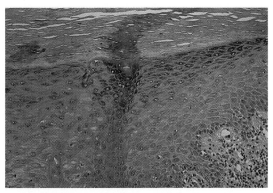

Figure 5–41. Skin lichen planus (high-power magnification of Figure 5–40). Compact orthokeratosis and wedge-shaped hypergranulosis are evident.

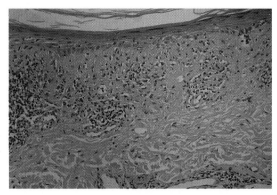

Figure 5–42. Skin lichen planus, resolving lesion. Note thinned epidermis, mild lichenoid lymphocytic infiltrate, and fibrosis in the thickened papillary dermis.

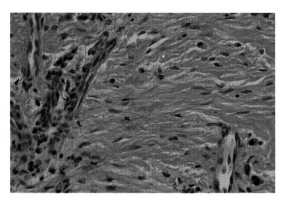

Figure 5–45. Nail lichen planus, resolving lesion (high-power magnification of Figure 5–44). Note that fibroblasts and collagen fibers are oriented parallel to the skin surface, whereas thick-walled vessels run perpendicular to it.

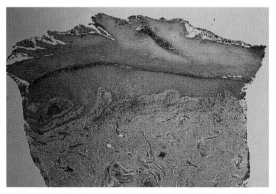

Figure 5–43. Nail lichen planus, resolving lesion. This lesion is differentiated from a fully developed lesion by having flattened rete ridges, sparse rather than dense bandlike infiltrate of lymphocytes, and considerable fibrosis of the upper dermis.

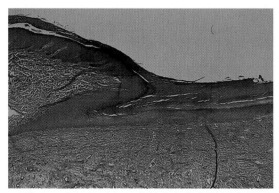

Figure 5–46. Pterygium. Atrophy of the nail matrix and nail bed epithelium devoid of rete ridges and scar in the underlying dermis is evident.

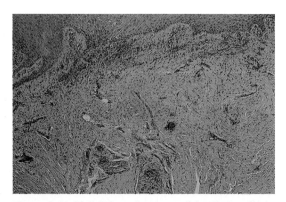

Figure 5–44. Nail lichen planus, resolving lesion (high-power magnification of Figure 5–43). A sparse, bandlike infiltrate of lymphocytes with marked fibrosis in the thickened papillary dermis and upper reticular dermis is evident.

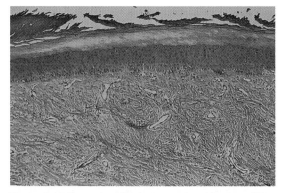

Figure 5–47. Pterygium (high-power magnification of Figure 5–46). Scar in the dermis is composed of scattered fibroblasts, altered collagen, and blood vessels.

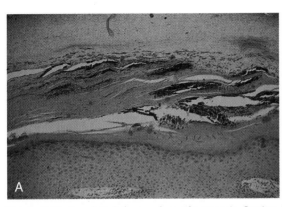
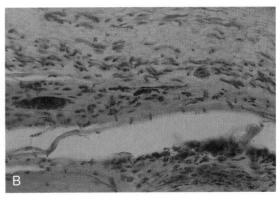

Figure 5–48. *A* and *B,* Subungual onychomycosis. Section demonstrates numerous hyphae in the thickened, cornified layer of the nail bed and lower nail plate.

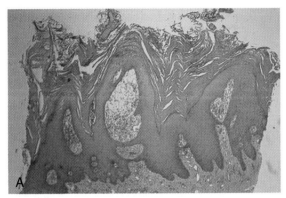
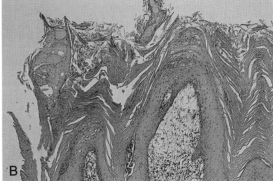

Figure 5–49. *A* and *B,* Subungual onychomycosis, acute lesion. Histologic changes show hyperkeratosis, spongiosis, acanthosis, papillomatosis, edema of the papillary dermis, and dense superficial perivascular infiltrate of lymphocytes and neutrophils that cannot be differentiated from nail psoriasis.

Figure 5–50. Subungual onychomycosis (high-power magnification of Figure 5–49). Scaly crusts and neutrophils within epidermis in spongiform are evident.

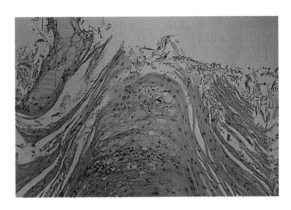

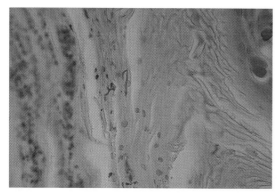

Figure 5–51. Subungual onychomycosis. Periodic acid–Schiff stain reveals hyphae that may not be easily discerned with hematoxylin and eosin stain.

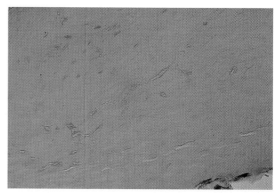

Figure 5–54. Subungual onychomycosis (high-power magnification of Figure 5–53). Numerous hyphae can be seen in orthokeratotic portion of cornified layer.

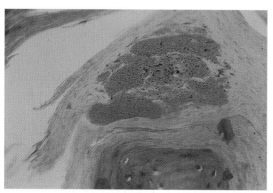

Figure 5–52. Subungual onychomycosis. Note the area of hemorrhage in the thickened, cornified layer that is not uncommon in onychomycosis.

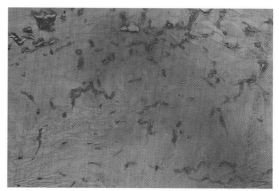

Figure 5–55. Subungual onychomycosis. Numerous hyphae are easily discerned with periodic acid–Schiff stain.

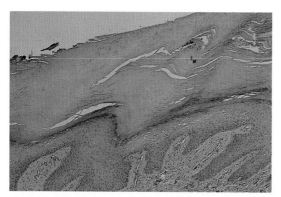

Figure 5–53. Subungual onychomycosis, chronic lesion. Compact hyperkeratosis, hypergranulosis, acanthosis, papillomatosis, and a sparse superficial perivascular infiltrate of lymphocytes are characteristic features.

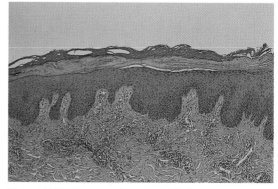

Figure 5–56. Dermatophytosis, scaly lesion. Diagnostic features are confluent parakeratosis beneath normal orthokeratosis, acanthosis, and dense perivascular infiltrate of lymphocytes and neutrophils.

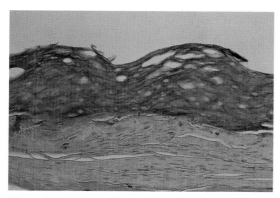

Figure 5–57. Dermatophytosis (high-power magnification of Figure 5–56). Hyphae at the junction between orthokeratosis and parakeratosis (sandwich sign) are evident.

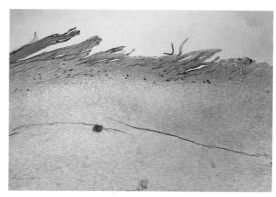

Figure 5–59. White superficial onychomycosis. Note the rough and irregular surface of the dorsal nail plate.

chomyosis of the toenails. Histologically, nondermatophytic onychomycosis is diagnosed when it shows invasion of fungal elements in the nail plate, with the typical histologic picture of onychomycosis in the nail bed and nail plate.

The histologic findings of superficial white onychomycosis reveal hyphae of dermatophytes or nondermatophytic fungi in the superficial portion of the nail plate, whereas the underlying nail bed is normal (Figs. 5–59 to 5–61). Furthermore, *Candida albicans* is a common cause of onycholysis and can be distinguished from psoriasis. The separation in candidal onycholysis occurs between the lytic nail plate and the nail bed, with organisms present in the fragment of the lytic nail plate and the cornified layer of the nail bed (Fig. 5–62).

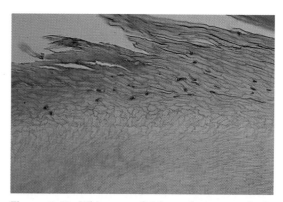

Figure 5–60. White superficial onychomycosis (high-power magnification of Figure 5–59). Hyphae of dermatophytes within the dorsal nail plate (periodic acid–Schiff stain) are evident.

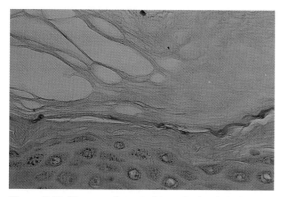

Figure 5–58. Dermatophytosis. Note the hyphal elements with periodic acid–Schiff stain.

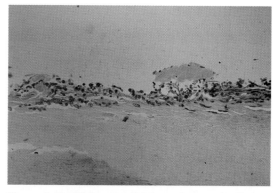

Figure 5–61. White superficial onychomycosis. Fungus consists of round, eroding bodies and hyphae of nondermatophytic fungi seen in the dorsal nail plate.

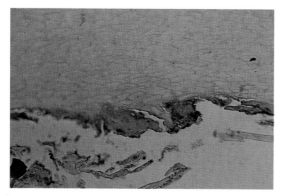

Figure 5–62. *Candida* onycholysis. Note hyphae and yeast within lytic nail plate and clusters of cornified cells at the undersurface of the nail plate.

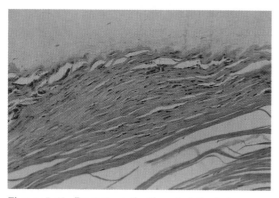

Figure 5–63. Psoriatic nail. Characteristic features are mounds of parakeratosis containing neutrophils and absence of hyphae beneath the nail plate.

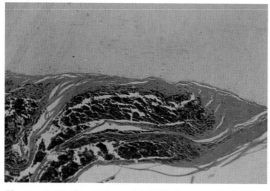

Figure 5–64. Psoriatic nail. Well-circumscribed intracorneal pustules are not uncommon findings in psoriasis.

Pityriasis Rubra Pilaris

Nail changes are seen in many of the disorders in the differential diagnosis of type I pityriasis rubra pilaris and include distal yellow-brown discoloration, subungual hyperkeratosis, nail plate thickening, and splinter hemorrhages. Histology from a nail biopsy demonstrates patchy parakeratosis in the nail plate and cornified layers of nail bed. The epithelium of the nail bed is slightly thickened. Granular cell layers are intermittently present. The dermal vessels are dilated in some areas but are not abnormally tortuous. A sparse perivascular infiltrate of lymphocytes is seen in the papillary dermis. These changes are more prominent in the nail bed than in the nail matrix. Orthokeratosis and parakeratosis are present at the hyponychium.[12]

Nail Clippings

When dermatologists are reluctant to perform a nail biopsy because of fear of causing permanent nail dystrophy, a nail plate clipping should be obtained.[13] This technique is simple, noninvasive, and effective for the diagnosis of distal subungual onychomycosis and psoriatic nail. The histologic findings of psoriatic nails from nail plate clippings include thick and confluent or mounds of parakeratosis with the nuclei of cells showing thin, elongated pyknosis arranged in dense aggregates. The parakeratotic cells are admixed with neutrophils (Fig. 5–63). Small pustules with a well-circumscribed collection of degenerated neutrophils and their exudate might be observed (Fig. 5–64). The histology of onychomycosis is indistinguishable from that of psoriasis except for the presence of a fungal element within the cornified layer of the nail bed or lower portion of the nail plate (Figs. 5–65 and 5–66). The nail change of pityriasis rubra pilaris is focal parakeratosis and orthokeratosis, horizontally and vertically, in the thick cornified layer of the nail bed (Fig. 5–67*A* and *B*). Idiopathic onycholysis usually shows a jagged sawtooth appearance of the undersurface of the nail plate when clusters of cornified cells have been shed (see Fig. 5–68).

Spongiotic Trachyonychia

Trachyonychia is a morphologic manifestation that can occur in different conditions. Definitive diagnosis of the specific disease that

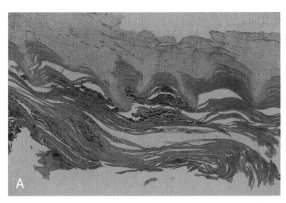
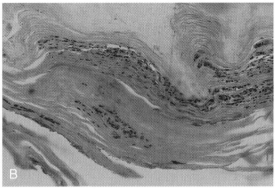

Figure 5–65. *A* and *B*, Onychomycosis. Mounds of parakeratosis containing neutrophils should prompt a search for fungi.

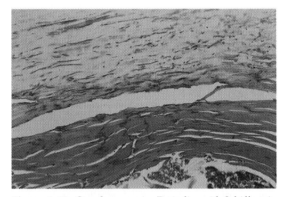

Figure 5–66. Onychomycosis. Periodic acid–Schiff stain demonstrates numerous hyphae in the cornified layer of the nail bed and the ventral nail plate.

causes trachyonychia requires a pathologic examination of the nail and cannot be determined clinically.

This clinicopathologic entity is thin, rough, friable, and opalescent, with excessive longitudinal striation and distal splitting (Fig. 5–68). There is no pterygium formation as a rule in spongiotic trachyonychia. It may involve a few nails or all 20 nails and present with the clinical features of 20-nail dystrophy.[14] This condition may be seen in patients with alopecia areata or atopy or may be apparently idiopathic.[14–16] The histologic changes of spongiotic trachyonychia show an inflammatory response confined to the epithelial component and superficial dermis of the nail matrix. Epithelial hyperplasia and spongiosis can occur, with an inflammatory infiltrate under and within the matrix epithelium. The degree of spongiosis varies from mild changes (Figs. 5–69 to 5–71) to most severe changes with intraepidermal microvesicles (Figs. 5–72 and 5–73). The inflammatory cells are composed of

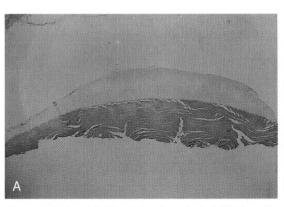
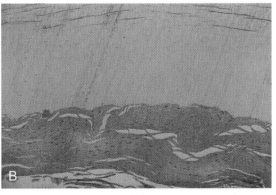

Figure 5–67. *A* and *B*, Pityriasis rubra pilaris. Nail plate clipping shows parakeratosis that alternates with orthokeratosis, both vertically and horizontally, in the cornified layer beneath the nail plate.

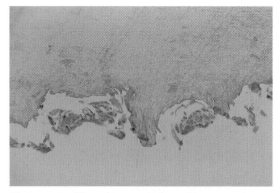

Figure 5–68. Idiopathic onycholysis. Note jagged saw-tooth appearance with clusters of cornified cells shed at the undersurface of the nail plate.

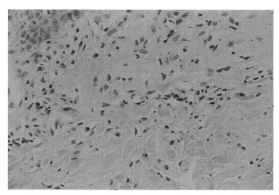

Figure 5–71. Spongiotic trachyonychia (high-power magnification of Figure 5–69). Inflammatory cell infiltrate of lymphocytes and eosinophils is evident.

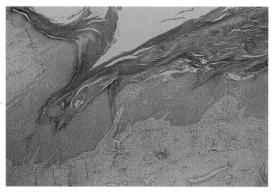

Figure 5–69. Spongiotic trachyonychia. Mounds of para-keratosis and scaly crust, spongiotic epidermal hyperplasia, and superficial perivascular inflammatory cell infiltrate are typical features. Note that the cornified layer stains pink with hematoxylin and eosin as does normal skin.

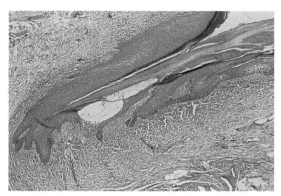

Figure 5–72. Spongiotic trachyonychia. Varying degrees of spongiosis, including spongiotic vesicles, can be seen in the severe lesion.

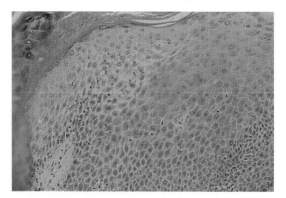

Figure 5–70. Spongiotic trachyonychia (high-power magnification of Figure 5–69). Foci of spongiosis associated with epidermal hyperplasia and hypergranulosis are evident.

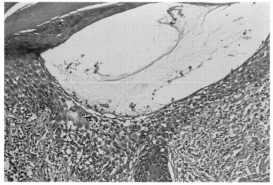

Figure 5–73. Spongiotic trachyonychia (high-power magnification of Figure 5–72). Evolution from spongiosis to spongiotic vesiculation within the nail matrix can be seen.

lymphocytes with a variable number of eosinophils. The nail plate overlying these inflamed areas shows focal parakeratosis with inflammatory cells. The nail plates stain pink with hematoxylin and eosin stain and are similar in appearance to the adjacent stratum corneum of the volar skin. The prominent granular cell layer is usually observed.[14]

Lichen Striatus

Lichen striatus is a self-limited linear eruption occurring in childhood. It may extend along a finger or a toe as far as the proximal nail fold and affect the nail plate. There are several types of onychodystrophy, including longitudinal splitting, punctate or transverse leukonychia, onycholysis, shredding, and total nail loss.[17] Histology shows a superficial perivascular and focal lichenoid infiltrate of lymphocytes and histiocytes. Lymphocytes may also be present at the dermal–epidermal junction, where there is vacuolar alteration. Lymphocytes usually predominate at the interface, especially in early lesions, but in the dermal papillae there may be a predominance of histiocytes, among them melanophages. The inflammatory infiltrate is usually also seen in and around some of the deeper vessels. The epidermal changes consist of spongiosis, dyskeratotic cells, and parakeratosis. In the old lesions, the infiltrate shows a focal lichenoid pattern under the spongiotic foci (Figs. 5–74 to 5–76). The same histologic changes are also observed in the dorsal surface of the proximal nail fold.

Histiocytosis X

Nail changes in histiocytosis X can be observed in both fingernails and toenails and include longitudinal grooves, purpuric striae, subungual hyperkeratosis, subungual pustules, onycholysis, chronic paronychia, deformation, and pitting of the nail plate.[18–20] Histologic study shows superficial perivascular and lichenoid infiltrate of atypical histiocytes (Figs. 5–77 and 5–78). The histiocytes possess large, kidney-shaped, eccentrically placed nuclei and well-defined eosinophilic cytoplasm (Fig. 5–79). Some histiocytes are usually present focally within the epidermis. The upper dermis is markedly edematous. A few scattered lymphocytes and varying numbers of eosinophils may be present. Extravasated

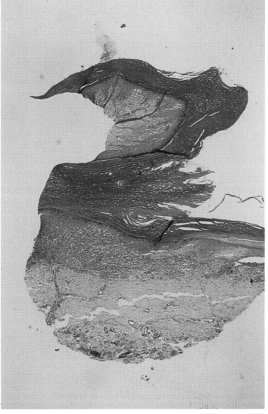

Figure 5–74. Lichen striatus. Diagnostic findings are foci of both spongiosis and vacuolar alteration in association with superficial perivascular and focal lichenoid infiltrate containing lymphohistiocytes.

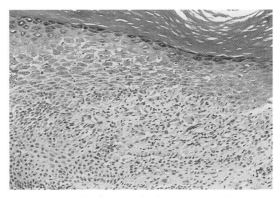

Figure 5–75. Lichen striatus (high-power magnification of Figure 5–74). Foci of both spongiosis and vacuolar alteration in association with dense lichenoid infiltrate of lymphocytes and histiocytes are evident.

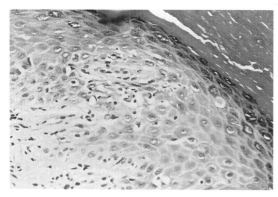

Figure 5–76. Lichen striatus. The subtle changes of both focal spongiosis and vacuolar alteration are also seen in the proximal nail fold.

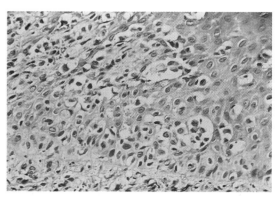

Figure 5–79. Histiocytosis X, proliferative lesion (high-power magnification of Figure 5–78). The histiocytes show bean- or kidney-shaped nuclei and abundant, well-demarcated cytoplasm.

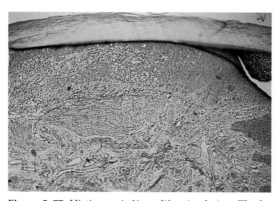

Figure 5–77. Histiocytosis X, proliferative lesion. The lesion shows dense lichenoid infiltrate of atypical histiocytes in the papillary dermis with epidermotropism.

erythrocytes frequently lie within the infiltrate of histiocytes. Electron microscopy confirms that these are Langerhans' cells, which possess Birbeck granules, and immunohistochemical investigations show that these cells are S-100 protein and CD1 positive.[21]

In persistent lesions, one may find extensive aggregates of Langerhans' cells extending deep into the dermis. Multinucleated giant cells are seen frequently. In addition, some eosinophils, neutrophils, lymphocytes, and plasma cells may be present (Figs. 5–80 and 5–81).

Darier-White Disease

The clinical nail manifestations of Darier-White disease include longitudinal, subungual red and white streaks associated with

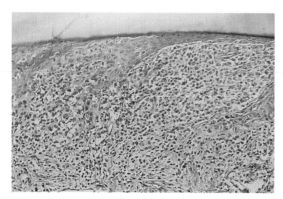

Figure 5–78. Histiocytosis X, proliferative lesion (high-power magnification of Figure 5–77). Dense infiltrate of atypical histiocytes in the papillary dermis and epidermis of the nail bed is evident.

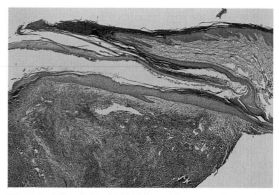

Figure 5–80. Histiocytosis X, granulomatous lesion. The lesion shows extensive aggregates of predominantly histiocytes in dermis of the nail bed.

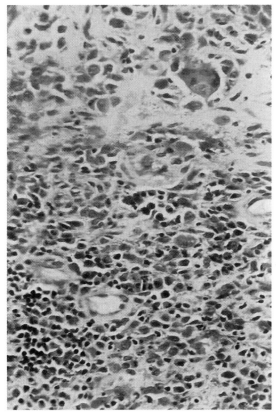

Figure 5–81. Histiocytosis X, granulomatous lesion (high-power magnification of Figure 5–80). Multinucleated giant cells, eosinophils, and plasma cells also lie within the aggregates of histiocytes.

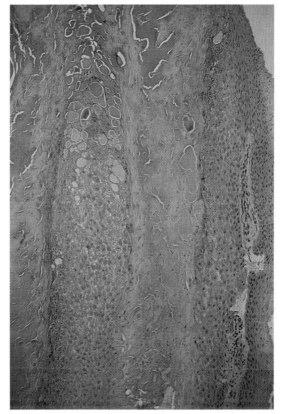

Figure 5–82. Pachyonychia congenita. There is pronounced hyperkeratosis with scaly crusts, hypergranulosis, and digitated epidermal hyperplasia of the nail bed epithelium.

distal wedge-shaped subungual hyperkeratosis. Rarely, Darier-White disease is limited to the nails. The histologic picture may show suprabasilar clefts containing acantholytic cells on the dorsal surface of the proximal nail fold, nail matrix, and epidermis of the volar skin. Additionally, the presence of numerous multinucleated epithelial cells with abundant eosinophilic cytoplasm throughout the length of the nail bed, the nail matrix, and the nail plate has been described.[22]

Pachyonychia Congenita

Pachyonychia congenita is characterized by three major features: subungual hyperkeratosis, keratosis palmaris et plantaris, and leukokeratosis of the oral mucosa. The abnormalities of the nail unit are mostly confined to the nail bed, whereas the nail plate itself is actually normal. The nail bed shows marked hyperkeratosis, papillomatous epidermal hyper-

plasia, and the presence of a granular cell layer. The hyperplastic nail bed and subungual hyperkeratosis push up the plate so that it grows out, angled away from the axis of fingers (Fig. 5–82). The distal matrix is also hyperplastic and papillomatous, producing large quantities of cornified material mixed with plasma.[23]

Keratosis Punctata

Nail involvement has occasionally been described in keratosis punctata. The presenting symptoms include onychogryphosis, nail thickening, subungual hyperkeratosis, longitudinal fissures, and onychomadesis.[24] Pathologic studies of the nail bed reveal a sharply limited column of parakeratosis associated with hypergranulosis and depression of the underlying nail bed epithelium. Similar changes may be seen in the distal nail matrix. No inflammatory infiltrate is observed.[25]

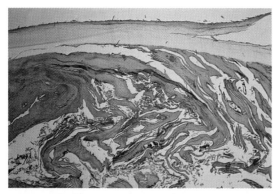

Figure 5–83. Keratotic scabies. Marked hyperkeratosis with focal parakeratosis beneath the nail plate is evident.

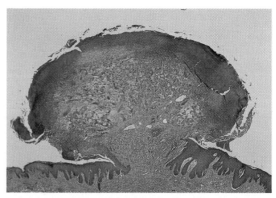

Figure 5–85. Pyogenic granuloma, acute stage. The lesion shows ulcerated exophytic granulation tissue. Note the characteristic collarettes of elongated epidermal rete ridges on both sides that point toward the center of lesion.

Keratotic Scabies

The nail unit is not usually involved in scabies infestation, except in keratotic scabies (Norwegian scabies). The persistence of mites subungually is generally due to resistance to treatment, unless the nails are cut short and the scabicide is vigorously brushed beneath them. Microscopically, the nail bed shows marked hyperkeratosis with focal parakeratosis. Ascarides can be seen in the cornified layer of the nail bed[26] (Figs. 5–83 and 5–84).

Yellow Nail Syndrome

In patients with yellow nail syndrome, results of light microscopy of the nail plate are normal, but electron microscopy reveals keratohyalin granules, which are not normally seen in the nail matrix and postulated to be associated with the slowed nail growth.[27]

Pyogenic Granuloma

Pyogenic granuloma of the nail unit occurs primarily along the lateral nail fold and can result from an ingrown nail. Histologic examination reveals a well-circumscribed lobular lesion characterized by a markedly increased number of widely dilated capillaries associated with edematous stroma, a scattered mixed inflammatory cell infiltrate, and an eroded surface (Figs. 5–85 and 5–86). In old lesions, the stroma is fibrotic, with thickened collagen bundles, increased numbers of fibroblasts, and prominent interlobular septa (Figs. 5–87 and

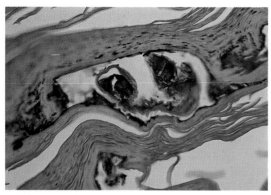

Figure 5–84. Keratotic scabies (high-power magnification of Figure 5–83). Ascarides in the thickened, cornified layer are evident.

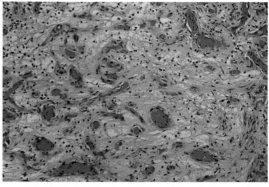

Figure 5–86. Pyogenic granuloma, acute stage (high-power magnification of Figure 5–85). One observes considerable proliferation of capillaries and venules lined by plump endothelial cells. The stroma is edematous and contains a mixed inflammatory cell infiltrate.

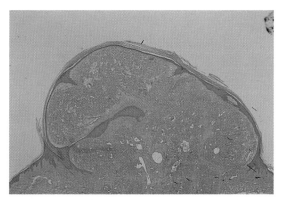

Figure 5–87. Pyogenic granuloma, chronic stage. This stage shows exophytic angiomatous mass with fibrous trabecula intersecting the angiomatous elements and prominent epidermal rete ridges.

5–88). The overlying epidermis has flattened rete ridges and a collarette of epithelium at the base of the lesion.

Epithelial Neoplasms

Most of the neoplasms of the epidermis that affect the skin may also occur in the nail unit. Solar keratosis and basal cell carcinoma seldom occur in the nail unit except on the proximal nail fold because this particular area is not protected by the nail plate against solar damage.

Subungual Basal Cell Carcinoma

Although basal cell carcinoma is the most common skin malignancy, usually occurring in actinically damaged skin, subungual basal cell carcinoma is extremely rare.[28–30] It usually presents as a chronic paronychia or periungual eczematous lesion often associated with ulceration, granulation tissue, and pain. Histologic findings include aggregations of atypical basal cells with large hyperchromatic pleomorphic and palisading nuclei protruding from the surface epithelium of nail bed or nail matrix and extending into the subadjacent dermis. An abundance of melanin and melanin-producing cells may be observed in some nests of tumor cells.

Squamous Cell Carcinoma

Squamous cell carcinoma is the most common malignant tumor found in the nail bed. The presenting symptoms of squamous cell carcinoma of the nail bed include paronychia, ingrown nail, nail separation, nail deformity, dyschromia of the nail plate, bleeding, and pain.[31–33] Histologically, squamous cell carcinoma in situ, or Bowen's disease, is diagnosed when there is a proliferation of atypical keratinocytes consisting of large, hyperchromatic, pleomorphic nuclei with eosinophilic cytoplasm involving the full thickness of the epidermis (Figs. 5–89 and 5–90). When the neoplasm extends into the reticular dermis, the diagnosis of squamous cell carcinoma can be rendered (Figs. 5–91 and 5–92). The features of preexisting verruca, including large parakeratotic cells, papillomatosis, hypergranulosis, and perinuclear vacuoles of keratinocytes, may be found in some lesions.[33]

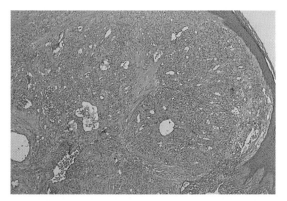

Figure 5–88. Pyogenic granuloma, chronic stage (high-power magnification of Figure 5–87). Note trabeculation by fibrous septum.

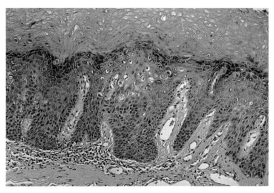

Figure 5–89. Bowen's disease. There are atypical keratinocytes with large hyperchromatic nuclei at all levels of the epidermis.

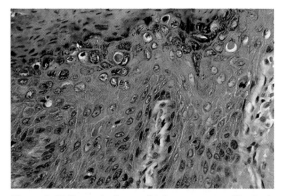

Figure 5–90. Bowen's disease (high-power magnification). Atypical keratinocytes, dyskeratotic cells, and mitotic figures in the thickened epidermis are evident.

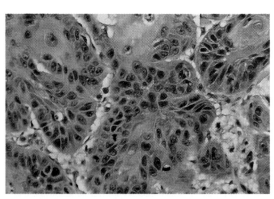

Figure 5–92. Squamous cell carcinoma (high-power magnification of Figure 5–91). Nuclear atypia and mitotic figures of squamous cells are evident.

Carcinoma Cuniculatum (Verrucous Carcinoma)

Carcinoma cuniculatum (verrucous carcinoma on volar skin) is a rare, low-grade variant of squamous cell carcinoma characterized by a local aggressive clinical behavior but a low potential of metastasis. The sole of the foot is the typical site of tumor development; however, reports in the literature of nail apparatus involvement are uncommon.[34] Histologically, carcinoma cuniculatum exhibits both exophytic and endophytic growth patterns. The tumor is characterized by an invaginated proliferation of well-differentiated keratinocytes, some of which have central crypts containing keratinous debris. The surface of the neoplasm shows diffuse parakeratosis and hypogranulosis with a papillated surface. The base of the neoplasm consists of bulbous islands of well-differentiated squamous epithelium infiltrat-

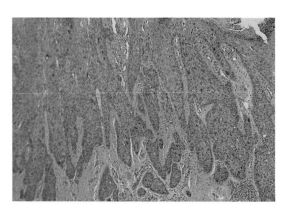

Figure 5–91. Squamous cell carcinoma. The lesion shows irregularly shaped aggregations of atypical squamous epithelium extending into the reticular dermis.

ing the dermis and deeper structure. The squamous cells have scant or no atypia. Mitotic figures are minimal and are usually confined to the basal cell layer (Figs. 5–93 to 5–95). The tumor may grow to involve the phalangeal bone.

Subungual Keratoacanthoma

Subungual keratoacanthoma is an uncommon distinctive tumor of the nail bed. It can easily be confused with well-differentiated squamous cell carcinoma and verrucous carcinoma. Distinctive features of subungual keratoacanthoma include pain, rapid growth, and early underlying bony destruction. Unlike keratoacanthoma arising on other parts of the skin, subungual keratoacanthoma seldom resolves spontaneously and is more locally destructive. Histologically,[35–37] the neoplasm is characterized by bulbous aggregations of squamous epithelium involving the dermis and underlying structures, with epithelial lips at the periphery and central crater filled with cornified debris. Keratinization is abrupt and without an intervening granular layer. Numerous eosinophilic dyskeratotic cells are scattered throughout the cell layers. There are infrequent mitoses in the basal cell layer, and atypia is minimal. The base of the neoplasm is somewhat wedge shaped, with a sparse lymphocytic infiltrate in the underlying stroma (Figs. 5–96 to 5–99). The tumor and associated inflammatory infiltrate are adjacent to the bone at the site of the cortical erosion. The bone marrow may show reactive fibrosis and increased osteoclastic activity. The major histologic feature that distinguishes subungual keratoacanthoma from squamous cell carcinoma or verru-

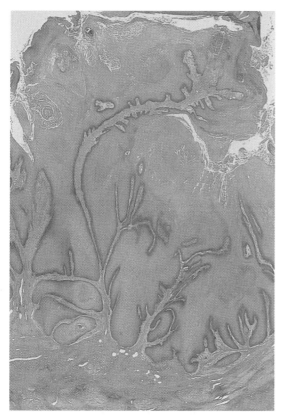

Figure 5–93. Carcinoma cuniculatum (verrucous carcinoma on volar skin). There is a papillated proliferation of well-differentiated squamous cells. The base extends into the deep reticular dermis.

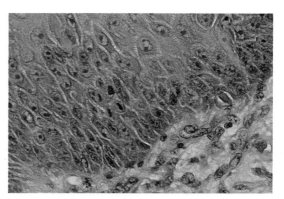

Figure 5–95. Carcinoma cuniculatum (high-power magnification of Figure 5–94). Nuclear atypia and mitotic figures at the base of the neoplastic epithelium are evident.

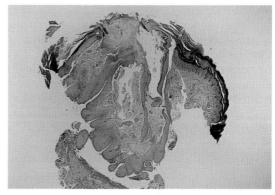

Figure 5–96. Subungual keratoacanthoma. The tumor is characterized by an endophytic growth of squamous epithelium with a central keratin-filled crater.

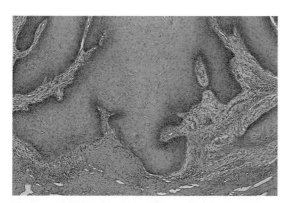

Figure 5–94. Carcinoma cuniculatum (high-power magnification of Figure 5–93). At the base of the neoplastic epithelium, there are bulbous aggregations in association with a dense mixed inflammatory cell infiltrate.

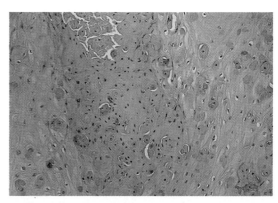

Figure 5–97. Subungual keratoacanthoma (high-power magnification of Figure 5–96). The central crater is filled with cornified debris and parakeratotic cells. The keratinization is abrupt, and there is no intervening granular layer.

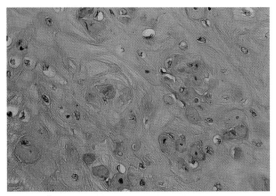

Figure 5–98. Subungual keratoacanthoma (high-power magnification of Figure 5–96). The neoplastic epithelium consists of keratinocytes with dark, small nuclei; glassy, pale eosinophilic cytoplasm; and numerous dyskeratotic cells.

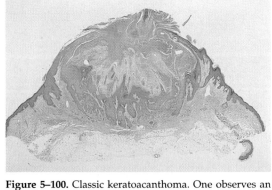

Figure 5–100. Classic keratoacanthoma. One observes an exophytic-endophytic neoplasm with a central keratin-filled crater surrounded by overhanging lips of epithelium.

cous carcinoma is the different and distinctive architectural patterns. Subungual keratoacanthoma differs from typical keratoacanthoma in that it occurs on non–hair-bearing skin and has more vertical orientation, less or no cytologic atypia, less associated inflammation, and much more dyskeratotic cells[35] (Figs. 5–100 to 5–102).

Wart

Common warts on the nail unit usually involve the proximal and lateral nail folds, so-called periungual warts. The warts that initially affect the hyponychium may grow toward the nail bed and eventuate into subungual warts. The histopathology of periungual and subungual warts is indistinguishable

from that of volar skin. The early lesion shows hyperkeratosis, hypergranulosis, papillomatous epidermal hyperplasia, and elongated and inward bending of the peripheral rete ridges with widely dilated capillaries in the papillary dermis (Fig. 5–103). There are perinuclear halos and coarse keratohyalin granules in the granular cell and upper spinous cell layers (Fig. 5–104). In old warts, in contrast to new warts, the surface is less papillated and more endophytic, with epidermal hyperplasia and hypergranulosis (Figs. 5–105 and 5–106). The changes in resolved lesions are characterized by hyperkeratosis above a cup-shaped hyperplastic epidermis with hypergranulosis and a collarette of epithelium at the periphery. The papillary dermis contains widely dilated capillaries, thickened collagen bundles, and plump fibroblasts (Fig. 5–107).

Deep palmoplantar warts occur not only on

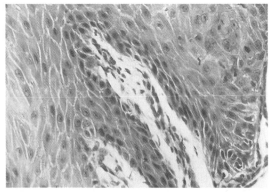

Figure 5–99. Subungual keratoacanthoma (high-power magnification). There is a sparse inflammatory cell infiltrate at the base of the neoplastic epithelium.

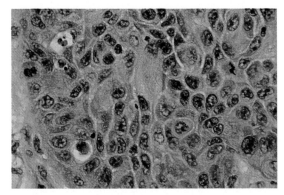

Figure 5–101. Classic keratoacanthoma (high-power magnification of Figure 5–100). A greater degree of nuclear atypia is seen than in subungual keratoacanthoma.

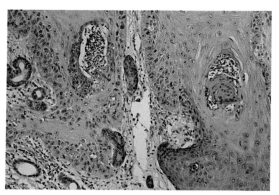

Figure 5–102. Classic keratoacanthoma (high-power magnification). Dense mixed inflammatory cell infiltrate with intraepithelial abscess within the neoplasm is evident.

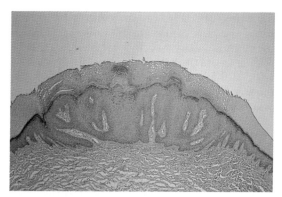

Figure 5–105. Verruca vulgaris, old lesion. The surface is less papillated. Note epithelial collarettes at the periphery.

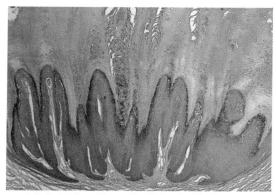

Figure 5–103. Verruca vulgaris, early lesion. There is thick, compact hyperkeratosis, acanthosis, and papillomatosis with collarettes of epithelium at the periphery of the lesion.

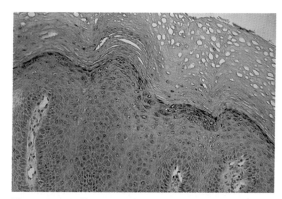

Figure 5–106. Verruca vulgaris, old lesion (high-power magnification of Figure 5–105). Focal parakeratosis, perinuclear halos, and coarse keratohyaline granules in the hyperplastic granular layer are evident.

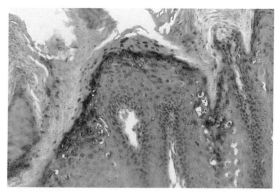

Figure 5–104. Verruca vulgaris, early lesion (high-power magnification of Figure 5–103). Focal parakeratosis at the tips of the epidermal digitation, hypergranulosis, perinuclear halos in the granular layer, and dilated blood vessels in the dermal papillae are evident.

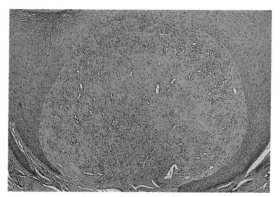

Figure 5–107. Verruca vulgaris, resolving lesion. The epidermis shows endophytic, club-shaped hyperplasia and epidermal collarettes; the papillary dermis is filled with dilated blood vessels, coarse collagen fibers, and fibroblasts.

the palms and soles but also on the lateral aspects and tips of the fingers and toes. Unlike the common wart, palmoplantar warts usually appear as deeply set keratotic papules covered with a thick callus. When the callus is removed, the wart appears as soft, granular, white, or yellow tissue.

Histologically, deep palmoplantar warts are characterized by endophytic growth of epidermis with hyperkeratosis, hypergranulosis, papillomatosis, and elongated and inward bending of the peripheral rete ridges (Figs. 5–108 and 5–109). There are numerous homogeneous eosinophilic bodies within the cytoplasm of keratinocytes in the upper malpighian layer. In addition to these bodies, some of the cells in the upper malpighian layer with vacuolar nuclei show a small intranuclear eosinophilic inclusion body. The keratinocytes in the granular layer show coarse keratohyalin granules and perinuclear vacuolization. The nuclei in the cornified layer persist, appearing as deeply basophilic round bodies surrounded by a clear zone (Fig. 5–110).

Subungual Epidermoid Cyst

Two types of subungual epidermoid cysts have been reported in the literature. The common variety are bone-located epidermoid cysts associated with osteolysis.[38–40] The usual symptoms are redness, pain, tenderness, and swelling of the terminal phalanx, resulting in clubbing or pincer nails. It is better referred to as an epidermoid implantation cyst. The other type of subungual epidermoid cyst is simply a cystic lesion with no bone involvement (Fig. 5–111). The clinical features are subungual hyperkeratosis associated with shortened and dystrophic nail plate.[41] The pathologic features of epidermoid implantation cyst include a round epidermal inclusion cyst in the bone filled with laminated cornified material and lined by stratified squamous epithelium with a granular layer,[38–40] whereas the histologic findings of subungual epidermoid cysts include a small keratinous cyst. The wall of the cysts is formed by nail bed epithelium[42,43] or nail matrix,[41] giving rise to a compact cornified material generally without a granular layer.[41] These histologic features resemble trichilemmal features of the hair follicle; therefore, they should also be defined as onycholemmal cysts. The overlying nail bed usually shows hyperkeratosis and acanthosis.

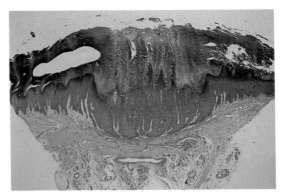

Figure 5–108. Deep palmoplanter wart. The lesion is characterized by endophytic growth of epidermis with hyperkeratosis, papillated epidermal hyperplasia, and collarettes of the rete ridges at the periphery.

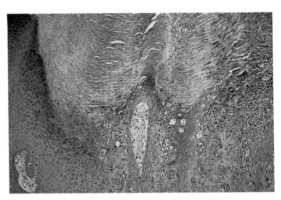

Figure 5–109. Deep palmoplantar wart (high-power magnification of Figure 5–108). Hypergranulosis with coarse keratohyaline granules and perinuclear halos in the upper malpighian layer are evident.

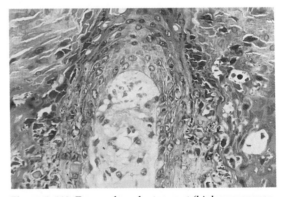

Figure 5–110. Deep palmoplantar wart (high-power magnification of Figure 5–109). Numerous homogeneous purplish inclusions within the cytoplasm and the nuclei in the upper malpighian layer are evident.

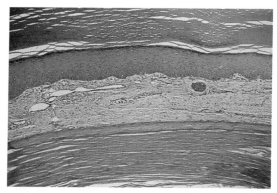

Figure 5–111. Subungual epidermal cyst. The wall of the cyst is a squamous epithelium resembling epidermis and is filled with compact, cornified layer.

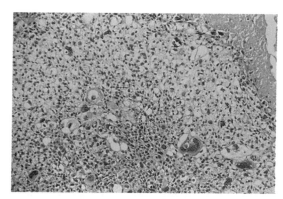

Figure 5–113. Malignant proliferating onycholemmal cyst (high-power magnification of Figure 5–112). Atypical squamous epithelium consisting of atypical nuclei and clear abundant cytoplasm is seen. Note the absence of the intervening granular layer.

Malignant Proliferating Onycholemmal Cyst

The malignant proliferating onycholemmal cyst is a slow-growing tumor of the nail unit that is regarded as the malignant analogue of the onycholemmal cysts arising from the nail bed epithelium[42,43] or nail matrix.[41] The growth of the tumor is infiltrative, and it may destroy the phalangeal bone. Histologically, the tumor is composed of cornified cysts and solid nests and strands of atypical keratinocytes. The cystic structure is filled with eosinophilic, amorphous cornified material and lined by atypical squamous epithelium devoid of a granular layer[44] (Figs. 5–112 and 5–113). Periodic acid–Schiff (PAS) stains reveal small amounts of glycogen in the epithelial nests associated with clear cell change. The histology is homologous to that of a follicular cyst, being comparable to the malignant proliferating trichilemmal cyst.

Eccrine Porocarcinoma

Eccrine porocarcinoma is a rare malignant neoplasm. Its most common localization is on the extremities, especially the lower limbs. Few cases of periungual porocarcinoma have been described, suggesting an origin at the proximal or lateral nail folds.[45,46] Histologic studies show irregular nests of epithelial cells that vary from a monomorphous poroid cell type that predominates in eccrine poroma to a highly pleomorphic large cell component (Figs. 5–114 to 5–117). In the solid tumor, there are small ductal cavities surrounded by cuticular cells. Some areas show en masse necrosis of neoplastic cells. Many cells are in mitosis. Some accumulation of acid mucopolysaccharides is observed between tumor cells and in small cystic spaces. The neoplasm shows a strongly infiltrative growth that even penetrates into the bone of the distal phalanx.

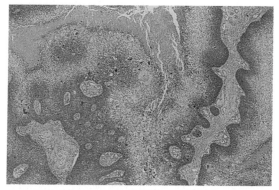

Figure 5–112. Malignant proliferating onycholemmal cyst. The tumor is composed of irregularly shaped lobules of squamous epithelium undergoing abrupt change into amorphous, cornified material.

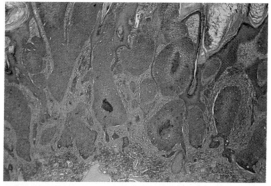

Figure 5–114. Eccrine porocarcinoma. The tumor consists of irregular bands and nests of neoplastic cells protruding into the deep reticular dermis.

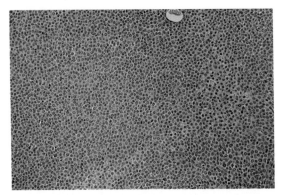

Figure 5–115. Eccrine porocarcinoma (high-power magnification of Figure 5–114). In some foci, the tumor has an appearance similar to that of eccrine poroma consisting of uniformly small, cuboidal cells. Note the ductal lumina at the top of this photomicrograph.

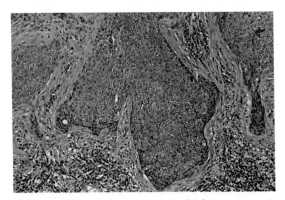

Figure 5–116. Eccrine porocarcinoma (high-power magnification of Figure 5–114). In some foci, the neoplastic aggregates consist of large, atypical cuboidal cells. A dense inflammatory infiltrate is present at the base of the lesion.

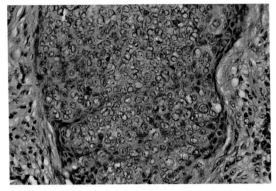

Figure 5–117. Eccrine porocarcinoma (high-power magnification of Figure 5–116). The malignant cells have large, hyperchromatic, irregularly shaped nuclei and may be multinucleated.

Onychomatrixoma

Onychomatrixoma, a hamartomatous lesion of the nail matrix described by Baran and Kint, is characterized clinically by a yellow discoloration along the entire length of the nail plate with splinter hemorrhage in its proximal portion, a tendency toward transverse overcurvature of the affected nails, and exposure of a matrix tumor after the nail has been avulsed and the proximal nail fold turned back.[47] Histologically, the tumor consists of epithelial cell strands emanating from the nail matrix and penetrating vertically into the dermis. In the central parts of the strands, the epithelial cells evolve to the parakeratotic cell layer, oriented along the long axis of the strands. Lacunae are observed in the center of some of these epithelial strands after elimination of the parakeratotic cells. The peritumoral stroma is sharply delineated from the underlying dermis and is composed of loose connective tissue with numerous fibroblasts and thin collagen bundles. The elastic fibers are sparse and thin. No mucin or inflammatory cell infiltrates are found.[47]

Mucinous Syringometaplasia

Mucinous syringometaplasia is a distinct pathologic entity that demonstrates mucin-laden cells in the eccrine duct epithelium. Most cases of mucinous syringometaplasia are solitary lesions on the plantar surface,[48–50] but it may present with verrucous lesions beneath the nail.[51] Histologic examination shows focal invagination of the epidermis lined by squamous epithelium, with some eccrine ducts leading into the invagination. The eccrine ductal epithelium contains mucin-laden goblet cells. There is also mucinous syringometaplasia of the underlying eccrine coils.

Pigmented Lesions

The pigmented lesions of the nail unit are similar to those elsewhere on the skin, except for the lesions within the nail matrix that cause longitudinal pigmented streaks or melanonychia striata in the longitudinum. The histologic spectrum ranges from epithelial hyperpigmentation to benign or malignant neoplasms, namely epithelial hyperpigmentations, simple lentigines, melanocytic nevi, or malignant melanomas.

Epithelial hyperpigmentation may occur secondary to inflammation, trauma, irradiation, drugs, and endocrine diseases. The histologic change of epithelial hyperpigmentation is characterized by increased melanin in the basal cell layer with or without the presence of melanophages in the papillary dermis (Fig. 5–118A and B). Microscopically, simple lentigine has a slightly increased number of melanocytes, some of them dendritic, and in-

creased melanin in the basal cell layer with or without corresponding elongated rete ridges (Fig. 5–119A and B). Junctional nevi consist of melanocytes in both nests and solitary units at the dermal–epidermal junction (Fig. 5–120A and B), whereas malignant melanoma of the nail matrix has the same histologic picture as malignant melanoma of the skin, namely

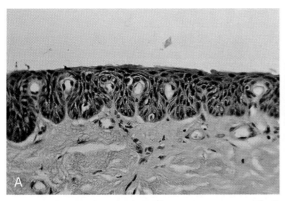
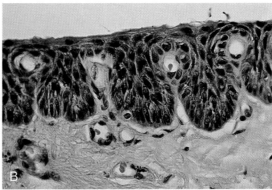

Figure 5–118. *A* and *B,* Epithelial hyperpigmentation. The lesion shows an increase in epidermal melanin in the nail matrix, most prominent in the basal layer. Note a solitary melanocyte at the basal layer.

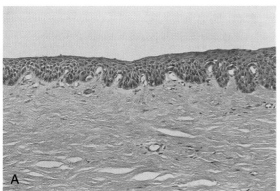
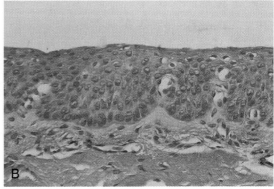

Figure 5–119. *A* and *B,* Simple lentigines. There is a marked increase in the number of typical melanocytes arranged as a solitary unit at the basal layer.

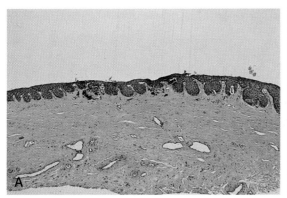
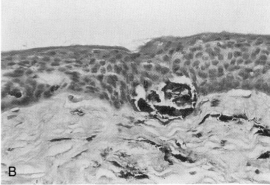

Figure 5–120. *A* and *B,* Junctional nevus. In contrast to simple lentigines, this lesion consists of melanocytes arranged both as solitary units and nests in the basal layer of nail matrix.

an asymmetric, poorly circumscribed lesion characterized by a proliferation of atypical melanocytes arranged both as solitary units and nests at all levels of the nail matrix (Fig. 5–121A and B). In addition to a melanocytic proliferation, epidermal hyperplasia, including subungual hyperkeratosis, hypergranulosis, and acanthosis of the nail bed and matrix, may be observed (Fig. 5–122A and B). Once in the dermis, however, atypical melanocytes tend to continue to descend progressively. The amount of inflammatory infiltrate in malignant melanoma varies. In malignant melanoma in situ and early invasive lesion, the papillary dermis shows bandlike infiltrate of lymphocytes, often intermingled with melanophages, at the base of the tumor (Fig. 5–123). In more advanced lesions, the inflammatory infiltrate is quite variable, but it is often only slight to moderate rather than pro-

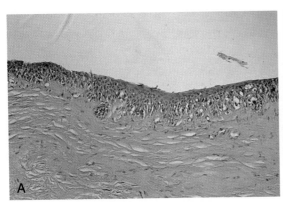
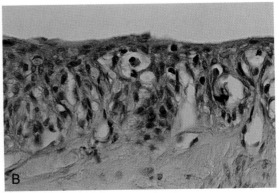

Figure 5–121. *A* and *B,* Malignant melanoma in situ. Many solitary melanocytes and nests of melanocytes are present at all layers of the nail matrix.

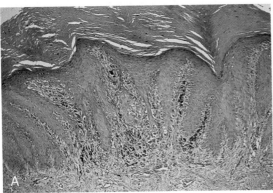
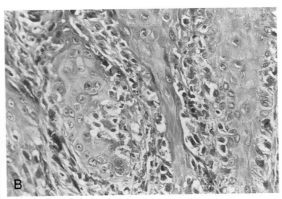

Figure 5–122. *A* and *B,* Malignant melanoma in situ. In addition to a proliferation of atypical melanocytes, the nail bed shows hyperkeratosis, hypergranulosis, and acanthosis.

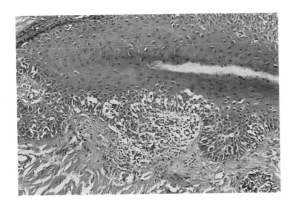

Figure 5–123. Malignant melanoma in situ. Atypical melanocytes are seen in the nail matrix epithelium. The upper dermis contains dense inflammatory infiltrate intermingled with melanophages.

nounced. In addition, the epidermal component is less prominent or even absent in contrast to that of early lesions or malignant melanoma in situ (Figs. 5–124 and 5–125).

Subungual Hemorrhage

Subungual hemorrhage is often seen in nail biopsy specimens because clinically it looks like a melanocytic lesion. Histologic findings shows collections of homogeneous eosinophilic and yellow-brown masses under the nail plate or within it (Figs. 5–126 and 5–127). These yellow-brown masses, consisting of lysed red blood cell hemoglobin, remain negative with prussian blue stain used for the demonstration of hemosiderin (Fig. 5–128) but positive (brown) with benzidine stain for hemoglobin.[52]

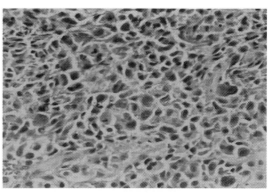

Figure 5–125. Malignant melanoma (high-power magnification of Figure 5–124). The tumor cells possess atypical nuclei and eosinophilic cytoplasm.

Soft Tissue Tumor

Focal Mucinosis (Myxoid Cyst)

Histologically, focal mucinosis does not show an epithelial lining[53,54] and therefore should not be termed a cyst. Microscopic change reveals a relatively well-circumscribed area of mucin in the upper dermis (Fig. 5–129). Spindle-shaped fibroblasts are usually seen interspersed among mucinous material. As large amounts of ground substance accumulate, a cavity forms, with marginal compression of the surrounding collagen (Fig. 5–130). In addition, the overlying surface epithelium shows compact hyperkeratosis with a collarette of hyperplastic epidermis. The mucinous material stains pale basophilic with hematoxylin and eosin and stains positive with alcian blue

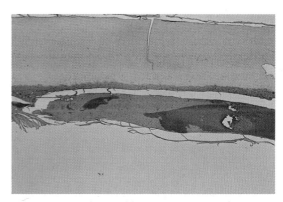

Figure 5–126. Subungual hematoma. Large collections of homogeneous eosinophilic and yellow-brown material beneath the nail plate are evident.

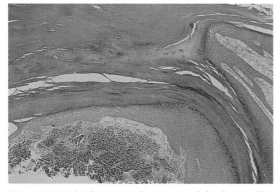

Figure 5–124. Malignant melanoma, nodular lesion. The upper dermis of nail unit contains dense aggregates of atypical melanocytes.

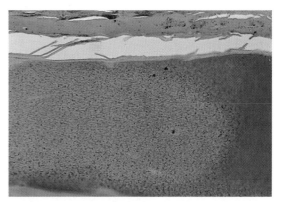

Figure 5–127. Subungual hematoma (high-power magnification of Figure 5–126). Homogeneous yellow-brown mass representing lysed red blood cells is evident.

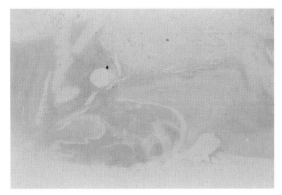

Figure 5–128. Subungual hematoma. The Perl stain for iron is negative.

or colloid iron for acid mucopolysaccharides.[53]

Glomus Tumor

The solitary type of glomus tumor is an extremely tender nodule usually located in the nail bed. Microscopic examination reveals a well-circumscribed vascular neoplasm characterized by a slightly increased number of dilated vascular spaces lined by a single layer of flattened, often elongated endothelial cells (Figs. 5–131 and 5–132). Peripheral to the endothelial cells is a row of cells with uniform round to oval nuclei and pale eosinophilic cytoplasm (glomus cells) (Fig. 5–133). The neoplasm is outlined by compressed collagen at the periphery. The stroma is edematous and rich in unmyelinated neural elements.[55]

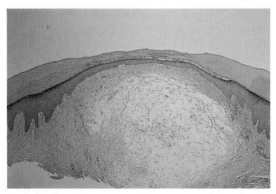

Figure 5–129. Myxoid cyst. The dermis contains a relatively well-defined collection of mucinous material.

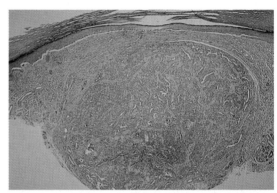

Figure 5–131. Glomus tumor. The tumor appears as well-circumscribed cellular aggregates compressing the surrounding collagen.

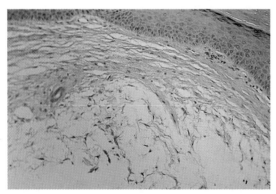

Figure 5–130. Myxoid cyst (high-power magnification of Figure 5–129). Scattered fibroblasts in the mucinous material are evident.

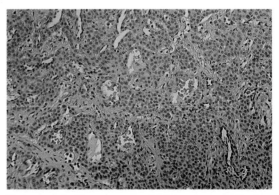

Figure 5–132. Glomus tumor (high-power magnification of Figure 5–131). Anastomosing aggregations of the cells around dilated, thick-walled blood vessels are evident.

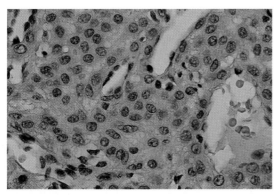

Figure 5–133. Glomus tumor (high-power magnification). The tumor cells are composed of round or oval nuclei and pale cytoplasm.

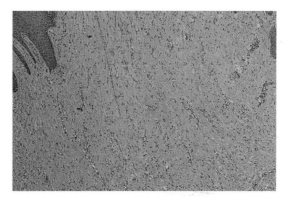

Figure 5–135. Acquired digital fibrokeratoma (high-power magnification of Figure 5–134). The central core is composed of interlacing fascicles of collagen bundles and plump fibroblasts.

Acquired Digital Fibrokeratoma

Histologically, acquired digital fibrokeratoma appears as a dense fibrous core with a surrounding epithelial envelope (Fig. 5–134). The central core is characterized by interlacing fascicles of thick collagen bundles predomi-

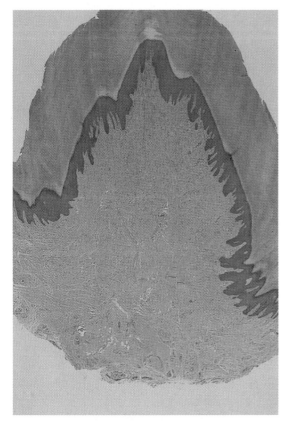

Figure 5–134. Acquired digital fibrokeratoma. The tumor is characterized by exophytic growth of fibrous tissues, which covered by hyperkeratotic and hyperplastic epidermis.

nantly oriented along the longitudinal axis and associated with increased number of plump fibroblasts and capillaries (Figs. 5–135 and 5–136). The tumor is devoid of epithelial adnexal structures, and elastic tissue is diminished. The paucity or absence of neural elements has also been described. The overlying epidermis is acanthotic and hyperkeratotic.[56,57]

Infantile Digital Fibromatosis (Recurrent Infantile Digital Fibroma)

Infantile digital fibromatosis is a smooth, dome-shaped, dermal nodule that is usually located on the dorsal surface of the fingers and toes. The lesion develops at birth or during infancy. On reaching the nail unit, the lesion may elevate the nail plate, leading to dystrophy. Histologically, the lesion is composed of

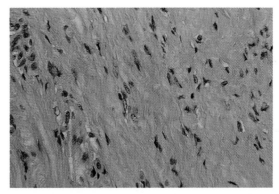

Figure 5–136. Acquired digital fibrokeratoma (high-power magnification). Fibroblasts markedly increasing in number are large and stellate.

interlacing fascicles of spindle-shaped fibro-blasts and collagen bundles (Fig. 5–137). A characteristic diagnostic feature is the presence of paranuclear eosinophilic inclusion bodies within some fibroblasts (Fig. 5–138). These inclusion bodies measure from 3 to 10 μm in diameter.[58] The inclusion bodies stain deep red with phosphotungstic acid–hematoxylin and purple with Masson trichrome.[59] Electron microscopic study shows that the tumor cells are typical myofibroblasts containing inclusion bodies and bundles of microfilaments. Immunohistochemistry shows the paranuclear inclusion consisting of actin fibers.[60]

Juvenile Hyaline Fibromatosis

Juvenile hyaline fibromatosis is characterized by skin nodules, muscle weakness, flexion contractures of large joints, and gingival hypertrophy. The nodules are found in the head and neck region, on the trunk, and at the tip of the digits, where acro-osteolysis and clubbing may be seen.[61] The histology of the skin nodules includes fibroblasts in homogeneous eosinophilic ground substance that are strongly PAS positive and diastase resistant[62] (Fig. 5–139). Clefts are seen between the fibroblast and the ground substance that give rise to the appearance of chondroid cells[63] (Fig. 5–140).

Periungual Fibroma (Koenen's Tumor)

Periungual fibroma is a rare benign fibrous tumor occurring around a nail plate and may be acquired or associated with tuberous sclero-

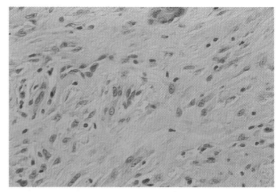

Figure 5–138. Infantile digital fibromatosis (high-power magnification of Figure 5–137). The presence of eosinophilic intracytoplasmic inclusion bodies within some fibroblasts is evident.

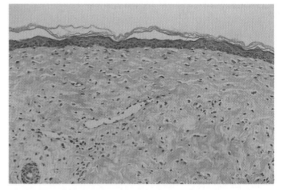

Figure 5–139. Juvenile hyaline fibromatosis. The nodule is composed of scattered fibroblasts among homogeneous eosinophilic ground substance.

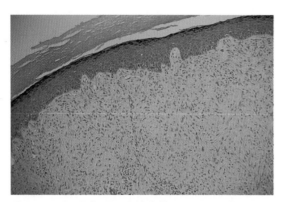

Figure 5–137. Infantile digital fibromatosis. The upper dermis shows numerous fibroblasts and collagen bundles arranged in interlacing fascicles.

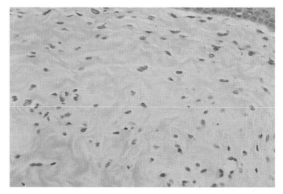

Figure 5–140. Juvenile hyaline fibromatosis (high-power magnification of Figure 5–139). Note clefts around the fibroblasts with the appearance of chondroid cells.

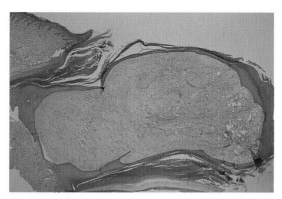

Figure 5–141. Periungual fibroma. The lesion appears as an exophytic mass protruding from the proximal portion of the ventral proximal nail fold.

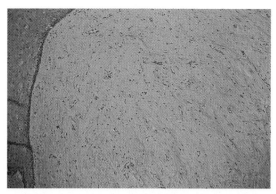

Figure 5–143. Periungual fibroma (high-power magnification of Figure 5–141). The proximal portion is composed of thinner collagen bundles and spindle-shaped fibroblasts.

sis. The tumor usually develops underneath the proximal or lateral nail fold and rests on the nail plate. The lesion may develop at the nail bed (subungual) and lift the nail plate distally. Histologically, the fibroma is similar to acquired digital fibrokeratoma, but areas of fibromatosis may have the large size and stellate shape of fibroblasts. The distal part of the tumor contains coarse collagen fibers, arranged haphazardly, and prominent capillaries (Figs. 5–141 and 5–142), whereas the proximal part is composed of thinner collagen fibers and seemingly arranged mostly parallel to the skin surface, fading into the contiguous dermis of the nail fold (Fig. 5–143). The lesion is usually elongated and covered with a slightly acanthotic epidermis, hyperkeratosis, and an epidermal collarette (see Fig. 5–141). No elastic fibers or neural structures are observed in the tumor.[64]

Invaginated fibrokeratoma, a histologic variant of periungual fibroma, with matrix differentiation,[65] usually occurs as a keratotic lesion simulating a rudimentary nail plate and fuses with the normal nail. The tumor is cone shaped, thickened proximally, and tapered distally. Histologically, it is characterized by a downward growth of a well-demarcated fibrous nodule lined between the ventral surface of the proximal nail fold and nail matrix. The fibrous mass consists of bundles of collagen densely packed with fibroblasts predominantly parallel to the longitudinal axis. The elastic tissue is absent. The epithelial envelope shows features of nail matrix with no granular layer that gives rise to a thick, homogeneous, orthokeratotic cornified layer (Figs. 5–144 and 5–145). Additionally, the cornified material is not stained by hematoxylin and eosin, the normal feature of the nail plate.

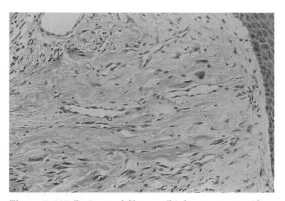

Figure 5–142. Periungual fibroma (high-power magnification of Figure 5–141). The distal portion of the tumor is composed of large stellate fibroblasts, coarse collagen bundles, and dilated, thick-walled blood vessels arranged haphazardly.

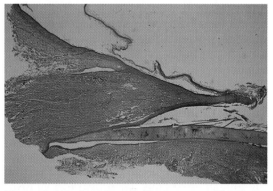

Figure 5–144. Invaginated fibrokeratoma. The lesion shows endophytic growth of the fibrous tissue at the junction of the ventral proximal nail fold and proximal nail matrix.

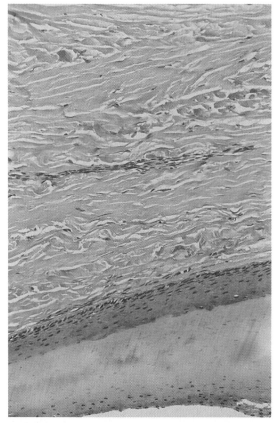

Figure 5–145. Invaginated fibrokeratoma (high-power magnification of Figure 5–144). The lower portion of the tumor is covered by nail matrix epithelium.

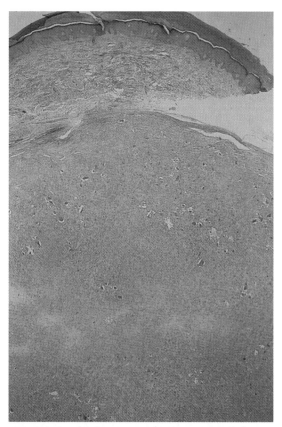

Figure 5–146. Giant cell tumor of tendon sheath. The lesion is characterized by a circumscribed cellular mass surrounded by dense collagen.

Giant Cell Tumor of Tendon Sheath

Giant cell tumor of the tendon sheath is one of the common soft tissue tumors of the hand. Sometimes it is seen around the nails. Its origin does not represent a component of the skin or nail unit, but it arises from the tendon sheath, joint ligament, or joint synovium, forming a firm nodule fixed deeply to the fibrous tissue of origin. Histologically, giant cell tumors of the tendon sheath are characterized by a circumscribed, lobulated mass surrounded by dense collagen. The appearance of the tumor varies depending on the proportion of mononuclear cells, giant cells, and collagen. The cellular area is composed of a sheet of round or polygonal cells that blend with hypocellular collagenized zones. Most cells in the cellular areas have the appearance of histiocytes and synovial cells (Figs. 5–146 and 5–147). Xanthoma cells are also frequent and often contain fine hemosiderin granules. Hypocellular areas show fibroblasts within a

fibrous or homogenized stroma[66] (Fig. 5–148). The characteristic multinucleated giant cells are found scattered randomly throughout both cellular and fibrous areas. Their cytoplasm is deeply eosinophilic and irregularly

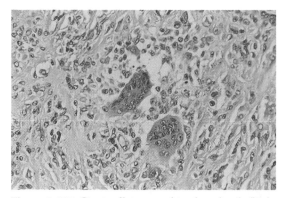

Figure 5–147. Giant cell tumor of tendon sheath (high-power magnification of Figure 5–146). In the cellular area, the cells are composed of histiocytes and multinucleated giant cells.

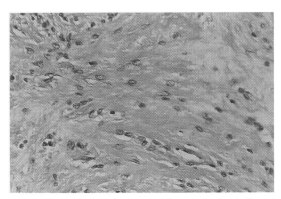

Figure 5–148. Giant cell tumor of tendon sheath (high-power magnification of Figure 5–146). In the hypocellular area, most of the cells are fibroblasts that are embedded in a hyalinized stroma.

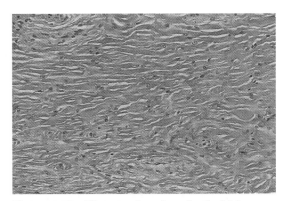

Figure 5–150. Fibroma of tendon sheath (high-power magnification). Scattered fibroblasts in a hyalinized collagenous stroma are evident.

demarcated and contains a variable number of haphazardly distributed nuclei (see Fig. 5–149). They resemble normal osteoclasts.[67]

Fibroma of Tendon Sheath

Fibroma of the tendon sheath is a slow-growing fibrous tumor firmly attached to the tendon sheath. It is found most frequently in the hands and feet; the thumb is the most common single site. Microscopically, it is characterized by a well-circumscribed lobular mass composed of scattered fibroblasts in a hyalinized collagenous stroma (Figs. 5–149 and 5–150). A gradual transition between the hyalinized hypocellular collagenous areas and more cellular areas is occasional found. In contrast to giant cell tumor of the tendon sheath, fibroma of the tendon sheath has no xanthoma cells or multinucleated giant cells. Foci of myxoid changes, rarely osseous or chondroid

metaplasia, may occur in a small portion of the lesions.

Osteochondroma

Osteochondroma is a benign, painful neoplasm that occurs on the terminal digit and nail unit. The tumor is loosely attached to bone and rarely may be soft tissue tumor with bony attachment.[68,69] Histologically, in the dermis there are islands of hyaline cartilage (Fig. 5–151). The mature cartilaginous cell is characterized by a dark, small, and uniform nucleus and is surrounded by a halo as a result of shrinkage of the cytoplasm[70] (Fig. 5–152). Along the margin of the hyaline cartilage, the cells flatten, simulating spindle-shaped fibroblasts so that there is no well-defined transition between the cartilage cells and surrounding connective tissue. Bone formation is seen in the center of the lesion, charac-

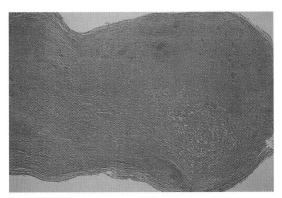

Figure 5–149. Fibroma of tendon sheath. The lesion appears as a well-circumscribed, lobular mass.

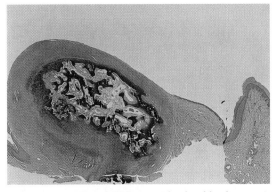

Figure 5–151. Osteochondroma. Islands of hyaline cartilage are found in the dermis.

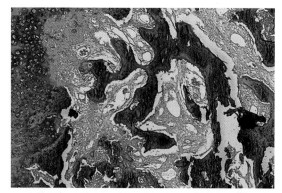

Figure 5–152. Osteochondroma (high-power magnification of Figure 5–151). The mature cartilagenous cells show dark, small nuclei and clefts around the cytoplasm.

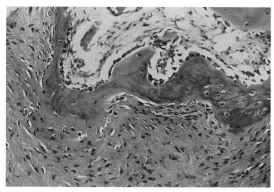

Figure 5–155. Subungual exostosis (high-power magnification of Figure 5–154). The bone is lined by osteoblasts and contains blood vessels and connective tissue.

terized by spicules of bone containing osteocytes (Fig. 5–153).

Subungual Exostosis

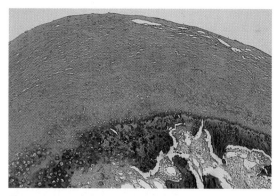

Figure 5–153. Osteochondroma (high-power magnification of Figure 5–151). Bone formation is seen in the center of the lesion.

Subungual exostosis is not a true neoplasm but rather an outgrowth of normal bone that is usually caused by antecedent trauma. The lesions mainly arise in the distal aspect of the terminal phalanx and radiologically are continuous with the tuft of the terminal phalanx. The histologic picture is similar to that of osteochondroma (i.e., a proliferation of bony spicules extending into the dermis[71]) (Fig. 5–154). The ossification or calcification in the lesion is relatively minimal. Its distal portion, however, is covered by fibrocartilage instead of hyaline cartilage (Fig. 5–155).

References

1. Hashimoto K: Ultrastructure of the human toenail: Proximal nail matrix. J Invest Dermatol 56:235, 1971.
2. Higashi N, Saito T: Horizontal distribution of the dopa-positive melanocytes in the nail matrix. J Invest Dermatol 53:163, 1969.
3. Higashi N: Melanocytes of nail matrix and nail pigmentation. Arch Dermatol 97:570, 1968.
4. Zaias N: The Nail in Health and Disease. S.P. Medical, New York, 1980.
5. Forslind B, Thyresson N: On the structure of the normal nail: A scanning electron microscope study. Arch Dermatol 251:199, 1975.
6. Hamilton JB, Terada H, Mestler GE: Studies of growth throughout the lifespan in Japanese: Growth and size of nails and their relationship to age, sex, hereditary, and other factors. J Gerontol 10:401, 1955.
7. Crawford GM: Psoriasis of the nails. Arch Dermatol Syphilology 38:583, 1938.
8. Alkiewicz J: Psoriasis of the nail. Br J Dermatol 60:195, 1948.

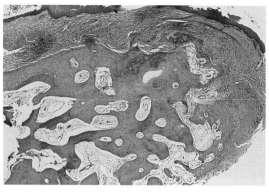

Figure 5–154. Subungual exostosis. The tumor appears as an outgrowth of bone spicules in the upper dermis.

9. Calvert HT, Smith MA, Well RS: Br J Dermatol 76:415, 1963.
10. Samman PD: The nails in lichen planus. Br J Dermatol 73:288, 1961.
11. Norton LA: Nail disorders: A review. J Am Acad Dermatol 2:451, 1980.
12. Sonnex TS, Douber RPR, Zachasy CB, et al: The nail in adult type I pityriasis rubra pilaris: A comparison with Sézary syndrome and psoriasis. J Am Acad Dermatol 15:956, 1986.
13. Suarez SM, Silvers DN, Scher RK, et al: Histologic evaluation of nail clippings for diagnosing onychomycosis. Arch Dermatol 127:1517, 1991.
14. Jerasutus S, Suvanprakorn P, Kitchawengkul O: Twenty nail dystrophy: A clinical manifestation of spongiotic inflammation of the nail matrix. Arch Dermatol 126:1068, 1990.
15. Wilkinson JD, Dowber RPR, Fleming K, et al: Twenty nail dystrophy. Arch Dermatol 115:369, 1979.
16. Tosti A, Fanti PA, Morelli R, et al. Trachyonychia associated with alopecia areata: A clinical and pathologic study. J Am Acad Dermatol 25:266, 1991.
17. Baran R, Dawber RPR: Diseases of the Nail and Their Management. Oxford, England, Blackwell Scientific, 1994.
18. Holzberg M, Wade TR, Buchanan ID, et al: Nail pathology in histiocytosis X. J Am Acad Dermatol 13:522, 1985.
19. Diestel Meier MR, Soden CE, Rodman OG: Histiocytosis X: A case of nail involvement. Cutis 30:483, 1982.
20. Timpatanapong P, Hathirat P, Isarangkura P: Nail involvement in histiocytosis X. Arch Dermatol 120:1052, 1984.
21. Alsina MM, Zamora E, Ferrando J, et al: Nail changes in histiocytosis X. Arch Dermatol 127:1741, 1991.
22. Zaias N, Ackerman AB: The nail in Darier-White disease. Arch Dermatol 107:193, 1973.
23. Su DWP, Chun S II, Hammond DE, et al: Pachyonychia congenita: A clinical study of 12 cases and review of the literature. Pediatr Dermatol 7:33, 1990.
24. Stone OJ, Mullin JF: Nail changes in keratosis punctata. Arch Dermatol 92:557, 1965.
25. Tosti A, Morelli R, Fanti PA, et al: Nail changes of punctate keratoderma: A clinical and pathological study of two patients. Acta Derm Venereol (Stockh) 73:66, 1993.
26. Scher PK: Subungual scabies. Am J Dermatopathol 5:187, 1983.
27. Pavlidaky GP, Hashimoto K, Blum D. Yellow nail syndrome. J Am Acad Dermatol 11:509, 1984.
28. Alpert LI, Zak FG, Werthamer S: Subungual basal cell epithelioma. Arch Dermatol 106:599, 1972.
29. Hoffman S: Basal cell carcinoma of the nail bed. Arch Dermatol 108:828, 1973.
30. Nelson LM, Hamilton CF: Primary carcinoma of the nail bed. Arch Dermatol 101:63, 1970.
31. Kouskoukis CE, Scher RK, Kopf AW: Squamous cell carcinoma of the nail bed. J Dermatol Surg Oncol 8:853, 1982.
32. Preaux J: Diagnostic problems related to lesions under and around finger nails. J Dermatol Surg 2:305, 1976.
33. Guitart J, Bergfeld WF, Tuthill RJ, et al: Squamous cell carcinoma of the nail bed: A clinicopathologic study of 12 cases. Br J Dermatol 123:215, 1990.
34. Tosti A, Morelli R, Fanti PA, et al: Carcinoma cuniculatum of the nail apparatus: Report of three cases. Dermatology 186:217, 1993.
35. Stoll DM, Ackerman AB: Subungual keratoacanthoma. Am J Dermatopathol 2:265, 1980.
36. Oliwiecki S, Peachey RDG, Bradfield JWB, et al: Subungual keratoacanthoma: A report of four cases and review of the literature. Clin Exp Dermatol 19:230, 1994.
37. Keeney GL, Banks PM, Linscheid RL: Subungual keratoacanthoma: Report of a case and review of the literature. Arch Dermatol 124:1074, 1988.
38. Fisher ER, Giruhn J, Skerrett P: Epidermal cyst in bone. Cancer 11:643, 1958.
39. Byers P, Mantle J, Salm R: Epidermal cyst of phalanges. J Bone Joint Surg 488:577, 1966.
40. Baran R, Broutart JC: Epidermal cyst of the thumb presenting as pincer nail. J Am Acad Dermatol 9:143, 1988.
41. Fanti PA, Tosti A: Subungual epidermoid inclusions: Report of 8 cases. Dermatologica 178:209, 1989.
42. Lewin K: The normal fingernail. Br J Dermatol 77:421, 1965.
43. Lewin K: Subungual epidermoid inclusion. Br J Dermatol 81:671, 1969.
44. Alessi E, Zorzi F, Gianotti R, et al: Malignant proliferating onycholemmal cyst. J Cutan Pathol 183, 1994.
45. Requena L, Sanchez M, Aguilar A, et al: Periungual porocarcinoma. Dermatologica 180:177, 1990.
46. Van Gorp J, Van der Putte SCJ: Periungual eccrine porocarcinoma. Dermatology 187:67, 1993.
47. Baran R, Kint A: Onychomatrixoma: Filamentous tufted tumor in the matrix of a funnel-shaped nail: A new entity (report of three cases). Br J Dermatol 126:510, 1992.
48. Kwitten J: Muciparous epidermal tumor. Arch Dermatol 109:554, 1974.
49. King DT, Barr RJ: Syringometaplasia: Mucinous and squamous variants. J Cutan Pathol 6:284, 1979.
50. Mehregan AH: Mucinous syringometaplasia. Arch Dermatol 116:988, 1980.
51. Scally K, Assad D: Mucinous syringometaplasia. J Am Acad Dermatol 11:503, 1984.
52. Hafner J, Hacnseler E, Ossent P, et al: Benzidine stain for the histochemical detection of hemoglobin in splinter hemorrhage (subungual hematoma) and black heel. Am J Dermatopathol 17:362, 1995.
53. Johnson WC, Graham JH, Heluig EB: Cutaneous myxoid cyst. JAMA 191:15, 1965.
54. Goldman JA, Goldman L, Jaffe MS, et al: Digital mucinous pseudocysts. Arthritis Rheum 20:997, 1977.
55. Shuguart RR, Soule BH, Johnson EW Jr: Glomus tumor. Surg Gynecol Obstet 117:334, 1963.
56. Bart RS, Andrade R, Kopf AW, et al: Acquired digital fibrokeratomas. Arch Dermatol 97:120, 1968.
57. Cahn RL: Acquired periungual fibrokeratoma: A rare benign tumor previously described as the garlic-clove fibroma. Arch Dermatol 113:1564, 1977.
58. Shapiro L: Infantile digital fibromatosis and aponeurotic fibroma. Arch Dermatol 99:37, 1969.
59. Santa Cruz DJ, Reiner EB: Recurrent digital fibroma of childhood. J Cutan Pathol 5:334, 1978.
60. Zina AM, Rampini E, Fulcheri E, et al: Recurrent digital fibromatosis of childhood: An ultrastructural and immunohistochemical study of 2 cases. Am J Dermatopathol 8:22, 1986.
61. Camarosa JG, Moreno A: Juvenile hyaline fibromatosis. J Am Acad Dermatol 16:881, 1987.
62. Kitano Y, Horiki M, Aoki T, et al: Two cases of juvenile hyaline fibromatosis. Arch Dermatol 106:877, 1972.
63. Remberger K, Krieg T, Kenze D, et al: Fibromatosis hyalinica multiplex (juvenile hyaline fibromatosis). Cancer 56:614, 1985.
64. Kint A, Baran R: Histopathologic study of Koenen tumors. J Am Acad Dermatol 12:816, 1955.

65. Perrin C, Baran R: Invaginated fibrokeratoma with matrix differentiation: A new histologic variant of acquired fibrokeratoma. Br J Dermatol 130:654, 1994.
66. King DT, Millman AJ, Gurevitch AW, et al: Giant cell tumor of the tendon sheath involving the skin. Arch Dermatol 114:944, 1978.
67. Cartens PHB: Giant cell tumors of tendon sheath. Arch Pathol 102:99, 1978.
68. Cahlin DC, Salvador AH: Cartilagenous tumors of the soft tissues of the hand and feet. Mayo Clin Proc 49:721, 1974.
69. Rosentfeld N, Kurzer A: Soft tissue "chondroma" of the hand. Hand 12:189, 1980.
70. Shelley WB, Ralston EL: Paronychia due to an enchondroma. Arch Dermatol 90:420, 1964.
71. Cohen HJ, Frank SB, Minkin W, et al: Subungual exostoses. Arch Dermatol 107:431, 1973.

SECTION 2

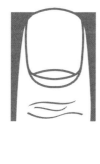 # The Abnormal Nail

CHAPTER 6

An Approach to Initial Examination of the Nail

C. Ralph Daniel, III

Adequate lighting without glare, natural sunlight being the preferred source, is a necessity when examining nails. All nail polish, lacquer, or other topical substances should be removed prior to examination. At times, the surface of the nail plate should be cleansed with a solvent such as alcohol or acetone, especially if a subtle change of the nail is being investigated. This may remove substances superficially adhering to the nail plate and will diminish glare. If this procedure or scraping the nail surface with a sharp object does not resolve an apparently superficial nail plate abnormality, the examiner should suspect a deeper or more inherent process.

Be sure to examine all of the nails. The pattern of nail involvement must be considered in each patient. Frequently, if only one or very few nails are affected, local factors such as fungus, trauma, tumors, circulation, and so forth are to blame for the abnormality. Keep in mind, however, that this is not always the case and that there are few hard and fast rules governing examination of the nails. In addition, note the portion of the nail unit manifesting the abnormality. Periungual location, nail bed, matrix, and plate all have certain disorders more common to each area. Yet certain conditions, for example, trauma, psoriasis, or lichen planus, can affect only one or all parts of the

nail unit concomitantly. Furthermore, as is discussed in future chapters, remember that the portion of the matrix affected often governs the site of clinical disease in different levels of the nail plate. The proximal portion of the matrix contributes mostly to the superficial nail plate and the distal portion mainly to the deeper nail plate.

When examining the nails, the patient's digits should be relaxed and not pressed against any surface. Failure to do this may alter the hemodynamics of the nail bed and change the appearance of the nails. If a subtle change in pigmentation is being examined, squeeze the tip of the digit to see if the appearance of the abnormality changes. In pigmented nail abnormalities, if a subtle vascular alteration is causative, it may be less visible with pressure on the nail unit.

Another clinical aid is a penlight. Shining a penlight up from distal digital pulp through the nail plate may be helpful. One should then observe the illuminated digit from all sides. This may help to localize an abnormality.

There are helpful rules to follow when examining nails for the effects of systemic disease or drugs and ingestants. See the systemic disease chapter. Physical examination of the nail is sometimes all that is required to make the proper diagnosis. Most of the time, however, other information is needed and simple physical examination alone is not adequate. A thorough history with particular attention to disease chronology, occupation, topical substance exposure, medical history, family history, drug history, and so forth will usually aid in obtaining the proper diagnosis. A screening questionnaire given to the patient prior to examination is often helpful and may aid in pinpointing your investigation (Fig. 6–1).

If the history and physical examination have not revealed the diagnosis, other measures are available. Some of these include x-ray films, potassium hydroxide preparation, fungal cultures, bacterial cultures, nail biopsy with appropriate stains and microscopy, fluorescence with a black light if porphyria or tetracyclines are suspected as factors, exfoliative cytology, nail composition studies (as when looking for arsenic content), and immunological testing (as for certain fungi).

After completing a proper history and physical examination, one should have a basic method of categorizing the problem. Again, there are no firm rules, and numerous classifications may overlap. Two general divisions separate conditions acquired after birth and familial or congenital problems. Here, too, there is some overlap because many dermatologic conditions, such as psoriasis, have associated hereditary factors. When assessing an acquired nail abnormality, mentally classify the problem according to the following categories:

1. Predominantly dermatologic conditions
2. Predominantly systemic disorders
3. Systemic drugs
4. Organisms (bacterial, fungal, viral, and so forth)
5. Local or topical agents in the vicinity of the nail
6. Tumors, either benign or malignant
7. Physical agents
8. Other

Once this is done, proceed with the investigation.

YOUR NAME: _____ AGE: _____ SEX: _____ DATE: _____

NAIL QUESTIONNAIRE

1. Were you born with this problem?
   When did you first ever have a problem like this?
2. Which nails were affected first? (Place a * by these)
   Which are affected now? (Place a √ by these)
3. How has this changed from beginning to now?
4. Describe your nails in general (hard, brittle, soft, etc.).
5. Have you ever traumatized any of the involved nails (stubbed your toe, hit the nail with a hammer, caught it in a door, etc.)?

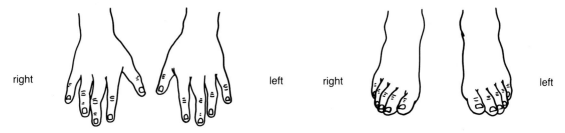

right   left   right   left

Figure 6-1.

6. What kind of work do you do? Do you do anything to affect your nails or the tips of your fingers or toes?

   Contact with chemicals or irritants, such as strong soaps, hair straightener, lye, etc.?

   Hands or feet in water a lot?

   Hands or feet moist because of sweating or other reasons?

7. List hobbies in which you might traumatize or otherwise affect your nails (tennis, jogging, basketball, racquetball, painting, playing the piano, etc.).

8. Did you in the past or have you recently
   a. Pick at your nails?
   b. Bite or suck on your nails?
   c. Tear your nails off?
   d. Have ingrown nails?
   e. Wear tight or pointed-toe shoes?
   f. Push the cuticle back (how often?)
   g. Remember "runarounds" or swelling around cuticles?
9. Personal nail care
   a. List any nail cosmetics or conditioners that you use:
      1. Base coat
      2. Top coat
      3. Enamel
      4. Nail strengtheners
      5. Nail hardeners
      6. Cuticle treatment
      7. Gloss
      8. Nail conditioners
      9. Other
      10. Please bring any of these products with you on your next office visit, along with list of ingredients, if possible.
   b. List any instruments that you use to care for your nails.
      What do you do with these instruments?
      How often do you do this?
   c. Do you go to a manicurist?   How often?   What is usually done to your nails?
   d. Have you ever had the following? (If so, how often and when was the last time?)
      1. Sculptured nails
      2. False or artificial nails or "gel" nails or nail tips
      3. Nail "wraps"
      4. Acrylic nails
      5. Other
10. Do you have any other skin or hair problems, or have you ever had any in the past?
   Lichen planus
   Psoriasis
   Ringworm
   "Jock itch"
   Athlete's foot
   Vaginal yeast infection or other yeast infection
   Other
11. List any medical problems that you have had in the past or have now (diabetes, heart trouble, thyroid problem, etc.).
12. List any medications that you have taken during the last year (sulfa, water pills, tetracycline, high-blood-pressure medicines, constipation medicine, chemotherapy, pain pills, vitamins, oral contraceptives, oral pills to help you tan, eye drops for glaucoma, pills for psoriasis therapy, retinoic acid, Neo-Synephrine, etc.).
13. What treatment (self and professional) have you had for your nail problem (past and present)?
   a. List pills and dates used.
   b. List topical treatments and dates used.
   c. List surgical treatment and dates performed.
14. Does anyone in your family have
   a. Nail problems
   b. Diabetes
   c. Skin problems (psoriasis, lichen planus, fungus, etc.)
   d. Thyroid problems
15. What do you think is the cause of your nail problem?

CHAPTER 7

Pediatric Disease

Robert A. Silverman

Nail diseases of infants and children compose a very small portion of a practice in pediatrics or dermatology. Except for periungual warts, an estimated 5 in 1000 visits to a pediatric dermatologist are for primary ungual disorders in children. The number of nail disorders in the pediatric population is as large as that of adults. Congenital and hereditary deformities, infections, tumors, ungual signs of systemic disease, and inflammatory and idiopathic problems all are a part of this wide spectrum.

Methods of diagnosis and therapy of pediatric nail diseases are limited by the cooperativeness of the patient and should be tempered by the potential morbidity of the primary problem as well as the invasiveness of whatever procedures are to be performed. This problem should be addressed with every parent or guardian during the initial patient evaluation. Truthful, age-appropriate explanations should be given to children before any procedure. For children ages 3 to 10 years, it frequently is helpful to demonstrate what is to be performed on yourself, a doll, or a puppet to allay any anxiety from unknown factors that he or she may fantasize (e.g., scraping, applying a tourniquet).

Local anesthesia of the nail unit in children may be preceded by application of 30 per cent

lidocaine cream for 15 to 30 minutes, or freon spray (Cryospray, Frigiderm). Tribeveled silicone-coated (e.g., Acuderm) 30-gauge needles reduce the pain of anesthetic administration. Serious consideration should be given to sedation and firm immobilization or general anesthesia of an uncooperative patient. Chloral hydrate (20 to 30 mg/kg/dose given 30 minutes before a procedure, less than 2 g total) and nitrous oxide (30 per cent O_2 to 70 per cent N_2O) analgesia administered in an outpatient surgical suite are excellent agents—again, provided that truthful, age-appropriate explanations of the procedures are given preoperatively to the patients and the operative atmosphere is quiet and comfortable. Physicians administering such agents should have at least one assistant present, and both should be trained in the use of anesthetic agents and for cardiopulmonary resuscitation in children.

THE NEWBORN NAIL AND ITS VARIANTS

Embryologic formation of the nail apparatus is completed by the end of the second trimester of pregnancy.[1] At birth, the nail plates are thin, transparent, and barely extend beyond the hyponychium. Superficial longitudinal ridges angulate centrodistally toward the midline of each plate. This pattern persists through infancy and has no known histologic or pathologic correlates. Terry's onychodermal band is quite prominent at birth. This transverse pale band, highlighted in pink, is located on the distal nail bed just proximal to the hyponychium. It becomes more prominent in cases of acrocyanosis or in children with congenital heart disease.

Evaluation of a newborn's gestational age may be made by observing nail length and texture.[2] The nails of postterm infants or those neonates that are large for gestational age (e.g., infants of diabetic mothers) may extend well beyond the hyponychium. The nail plates of premature infants and some term infants may be shorter than the distal digital pulp and give an ingrown appearance (Fig. 7–1).[3] This is particularly true of the toenails because their development lags behind that of the fingernails. Newborn maturity has also been correlated with the presence or absence of visible proximal nail fold capillary loops.[4] However, this observation is not routinely used in the scoring of gestational age. X-ray microanalysis of fingernails in term and preterm infants indicates that the elemental composition changes with gestational age. It has been suggested that ungual mineral content may be reflective of bone mineral content in neonates and that x-ray microanalysis may be useful in the eval-

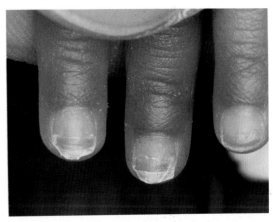

Figure 7–2. Beau's lines. Transverse grooves in nail plates of an infant born prematurely who survived a difficult delivery and neonatal period.

uation of osteopenia in the chronically ill premature newborn.[5]

Temporary koilonychia may be noted in some infants, as can Beau's lines. Koilonychia usually improves as the size and shape of the distal phalanx change.[6] Persistent congenital and autosomal dominant hereditary koilonychia has also been reported.[7,8] Beau's lines appear at about 1 month of age and grow out by 4 months (Fig. 7–2).[9] This infrequently observed transient arrest in nail growth is probably similar to telogen effluvium noted on many infants during the same time period and is probably related to the stress of adapting to extrauterine life. Correlations with intrauterine malnutrition, birth asphyxia, or breast versus bottle feeding have not been made. Onychomadesis from intrauterine asphyxia has been reported only once.[10]

Nail growth has not been measured in newborns. The average length of the newborn fingernail is 5 mm, so one could calculate a growth rate of 0.5 mm per week based on the report of Turano.[9] Few older children have been included in larger studies of nail growth.[11,12] The growth velocity of 0.7 mm per week is not significantly different from that of adults.

CONGENITAL MALFORMATIONS OF THE NAIL APPARATUS

Numerous congenital malformations of the nail apparatus have been described. These may be isolated defects or associated with other abnormalities such as ectodermal dysplasias, chromosomal abnormalities, or teratogen syndromes.

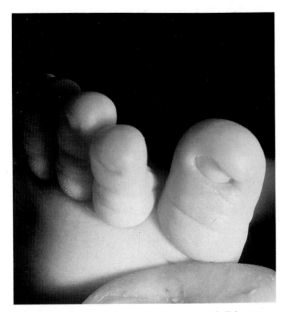

Figure 7–1. Congenital pseudo-ingrown nail. Edematous digital pulp regresses as growth of the phalanx occurs.

Isolated Nail Defects

Congenital malalignment of the great toe-nails was first reported by Samman in 1978 and was reviewed by Baran and Bureau (Fig. 7–3).[13] It is commonly observed as an isolated finding but has been reported as an autosomal dominant condition and as a disorder affecting twins.[14-16] In congenital malalignment, the nail plate laterally deviates from the longitudinal axis of the distal phalanx. A case of medial deviation has also been reported.[17] Transverse ridging from intermittent trauma to the matrix is regularly observed. Bacterial and candidal paronychia, ingrown nails, and latent onychomadesis may result if it is not corrected early. The surgical approach involves a crescent, wedge-shaped resection below the nail bed and matrix. The free, overlying nail unit can then be realigned over the phalanx similar to a rotation flap. Some authors recommend a conservative approach to caring for patients with congenital malalignment. Spontaneous improvement has been reported in several cases.[18] In addition, reports of postoperative epidermoid cyst formation at the site of realignment have tempered the surgical approach to this disorder.[19] Congenital malalignment should be differentiated from isolated congenital hypertrophy of the lateral nail folds of the hallux.[21]

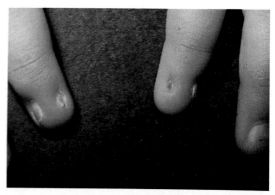

Figure 7–4. Congenital onychodysplasia of the index fingers (COIF)—polyonychia and micronychia (courtesy of Ichiro Kikuchi, MD). From Schachner L (ed): Advances in Dermatology. Year Book Medical, Chicago, in press.

Congenital anonychia without accompanying ectodermal defects has appeared sporadically and has been reported with autosomal dominant or recessive inheritance.[22,23] The underlying digits may be normal or are more often associated with phalangeal deformities or complete absence of the digit (ectrodactyly).[24] Amniotic bands may be the cause of anonychia with ectrodactyly.[25] Anonychia with bizzare flexural pigmentation (hyper- and hypopigmented macules) in one large kindred has been described.[26] Several affected individuals also had coarse, sparse hair and dry, fissured palms and soles, suggesting an unusual ectodermal dysplasia. However, sweating was not affected and consistent dental abnormalities were not present.

Congenital onychodysplasia of the index fingers (COIF) was first described in 1969 by Iso (Fig. 7–4).[20] Most of the 60 cases reported so far have been sporadic, but autosomal dominant inheritance of the disorder has been recognized in one family.[27] COIF affects both sexes equally, and it has been reported in many races and ethnic groups.[28] COIF may be unilateral or bilateral. It may present with anonychia, but micronychia is the rule. The nail plates are usually thin, but a rolled appearance, partial onychogryphosis, and malalignment are observed as well. Asymmetric polyonychia on the index fingers with the larger plate localized to the ulnar aspect of the distal phalanx is also not unusual. Rarely, deformities of other fingers are present, including brachydactyly or distal phalangeal enlargement. Because minor abnormalities are found on digits other than the index fingers, Baran and Stroud suggested that COIF be termed the Iso and Kikuchi syndrome.[29] The fact that toenails are never in-

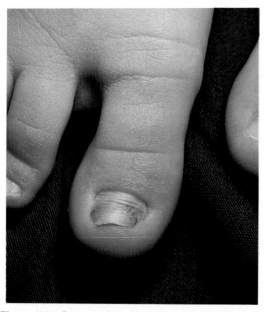

Figure 7–3. Congenital malalignment of the great toe nails. A thickened discolored nail plate is angulated from the axis of the phalanx. From Schachner L (ed): Advances in Dermatology. Year Book Medical, Chicago, in press.

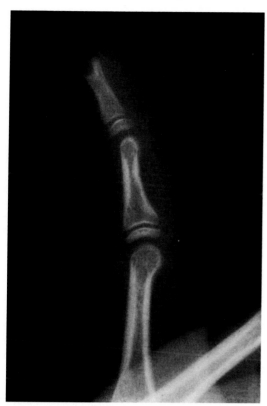

Figure 7–5. COIF. Y-type bifurcation of the distal phalanx observed on lateral radiographs (courtesy of Ichiro Kikuchi, MD). From Schachner L (ed): Advances in Dermatology. Year Book Medical, Chicago, in press.

volved distinguishes COIF from the ectodermal dysplasias, nail-patella syndrome, or Poland's syndrome. Initial cases of COIF were described without mention of underlying bone deformities. However, anteroposterior radiographs will frequently uncover a Y-type bifurcation or sharpened tip of the distal phalanx (Fig. 7–5).

Polyonychia without polydactyly is an infrequent occurrence. It may be observed in COIF or acquired as a result of pterygium formation from trauma or an inflammatory disorder.[30] True ectopic nails (onychoheterotopia) probably result from a hamartomatous rest of tissue, because their location on digits is most often reported on the dorsal or palmar surfaces.[31] A circumferential nail also localized to the palmar aspect of a finger has been reported.[32] Sessile keratotic papules of the lateral aspects of the fifth fingers may frequently be misinterpreted as ectopic nails. However, excision of such lesions will more often reveal a stump neuroma or digital remnant.

Onychia With Skeletal Dysplasias

Nail dystrophies frequently accompany skeletal dysplasias; for instance, patients with short stature exhibit short stubby nails, called racket nails. Pseudoclubbing occurs if the underlying distal phalanges are broad. These and other ungual deformities are found in many conditions (Table 7–1).[33–52]

A description of nail dysplasia and absent patellas can be found as early as 1897.[53] The nail-patella syndrome (Fig. 7–6) or hereditary onycho-osteodysplasia (HOOD) is an autosomal dominant disorder with variable expressivity and high penetrance.[54] The gene locus is thought to be on chromosome 9. Recognition of the disorder is important because of the crippling degenerative joint disease and renal failure that develop as the patient ages.

The ungual deformities of the nail-patella syndrome are present at birth. Hypoplasia or complete absence of the fingernails is characteristic.[55] The thumb and index fingers are usually most severely affected, with lesser deformities on the third through fifth fingers and toes. A triangle-shaped lunula present in most instances is nearly pathognomonic for this disorder.[56] Other ungual abnormalities include thinning, koilonychia, roughness, onychorrhexis, a median groove or cleft, and chromonychia.

Patients with the nail-patella syndrome may come to a physician's attention in later childhood when knee pain and gait impediments develop during vigorous exercise in school sports. Frequent dislocations result in the early onset of degenerative osteoarthritis.

Renal dysplasia affects middle-aged patients with nail-patella syndrome and is usually discovered as asymptomatic proteinuria.

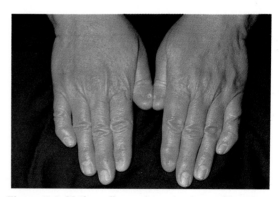

Figure 7–6. Nail-patella syndrome—micronychia, triangular lunulae, and clinodactyly (courtesy of Boni Elewski, MD).

Table 7–1. **NAIL DYSTROPHIES AND SKELETAL DEFORMITIES***

Name	Nail Deformity	Skeletal Defects	Other Findings
Absence of middle[33] phalanges with nail dysplasia	Hypoplasia	Absent phalanges, syndactyly, double of thumbs	AD
Acrodysostosis[34]	Broad, short	Peripheral dysostosis, short stature	Sporadic, nasal hypoplasia, retardation
Acro-osteolysis[35]	Short, elliptical	Multiple wormian bones, bathrocephaly, phalangeal osteolysis, loss of sensation	Short stature, early loss of teeth, AD
Apert's syndrome[36]	Broad, short fused nails and micronychia	Craniosyostosis, frontal bossing, syndactyly	Mental retardation, narrow palate
Brachydactyly[37] type[3]	Anonychia on 4th digit, others dysplastic	Asymmetric short phalanges	AD
Cartilage hair[38] hypoplasia (McKusick)	Short, broad	Short limbs, bowed legs	AR, fine hair, short stature, immunodeficient, malabsorption
CHILD syndrome[39]	Brittle, chipping onychogryphosis on affected side	Hemidysplasia of limbs	XD, deafness unilateral, ichthyosis
Cleidocranial[40] dysostosis	Down-curved small	Clavicular aplasia, variable phalangeal length	Short stature, delayed tooth eruption
Frontometaphaseal[41] dysplasia	Short	Marked supraorbital ridges	AD, AR, deaf, large nose, peculiar facies
Larsen's syndrome[42]	Short, broad	Spatulate thumbs, multiple dislocations	AR, flat face, hypertelorism
Pachydermoperiostosis[43]	Clubbing, thin, yellow	Periosteal new bone at puberty, thin tubular bones, ovoid vertebrae, clavicular	AD, cutis verticis gyrata, short stature
Poland anomaly[44]	Unilateral hypoplasia	Rib defect	Unilateral syndactyly, absent pectoralis muscles
Progeria[45] (Hutchinson-Gilford)	Thin, yellow	Thin tubular delayed ossification, premature osteoporosis	Birdlike facies, subcutaneous atrophy, atherosclerosis, premature death
Puretic syndrome[45]	Broad, pseudoclubbing, lysis, scleroderma-like skin	Phalangeal osteocontractures	Short stature
Pycnodysostosis[47]	Short, brittle pseudoclubbing or platyonychia	Osteosclerosis, fractures	AR, short stature, dental dysplasia
Seckel's syndrome[48]	Clubbing	Clinodactyly, absent phalangeal epiphyses, 11 ribs, proximal long-bone hypoplasia	AR, growth and mental retardation, "bird head"
Sclerosteosis[49]	Absent or dysplastic nails of 2nd & 3rd fingers	Hyperostosis of skull and tubular bones	Hypertelorism, broad mandible
Taybi syndrome[50]	Short	Irregular digit length, pectus, carpal fusions, deaf	AR, XR, short stature, facial hypoplasia, cleft palate
Williams syndrome[51]	Hyponychia	Coarse facies, depressed nasal bridge, clinodactyly	Growth & mental retardation, supravalvular aortic stenosis, stellate iris, hypercalcemia

*This list does not include ectodermal dysplasias.

AD, autosomal dominant; AR, autosomal recessive; XD, X-linked dominant; XR, X-linked recessive; CHILD, congenital hemidysplasia with ichthyosiform erythroderma and limb defects.

Table 7–2. **FINDINGS IN THE NAIL-PATELLA SYNDROME**

System	Findings
Skeletal	Patellar hypoplasia or aplasia
	Iliac horns
	Radial head hypoplasia
	Thick scapulae
	Scoliosis
	Cleft palate
	Spina bifida occulta
Ocular	Heterochromic irides
	Keratoconus
	Microcornea
	Microphakia
	Cataracts
Cardiovascular	Arterial aneurysms
Miscellaneous	Retardation
	Psychoses
	Stroke

A chronic glomerulonephritis-like picture then develops, resulting in renal failure, which is now amenable to kidney transplantation.

Many other abnormalities have been described in the nail-patella syndrome (Table 7–2).[57] The ungual deformities may be minimized by the patient, and indeed, their extent does not correlate with the severity of any other symptom. However, early diagnosis, counseling about appropriate physical activities, and frequent medical checks could avert many complications of this disorder.

Brachyonchia, hyponychia, and pencil-shaped digits have been associated with aplasia cutis congenita. The absence of skin may occur on the scalp, trunk, or other body sites. Amniotic bands and fetal vascular insufficiency have been etiologic considerations in those cases.[58]

Nail Deformities With Chromosome Disorders

Evidence of chromosomal abnormalities should be sought in patients with ungual dystrophy and unusual phenotypic features. Varying degrees of hypoplasia or hyperconvexity of the nail plates are most common (Table 7–3).[59–69]

Table 7–3. **CHROMOSOMAL ABNORMALITIES ASSOCIATED WITH NAIL DYSTROPHY**

Chromosome Defect	Identifying Features	Nail Findings
Down's syndrome[59]	Upward slanted palpebral fissures, Brushfield's spots, hypotonia, simian creases, cardiac defects, cutis marmorata, short broad digits	Clubbing with cardiac defects or macronychia
Trisomy 18[60]	Hypertonic, clenched hands with overlapped fingers, short sternum, abnormal dermatoglyphic pattern	Hypoplasia—especially 5th fingers and toes
Trisomy 13[61]	Cleft lip/palate, aplasia cutis, polydactyly, ambiguous genitalia, hemangiomas, microcephaly, cardiac defects	Narrow, hyperconvex or hypoplastic
Trisomy 9p[62]	Downward slanted palpebral fissures, microcephaly, hypertelorism, retardation, short digits	Dystrophy, clawlike
Monosomy 9p[63]	Upslanting palpebral fissures, trigonocephaly, midface hypoplasia, retardation, abnormal dermatoglyphics	Square shaped, wide, and convex
Trisomy 8p[64]	Retardation, abnormal facies	Hypoplasia or anonychia
Trisomy 7q[65]	Retardation, abnormal facies	Hyperconvex
Monosomy 4p[66]	Cleft lip/palate, fishlike mouth, cranial asymmetry, retardation, preauricular dimple	Hyperconvex
Group G ring chromosome[67]	Retardation, abnormal facies	Pachyonychia
Turner's syndrome (XO)[68]	Webbed neck, congenital lymphedema, ovarian dysgenesis, cubitus valgus, nevi	Narrow, hyperconvex, or deep set
Trisomy 3q[69]	Hirsutism, synophrys (converging eyebrows), ocular abnormalities, short neck, wide-spaced nipples	Hypoplasia or anonychia

Fetal Teratogen Syndromes

Several syndromes in children who have been exposed to systemic medicinal or recreational drugs early in their fetal development have been well described. There is wide phenotypic variation depending on the timing of fetal exposure and dose of teratogen. Nails are infrequently affected, except in complete expression of each syndrome (Table 7–4).[70–73]

Ectodermal Dysplasias

The ectodermal dysplasias are a diverse group of inherited disorders characterized by generalized anatomic or functional defects in one or more derivatives of the primordial ectodermal germ layer.[74] The derivatives or appendages that are commonly affected have been used by Freire-Maia to classify these disorders.[75] They include hair (subclass 1), teeth (subclass 2), nails (subclass 3), and eccrine sweat glands (subclass 4). According to Freire-Maia, a type A ectodermal dysplasia contains at least two abnormalities of appendages in subclasses 1 through 4. A type B ectodermal dysplasia contains one abnormality from any of those subclasses and one from a fifth subclass that contains all of the other ectodermal derivatives: apocrine and sebaceous glands, keratinocytes, melanocytes, the ocular lens, the anterior pituitary gland, the adrenal medulla, and the orofacial mucosa. The Freire-Maia taxonomic system does not distinguish between one abnormality of an appendage and another. Therefore, dysplasias with any nail abnormality would be included in subclass 3 (i.e., hypertrophy, atrophy, brittleness, chromonychia). For instance, both Christ-Siemens-Touraine and Rapp-Hodgkin anhidrotic ectodermal dysplasias would be classified as A, 1–2–3–4. Because morphologic development in the embryo is so dependent on close interactions between germ layers, malformations of mesodermal structures may also be present, although not sufficient for the diagnosis of an ectodermal dysplasia.

At least 177 syndromes have been classified as ectodermal dysplasias since the original descriptions in the 19th and early 20th centuries.[76–80] Ungual involvement has been found in at least 75 of these, but no uniform abnormality has been noted. The nail plates may be small, brittle, discolored, ridged, or in some cases thickened.

Table 7–5 lists many of the ectodermal dysplasia syndromes in which the nails are affected.[79–112]

THICKENED NAILS IN CHILDREN

Hypertrophy of the nail apparatus may assume several forms, which are as cosmetically displeasing in children as in adults (Table 7–6).[113] Such deformities are quite obvious, even to the casual observer. During childhood, they may serve as a focus of peer ridicule, as may other physical deformities, and this may in turn have an effect on psychosocial development. The approach to correcting nail hypertrophy depends on the type of thickening that is present.

Pachyonychia congenita (Fig. 7–7) is an autosomal dominant genodermatosis (Freire-Maia A,1–2–3–4) with high penetrance and variable expressivity in which the nails begin to thicken soon after birth.[114] One of the earliest descriptions was by Jadassohn and

Table 7–4. **TERATONGENIC AGENTS AFFECTING NAIL MORPHOLOGY**

Agent	Nail Findings	Phenotypic Features
Phenytoin[70]	Hypoplasia, longitudinal pigmented bands	Cleft lip/palate, coarse hirsutism, low-set ears, hypertelorism, depressed nasal bridge, wide-spaced nipples, wide mouth, short neck, finger-like thumbs, short tapered digits
Alcohol[71]	Hypoplasia with occasional anonychia on 5th digits, or hyperconvex and narrow philtrum	Microcephaly, retardation, short palpebral fissures, epicanthal folds, short nose, shallow philtrum
Trimethadione and related medications[72]	Hypoplasia	Microcephaly, V-shaped eyebrows and synophrys, epicanthal folds, ptosis, dysplastic ears, deaf, small flat nose
Warfarin[73]	Hypoplasia	Nasal hypoplasia, hypertelorism, short neck, brachydactyly, stippled epiphyses

Table 7–5. **ECTODERMAL DYSPLASIAS (ED)**

Type	Nail Morphology	Inheritance	Distinguishing Features
	Freire-Maia A, 1–2*		
Christ-Siemens-Touraine syndrome,[79] hypohidrotic ED	Normal or occasionally brittle	XR	Lacrimal hypoplasia, photophobia, periocular pigmentation, frontal bossing, saddle nose, eczema
Hypohidrotic ED[80]	Normal, rarely small	AR	As in Christ-Siemens-Touraine syndrome
Goltz-Gorlin syndrome,[81] focal dermal hypoplasia	Thin, spooned, narrow, often with digit deformities (syndactyly, etc.)	XD	Focal absence of skin, generally hypohidrotic with palmoplantar hyperhidrosis, oral papillomas, ocular and skeletal defects, hypo- and hyperpigmentation, hypotrichosis
Rosselli-Gulienetti syndrome[82] (ED-cleft lip and palate popliteal pterygia syndrome)	Subungual hyperkeratosis, longitudinal striations, distal plate chipping	AR	Woolly hair, popliteal and perineal pterygia pityriasis, cleft lip/palate
Dyskeratosis congenita[83]	Hyponychia, recurrent childhood paronychia resulting in anonychia	XR, AD, AR	Reticulate hyper-/hypomelanosis, Fanconi-like pancytopenia, premalignant leukoplakia, deafness
Rapp-Hodgkins syndrome,[84] anhidrotic ED	Small, narrow	AD, AR(?)	Dry skin, absent dermatoglyphics, epiphora, ectropion, cleft lip/palate, coarse scalp hair
EEC† syndrome[85]	Thin, brittle, striate, occasionally pitted	AD	ED with ectrodactyly (claw hand), cleft lip/palate retardation, blepharitis, speckled irides
AEC† syndrome[86]	Severe dystrophy to anonychia	AD	Ankyloblepharon, ED, cleft lip/palate, palmoplantar hyperkeratosis, supernumerary nipples, reticulate pigmentation
TOD[87] (tricho-odontodental syndrome)	Thin, longitudinal ridges; central nail bed; elevation of toes more than fingers	AD	Taurodontic molars, persistent deciduous teeth
KID[88] (keratitis icthyosis deafness syndrome)	Congenital anonychia, delayed development, onychauxis, leukonychia	AR	Palmoplantar hyperkeratosis, icthyosiform erythroderma, sensorineural deafness, blindness from keratitis
Papillon-Lefevre syndrome[89]	Spoon-shaped, striated, onychogryphosis	AR	Periodontosis with premature loss of teeth, palmoplantar hyperkeratosis extending onto dorsum of feet and up to elbows, palmoplantar hyperhidrosis, dura mater calcifications
Hypomelanosis of ITO[90] (incontinentia pigmenti achromians)	Transverse ridging	AD	Relative hyperhidrosis in hypopigmented areas, linear guttate and whorled hypopigmentation (generalized), conductive hearing loss, multiple ocular abnormalities, retardation, seizures, skeletal deformities, mostly females
Basan's syndrome[91]	Short, thick longitudinal ridges	AD	Fine dermal ridges, single flexion crease, xerosis, long philtrum, thin upper lip

Table continued on following page

Table 7–5. **ECTODERMAL DYSPLASIAS (ED)** (Continued)

Type	Nail Morphology	Inheritance	Distinguishing Features
Clouston's hidrotic ED[92–94]	Onychauxis, longitudinal striations, paronychia, convex curvature, anonychia	AD	Rough xerotic skin, palmoplantar hyperkeratosis, clubbing, eccrine poromas, French Canadian kindreds
Rothmund-Thompson syndrome[95]	Rough, ridged, "heaped-up"	AR	Photosensitivity, supernumerary teeth, skin atrophy, telangiectasia, hypo- and hyperpigmentation, palmoplantar hyperkeratosis, cataracts, short stature, skeletal anomalies
Coffin-Siris syndrome[96]	Absent or hypoplastic 5th fingernails and toenails	AD	Retardation, clinodactyly, sporadic syndactyly or hyperplastic 5th digits, lax joints, simian crease, blepharoptosis, hypotonia
TDO syndrome[97] (trichodentoosseous syndrome)	Flat, thick striate, onychoschizia	AD	Sclerostosis; pitted discolored teeth (amelogeneses imperfecta); thick, progressively curling hair; taurodontism
Fried's tooth and nail syndrome[98]	Thin, small, concave	AR	Prominent lips and chin
Dento-oculo syndrome[99]	Horizontal ridges, onychoschizia	AD	Pseudoknuckle pads, cutaneous deafness, glaucoma
Trichorhinophalangeal syndrome[100]	Thin, short, longitudinal grooves, koilonychia, racket thumbs	AD	Pear-shaped nose, wide philtrum, short stature, short phalanges
Ellis-van Creveld syndrome,[101] chondroectodermal dysplasia	Brittle, furrowed, hypoplastic	AR	Natal teeth, broad nose, hypertelorism, thick short limb bones, postaxial polydactyly carpal fusions, congenital heart disease, acromelic dwarfism
Freire-Maia A, 1–3–4*			
Freire-Maia syndrome[102] hypohidrotic ED	Onychogryphosis		? Upswept hair, scalp follicular keratosis, frontal bossing, cataracts
HEDH[103] (hypohidrotic ED with hypothyroidism)	Ridged, shriveled	AR	Haylike hair, hyperthermia, mottled brownish skin, short stature, hypothyroidism, respiratory infections from abnormal cilia
Freire-Maia 2–3–4*			
Amelo-onychohypohidrotic dysplasia[104]	Onycholysis and subungual keratosis	AD	Pitted, thin enamel; xerosis; keratosis pilaris
Naegli-Franceschetti-Jadassohn syndrome[105]	Onycholysis, subungual hyperkeratosis	AD	Hyperpigmentation, punctate palmar/plantar keratosis
Freire-Maia A, 1–3*			
Sabinas syndrome[106]	Dystrophy	AR	Brittle hair, retardation, xerosis, ocular dysplasia
CHANDU† syndrome[107]	Hyponychia	AR	Curly hair, ankyloblepharon, nail dysplasia
Onychotrichodysplasia with neutropenia[108]	Hyponychia, koilonychia, onychorrhexis	AR	Neutropenia, recurrent infections
BIDS†[109] (trichothiodystrophy)	Onychauxis, subungual keratosis, onychoschizia, longitudinal groove, koilonychia		Brittle hair, ichthyosis, deafness

Table 7–5. **ECTODERMAL DYSPLASIAS (ED)** (Continued)

Type	Nail Morphology	Inheritance	Distinguishing Features
	Freire-Maia (A) 2–3*		
DOOR syndrome[110] (deafness, onychosteodystrophy with retardation)	Hypoplasia, anonychia	AD, AR	Deafness, triphalangeal thumbs, retardation, seizures
Curry-Hall syndrome[111]	Short, thick vertical striations	AD	Short limbs, polydactyly
	Freire-Maia A, 3–4*		
Absence of dermal ridge patterns[112]	Rough, horizontal and vertical grooves; onycholysis; adherent hyponychium	AD	Anhidrosis of palms and soles with blisters at birth, milia on chin

*1. Generalized hypotrichosis usually includes brows, lashes, and body hair; may be coarse, fine, thin, brittle, short, or totally absent.

2. Hypodontia: pegged, conical, small or absent teeth, with enamel hypoplasia, caries, premature loss or delayed eruption.

3. Nail changes (listed).

4. Hypohidrosis: generalized; more severe cases accompanied by heat intolerance and recurrent fever.

†See column four for the characteristics that explain these acronyms. AD, autosomal dominant; AR, autosomal recessive; XD, X-linked dominant; XR, X-linked recessive.

Table 7–6. **HYPERTROPHY OF THE NAIL APPARATUS IN CHILDREN**

Generalized

Pachyonychia (thick with smooth surface)
　Pachyonychia congenita
　Keratitis ichthyosis deafness (KID) syndrome (and other ectodermal dysplasias)
Onychogryphosis (overcurved and laterally deviated)
　Neglect
　Hereditary
　Skeletal deformity
Onychauxis (brittle with distorted rough surface)
　Mucocutaneous candidiasis
　Atopic erythroderma, alopecia totalis
　Alopecia totalis, vitiligo,[113] recurrent infections
　Hayden's syndrome—alopecia universalis, hypohidrosis, icthyosiform hyperkeratosis, infections

Localized

Pachyonychia
　Dermatophytes
　Psoriasis
　Tumors (neurofibroma, myxoma)
　Exostoses

Lewandowsky, who in 1906 reported familial ungual thickening accompanied by several other ectodermal defects.[115] Three variants of pachyonychia congenita are currently recognized (Table 7–7). Ungual deformities are consistent between pedigrees. Biochemical evidence suggests that there is a dramatically increased expression of "soft" keratins in at least one family affected with the Jackson-Lawler type of pachyonychia congenita.[116]

The nails of patients with pachyonychia congenita are normally shaped at birth but exhibit proximal brown chromonychia and centrodistal leukonychia. Within 2 to 8 weeks, the lateral nail margins curve inwardly in a pincer motion and the distal nail plate begins to thicken in an upward direction to produce a conelike deformity. The nail plate surface remains relatively smooth or longitudinal striations develop. Spontaneous shedding secondary to trauma or underlying bullae occasionally occurs. The plates themselves are extremely hard and are very difficult to trim.

Numerous attempts at correcting the deformities and complications of pachyonychia congenita have been made. Callosities have been transiently diminished by keratolytic agents containing salicylic acid, lactic acid, or urea. Specially constructed orthopedic shoes may aid in ambulation. Most recently, oral

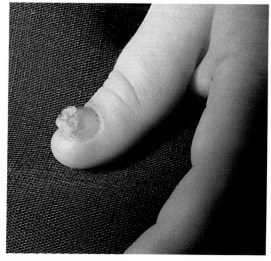

Figure 7–7. Pachyonychia congenita—rock-hard thickening of the ventral and medial nail plate.

Table 7–7. ECTODERMAL DEFECTS IN PACHYONYCHIA CONGENITA

Type I

Follicular keratosis most prominent over knees and elbows
Palmoplantar hyperkeratosis
    Hyperhidrosis
    Friction blister formation
Laryngeal keratosis—hoarseness
Hair with irregular shaft diameter, thick brows
Leukokeratosis oris (present at birth)

Type II

Natal teeth (present at birth) and premature anodontia
Steatocystoma multiplex
Follicular and palmoplantar keratosis without oral leukokeratosis

Type III

Corneal dystrophy
Mucocutaneous keratosis (as with type I)

retinoids have reduced the follicular, palmoplantar, and mucosal hyperkeratosis.[117,118] Bullae have been diminished by phenytoin, as in dystrophic epidermolysis bullosa.[119] Hoarseness and laryngeal stridor, when life threatening, have been circumvented with tracheostomies. The nail thickening of pachyonychia congenita has not been affected by high-dose vitamin A, retinoids, or x-ray therapy. Surgical avulsion has yielded the best cosmetic results.[120–122] Scarification of the nail bed after proximal or distal avulsion without matrix destruction results in regrowth of distorted plates. Also, destruction of the matrix without attention to the nail bed produces unacceptable ungual hyperkeratosis. Radical excision of the entire affected nail unit followed by full- or partial-thickness grafting has even been performed in some cases. A similar approach to correcting the pachyonychia in other dyskeratotic syndromes such as the keratitis icthyosis deafness (KID) syndrome[123] may also be undertaken.[114]

Pachyonychia localized to one or a few nail plates in children should be scraped and cultured for dermatophytes, particularly *Trichophyton rubrum*, which may be acquired from parents, or *Epidermophyton floccosum*, which can be contracted in the summer months when bare feet are in contact with soil. A 3- to 6-month course of microsized griseofulvin (15 mg/kg BID) given with milk and application of ciclopirox olamine (Loprox) is usually adequate therapy.

Children with psoriasis may have nail dystrophy in up to 21 per cent of cases.[124] Pitting, onycholysis (Fig. 7–8), and yellow oil-spot dis-

coloration are most common, whereas ungual thickening is unusual. The thickening, when present, involves one or more nails and resembles pachyonychia, because it results from accumulation of loose subungual debris that pushes the nail plate in an upward direction. Differentiation from fungual pachyonychia is important. Treatments other than frequent manicuring have been unsatisfactory.

Benign tumors of the region surrounding the nail matrix may also cause pachyonychia. Examples include isolated neurofibromas or bony exostoses. The latter may be suspected if a slightly painful, fixed, firm nodule is present in the phalangeal tissues adjacent to the thickening. X-ray film can confirm the osseous overgrowth. Curettage of the phalangeal cortex after nail avulsion is the treatment of choice.[125]

Onychogryphosis in children may be a result of neglect. Failure to thrive and an ill-kept appearance usually accompany those cases. Onychogryphosis may also arise in nails whose matrices are distorted by congenital malalignment, traumas, or external pressure from an infant's first pair of poorly fitting shoes.[126] Acquired and congenital onychogryphoses, inherited in an autosomal dominant fashion, have been reported.[127,128] Congenital clawlike nails may be confused with onychogryphosis, but in that deformity, the distal digital pulp forms only an abortive nail bed and hyponychium.[129] Clipping the nails after careful overnight application of 40 per cent urea paste under occlusion will allow a more thorough evaluation of any underlying deformity.

Chronic mucocutaneous candidiasis is characterized by massively thickened nails caused by *Candida albicans* as well as widespread involvement of the skin and oral mucosa. This

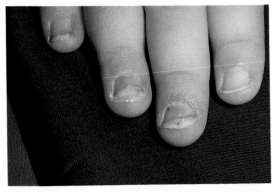

Figure 7–8. Psoriasis. Distal onycholysis and oil-spot discoloration of nails of a teenaged boy with sausage-shaped digits caused by psoriatic arthritis.

Table 7–8. **CONDITIONS ASSOCIATED WITH CHRONIC MUCOCUTANEOUS CANDIDOSIS**

Primary immunodeficiency
    DiGeorge's
    Nezelof's
    Common variable immunodeficiency
    Hyper IgE syndromes (Job's, Buckley's)
    Myeloperoxidase deficiency

Secondary immunosupression
Medical conditions
    Multiple endocrinopathies
        Parathyroid, adrenal, thyroid, and diabetes
        Polyendocrinopathy and vitiligo
    Iron-deficient states
    Thymoma, myasthenia, hypogammoglobulinemia
    EEC syndrome (ED with ectrodactyly, cleft lip/palate)
    Dental enamel dysplasia syndrome

IgE, immunoglobulin E; ED, ectodermal dysplasia.

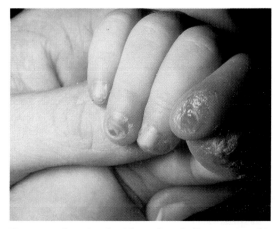

Figure 7–9. Junctional epidermolysis bullosa—anonychia and subungual blister formation.

disseminated infection occurs in a wide variety of circumstances in which immune responsiveness to *Candida* and other fungal organisms is diminished (Table 7–8). Ungual involvement may begin soon after birth in hereditary forms of the disorder or in later childhood if acquired immunodeficiency occurs. A few or all 20 nails may be involved. Paronychia, subungual hyperkeratosis, and onycholysis are initially evident. A bulbous digital tip results from chronic inflammation. Invasion of organisms from the hyponychium gradually envelops the entire nail plate and results in onychauxis, chipping, brittleness, and a yellow-brown discoloration. *Candida* pseudohyphae are readily identified in potassium hydroxide examinations of nail scrapings from these patients.

Sustained remissions are now reported in mucocutaneous candidiasis with oral ketoconazole (Nizoral).[130–134] Oral itraconazole (Sporanox) and fluconazole (Diflucan) have also been used. Ungual deformities resolve slowly over a period of 3 to 4 months, and oral and cutaneous findings disappear within 1 month of therapy. Dosages of 6 mg/kg up to 400 mg/day have been used for initial therapy. Discontinuing the drug leads to rapid recurrence of lesions. Failure to respond may be due to concomitant infections with dermatophytes that may be relatively resistant to the drug. Adverse reactions that include nausea, headaches, dizziness, and pruritus are infrequent. Careful monitoring of side effects such as drug-induced hepatitis and alterations in serum lipid levels, hematologic, and renal parameters should be performed. Potentially childbearing female adolescents should be monitored for pregnancy because ketoconazole is teratogenic.

BLISTERING DISEASES AND THE NAIL

Vesicobullous lesions involving the nail unit are infrequent in newborns and very young infants. Blisters involving the distal digital pulp from intrauterine finger sucking have been reported.[135] Sterile puncture for Gram stain, Tzanck preparation, and bacterial and viral culture should be performed to rule out staphylococcal or herpetic infections, both of which carry a high mortality rate during the neonatal period if left untreated. Epidermolysis bullosa (Fig. 7–9) may present at birth, with periungual or subungual bullae resulting in onychomadesis (Fig. 7–10) or lesser deformities (Table 7–9).[136–151] Subungual collections of fluid in neonates should also be cultured for anaerobes. *Veillonella*, a small gram-negative coccal organism, may localize under the nail plates. This suspected pathogen is frequently

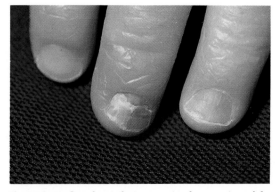

Figure 7–10. Onychomadesis—proximal separation of the nail plate from the nail bed.

Table 7–9. **NAIL FINDINGS IN HEREDITARY EPIDERMOLYSIS BULLOSA**

Eponym	Genetics	Nails	Blister Location	Blisters at Birth	Other Findings
Epidermolytic (Simplex)					
Koebner-Weber[136]	AD	NL	G	Yes	Oral lesions
Cockayne[137]	AD	NL	L	No	Palm-sole involvement
With mottled pigment[138]	AD	Curved	G	Yes	Bruising, atrophy
Ogna[139]	AD	Onychogryphosis	G	No	RBC-GPT linkage
Dowling-Meara[140] (herpetiformis)	AD	Onychomadesis with frequent permanent deformity		Yes	Circinate distal milia, palmoplantar keratosis
Junctional					
Hurlitz-EB[141] atrophicans (Gravis)	AD	Absent, hypoplastic, easily shed, heaped up in adults	G	Yes	Blisters with erosions, especially fingers and toe tips
Schnyder-Anton[142]	AD	Dystrophy	G	Yes	Caries, gastrointestinal involvement, improves with age
Lamprecht (mitis) Schnyder-Anton[143]	AD	Dystrophy from birth	L	No	Soles and lower legs minor scarring
Lamprecht Gedde-Dahl[136] (inversal)	AR	Dystrophy	G	Yes	Albostriate atrophy; trunkal distribution; caries; gastrointestinal/respiratory involvement
Gedde-Dahl[144] (progressiva)	AR	Onychomadesis during childhood results in anonychia, usually first symptom	L	No	Hypoacusis; hands, feet, elbows, knees involved; loss of dermatoglyphics
Dermatolytic (Dystrophic)					
Cockayne-Touraine[145]	AD	Dystrophy, anonychia, onychogryphosis	G	No	Milia, hypertrophic scars, extensor surfaces and oral mucosa involved
Pasini[146]	AD	Dystrophy; anonychia; thick, short, split frequently	G	Yes	Milia, atrophic scars (albopapuloid)
Hallopeau-Siemens[147]	AR	Onychomadesis common, pterygium anonychia	G	Yes	Milia; atrophic scars; syndactyly with mitten deformity; gastrointestinal, respiratory, oral involvement
Inversa[148]	AR	Dystrophy variable	L	Yes	Axillae, neck, groin, and oral mucosa albostriate scars, without milia
Kindler's[149]	?	Dystrophy	L	Yes	Hands and feet, poikiloderma, photosensitivity, syndactyly, palmoplantar keratosis

Table 7–9. **NAIL FINDINGS IN HEREDITARY EPIDERMOLYSIS BULLOSA** (Continued)

Eponym	Genetics	Nails	Blister Location	Blisters at Birth	Other Findings
Bart's	AD	Anonychia or dystrophy at birth; split, short, onychogryphotic, especially great toe and thumb	G	No	Congenital localized absence of skin, nonscarring
Fine-Osment[151]	?	Dystrophy	G	No	Progressive, arcuate, symmetric, centripital bullae with scars and milia

AD, autosomal dominant; AR, autosomal recessive; G, general; GPT, glutamate pyruvate transaminase; L, localized; RBC, red blood cells.

isolated from the maternal vaginal vault. Soon after birth, a turbid vesicle elevates the nail plate.[152] It rapidly becomes purulent and may drain onto the digital pulp, producing erythema and desquamation. Within 4 days, the nail bed appears brownish, signaling inflammatory resorption, which lasts up to 6 weeks. Antibiotic treatment did not affect the course of the disorder in one nursery epidemic.

Two acquired bullous disorders that may involve the nail unit of older infants and children are blistering distal dactylitis and herpetic whitlow.

Blistering distal dactylitis (Fig. 7–11) is a nontender localized bacterial infection of the distal volar fat pad of one or more digits.[153] When the blister is incised, the thin, turbid exudate contains gram-positive cocci that invariably are group A β-hemolytic streptococci. *Staphylococcus aureus* and *Staphylococcus epidermidis* are isolated less frequently.[154] In many instances, the blister dissects dorsally to the nail folds and may potentially result in paronychia or latent onychomadesis. Treatment includes incision and drainage of the exudate, frequent soaks with Burow's or antibacterial solutions, and oral penicillin or erythromycin. Systemic complications have not been reported, but streptococcal organisms have been isolated from other body sites concurrently with the infection.[155]

Herpetic whitlow (Fig. 7–12) is the major diagnostic consideration when a painful blister forms around the nail unit in children.[156] This

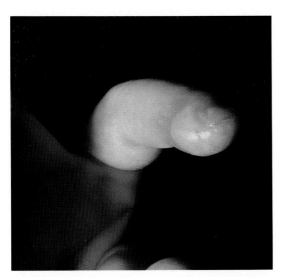

Figure 7–11. Blistering dactylitis. A single large distal phalangeal bulla develops from infection with group A β-hemolytic streptococci.

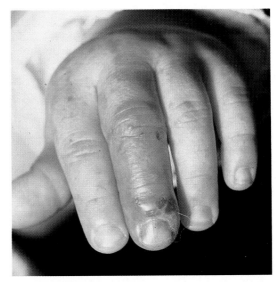

Figure 7–12. Herpetic whitlow—clustered vesicopustules and crust of periungual tissues.

localized viral infection presents with pain of the distal phalanx followed shortly by swelling and redness. A coalescent cluster of vesicles then develops. These lesions contain clear fluid that becomes turbid but rarely purulent over a 10-day period. The lack of frank purulence helps to distinguish herpetic whitlow from blistering dactylitis. Crusting and desquamation occur within 3 weeks. When whitlow involves the nail unit, paronychia, onycholysis, or onychomedesis may occur. Recurrent herpes labialis or primary gingivostomatitis is frequently concurrent. As with other herpes infections, Tzanck preparations reveal multinucleated giant cells early in the course of the illness. Aspiration of vesicular fluid, wet to dry dressings, and analgesics are standard treatment. The efficacy of topical and systemic antiviral agents (Acyclovir, idoxuridine) has not been studied in children with this disorder, but the potential benefits of decreased viral shedding, diminution of pain, and acceleration of healing time make these agents logical first-line therapy.

INFLAMMATORY DISORDERS OF NAILS IN CHILDREN

Severe erythema multiforme, or Stevens-Johnson syndrome, may involve the nails of affected individuals. If the nails are shed early in the illness along with surrounding phalangeal skin, anonychia may result.[157] Meticulous care and protection of the ungual tissues may promote regrowth of shed nails in 4 to 6 months.

Kawasaki syndrome, or mucocutaneous lymph node syndrome, is a sporadic disorder that may occur in miniepidemics throughout the world.[158] It affects children from 6 months to 10 years of age and is characterized by an acute stage of fever for more than 5 days unresponsive to antibiotics; conjunctival injection; erythema of the lips, tongue, or pharynx; erythema or edema of the hands and feet; and generalized adenopathy. A polymorphous, multiforme, or urticarial eruption may also be present. Ten to 14 days after the onset of the illness, a characteristic desquamation of the palms and soles begins at the hyponychium. Desquamation may also occur at other body sites such as the groin. Serious complications include coronary artery aneurysms (at least 20 per cent of affected individuals), iritis, gallbladder hydrops, and thrombosis of acral vessels leading to gangrene. Fatal coronary artery

rupture or myocardial infarction is reported in 2 to 5 per cent of severely affected individuals at the end of the acute phase of the illness. As with any acute febrile disease, Beau's lines may appear during convalescence, 1 month after resolution of symptoms.[159] Rarely, a persistent eczematous eruption occurs around the nails after recovery. Treatment is supportive. High doses of aspirin and immediate administration of intravenous immunoglobulin may reduce fever and the development of coronary artery complications.[160]

Nail findings in childhood atopic dermatitis are quite common.[161] The polished, shiny parrot-beaked deformities that reflect chronic rubbing with the dorsal nail plate surface and irregularly shaped pits from inflammation of the proximal nail folds are observed most frequently.

Persistent scratching of heavily infected skin in children with atopic dermatitis can result in the insidious onset of osteomyelitis of the distal phalanges.[165] The affected digits develop a characteristic triangle-shaped subungual black macule with its base at the distal free edge and the apex directed proximally. The macule is accompanied by edema, erythema, and pain. Roentgenographic and scintigraphic evidence of bony destruction may be uncovered despite the absence of fever, systemic symptoms, and abnormal laboratory parameters. *Staphylococcus aureus* is the most common etiologic agent, but other bacteria have been isolated as well. Initial treatment with intravenous antibiotics should be considered until objective improvement is noted.

Parakeratosis pustulosa (Fig. 7–13), a benign inflammatory condition of the distal phalanx, has been reported only in children.[162,163] It primarily affects one to several digits of both hands and feet. Typically, patients are girls younger than 5 years. No consistent history of preceding trauma, onychophagia, or finger sucking can be elicited. Examination reveals a well-demarcated, bright red, somewhat swollen distal phalanx that is nontender. At the onset, a good parental observer may detect a few periungual pustules. Swollen nail folds and absent cuticles also suggest an early paronychia, but cultures for bacteria and fungi do not reveal any consistent pathogens or saphrophytes. The nail plate becomes chipped and brittle. Onycholysis and subungual debris may accumulate enough to result in onychomadesis. Biopsies of parakeratosis pustulosa have disclosed changes consistent with psoriasis and eczema, but the cause remains

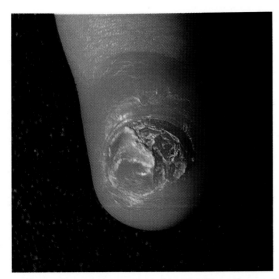

Figure 7–13. Parakeratosis pustulosa. Bright erythema of the distal plalanx associated with dissolution of the nail plate most often seen on one or two fingers of young girls.

unclear. Treatment with clotrimazole solution and/or a topical corticosteroid solution has been ineffective. Parakeratosis pustulosa resolves spontaneously over several years.

NAIL CHANGES IN CHILDHOOD CANCER CHEMOTHERAPY

Children who have cancer and who undergo chemotherapy and bone marrow transplantation frequently have evidence of Beau's lines or transverse leukonychia that indicates the time antimitotic agents were given.[164] A lichen planus–like eruption or sclerodermoid changes are characteristic of chronic graft-versus-host disease following allogeneic bone marrow transplantation. In each case, inflammation of the nail unit may result in ungual changes similar to those in the primary disorders: trachyonychia and pterygium or periungual erythema with anonychia.[165,166] Finally, onychophagia or the seemingly trivial trauma from overzealous nail trimming may result in dactylitis and serve as a source of sepsis in these immunocompromised individuals.[167]

NAIL DYSTROPHY WITH LINEAR DISORDERS AFFECTING LIMBS

Nail dystrophy has been reported in many "linear" disorders commonly found in children, including inflammatory linear verrucous epidermal nevi (ILVEN),[168] incontinentia pigmenti,[169] lichen striatus,[170] lichen niditus,[171] and linear porokeratosis.[172] Longitudinal depressions distal to areas where inflammatory cells disrupt the nail matrix architecture are the most common finding, although subungual tumors and pitting have also been noted. Successful treatments have not been reported, but nails return to normal if the inflammatory process is transient (e.g., lichen niditus).

TWENTY-NAIL DYSTROPHY

The term *20-nail dystrophy of childhood* (Fig. 7–14) was popularized by Hazelrigg and colleagues in a report of children with acquired trachyonychia of all 20 nails.[173] The authors acknowledged Samman's prior observations of exaggerated closely spaced longitudinal striations several years earlier[174] and suggested that when the sign is found in children it could represent a distinct clinical entity. The original six cases were characterized not only by excess longitudinal ridging but also by onychorrhexis, onychoschizia, distal chipping, a dull opalescent appearance of the thin nail plates, and a yellowish onychauxis of the great toenails. The onset of these asymptomatic changes was insidious and was noted to occur either in all nails simultaneously or in individual nails gradually over many months. Onychomycosis was absent, and mucocutaneous signs of other diseases such as alopecia areata, lichen planus, psoriasis, or ectodermal dysplasias were not present on examination. However, biopsies of the nail unit and prospective follow-up were not reported. Thus, subsequent investigators suggested that

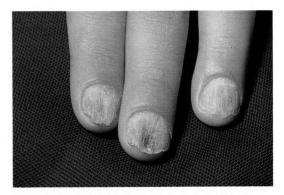

Figure 7–14. Twenty-nail dystrophy of childhood—trachyonychia without distinct pitting. From Schachner L (ed): Advances in Dermatology. Year Book Medical, Chicago, in press.

the 20-nail dystrophy of childhood represents one or more recognizable disease states. Scher and colleagues, Zaias, and Donofrio and Ayala performed biopsies on several patients and uncovered histopathologic findings of lichen planus.[175–177] Silverman and Rhodes also discovered biopsy-proven oral lichen planus in a child with a long-standing dystrophy of all 20 nails.[178] Baran and Dupre observed several cases of "vertical striated sandpaper nails" with identical morphology and alopecia areata.[179] Nail dystrophy of alopecia areata may persist long after the effluvium has resolved or may precede hair loss by many months.[180–182] Biopsies of other patients have revealed eczematous changes.[183] Additional associations include immunoglobulin A deficiency[184] and ichthyosis vulgaris.[185] Twins, familial and congenital 20-nail dystrophy, and similar findings in adults have also been reported.[186–189]

Most cases of idiopathic 20-nail dystrophy in children gradually resolve spontaneously over several years, although a few cases have persisted into adulthood.[190] Treatment with topical corticosteroid solutions applied to the proximal nail fold may be attempted, although premature closure of underlying epiphyses is a risk. Intramatrix injections with triamcinolone are reportedly beneficial,[176] but the pain of the procedure and the need for repetitive injections limit its usefulness in small children. Close clipping of the distal nail plate minimizes traumatic onychorrhexis. Clear nail hardeners may improve appearance.

PARONYCHIA

Paronychia is one of the more common ungual disorders confronting pediatricians and family physicians. Traumatic disruption of the cuticle leads to proliferation of infecting organisms in the open nail fold sulcus. The folds become red, rounded, tender, and retracted, preventing readhesion of the cuticle.[191] Purulent material may not collect in a child's paronychia because of thumb sucking and mouthing of digits, which reduces associated pain. This habit unfortunately results in further maceration and perpetuation of the moist environment that promotes infection. Paronychia may be accompanied by an undulating nail plate dystrophy, because sucking injures the nail matrix intermittently over several months.

Mouthing of digits of the hands and feet is a normal developmental response that begins about 6 months of age and peaks after 1 year of age. This activity may be a response to teething or may be pleasurable in itself.[192] Substitutes for this extranutritional sucking may be sought to promote the healing of paronychia that has already been established. However, local therapy and education of the concerned parents regarding the transient nature of the problem should be all that is needed.

Thumb sucking or mouthing of digits may occur at bedtime or naptime until 4 years of age. Daytime sucking past that age is considered pathologic by some development or behavior specialists. Substitution of a bottle or a pacifier may alleviate paronychia but may produce unwanted dental caries or dental malalignment.

Therapy for childhood paronychia should be directed at drying the affected digits as well as killing any *Candida* or bacteria that may be present. Applications of thymol (4 per cent) in chloroform to the nail will dry out the moist areas.[193] Mycostatin or clotrimazole drops several times daily should inhibit any fungal growth. Concurrent oral treatment may be helpful in some situations. Topical clindamycin (Cleocin T) solution applied to the fingers several times daily has been successful in many cases. This preparation kills bacteria, has a bitter taste to discourage sucking, and has an alcohol–propylene glycol vehicle that dries out residual moisture. Side effects from oral absorption of these medications have not been reported. Comparative studies have also not been performed. Attempts at behavior modification to control pathologic thumb sucking have been disappointing.[194] Gloves or other inhibitory devices can be taken off. Digital splints to attenuate the pleasurable sensory input from the activity have been reported to be transiently effective. Other behavior modification programs that substitute positive reinforcers for the sucking activity need to be developed.[195]

Simultaneous paronychia on digits of the hands and feet of a child who is failing to thrive, is suffering from recurrent infections (e.g., otitis, pneumonia), or has a cutaneous eruption that is unresponsive to topical therapy should prompt careful examination for underlying systemic disease (Table 7–10).[196–198] Clinical signs of brittleness, trachyonychia, onycholysis, or subungual hyperkeratosis are nonspecific signs of direct nail matrix involve-

Table 7–10. SYSTEMIC DISEASES ASSOCIATED WITH CHILDHOOD PARONYCHIA

Disease	Diagnostic Procedure
Mucocutaneous candidiasis	Potassium hydroxide (KOH) scraping
Acrodermatitis enteropathica[196]	Plasma zinc level
Histiocytosis X[197]	Biopsy
Reiter's syndrome[198]	HLA typing

HLA, human leukocyte antigen.

ment by these processes. Paronychia with subungual purpura is quite specific for histiocytosis X. The capillary nail fold telangiectasis of lupus erythematosus and dermatomyositis should be differentiated from true paronychia of other disease states.

INGROWN NAILS

Ingrown nails in children have generally been attributed to similar factors found in adults. Poorly fitted shoes, overzealous manicuring, or onychopagia of the nail plate so that the lateral free edge grows into the nail fold are blamed most often.[199] Congenital malalignment of the great toenails[200] as well as trauma from repetitive bicycling movements while lying prone in tight-fitting occlusive jumpsuits have also been suggested to play an etiologic role.[201] As mentioned earlier, the relative shortness of some infants' toenails that seem to bury into the distal digital pulp should not be confused with true ingrown nails.[202] Methods for treatment of ingrown nails in children are not unlike procedures used in adults. Early ingrown nails caused by improper cutting may be packed with gauze under the lateral hyponychium. This and applications of an anti-inflammatory solution may be all that is needed. In other circumstances, surgical or chemosurgical ablation of the offending lateral matrix may be necessary.[203,204] The Zadik procedure of nail bed ablation has been reported to result in a low recurrence rate in the hands of some surgeons.[205]

NAIL BITING IN CHILDREN

It has been estimated that at least 50 per cent of children exhibit onychophagia for short periods of time.[206] Fortunately, this behavior diminishes during adolescence when body image becomes of primary concern. Ony-

chophagia in early childhood should alert the physician to check for Lesch-Nyhan syndrome.[207] It may also serve as a means of spread of warts or other infectious agents. For girls, application of colored nail polish highlights damage and may heighten awareness of the activity, thus making the activity consciously unpleasant to perform. The habit in some children may be amenable to behavior modification or hypnosis.[208,209]

CHROMONYCHIA

It is unusual for parents to complain of the color of their child's nails. Leukonychia punctata resulting from trauma is quite common. Exogenous staining from dyes used in crayons and fingerpaints and ink may also be a nuisance.

Familial total or partial leukonychia has been reported to occur in both an autosomal dominant and recessive pattern.[210,211] It has been associated with pili torti,[212] multiple sebaceous cysts with renal calculi,[213] knuckle pads with deafness,[214] and duodenal ulcers with gallstones.[215]

Yellow nails may also be observed in children.[216] Familial lymphedema of the Meige type is associated with swelling and yellow nails developing around puberty, whereas Milroy's disease has its onset during the neonatal period.[217] Treatment with oral alpha-tocopherol, reported to be effective in adults, has not been attempted in children.[218] A yellowish-brown discoloration of nail plates may also be noted in the 20-nail dystrophy of childhood.[173,219]

TUMORS OF THE NAIL APPARATUS IN CHILDREN

Periungual warts are the most common tumor impinging on the nail unit in children. Therapy for these virus-induced lesions should be tailored for the age of the patient and the amount of disability that is present. An attempt to cover the wart should be made, because children frequently bite the wart and spread virus to the lips and face. An atraumatic approach to the treatment of warts in young children is important. A calm explanation of the benign and limited nature of this cutaneous viral infection is most important. Electrosurgery, cryotherapy, or other painful office procedures may result only in antago-

Table 7–11. **TUMORS OF THE NAIL APPARATUS IN CHILDREN**

Koenen's tumors (angiofibromas of tuberous sclerosis)[220]
Exostoses[221]
Digital fibromas[222]
Pyogenic granulomas
Angiokeratomas[223]
Enchondromas of Maffucci's syndrome
Hemangiomas of blue rubber bleb nevus or Klippel-
   Trenaunay-Weber syndrome
Osteochondromas[224]
Juvenile xanthogranuloma[225]
Incontinentia pigmenti[226]

nizing parents of a fearful, crying, struggling young infant. In addition, the infant patient will then be unaccepting of such treatments in later years when office surgery may be necessary.

Other tumors are infrequently observed in children (Table 7–11).[220] They may present as tender, firm, dusky red to blue subcutaneous nodules located adjacent to the proximal nail folds or as flesh-colored papules that extend out from under the nail folds. X-ray films should be obtained on all suspected tumors to rule out osseous involvement. Narrow or wide longitudinal grooves may be produced by tumors compressing the matrix. Careful surgical excision may result in regrowth of a normal nail plate.

References

1. Zaias N: Embryology of the human nail. Arch Dermatol 87:37, 1963.
2. Lamberti G, et al: The role of skin and its appendages in the assessment of a newborn's maturity. J Perinat Med [Suppl] 9:147, 1981.
3. Honig PJ, Spitzer A, Bernstein R, et al: Congenital ingrown toenails. Clinical significance. Clin Pediatr 21:424, 1982.
4. Syme J, Riley ID: Nail-fold capillary loop development in the infant of low birth weight. Br J Dermatol 83:591, 1970.
5. Sirota L, Straussberg R, Fishman P, et al: X-ray microanalysis of the fingernails in term and preterm infants. Pediatr Dermatol 5:184, 1988.
6. Baran R, Dawber RPR: Diseases of the Nails and Their Management. Blackwell Scientific Publications, Oxford, England, 1984, p 33.
7. Almagor G, Haim S: Familial koilonychia. Dermatologica 162:400, 1981.
8. Bergeron JR, Stone OJ: Koilonychia. A report of familial spoon nails. Arch Dermatol 95:351, 1967.
9. Turano AF: Transverse nail ridging in early infancy. Pediatrics 41:996, 1968.
10. Wolf D, Wolf R, Goldberg MD: Beau's lines. A case report. Cutis 29:191, 1982.
11. Hillman RW: The fingernail growth in the human subject. Rates and variations in 300 individuals. Hum Biol 27:274, 1955.
12. Hamilton JB, Terda H, Mestler GE: Studies of growth throughout the lifespan in Japanese: Growth and size of nails and their relationship to age, sex, heredity and other factors. J Gerontol 10:401, 1955.
13. Baran R, Bureau H: Congenital malalignment of the big toenail as a cause of ingrowing toenail in infancy. Pathology and treatment (a study of 30 cases). Clin Exp Dermatol 8:619, 1983.
14. Dawson TAJ: An inherited nail dystrophy principally affecting the great toe nails. Clin Exp Dermatol 4:309, 1979.
15. Harper KJ, Beer WE: Congenital malalignment of the great toe nails—An inherited condition. Clin Exp Dermatol 11:514, 1986.
16. Barth JH, Dawber RPR: Congenital malalignment of great toenails in two sets of monozygotic twins. Arch Dermatol 122:379, 1986.
17. Baran R: Congenital malalignment of the big toenail: A new subtype. Arch Dermatol 123:437, 1987.
18. Handfield-Jones SE, Harman RRM: Spontaneous improvement of congenital malalignment of the great toe nails. Br J Dermatol 118:305, 1988.
19. Baran R, Bureau H: Two post-operative epidermoid cysts following realignment of the hallux nail. Br J Dermatol 119:245, 1988.
20. Iso R: Congenital nail defects of the index finger and reconstructive surgery. Orthop Surg 20:1383, 1969.
21. Hammerton MD, Shrank AB: Congenital hypertrophy of the lateral nail folds of the hallux. Pediatr Dermatol 5:243, 1988.
22. Hopeu-Havru VK, Jansen CT: Anonychia congenita. Arch Dermatol 107:752, 1973.
23. Timerman I, Miseteanu C, Simionescu NN: Dominant anonychia onychodystrophy. J Med Genet 6:105, 1969.
24. Rahbari H, Heath L, Chapel TA: Anonychia with ectrodactyly. Arch Dermatol 111:1482, 1975.
25. Torpin R: Fetal Malformations Caused by Amnion Rupture. Charles C Thomas, Springfield, IL, 1965, p 120.
26. Verbov J: Anonychia with bizarre flexural pigmentation: An autosomal dominant dermatosis. Br J Dermatol 92:469, 1975.
27. Millman AJ, Strier RP: Congenital onychodysplasia of the index fingers. Report of a family. J Am Acad Dermatol 7:57, 1982.
28. Kitayama Y, Tsukada S: Congenital onychodysplasia. Report of 11 cases. Arch Dermatol 119:8, 1983.
29. Baran R, Stroud JD: Congenital onychodysplasia of the index fingers—Iso and Kikuchi syndrome. Arch Dermatol 120:243, 1984.
30. Kikuchi I: Congenital polynychias, reduction versus duplication digit malformations. Int J Dermatol 24:211, 1985.
31. Katayama I, Maeda M, Nishioka K: Congenital ectopic nail of the fifth finger. Br J Dermatol 111:231, 1984.
32. Kalisman M, Kleinert HE: A circumferential fingernail: Fingernail on the palmar aspect of the finger. J Hand Surg 8:58, 1983.
33. Bass HN: Familial absence of middle phalanges with nail dysplasia: A new syndrome. Pediatrics 42:318, 1968.
34. Robinow M, Pfeiffer RA, Gorlin RJ, et al: Acrodystosis, a syndrome of peripheral dysostosis, nasal hypoplasia and mental retardation. Am J Dis Child 121:195, 1971.

35. Cheney WD: Acro-osteolysis. Am J Roentgenol 94:595, 1965.
36. Blank CE: Apert's syndrome (a type of acrocephalosyndactyly): Observations on British series of 39 cases. Ann Hum Genet 24:151, 1960.
37. Schott GD: Heredity bradydactyly with nail dysplasia. J Med Genet 15:119, 1978.
38. McKusick VA, Eldridge R, Hostetler JA, et al: Dwarfism in the Amish: II. Cartilage-hair hypoplasia. Bull Johns Hopkins Hosp 116:285, 1965.
39. Happle R, Koch H, Zenz W: The C.H.I.L.D. syndrome. Congenital hemidysplasia with ichthyosiform erythroderma and limb defects. Eur J Pediatr 134:27, 1980.
40. Spranger JW, Langer LO, Wiedemann HR: Bone Dysplasias: An Atlas of Constitutional Disorders of Skeletal Development. WB Saunders, Philadelphia, 1974, pp 254–257.
41. Gorlin RJ, Cohen MM: Frontometaphaseal dysplasia: A new syndrome. Am J Dis Child 118:487, 1969.
42. Latta RJ, Graham CB, Aase J, et al: Larsen's syndrome: A skeletal dysplasia with multiple joint dislocations and unusual facies. J Pediatr 78:291, 1971.
43. Hambrick GW, Carter MD: Pachydermoperiostosis. Arch Dermatol 94:594, 1966.
44. Mace JW, Kaplan JM, Schamberger JE, et al: Poland's syndrome. Clin Pediatr 11:98, 1972.
45. DeBusk FL: The Hutchinson-Gilford progeria syndrome. J Pediatr 80:697, 1972.
46. Puretic S, Puretic B, Fiser-Herman M, et al: A unique form of mesenchymal displasia. Br J Dermatol 74:8, 1962.
47. Elmore SM: Pycnodysostosis: A review. J Bone Joint Surg 49A:153, 1967.
48. McKusick VA, Mahloudji M, Abbott MH, et al: Seckel's bird-headed dwarfism. N Engl J Med 277:279, 1967.
49. Sugiura Y, Yashuhare T: Sclerosteosis. J Bone Joint Surg 57A:273, 1975.
50. Dudding BA, Gorlin RJ, Langer LO: The oto-palatodigital syndrome. A new symptom complex consisting of deafness, dwarfism, cleft palate, characteristic facies and a generalized bone dysplasia. Am J Dis Child 113:214, 1967.
51. Jones KL, Smith DW: The Williams elfin facies syndrome. A new perspective. J Pediatr 86:718, 1975.
52. Kucirka SJ, Scher RK: Heritable nail disorders. *In* Alper JC (ed): The Genodermatoses. Dermatol Clin 5:179, 1987.
53. Little EM: Congenital absence or delayed development of the patella. Lancet 2:781, 1897.
54. Lucas GL, Opitz JM: The nail-patella syndrome: Clinical and genetic aspects of 5 kindreds with 38 affected family members. J Pediatr 68:273, 1966.
55. Burkhart CG, Bhumbra R, Iannone AM: Nail-patella syndrome: A distinctive clinical and electron microscopic presentation. J Am Acad Dermatol 3:251, 1980.
56. Daniel CR, Osment LS, Noojin RO: Triangular lunulae: A clue to the nail-patella syndrome. Arch Dermatol 116:448, 1980.
57. Carbonara P, Alpert M: Hereditary osteo-onychodysplasia (HOOD). Am J Med Sci 248:139, 1964.
58. Sybert VP: Aplasia cutis congenita: A report of 12 new families and review of the literature. Pediatr Dermatol 3:1, 1985.
59. Smith DW, Jones KL: Recognizable Patterns of Human Malformation, ed 3. WB Saunders, Philadelphia, 1982, pp 10–13.
60. Warkany J, Rissarge E, Smith LB: Congenital malformation in autosomal trisomy syndromes. Am J Dis Child 112:502, 1966.
61. Smith DW, Jones KL: Recognizable Patterns of Human Malformation, ed 3. WB Saunders, Philadelphia, 1982, pp 18–23.
62. DeGrouchy J, Turleau C: Clinical Atlas of Human Chromosomes, ed 2. John Wiley & Sons, New York, 1984, pp 148–154.
63. Smith DW, Jones KL: Recognizable Patterns of Human Malformation, ed 3. WB Saunders, Philadelphia, 1982, pp 158–163.
64. Clark CE, Telfer MA, Cowell HR: A case of partial trisomy 8p resulting from a maternal balanced translocation. Am J Med Genet 7:21, 1980.
65. Schmid M, Wolf J, Nestler H, et al: Partial trisomy of the long arm of chromosome 7 due to familial balanced translocation. Hum Genet 49:283, 1979.
66. Guthrie RE, Case JM, Asper AC, et al: The 4 p-, a clinically recognizable chromosome deletion syndrome. Am J Dis Child 122:421, 1971.
67. Dubowitz V, Cooke P, Colver D, et al: Mental retardation, unusual facies and abnormal nails associated with a group G ring chromosome. J Med Genet 8:195, 1971.
68. Lemli L, Smith DW: The XO syndrome: A study of the differential phenotype in 25 patients. J Pediatr 63:577, 1963.
69. Smith DW, Jones KL: Recognizable Patterns of Human Malformation, ed 3. WB Saunders, Philadelphia, 1982, pp 134–141.
70. Johnson RB, Goldsmith LA: Dilantin digital effects. J Am Acad Dermatol 5:191, 1981.
71. Crain LS, Fitzmaurice NE, Mondry C: Nail dysplasia and fetal alcohol syndrome. Case report of a heteropaternal sibship. Am J Dis Child 137:1069, 1983.
72. Kosem RC, Lightner ES: Phenotypic malformations in association with maternal trimethadione therapy. J Pediatr 92:240, 1978.
73. Pettifor JM, Benson R: Congenital malformations with the administration of oral anticoagulants during pregnancy. J Pediatr 86:459, 1975.
74. Solomon LM, Keuer EJ: The ectodermal dysplasias: Problems of classification and some newer syndromes. Arch Dermatol 116:1295, 1980.
75. Freire-Maia N: Ectodermal dysplasias. Hum Hered 21:309, 1971.
76. Freire-Maia N, Penheiro M: Ectodermal Dysplasias: A Clinical and Genetic Study. Alan R Liss, New York, 1984.
77. Thurman J: Two cases in which the skin, hair and teeth were very imperfectly developed. Proc R Med Chir Soc 31:71, 1848.
78. Weech AA: Hereditary ectodermal dysplasia, congenital ectodermal defect: A report of 2 cases. Am J Dis Child 37:766, 1929.
79. Reed WB, Lopez DA, Landing B: Clinical spectrum of anhidrotic ectodermal dysplasia. Arch Dermatol 102:134, 1979.
80. Crump IA, Danks DM: Hypohidrotic ectodermal dysplasia. J Pediatr 78:466, 1971.
81. Goltz RW, Henderson RR, Hitch JM, et al: Focal dermal hypoplasia syndrome. A review of the literature and report of 2 cases. Arch Dermatol 101:1, 1970.
82. Rosselli D, Gulienetti R: Ectodermal dysplasia. Br J Plast Surg 14:190, 1961.
83. Gutman A, Frunskin A, Adam A, et al: X-linked dyskeratosis congenita with pancytopenia. Arch Dermatol 114:1667, 1978.

84. Stasiowska B, Sartous S, Goitre M, et al: Rapp-Hodgkin ectodermal dysplasia syndrome. Arch Dis Child 56:793, 1981.
85. Rudiger RA, Haase W, Passarge E: Association of ectrodactyly, ectodermal dysplasia and cleft lip-palate: The EEC syndrome. Am J Dis Child 120:160, 1970.
86. Hay RJ, Wells RS: The syndrome of ankyloblepharon, ectodermal defects and cleft lip and palate. An autosomal dominant condition. Br J Dermatol 94:277, 1976.
87. Koshiba H, Kimura O, Nakata M, et al: Clinical, genetic and histologic features of trichoonychodental (TOD) syndrome. Oral Surg 46:376, 1978.
88. Cram DL, Resneck JS, Jackson WB: A congenital icthyosiform syndrome with deafness and keratitis. Arch Dermatol 115:467, 1979.
89. Gorlin RJ, Sedano H, Anderson VE: The syndrome of palmar-plantar hyperkeratosis and premature periodontal destruction of the teeth. A clinical and genetic analysis of Papillon-Lefevre syndrome. J Pediatr 65:895, 1964.
90. Takematsu H, Sato S, Igarashi M, et al: Incontinentia pigmenti achromians (Ito). Arch Dermatol 119:391, 1983.
91. Bergasma D: Birth Defects Compendium, ed 2. Alan R Liss, New York, 1979, p 138.
92. Rajagopalan K, Tay CH: Hidrotic ectodermal dysplasia. Study of a large Chinese pedigree. Arch Dermatol 113:481, 1977.
93. Wilkinson RD, Schopflocher P, Rozenfeld M: Hidrotic ectodermal dysplasia with diffuse eccrine poromatosis. Arch Dermatol 113:472, 1977.
94. Hazen P, Zamora I, Bruner WE, et al: Premature cataracts in a family with hidrotic ectodermal dysplasia. Arch Dermatol 116:1385, 1980.
95. Taylor WA. Rothmund's syndrome: Thomson's syndrome. Arch Dermatol 75:236, 1957.
96. Carey JC, Hall BD: The Coffin-Siris syndrome. Five new cases including two siblings. Am J Dis Child 132:667, 1978.
97. Shapiro SD, Quattromani FL, Jorgenson RJ, et al: Tricho-dento-osseous syndrome: Heterogeneity or clinical variability. Am J Med Genet 16:225, 1983.
98. Fried K: Autosomal recessive hidrotic ectodermal dysplasia. J Med Genet 14:137, 1977.
99. Ackerman JL, Ackerman AL, Ackerman AB: A new dental, ocular and cutaneous syndrome. Int J Dermatol 12:285, 1973.
100. Gidion A, Burdea M, Fruchter Z, et al: Autosomal dominant transmission of tricho-rhino-phalangeal syndrome: Report of 4 unrelated families, review of 60 cases. Helv Pediatr Acta 28:249, 1973.
101. McKusick VA, Egeland JA, Eldrige R, et al: Dwarfism in the Amish. I. The Ellis-van Creveld syndrome. Bull Johns Hopkins Hosp 115:306, 1964.
102. Smith DW, Knudson RW: Aberrant scalp hair patterning in hypohidrotic ectodermal dysplasia. J Pediatr 90:248, 1977.
103. Pabst HF, Groth O, McCoy EE: Hypohidrotic ectodermal dysplasia with hypothyroidism. J Pediatr 98:223, 1981.
104. Witkop CJ, Brearly LJ, Gentry WC: Hypoplastic enamel onycholysis and hypohidrosis inherited as autosomal dominant trait: A review of ectodermal dysplasia syndromes. Oral Surg 39:71, 1975.
105. Sparrow GP, Samman PD, Wells RS: Hyperpigmentation and hypohidrosis (the Naegli-Franceschetti-Jadassohn syndrome): Report of a family and review of the literature. Clin Exp Dermatol 1:127, 1976.
106. Howell RR, Arbeser AI, Parsons DS, et al: The Sabinas syndrome. Am J Hum Genet 33:957, 1981.
107. Touriello HV, Lindstrom JA, Waterman DF, et al: Re-evaluation of CHANDS. J Med Genet 16:316, 1979.
108. Cantu JM, Arias J, Foncerrada M, et al: Syndrome of onychotrichodysplasia with chronic neutropenia in an infant from consanguineous parents. Birth Defects II:63, 1975.
109. Price VH, Odom RB, Ward WH, et al: Trichothiodystrophy. Arch Dermatol 116:1375, 1980.
110. Nevin NC, Thomas PS, Calvert J, et al: Deafness, onycho-osteodystrophy, mental retardation (DOOR) syndrome. Am J Med Genet 13:325–332, 1982.
111. Shapiro SD, Jorgenson RJ, Salinas CF: Brief clinical report: Curry-Hall syndrome. Am J Med Genet 17:579, 1984.
112. Reed T, Schreiner RL: Absence of dermal ridge patterns: Genetic heterogeneity. Am J Med Genet 16:81, 1983.
113. Milligan A, Graham-Brown RAC: Vitiligo and nail dystrophy. Clin Exp Dermatol 14:175, 1989.
114. Schonfeld PHIR: The pachyonychia congenita syndrome. Acta Derm Venereal (Stock) 60:45, 1980.
115. Jadassohn J, Lewandowsky F: Pachyonychia congenita. Ikonograph Dermatol 1:29, 1906.
116. Hordinsky M, LaVilla S, Panter S, et al: Differential nail protein expression in two ectodermal dysplasias (abstract). Clin Res 37:706, 1989.
117. Thomas DR, Jorizzo JL, Brysk MM, et al: Pachyonychia congenita: Electron microscopic and epidermal glycoprotein assessment before and during isotret-inoin treatment. Arch Dermatol 120:1475, 1984.
118. Hoting E, Wassilew SW: Systemische Retinoidtherapie mit Etretinate bei Pachyonychia congenita. Hautarzt 36:526, 1985.
119. Blank H: Treatment of pachyonychia congenita with phenytoin. Br J Dermatol 106:21, 1982.
120. Cosman B, Symonds FC, Crukelair GF: Plastic surgery in pachyonychia congenita and other dyskeratoses: Case report and review of the literature. J Plast Reconstr Surg 33:229, 1964.
121. White RR, Noone RB: Pachyonychia congenita (Jadassohn-Lewandowski syndrome). Case report. J Plast Reconstr Surg 59:855, 1977.
122. Thomasen RJ, Zuchlke RL, Beckman BI: Pachyonychia congenita: Surgical management of the nail changes. J Dermatol Surg Oncol 8:24, 1982.
123. Harms M, Gilardi S, Levy PM, et al: KID syndrome (keratitis, ichthyosis, and deafness) and chronic mucocutaneous candidiasis: Case report and review of the literature. Pediatr Dermatol 2:1, 1984.
124. Menter MA, Whiting DA, McWilliams J: Resistant childhood psoriasis: Analysis of patients seen in a day care center. Pediatr Dermatol 2:8, 1984.
125. Woo TY, Rasmussen JE: Subungual osteocartilaginous exostosis. J Dermatol Surg Oncol 11:534, 1985.
126. Gibbs RC: Toe nail diseases secondary to poorly fitting shoes or abnormal biomechanics. Cutis 36:399, 1985.
127. Vidabaek H: Hereditary onychogryphosis. Ann Eugen 14:139, 1948.
128. Lubach D: Erbliche onychogryphosis. Hautarzt 33:331, 1982.
129. Eqawa T: Congenital claw-like fingers and toes. Plast Reconstr Surg 59:569, 1977.
130. Graybill JR, Herndon JH, Knicker WT, et al: Ketoconazole treatment of chronic mucocutaneous candidiasis. Arch Dermatol 116:1137, 1980.

131. Hay RJ, Clayton YM: The treatment of patients with chronic mucocutaneous candidiasis and candida onychomycosis with ketoconazole. Clin Exp Dermatol 7:155, 1982.

132. Fanconi S, Seger R, Joller P, et al: Intermittent ketoconazole therapy in chronic mucocutaneous candidiasis in childhood. Eur J Pediatr 139:176, 1982.

133. Horsburgh CR, Kirkpatrick CH: Long-term therapy of chronic mucocutaneous candidiasis with ketoconazole: Experience with twenty-one patients. Am J Med [Suppl] 74:23, 1983.

134. Roberton DM, Hosking CS: Ketoconazole treatment of nail infection in chronic mucocutaneous candidiasis. Aust Paediatr J 19:178, 1983.

135. Murphy WF, Langley AL: Common bullous lesions, presumably self-inflicted, occurring in utero in the newborn infant. Pediatrics 32:1099, 1963.

136. Haber RM, Hanna W, Ramsay CA, et al: Hereditary epidermolysis bullosa. J Am Acad Dermatol 13:252, 1985.

137. Schachner LA, Press S: Vesicular, bullous and pustular disorders. In Schachner LA, Hansen RC (eds): Pediatric Dermatology. Churchill Livingstone, New York, 1988.

138. Fischer T, Gedde-Dahl T Jr: Epidermolysis bullosa simplex and mottled pigmentation: A new dominant syndrome. Clin Genet 15:228, 1979.

139. Olaisen B, Gedde-Dahl T Jr: GPT-epidermolysis bullosa simplex (EBS Ogna) linkage in man. Hum Hered 23:189, 1973.

140. Anton-Lamprecht I, Schnyder VW: Epidermolysis bullosa herpetiformis Dowling Meara. Dermatologica 164:221, 1982.

141. Pearson RW, Potter B, Strauss F: Epidermolysis bullosa hereditaria letalis. Arch Dermatol 109:349, 1974.

142. Hintner H, Wolff K: Generalized atrophic benign epidermolysis bullosa. Arch Dermatol 118:375, 1982.

143. Schnyder VW, Anton-Lamprecht I: Zur Klinik der epidermolysa mit junkionaler blasenbiddung. Dermatologica 159:402, 1979.

144. Gedde-Dahl T Jr: Epidermolysis bullosa: A clinical, genetic and epidemiological study. Johns Hopkins University Press, Baltimore, 1971.

145. Oakley CA, Gawkrodger DR, Ross JA, et al: The Cockayne-Touraine type of dominant dystrophic epidermolysis bullosa: Ultrastructural similarities to the Pasini variant. Acta Dermatol Venereol (Stockh) 64:253, 1983.

146. Sasai Y, Saito N, Seji M: Epidermolysis bullosa dystrophica et albo-papuloidea. Arch Dermatol 108:554, 1973.

147. Pearson RW: Studies on the pathogenesis of epidermolysis bullosa. J Invest Dermatol 52:449, 1969.

148. Hashimoto I, Anton-Lamprecht I, Haufbauer M: Epidermolysis bullosa dystrophica inversa. Hautarzt 27:532, 1976.

149. Kindler T: Congenital poikiloderma with traumatic bulla formation and progressive cutaneous atrophy. Br J Dermatol 66:104, 1954.

150. Bart BJ, Gorlin RJ, Anderson VE, et al: Congenital localized absence of skin and associated abnormalities resembling epidermolysis bullosa. Arch Dermatol 93:296, 1966.

151. Fine JD, Osment LS, Gay S: Dystrophic epidermolysis bullosa: A new variant characterized by progressive symmetrical centripital involvement with scarring. Arch Dermatol 121:1014, 1985.

152. Sinniah D, Sandeford BR, Dugdale AE: Subungual infection in the newborn: An institutional outbreak of unknown etiology, possibly due to Vielonella. Clin Pediatr 11:690, 1972.

153. Hays GC, Mullard JE: Blistering distal dactylitis: A clinically recognizable streptococcal infection. Pediatrics 56:129, 1975.

154. McCray MK, Esterly NB: Blistering distal dactylitis. J Am Acad Dermatol 5:592, 1981.

155. Schneider JA, Parlette HL: Blistering distal dactylitis: A manifestation of group A β-hemolytic streptococcal infection. Arch Dermatol 118:879, 1982.

156. Feder HM, Long SS: Herpetic whitlow, epidemiology, clinical characteristics, diagnosis and treatment. Am J Dis Child 137:861, 1983.

157. Hansen RC: Blindness, anonychia and oral mucosal scarring at sequelae of the Stevens-Johnson syndrome. Pediatr Dermatol 1:298, 1984.

158. Melish ME: Kawasaki syndrome (mucocutaneous lymph node syndrome). Pediatr Rev 2:107, 1980.

159. Kawasaki T, Kosaki F, Okawa S, et al: A new infantile acute febrile mucocutaneous lymph node syndrome (MLNS) prevailing in Japan. Pediatrics 54:271, 1974.

160. Rowley AH, Duffy CE, Shulman S: Prevention of giant coronary artery aneurysms in Kawasaki disease by intravenous gamma globulin therapy. J Pediatr 113:290, 1988.

161. Boiko S, Kaufman RA, Lucky AW: Osteomyelitis of the distal phalanges in three children with severe atopic dermatitis. Arch Dermatol 124:418, 1988.

162. Hjorth N, Thomsen KZ: Parakeratosis pustulosa. Br J Dermatol 79:527, 1967.

163. deDulanto F, Armujo-Moreno M, Camacho-Martinez F: Parakeratosis pustulosa: Histological findings. Acta Dermatovenereol 54:365, 1974.

164. Daniel CR, Scher RK: Nail changes secondary to systemic drugs or ingestants. J Am Acad Dermatol 10:250, 1984.

165. Saurat JH, Glickman E: Lichen planus-like eruption following bone marrow transplantation: A manifestation of the graft-versus-host disease. Clin Exp Dermatol 2:325, 1977.

166. Saurat JH: Cutaneous manifestations of graft-versus-host disease. Int J Dermatol 20:249, 1981.

167. Gutjahr P, Schmitt HJ: Caring of the nails and anticancer treatment. Eur J Pediatr 143:74, 1984.

168. Landwehr AJ, Starink TM: Inflammatory linear verrucous epidermal nevus: Report of a case with bilateral distribution and nail involvement. Dermatologica 166:107, 1983.

169. Mascaro JM, Palou J, Vives P: Painful subungual keratotic tumors in incontinentia pigmenti. J Am Acad Dermatol 131:913, 1985.

170. Meyers M, Storino W, Barsky S: Lichen striatus with nail dystrophy. Arch Dermatol 114:964, 1978.

171. Kellett JK, Beck MH: Lichen niditus associated with distinctive nail changes. Clin Exp Dermatol 9:201, 1984.

172. Rahbari H, Cordero AA, Mehregan AH: Linear porokeratosis: A distinctive clinical variant of porokeratosis of Mibelli. Arch Dermatol 109:526, 1974.

173. Hazelrigg DE, Duncan WC, Jarratt M: Twenty-nail dystrophy of childhood. Arch Dermatol 113:73, 1977.

174. Samman PD: The Nails in Disease. William Heinemann, London, 1965, p 122.

175. Scher RK, Fischbein R, Ackerman AB: Twenty-nail dystrophy a variant of lichen planus. Arch Dermatol 114:612, 1978.

176. Zaias N: The Nail in Health and Diseases. Spectrum Publications, New York, 1980, p 126.

177. Donofrio P, Ayala F: Twenty-nail dystrophy: Report of a case and review of the literature. Acta Derm Venereol (Stockh) 64:180, 1984.

178. Silverman RA, Rhodes AR: Twenty-nail dystrophy of childhood: A sign of localized lichen planus. Pediatr Dermatol 1:207, 1984.

179. Baran R, Dupre A: Vertical striated sandpaper nails. Arch Dermatol 113:1613, 1977.

180. Wilkinson JD, Dawber RPR, Bowers RP, et al: Twenty-nail dystrophy of childhood: Case report and histopathological findings. Br J Dermatol 100:217, 1979.

181. Braun-Falco O, Dorn M, Neubert V, et al: Trachyonychie: 20-nagel dystrophie. Hautarzt 32:17, 1981.

182. Horn RT, Odom RB: Twenty-nail dystrophy of alopecia areata. Arch Dermatol 116:573, 1980.

183. Samman PD: Trachyonychia (rough nails). Br J Dermatol 101:701, 1979.

184. Leong AB, Gange RW, O'Connor RD: Twenty-nail dystrophy (trachyonychia) associated with selective IgA deficiency. J Pediatr 100:418, 1982.

185. James WD, Odom RB, Horn RT: Twenty-nail dystrophy and icthyosis vulgaris. Arch Dermatol 117:316, 1981.

186. Pavone L, Volti SL, Guarneri B, et al: Hereditary twenty-nail dystrophy in a Sicilian family. J Med Genet 19:337, 1982.

187. Arias AM, Yung CW, Rendler S, et al: Familial severe twenty-nail dystrophy. J Am Acad Dermatol 7:349, 1982.

188. Bruynzeel DP, Frankenmolen-Witkiewicz IM: Twenty-nail dystrophy in adults. Arch Dermatol 116:862, 1980.

189. Commens CA: Twenty nail dystrophy in identical twins. Pediatr Dermatol 5:117, 1988.

190. Civatte MJ: Ongles greses et "twenty-nail dystrophy of childhood" a propos de 2 cas. Dermatologica 168:242, 1984.

191. Stone OJ, Mullins JF: Chronic paronychia in children. Clin Pediatr 7:104, 1968.

192. Brazelton TB: Infant thumbsucking. JAMA 252:945, 1984.

193. Wilson JW: Paronychia and onycholysis, etiology and therapy. Arch Dermatol 92:726, 1965.

194. Lewis M, Shelton P, Fuqua RW: Parental control of nocturnal thumbsucking. J Behav Ther Exp Psychiatry 12:87, 1981.

195. Schloss PJ, Johann M: A modeling and contingency management approach to pacifier withdrawal. Behav Ther 13:254, 1982.

196. Shaw JCL: Trace elements in the fetus and young infant: I. Zinc. Am J Dis Child 133:1260, 1979.

197. Timpatanapong P, Hathirat P, Isarangkura P: Nail involvement in histiocytosis X: A 12-year retrospective study. Arch Dermatol 120:1052, 1984.

198. Pajarre R, Kero M: Nail changes as the first manifestation of the HLA-B27 inheritance. Dermatologica 154:350, 1977.

199. Bently Phillips B, Cole I: Ingrowing toenails of infancy. Int J Dermatol 22:113, 1983.

200. Baran R, Bureau H: Congenital malalignment of the big toenail as a cause of ingrowing toenails in infancy: Pathology and treatment (a study of 30 cases). Clin Exp Dermatol 8:619, 1983.

201. Walker S: Paronychia of the great toe of infants. Clin Pediatr 28:247, 1979.

202. Honig PJ, Spitzer A, Bernstein R, et al: Congenital ingrown toenails: Clinical significance. Clin Pediatr 21:424, 1982.

203. Herold HZ, Barueshin AM, Shmueli G, et al: Radical wedge resection for ingrown toenail: Long-term results. J Dermatol Surg Oncol 11:513, 1985.

204. Brown FC: Chemocautery for ingrown toenails. J Dermatol Surg Oncol 7:331, 1981.

205. Robb JE: Surgical treatment of ingrowing toenails in infancy and childhood. Z Kinderchir 36:63, 1982.

206. Baran R, Dawber RPR: Diseases of the Nails and Their Management. Blackwell Scientific Publications, Oxford, England, 1984, pp 377–379.

207. Kelly WN, Wyngaarden VB: Clinical syndromes associated with hypoxanthine-guanine phosphoribosyltransferase deficiency. In Stanbury JB, Wyngaarden JB, Fredrickson DS (eds): The Metabolic Basis of Inherited Disease, ed 5. McGraw-Hill, New York, 1983, pp 1116–1117.

208. Horne DJ, Wilkinson J: Habit reversal treatment for fingernail biting. Behav Res Ther 18:287, 1980.

209. Bornstein PH, Rychtarik RG, McFall ME, et al: Hypnobehavioral treatment of chronic nail biting: A multiple baseline analysis. Int J Clin Exp Hypn 28:208, 1980.

210. Juhlin L: Hereditary leukonychia. Acta Derm Venereol (Stockh) 43:136, 1963.

211. Albright SD, Wheeler CE: Leukonychia—Total and partial leukonychia in a single family with a review of the literature. Arch Dermatol 90:392, 1964.

212. Giustina TA, Woo TY, Campbell JP, et al: Association of pili torti and leukonychia. Cutis 32:533, 1985.

213. Bushkell LL, Gorlin RJ: Leukonychia totalis, multiple sebaceous cysts and renal calculi: A syndrome. Arch Dermatol 111:899, 1975.

214. Bart RS, Punphyre RE: Knuckle pads, leukonychia and deafness. A dominantly inherited syndrome. N Engl J Med 276:202, 1967.

215. Ingegaro AD, Yatto RP: Hereditary white nails (leukonychia totalis) duodenal ulcer and gallstones. Genetic implications of a syndrome. NY State J Med 82:1797, 1982.

216. Magid M, Esterly NB, Prendiville J, et al: The yellow nail syndrome in an 8 year old girl. Pediatr Dermatol 4:90, 1987.

217. Goodman RM: Familial lymphedema of the Meige's type. Am J Med 32:651, 1962.

218. Norton L: Further observations on the yellow nail syndrome with therapeutic effects or oral alphatocopherol. Cutis 32:457, 1985.

219. Hazelrigg DE, Duncan WC, Jarratt M: Twenty-nail dystrophy of childhood. Arch Dermatol 113:73, 1977.

220. Gomers MR: Neurocutaneous Diseases: A Practical Approach. Butterworths, Boston, 1987, p 36.

221. Woo TY, Rasmussen JE: Subungual osteocartilagenous exostosis. J Dermatol Surg Oncol 4:534, 1985.

222. Beckett JH, Jacobs AH: Recurring digital fibrous tumors of childhood: A review. Pediatrics 59:401, 1977.

223. Dolph JL, Demuth RJ, Miller SH: Angiokeratoma circumscriptum of the index fingers in a child. Plast Reconstr Surg 67:221, 1981.

224. Appelberg DB, Drucker D, Maser MR, et al: Subungual osteochondroma differential diagnosis and therapy. Arch Dermatol 115:472, 1979.

225. Frumkin A, Roytman M, Johnson S: Juvenile xanthogranuloma underneath a toenail. Cutis 40:244, 1987.

226. Simmons DA, Kegel MF, Scher RK, et al: Subungual tumors in incontinentia pigmenti. Arch Dermatol 122:1431, 1986.

CHAPTER 8

The Nail in Older Individuals

Philip R. Cohen and Richard K. Scher

A large and rapidly growing segment of the population is composed of elderly individuals. Nail changes and disorders occur in these patients (Table 8–1).[1,2] The color, contour, histology, growth, surface, and thickness of the nail unit may change as people age (Table 8–2).[3–13] Acquired nail disorders in the elderly population may represent changes of the nail unit associated with aging and altered biomechanics, may be related to either concurrent dermatologic or systemic diseases and their treatments, or might be secondary to tumors of the nail and surrounding structures. Some of these conditions include brittle nails, dystrophies secondary to faulty biomechanics and trauma, infections, onychauxis, onychoclavus, onychogryphosis, onychophosis, splinter hemorrhages, subungual hematomas, and subungual exostosis. Appropriate assessment and management of these onychologic concerns in this group of patients are reviewed.

AGING-ASSOCIATED NAIL CHANGES

Color

The color of the normal nail plate varies. The region of the nail plate overlying the lunula is white. The nail plate overlying the nail bed is pink. A slightly paler, pink-amber–tinged onychodermal band is found on the nail plate overlying the area just before and including the hyponychium. Overlying the distal nail groove, the nail plate is white.

The color of the nail plate may change as individuals age. The nails can be dull and opaque in appearance. Their color varies from shades of yellow to gray (Fig. 8–1). The lunula is often decreased in size or absent in older people.[14,15]

Horan and colleagues[16] evaluated the fingernails and toenails of 258 individuals older than 70 years. Nail changes were observed in 19 per cent of these patients and included the loss of the lunula, a white appearance of the proximal portion of the nail, a more normal pink band, and an opaque free edge of the nail. These changes were identical to those described by Lindsay[17] in patients with associated renal failure and similar to those observed by Terry[18] in patients with hepatic cirrhosis; however, none of the elderly individuals had evidence of renal or hepatic disease.

Horan and associates[16] speculated that these age-related color changes in the nails might represent an underlying disturbance of collagen. These color changes did not progress with nail growth and were not eliminated after engorging the nail bed with blood. Interestingly, in some of the patients who had previously had strokes, the neapolitan nails oc-

Table 8–1. **AGING-ASSOCIATED NAIL CHANGES
AND DISORDERS**

Changes
Color
Contour
Histology
Linear growth
Surface
Thickness
Disorders
Brittle nails
Faulty biomechanics and traumatic
Infections
Onychauxis
Onychoclavus
Onychocryptosis
Onychogryphosis
Onychophosis
Splinter hemorrhages and subungual hematomas
Subungual exostosis

curred only unilaterally on the hemiparetic side. The authors introduced the term *neapolitan nails* to describe these color changes, because there were three distinctive color bands on the nails analogous to those of Neapolitan ice cream.

Contour

The normal nail plate has a smooth surface and a double curvature: longitudinal and transverse. The double curvature of the nor-mal nail plate is frequently altered in the elderly. Typically, the transverse convexity is increased and the longitudinal curvature is decreased. However, flattening of the nail plate (platyonychia), spooning of the nail plate (koilonychia), and clubbing of the digit have also been noted in elderly individuals.[19–22] A "ram's horn" deformity (onychogryphosis), often primarily restricted to the great toenails, may occur.[23,24] In addition, modifications in the contour of the nail plate in aged patients can be secondary to an associated cutaneous or systemic disease (Fig. 8–2).

Histology

The nail unit consists of a cuticle, matrix, bed, hyponychium, plate, and surrounding proximal and lateral folds, or perionychium. The distal skin on the dorsal digit forms the proximal nail fold. The cuticle extends from the proximal nail fold onto the nail plate. Beneath the proximal nail fold is the nail matrix, which extends about 5 mm proximally. Melanocytes are present in the nail matrix, in greater number distally than proximally. However, the granular layer, with keratohyalin granules, is absent not only in the nail matrix but also in the nail bed.

The lunula represents the nail matrix, which extends distally beyond the proximal nail fold. The nail bed begins where the lunula ends. The nail bed extends distally to where the nail plate begins to separate from the underlying epithelium: the hyponychium. The nail plate begins in the groove between the proximal

Table 8–2. **CHARACTERISTICS OF NAIL CHANGES ASSOCIATED WITH AGING**

Characteristics	Changes	Study
Color	Yellow to gray with a dull, opaque appearance	3, 4
	"Neapolitan" nails: nails with a loss of the lunulae and a white proximal portion, a normal pink central band, and an opaque distal free edge	
Contour	Increased transverse convexity	3, 5
	Decreased longitudinal curvature	
Histology	Nail plate keratinocytes	6, 7
	Increased size	
	Increased number of pertinax bodies (keratinocyte nuclei remnants)	
	Nail bed dermis	8
	Thickening of the blood vessels	
	Degeneration of elastic tissue	
Linear growth	Decreases	9, 10
Surface	Increased friability with splitting and fissuring	11, 12
	Longitudinal furrows that are superficial (onychorrhexis) and deep (ridges)	
Thickness	Variable: normal, increased, or decreased	8, 13

Adapted with permission from Cohen PR, Scher RK: Geriatric nail disorders: Diagnosis and treatment. J Am Acad Dermatol 26:521, 1992. Copyright 1992, Mosby-Year Book, Inc, St. Louis, Missouri.

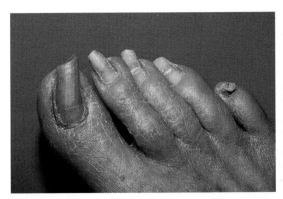

Figure 8–1. The great toe nail is yellow and thickened. The transverse convexity is increased, and there are early changes of onychogryphosis. Reprinted with permission from Cohen PR, Scher RK: Nail changes in the elderly. Geriatric Dermatol 1:45–53, 1993. Copyright 1993, Hospital Publications, King of Prussia, PA.

nail fold and the matrix and continues over the entire nail bed and slightly distal to the hyponychium. Normal ventral digital epidermis begins at the distal groove, a subtle depression that represents the end of the hyponychium.

Histologic changes in the aging nail plate and nail bed have been described. The cause of some of these changes is multifactorial. One pathogenic cause is a diminished local blood supply. In elderly individuals, there is thickening of the subungual blood vessels and alteration of the nail bed connective tissue characterized by degeneration of the elastic tissue.[25] These changes in elastic tissue were most severe in the dermis beneath the pink nail bed, less marked beneath the lunula, and absent in the matrix area beneath the proximal nail fold. The alteration of elastic tissue in the nail bed is more pronounced than that observed in the adjacent paronychial skin.

On the basis of the distribution of altered nail bed elastic tissue, Lewis and Montgomery postulated that the nail plate provided poor protection of the nail bed from exposure to sunlight. Subsequent investigators even recommended the use of a sunscreen nail varnish to protect the nail plate from the effects of solar radiation. An evaluation of the transmission of optical radiation through human toenails revealed that relatively little ultraviolet A radiation actually reaches the nail bed.[26] The authors also concluded that the nail plate permits a very low transmission of ultraviolet B radiation and, therefore, acts as a very efficient sunscreen for the underlying nail bed.

Morphologic factors of the keratinocytes from the superficial layers of human nail plates also vary with age. Germann and coworkers[27]

evaluated keratinocytes from normal fingernail and toenail plates of healthy infants (from birth to 1 year of age), adults (16 to 36 years of age), and elderly (older than 75 years). The size of nail plate keratinocytes significantly increased as individuals aged. These observations correlated with nail plate growth and showed that cell proliferation had a measurable effect on the size of keratinocytes from the nail plate surface. Specifically, slowed epidermopoiesis resulted in larger cells. Another histologic alteration in the nail plate keratinocytes was an increased number of pertinax bodies. These bodies are interpreted to be remnants of keratinocyte nuclei and consist of perinuclear eosinophilic material or material undergoing vacuolation or both.[28]

Linear Growth

The linear nail growth rate varies among individuals and among digits. Normal fingernail growth can range from 1.8 to 4.5 mm per

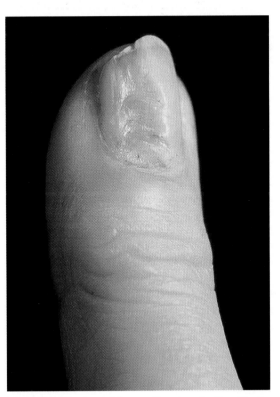

Figure 8–2. The normal fingernail contour is altered by focal mucinosis (a myxoid cyst), which presses against the proximal nail matrix and results in a groove in the nail plate. Reprinted with permission from Cohen PR, Scher RK: Nail changes in the elderly. Geriatric Dermatol 1:45–53, 1993. Copyright 1993, Hospital Publications, King of Prussia, PA.

month. An average growth rate of the fingernails is 0.1 mm per day or 3.0 mm per month. Thus, it takes approximately 6 months for a fingernail to grow from the matrix to the free edge. Toenails grow at one half to one third the fingernail rate: 0.3 mm per day or 1.0 mm per month. Hence, it may take as long as 12 to 18 months for a toenail to grow from the cuticle to the distal free edge.

In addition to aging, many other factors influence the linear nail growth rate (Table 8–3).[10–12] For example, the rate of growth is proportional to the length of the digit and is more rapid on the dominant hand. Alterations in temperature, hormonal status, circulation, and activity can increase or decrease nail growth. Although certain dermatologic disorders that involve the nail unit may stimulate the growth rate, many systemic diseases or infections slow nail growth.

Aging tends to decrease the rate of linear nail growth.[13,29,30] One study evaluating thumb nails revealed that linear nail growth was most rapid in the first and second decades of life. It decreased steadily thereafter.[13,29]

Orentreich and Scharp[31] measured thumbnail growth in 257 individuals; they also observed that the rate of linear nail growth increased not only during the first and second decades but also well into the third decade of life. On reaching the ninth decade of life, the linear nail growth rate had decreased by approximately 38 per cent from the average linear growth rate of 0.9 mm per week during the third decade. Specifically, the linear nail growth rate decreased approximately 0.5 per cent per year from 25 to 100 years of age. The rate of decrease was greater for women until the sixth decade and greater for men after the eighth decade; between the sixth and eighth decades, the rate of decreased nail growth was similar for both sexes.

In a later study, Orentreich and others[12] evaluated the effect of aging on the rate of linear nail growth in 171 people ranging in age from 10 to 100 years. They demonstrated a multiple-year biorhythm. There were 7-year periods of slow decline of linear nail growth alternating with 7-year periods of rapid decline.

Individual investigators have also studied the linear nail growth rate on their own nails. During a 35-year period, Bean observed that the average daily growth of his left thumbnail decreased from 0.123 mm a day at 32 years of age to 0.095 mm a day at 67 years of age.[13] Similarly, Dawber noticed a 10.4 per cent decline in the rate of linear nail growth of his right index finger during a 12-year period.[10] When treating

Table 8–3. **FACTORS THAT INFLUENCE LINEAR NAIL GROWTH RATE**

Increase	Decrease
Dominant hand	Acute infection
Hyperpituitarism	Aging
Hyperthyroidism	Antimitotic drug therapy
Increased blood supply (arteriovenous shunt)	Colder temperatures
Localized trauma (piano playing or typing)	Congestive heart failure
Longer digits	Decreased circulation (atherosclerosis)
Males	Females
Onycholysis	Hypothyroidism
Periungual inflammation	Immobilization or paralysis
Pregnancy	Lactation
Premenstrual	Malnutrition
Psoriasis	Measles
Regeneration after avulsion	Mumps
Warmer temperatures	Night
	Peripheral neuropathy
	Pneumonia
	Smoking
	Systemic diseases
	Yellow nail syndrome

elderly patients for onychomycosis with systemic antifungals, the decreasing linear nail growth has markedly important clinical significance. The necessary duration of treatment in older patients (with its associated risk of side effects) is often much longer than that in younger individuals with tinea unguium.

Surface

Nail plate friability, splitting, fissuring, and superficial longitudinal striations (onychorrhexis) frequently develop with advancing age.[32,33] Deeper longitudinal lines (ridging) also become more numerous and pronounced in elderly individuals and have been described as "sausage-shaped" ridges or "sausage link" ridges[34] (Fig. 8–3). These surface changes may be localized or diffuse. They reflect the relative depth of the indented grooves and the prominence of their adjacent projection ridges. Earlier investigators postulated that the production of the ridges might be secondary to the whorls of generative cells in the proximal matrix region or caused by variations in the turnover rate of the matrix cells.

The development of onychorrhexis and ridging is not limited to the elderly. Disorders in which onychorrhexis has also been described include gout, hemochromatosis, hypothyroidism, lichen planus, peripheral vascular disease, psoriasis vulgaris, Reiter's syndrome, and scleroderma.[35–40] In addition to its presence in older individuals, longitudinal ridging of the nail plates has been observed in patients with hypothyroidism, lichen planus, lupus erythematosus, radiodermatitis, Raynaud's disease, and rheumatoid arthritis.[41–45]

Onychorrhexis, or longitudinal ridging, is rarely a functional problem. However, it may be a source of cosmetic concern for the elderly individual. A practical and safe treatment for these patients is daily buffing of the nail plates. Buffing powder, paste, or cream contains (1) waxes for enhancing nail surface gloss and (2) finely ground pumice (particles of kaolin, precipitated chalk, silica, stannic acid, and talc) as an abrasive.[46] After the buffing agent has been applied, a chamois-covered buffer is used to polish each nail plate until it shines.[47]

Thickness

The length of the nail matrix determines the thickness of the nail plate. The nail plate thickness varies with the sex of the individual and with each digit. The nail plate is approximately 0.6 mm thick in men and 0.5 mm thick in women. The nail plate of the thumb is the thickest and that of the little finger is the thinnest. For the remaining digits of the hand, the nail plate of the index finger is thicker than that of the middle finger, which is thicker than that of the ring finger.[6–9]

The clinical observations regarding the relationship between nail plate thickness and aging have been variable. The thickness of the nail plate has been described to be normal, increased, or decreased with advancing age. One group of investigators found that the thickness of the left thumb nail increased rapidly during the first two decades of life and then more slowly thereafter.[29] They observed little change in the volume of nail growth per day as the patients aged because the increase in nail plate thickness counterbalanced the decrease in linear nail plate growth.[29] Other authors implied that there is a difference between the thickness of the fingernail and toenail plates as a given individual ages: the

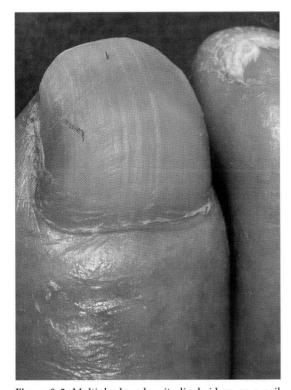

Figure 8–3. Multiple deep longitudinal ridges on a nail plate that also has increased longitudinal curvature. Reprinted with permission from Cohen PR, Scher RK: Nail changes in the elderly. Geriatric Dermatol 1:45–53, 1993. Copyright 1993, Hospital Publications, King of Prussia, PA.

fingernails often become soft and fragile, whereas the toenails are usually thicker and harder.[22,48]

Pachyonychia refers to thickening of the entire nail plate, whereas onychauxis describes localized nail plate hypertrophy. Pachyonychia and onychauxis are not only found as idiopathic, age-associated nail plate changes. They also can develop secondary to several conditions that may occur in elderly individuals. Thickening of the nail plate has been described in patients with acanthosis nigricans, acromegaly, arteriosclerosis, dermatitis, inflammation, ischemia, local infection, nutritional disturbances, pityriasis rubra pilaris, Raynaud's disease, repeated trauma, rheumatoid arthritis, and sarcoidosis.[49–54] In addition, it is important clinically to differentiate thickened nail plates from subungual hyperkeratosis; the latter has been observed in many disorders affecting older patients such as bullous pemphigoid, onychomycosis, pemphigus vulgaris, pityriasis rubra pilaris, psoriasis vulgaris, radiodermatitis, and Reiter's syndrome.

Daily buffing may cosmetically improve thickened nail plates. Alternatively, an abrasive disk attached to an electric drill can be used to mechanically thin the superficial surface of the nail plate. Severe nail plate thickening may require mechanical or chemical avulsion of the nails[55–61] (Table 8–4). In some instances, concurrent destruction of the nail matrix may be elected to prevent subsequent recurrences.

AGING-ASSOCIATED NAIL DISORDERS

Incidence

A 1987 survey of skin problems and skin care regimens discovered that 12 per cent of 68 noninstitutionalized volunteers aged 50 to 91 years did not practice regular fingernail care. Only 34 of the 68 individuals cut their own toenails. In 85 per cent of these individuals, onychorrhexis (superficial longitudinal striations of the nail plate) was observed.[3]

Table 8–4. **SUMMARY OF CHEMICAL MODALITIES FOR NAIL AVULSION**

Reagents	%	Comments	Study
		Compound A	
Urea	22.25	The normal skin was treated with tincture of benzoin and cloth	55
Anhydrous lanolin	22.25	adhesive tape. Compound A or B was generously applied to the	
White wax	5.50	nail plate; adhesive tape or plastic (vinyl) glove occluded the	
White petrolatum	50.00	plastic film wrap that covered the ointment. The area was kept	
Total	100.00	absolutely dry.	
		Compound B	
Urea	40.00	Results: (1) Average occlusion duration for successful avulsion was	
Anhydrous lanolin	20.00	9.4 (days) (range, 3–8) for Compound A and 7.2 days (range,	
White wax	5.00	4–10) for Compound B. (2) Only the abnormal nail was affected.	
White petrolatum	35.00		
Total	100.00		
Urea	40.00	New preparation used instead of Compounds A and B by the same	56
White beeswax (or paraffin)	5.00	investigators. Similar treatment protocol was used. After 7 days	
Anhydrous lanolin	20.00	of occlusion, treated nail was removed without anesthesia	
White petrolatum	25.00	followed by curettage of nail bed. Easily controlled, pinpoint	
Silica gel type H	10.00	bleeding occurred in 25% of patients.	
Total	100.00		
Urea 57	20.00	Painless avulsion of *non*dystrophic nails occurred after a period of	
Salicylic acid	10.00	2 weeks of occlusive application. There is a single detailed case	
Distilled water	15.00	report and reference to three additional patients whose nondys-	
Aquaphor[a]	55.00	trophic nails were successfully treated.	
Total	100.00		
Potassium iodide	50.00	Using this preparation, the patients themselves (N = 250) success-	58
Anhydrous lanolin	45.50	fully removed onychomycotic fingernails or toenails (N = 1500)	
Iodochlorhydroxyquine	0.50		
Total	100.00		
Urea ointment	40.00	Occlusive treatment was followed by antifungal cream alone.	59–61
Bifonazole cream	1.00	Mycologic cure rates of 60 to 90% were achieved.	

[a]Aquaphor contains 10% lanolin, 20% petrolatum, 30% mineral oil, and 40% water.

Table 8–5. AGING-ASSOCIATED NAIL DISORDERS

Brittle Nails

Clinical: excessive longitudinal ridging, horizontal layering (lamellar separation) of the distal nail plate, roughness (trachyonychia) of the nail plate surface, and irregularity of the distal edge of the nail plate.

Therapy: eliminate exacerbating factors and rehydrate the nail plate, cuticle, and surrounding nail folds. Oral biotin may be useful. Weekly applications of nail enamel may be helpful when preliminary measures are unsuccessful or in extreme cases.

Faulty Biomechanics- and Trauma-Induced Onychodystrophies

Clinical: present as onychauxis, onychoclavus, onychocryptosis, onychogryphosis, onychophosis, splinter hemorrhages, subungual exostoses, subungual hematoma, or subungual hyperkeratosis.

Therapy: treatment of the underlying limb function or gait cycle abnormality, correction of the associated bony deformity, or use of a molded shoe or an orthotic insert.

Infections

Clinical: (1) onychomycosis (distal subungual, white superficial, proximal subungual, and *Candida*); (2) paronychia: acute (the nail fold is red and tender and contains pus) or chronic (the cuticle is absent and the nail fold is swollen and uncomfortable).

Treatment: (1) onychomycosis: medical (topical or systemic antifungals) surgical (nail avulsion); (2) paronychia: acute (lancing, warm soaks, oral or topical antibiotics) or chronic (keeping the nail fold dry and applying topical antifungal or antiseptic agents).

Onychauxis

Clinical: localized hypertrophy of the entire nail plate characterized by a hyperkeratotic, discolored, nontranslucent nail plate; subungual keratosis and debris are often present.

Treatment: periodic partial or total debridement of the thickened nail plate: nail thinning using electric drills and burs; nail avulsion chemically (40% urea paste) or surgically; and, if necessary, matricectomy chemically (phenol) or surgically.

Onychoclavus (Subungual Heloma, Subungual Corn)

Clinical: a sometimes painful, hyperkeratotic process that is most commonly located under the distal nail margin of the great toenail.

Treatment: (1) removal of the lesion and (2) prevention of recurrence by modifying footwear and using protective pads or tube foam to eliminate the causative pressure.

Onychocryptosis (Ingrown Nail)

Clinical: the nail plate pierces the lateral nail fold and causes inflammation with or without accompanying granulation tissue, tenderness at rest, and pain on ambulation or with pressure to the digit.

Treatment: (1) correct predisposing factors and proper nail trimming, (2) elevate the lateral nail border by placing a small wisp of cotton beneath the edge of the nail plate, (3) provide local care consisting of warm soaks and topical antibiotics, (4) surgically remove the nail plate with or without partial or total ablation of the nail matrix, or (5) use alternative modalities such as a liquid nitrogen spray cryotherapy or (b) an orthonyx technique using a stainless steel wire nail brace.

Onychogryphosis

Clinical: an exaggerated, oyster- or ram's horn–like nail plate enlargement primarily only involving the great toenails.

Treatment: (1) proper nail plate trimming and foot care by filing the thickened nail plate using an electric drill and bur and removing the subungual hyperkeratosis, and (2) nail avulsion with or without ablation of the nail matrix.

Onychophosis

Clinical: localized or diffuse hyperkeratotic tissue of varying degree that develops on the lateral or proximal nail folds, in the space between the nail folds and the nail plate, or even subungually.

Treatment: (1) initially, debriding the hyperkeratotic tissue; (2) additional management may also include thinning of the nail plate, packing of the nail, or surgical intervention similar to that described for onychocryptosis.

Splinter Hemorrhages

Clinical: idiopathic or trauma-induced lesions that are black in color and located in the middle or distal third of the nail.

Treatment: avoidance of trauma.

Subungual Exostosis

Clinical: a benign tender bony proliferation, most commonly on the great toe, which usually produces hypertrophy of the entire nail bed such that the appearance of the nail is an inverted U with incurvation of the medial and lateral aspects of the nail plate.

Treatment: nail plate avulsion and aseptic removal of the excess bone.

Subungual Hematomas

Clinical: (1) acute (recent hemorrhage may be red and painful); (2) chronic (older lesions with residual hematoma may appear dark blue and are usually nontender).

Treatment: (1) acute: (a) a roentgenogram if a fracture of the underlying phalanx is suspected and (b) piercing the nail plate with either a needle or electric drill to relieve the underlying pressure; (2) chronic: if the patient cannot remember an associated traumatic incident, it may be necessary to rule out a pigmented lesion (melanoma) with microscopic evaluation of the nail plate and a biopsy specimen from the underlying nail matrix and/or nail bed.

Adapted with permission from Cohen PR, Scher RK: Nail changes in the elderly. Geriatric Dermatol 1:45, 1993. Copyright 1993, Hospital Publications, Inc, King of Prussia, Pennsylvania.

Another study evaluated foot problems in elderly patients. Nail or skin problems were identified by the investigators in 36 per cent of 426 patients 65 years of age or older encountered over a 3-year period in an outpatient foot clinic.[4]

In a third study, footwear was evaluated in 274 consecutive elderly patients who were admitted to a geriatric medical unit during a 3-month period. Foot problems were identified in 106 patients. An associated nail disorder was present in 70 per cent of these individuals.[5]

These preliminary observations confirm that nail abnormalities are frequently observed during the mucocutaneous examination of patients. However, it is difficult to estimate the exact incidence of nail disorders in the elderly because a prospective, age-controlled study that specifically addresses this issue remains to be performed. Additional investigation to clarify the prevalence of onychodystrophy in the elderly is warranted. Nail disorders that may occur in older individuals are summarized in Table 8–5.

Brittle Nails

The hardness of the nail plate is related to its state of hydration. The normal water content of the nail plate is approximately 18 per cent and varies between 10 and 30 per cent.[62,63] Brittle nails appear in dry environments, when the water content decreases below 16 per cent. In contrast, softness of the nail plate occurs in humid environments when the water content level of the nail plate is greater than 25 per cent.[64]

Brittle nails are characterized clinically by excessive longitudinal ridging, horizontal layering (lamellar separation) of the distal nail plate, roughness (trachyonychia) of the nail plate surface, and irregularity of the distal edge of the nail plate (Fig. 8–4). A 1986 study evaluating several groups of individuals (a total of 1584 participants) showed that approximately 20 per cent of the participants had brittle nails.[65] One group consisted of 79 residents of a senior citizens home in which 18 individuals (23 per cent) had brittle nails. The data from three other groups were combined before evaluating the incidence of brittle nails on these 1204 patients; 56 of the 161 individuals older than 60 years (35 per cent) had this problem.

Brittle nails therefore may be observed in aging patients.[48] In addition, several endogenous and exogenous causes can result in im-

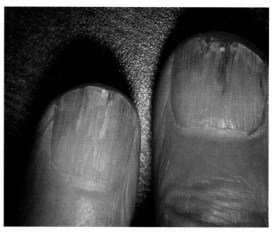

Figure 8–4. Onychorrhexis and trachyonychia with irregularity and lamellar separation of the distal nail plate are noted on these brittle fingernails. Reprinted with permission from Cohen PR, Scher RK: Geriatric nail disorders: diagnosis and treatment. J Am Acad Dermatol 26:521–531, 1992. Copyright 1992, Mosby-Year Book, St. Louis, MO.

pairment of either the nail plate or the nail matrix with subsequent development of brittle nails.[66] Many elderly individuals acquire brittle nails secondary to repetitive hydration and dehydration cycles or from excessive use of dehydrating agents such as nail enamels and remover and cuticle removers.[67]

The initial treatment of brittle nails involves the elimination of exacerbating factors. Hence, successful management of an existing brittle nail–associated systemic disorder may improve the onychodystrophy. When a causative condition is not readily identifiable, precipitating habits and agents should be eliminated.

The next intervention for treating brittle nails is the inauguration of local measures to rehydrate the nail plate, cuticle, and surrounding nail folds. A moisturizer (such as 12 per cent alpha-hydroxy acid [lactic acid] lotion, mineral oil, phospholipid, or urea cream) should be applied after the nails have been soaked for 10 to 20 minutes in lukewarm water. Optimally, the moisturizing agent should be used under occlusion. For this purpose, light cotton glove liners or white cotton socks are excellent.

In extreme cases or when preliminary measures for treating brittle nails are unsuccessful, the use of nail enamel may be helpful because it slows the evaporation of water from the nail plate. If a nail enamel is used, it should not be removed and reapplied more often than once a week. Although formaldehyde-containing lacquers may be used for intractable cases, some individuals may acquire an allergic contact dermatitis or onycholysis. Hence, the potential possibility of these adverse sequelae makes treatment with formaldehyde-containing lacquers less appealing. Oral biotin has been reported as an effective agent for the management of brittle nails.[68,69]

Faulty Biomechanics and Trauma

Acute trauma to the nail unit can result in onychodystrophy. These nail dystrophies include clubbing, koilonychia (after frostbite or thermal burns), leukonychia, longitudinal melanonychia striata (Fig. 8–5), onycholysis, ridging and splitting of the nail plate, splinter hemorrhages, and subungual hematomas (with or without a fracture of the underlying digit).[70–76] Depending on the cause, the nail changes may be temporary or permanent.

Chronic trauma to the nail unit can result from faulty biomechanics. The normal gait cycle is composed of a stance phase (60 per cent) and a swing phase (40 per cent); the stance phase is divided into contact, midstance, and propulsion periods.[77,78] Disease, abnormal development, or trauma can alter the normal biomechanical function of the limb and the gait cycle. Some of the bony deformities that can result in a biomechanical abnormality are listed in Table 8–6 (Fig. 8–6). The onychodystrophies observed in elderly patients secondary to faulty ambulatory biomechanics are summarized in Table 8–7 (Fig. 8–7).

Shoe-induced biomechanical abnormalities secondary to incompatibility between the foot, its digits, and the shoe can also result in trauma to the toenails and subsequent onychodystrophy. Onychauxis and onychogryphosis may develop from the abnormal growth of the toenails secondary to pressure from the shoes. Subungual hematoma and

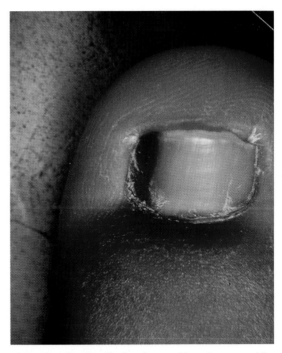

Figure 8–5. Longitudinal melanonychia striata caused by benign melanocytic hyperplasia.

subsequent onycholysis of that nail may occur in individuals who wear rigid platform shoes or footwear that is too short because of the repeated trauma to the nail unit during walking. Onychoclavus of the fifth toe and onychocryptosis may also be caused by inappropriate, poorly fitting footwear. In addition, if the distal nail plate becomes worn by continually rubbing against the inside of the shoe, elderly patients may mistakenly believe that their toenails do not grow.

Treatment of onychodystrophy secondary to biomechanical abnormalities should be directed toward (1) the underlying bony abnormality and (2) elderly patients' foot care and footwear. Visual and arthritic difficulties are

Table 8–6. **BONY DEFORMITIES OF THE FOOT THAT CAN RESULT IN BIOMECHANICAL ABNORMALITY AND SUBSEQUENT NAIL DYSTROPHY**

Bony Deformity	Comment
Digiti flexus	Contracted or hammer toes, in which the toes buckle because the muscles controlling the digits are shortened
Hallux rigidus	The distal phalanx is dorsiflexed, and there is excessive motion of the interphalangeal joint secondary to a loss of motion in the metatarsal phalangeal joint of the great toe
Hallux valgus	Shifting and rotation of the great toe toward the second toe
Overlapping and underlapping toes	
Rotated fifth toe	The digit is oriented such that the patient ambulates on the lateral portion of the nail plate

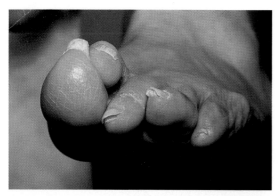

Figure 8–6. Overlapping and underlapping toes that caused faulty ambulatory biomechanics and subsequent onychauxis. Reprinted with permission from Cohen PR, Scher RK: Geriatric nail disorders: diagnosis and treatment. J Am Acad Dermatol 26:521–531, 1992. Copyright 1992, Mosby-Year Book, St. Louis, MO.

not uncommon in older individuals. These patients not only may have difficulty seeing their shoe laces but also may be unable to bend over and reach the shoes or tie the laces. Footwear with Velcro closures may be used instead of laced shoes. A molded shoe or an orthotic insert that conforms to the shape of the foot is helpful in the nonsurgical management of bony deformities. These modalities can provide adequate shoe fit by comfortably accommodating the existing deformity, by relieving pressure from the deformed joints, and by evenly distributing that pressure over the foot. Soft athletic shoes or sneakers are a less expensive (though less desirable) footwear alternative for elderly patients with bony deformities of the feet.

Other causes of chronic trauma to the nail unit include self-induced habits such as onychotillomania. Onychotillomania is an uncommon disorder in which the patient picks off pieces of the nail plate, nail bed, and nail folds.

Table 8–7. ONYCHODYSTROPHY SECONDARY TO FAULTY BIOMECHANICS

Onychauxis (Nail Plate Hypertrophy)

Digiti flexus
Foot-to-shoe incompatibility
Hallux rigidus
Hallux valgus
Overlapping and underlapping toes

Onychoclavus (Subungual Corn)

Digiti flexus
Foot-to-shoe incompatibility
Hallux valgus
Rotated fifth toes

Onychocryptosis (Ingrown Toenails)

Foot-to-shoe incompatibility
Hallux valgus

Onychogryphosis

Foot-to-shoe incompatibility

Subungual exostosis

Hallux rigidus
Hallux valgus

Subungual hematoma

Foot-to-shoe incompatibility
Hallux rigidus
Hallux valgus
Overlapping and underlapping toes

Subungual hyperkeratosis

Digiti flexus
Hallux rigidus
Rotated fifth toes

Modified and republished with permission from Cohen PR, Scher RK: Geriatric nail disorders: Diagnosis and treatment. J Am Acad Dermatol 26:521, 1992. Copyright 1992, Mosby-Year Book, Inc, St. Louis, Missouri.

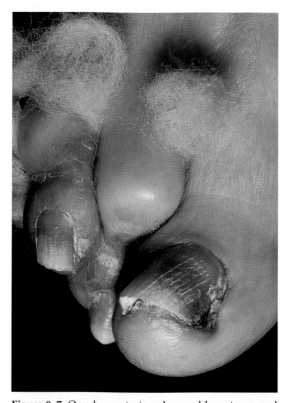

Figure 8–7. Onychocryptosis, subungual hematoma, and subungual hyperkeratosis that resulted from altered pedal function secondary to bony deformities of the toes. Reprinted with permission from Cohen PR, Scher RK: Geriatric nail disorders: diagnosis and treatment. J Am Acad Dermatol 26:521–531, 1992. Copyright 1992, Mosby-Year Book, St. Louis, MO.

One elderly woman claimed that she was "merely dissecting and removing tissue which had been destroyed by 'minute organisms.'"[79] Short, irregular nails that grow faster than normal, periungual verrucae, and hangnails (in which small, superficial portions of skin have split away from the lateral nail folds) with secondary bacterial infections may occur in patients with onychophagia who bite the free edge of their nails. Recurrent paronychia and leukonychia striata have also been observed after biting or pushing back the cuticles, respectively. Occlusive dressings may be helpful as an adjunctive measure in the management of these patients with onychotillomania and onychophagia. Referral for psychiatric counseling and treatment should be considered for these individuals.

A habit tic deformity is the result of another, consciously or inadvertently, self-induced habit that causes chronic trauma to the nail plate. This condition involves the thumbnails and develops after the individual rubs the central portion of the proximal nail fold of the thumb with the ipsilateral index fingernail. This onychodystrophy can be unilateral or bilateral, appears as central transverse Beau's lines of the thumbnail plate, and may resolve spontaneously if the patient stops injuring the corresponding nail matrix.[80,81] A habit tic nail deformity should be distinguished from dystrophia unguis mediana canaliformis (median nail dystrophy), which consists of an inverted fir tree–like split or canal in the nail plate that is slightly off center, extends from the cuticle to the free edge of the nail, and may occur on any fingernail but frequently involves those of the thumbs.[82]

Infections

Onychomycosis

The nail structures may be the target of a primary infection or may be the innocent bystander secondarily involved in an infectious process localized to that area. Onychomycosis is more common in elderly patients and frequently involves both toenails and fingernails. The diagnosis of onychomycosis can be confirmed by (1) observing a fungal organism after a potassium hydroxide preparation has been performed, (2) culturing the organism from specimens taken (preferably) from the nail bed or (less optimally) from the nail plate, or (3) detecting fungi on sections (preferably periodic acid–Schiff stained) prepared from a biopsy specimen of the nail bed and nail plate.[83] Even in the presence of bona fide onychomycosis, the potassium hydroxide preparation and culture may be negative. Therefore, a biopsy for histology, culture, or both may be necessary to establish definitively the presence of fungal organisms.[84]

In a study of onychomycosis by English and Atkinson[85] of 168 patients older than 60 years attending a podiatry clinic, 68 individuals (41 per cent) tested microscopically positive; yet the organism could not be cultured in 12 per cent of these patients. Among the remaining individuals, 20 (12 per cent) were infected by dermatophytes and 42 (25 per cent) by molds. In a more recent evaluation of fungal flora in 205 elderly individuals from Alexandria, Egypt, onychomycosis was demonstrated in 65% of the people investigated: pathogenic yeast (10 per cent), dermatophytes (3 per cent), and saprophytic filamentous fungi (51 per cent).[86]

Onychomycosis has been divided into four types: (1) distal subungual onychomycosis, (2) proximal subungual onychomycosis, (3) white superficial onychomycosis, and (4) *Candida* onychomycosis.[87,88] In addition, in the elderly, organisms previously considered to be saprophytic may also behave as nail pathogens: *Scytalidium dimidiatum* (previously called *Hendersonula toruloidea*), *Scytalidium hyalinum*, and *Scopulariopsis brevicaulis*.[89]

Distal subungual onychomycosis is the most common dermatophyte type. It is most often caused by *Trichophyton rubrum* and manifests clinically by subungual hyperkeratosis and uplifting of the nail plate. In contrast, proximal subungual onychomycosis is the least common type of onychomycosis. In proximal subungual onychomycosis, the point of fungal entry is the proximal nail fold region, and a white area extends distally from this site.

White superficial onychomycosis shows coalescing, opaque to white islands of fungi on the surface of the toenails. *T. mentagrophytes* is usually the causative organism of white superficial onychomycosis. Treatment merely requires scraping the fungi from the nail plate surface (Fig. 8–8).

Several possible treatment alternatives for onychomycosis exist.[90] Topical therapy has minimal associated toxicity. As an individual therapeutic approach, topical treatments are helpful in containing fungal infections of the nail and yet are unable—to date—to cure onychomycosis. Topical agents are available in several galenical forms: creams, gels, lacquers,

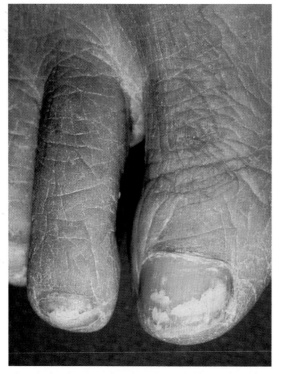

Figure 8–8. White superficial onychomycosis located on the surface of the toenails. Reprinted with permission from Cohen PR, Scher RK: Geriatric nail disorders: diagnosis and treatment. J Am Acad Dermatol 26:521–531, 1992. Copyright 1992, Mosby-Year Book, St. Louis, MO.

lotions, ointments, solutions, sprays, and tinctures. The types of topical antifungal agents currently available include allylamines, fungoid tincture, imidazoles, iodinated trichlorophenols (haloprogin), morpholines, polyenes, pyridone-ethanolamine salt (ciclopirox olamine), and miscellaneous agents. In addition to antifungal preparations, the topical agents that have been used to manage onychomycosis include desiccating solutions, disinfectants, keratolytics, and vital dyes[84,91–104] (Table 8–8).

Once the decision has been made to treat fungal infection of the nail with a topically applied agent, the patient should apply the medication two to three times each day. Using topical antifungal medications under occlusion may help to expedite improvement. The patient should be re-evaluated approximately every 3 to 4 weeks. At each visit, the nail plate should be trimmed back and the underlying nail bed treated with vigorous curettage. The anticipated duration of topical monotherapy for onychomycosis is typically prolonged (ranging from 6 to 12 months) if not lifelong.

Several systemic therapies have been used to treat patients with onychomycosis. Griseofulvin is effective only for dermatophytes. Ketoconazole and fluconazole (Diflucan) have also been used. Oral terbinafine for treating fingernail onychomycosis demonstrated significant efficacy with minimal to no drug-related toxicity. The approved dose is 250 mg once a day for 3 months for toenails.[105]

Itraconazole is a synthetic triazole. It exerts its antifungal activity by interfering with the synthesis of ergosterol (a component of fungal cell membranes).[106] Itraconazole (200 mg once daily for 3 consecutive months) has been approved by the Food and Drug Administration for use in treating onychomycosis resulting from dermatophytes of the toenails with or without fingernail involvement. Studies have also shown that pulse therapy with intraconazole (400 mg for 7 consecutive days each month for 3 sequential months) is effective in achieving mycologic cures in patients with onychomycosis of the toenails[107]—probably with better efficacy than with continuous therapy.

Several factors may preclude the use of systemic antifungals in elderly patients. All of the oral medications available for onychomycosis can have drug-associated adverse side effects, including multiple interactions with other systemic drugs. In addition, with the exception of itraconazole, prolonged duration of therapy is typically required. Therefore, it is recommended to have a culture-confirmed diagnosis of onychomycosis before initiating therapy with these agents.

Nail avulsion may be a useful adjuvant therapy when the onychomycosis is limited to only one or two markedly dystrophic nails.[103,108] After removal of the infected nail, the course of antifungal therapy may be shortened, the duration of remission may be increased, and the opportunity to prevent recurrence of infection may be enhanced.[102] In addition to dermatophyte nail infections, nail plate avulsion is also helpful in treating onychomycosis secondary to saprophytes.

Nail avulsion may be performed nonsurgically (see Table 8–4)[55–61] or surgically (reviewed by Daniel[109]). The advantages and disadvantages of using urea ointment for the chemical "avulsion" of dystrophic nails are summarized in Table 8–9.[55,56] Either surgical instruments or the carbon dioxide laser can be used for the surgical treatment of onychomycosis.[110–113]

Table 8–8. **TOPICAL AGENTS USED IN THE MANAGEMENT OF ONYCHOMYCOSIS**

Type of Topical Medication	Drug	Galenical Form
Allylamines	Naftifine	C, G
	Terbinafine	C
Imidazoles	Bifonazole	C
	Butoconazole	C
	Clotrimazole	C, Lo, So
	Econazole	C
	Ketoconazole	C
	Miconazole	C
	Oxiconazole	C
	Sulconazole	C, So
	Terconazole	C
	Tioconazole	So
Miscellaneous[a]	Castellani Paint	So
	Ciclopirox olamine	C, Lo
	Fungi-Nail	T
	Fungoid	C, So, T
	Gentian violet	So
	Glutaraldehyde	So
	Gordochom	So
	Haloprogin	C, So
	Iodochlorhydroxyquin	C, O
	Ony-Clear Nail	Sp
	Propylene glycol urea lactic acid	So
	Thymol	So
	Whitfield's ointment	C, O
Morpholines	Amorolfine	La
Polyenes	Amphotericin B	C, Lo, O
	Nystatin	C, O

C, cream; G, gel; La, lacquer; Lo, lotion; O, ointment; So, solution; Sp, spray; T, tincture.

[a]Castellani paint (10% resorcinol, 4.5% phenol, alcohol, acetone, purified water, with or without basic fuchsin); Fungi-Nail (10% undecylenic acid, 5% salicylic acid, 70% vol/vol isopropyl alcohol); Fungoid (the cream contains miconazole; the solution contains triacetin, chloroxylenol, and cetylpyridinium chloride in propylene glycol and benzalkonium chloride; the tincture contains miconazole in a vehicle that contains water, acetone, isopropyl and benzyl alcohols, glacial acetic acid, and laureth 4); gentian violet (triphenylmethane [rosaniline] dye); glutaraldehyde (10%); Gordochom (25% undecylenic acid, 3% chloroxylenol in a penetrating oil base); Ony-Clear Nail (triacetin, cetylpyridinium chloride, chloroxylenol); propylene glycol urea lactic acid (a solution containing 10 g urea, 15 g lactic acid, 4 g sodium hydroxide, 50 g propylene glycol, and 21 g purified water); thymol (3 to 5% in either chloroform or 95 to 100% alcohol); Whitfield's ointment (12% benzoic acid, 6% salicylic acid).

Table 8–9. **ADVANTAGES AND DISADVANTAGES OF UREA OINTMENT FOR CHEMICAL NAIL AVULSION**

Advantages	Disadvantages
1. Nonsurgical method	1. Time consuming for the physician
2. Less expensive for the patient	2. Inconvenient to keep dressings *absolutely* dry for duration of occlusion (approximately 7 days)
3. Multiple abnormal nails can be treated in one session	3. Because commercial preparation is not available, the formulation must be compounded by a skilled pharmacist
4. Essentially a painless procedure	
5. The procedure is without risk of hemorrhage or infection	4. The preparation has a 4- to 6-month shelf life.

6. The procedure is optimal for patients
    With diabetes mellitus
    With vascular insufficiency
    With digital neuropathy
    Receiving anticoagulants
    With immune suppression
	5. Treatment failures secondary to
	    Lack of gross nail dystrophy
	    Dressing inadequately occluded
	    Immersion of the dressing into water
	    Outdated urea preparation

Adapted with permission from Cohen PR, Scher RK: Topical and surgical treatment of onychomycosis. J Am Acad Dermatol 31:S74, 1994. Copyright 1994, Mosby-Year Book, Inc, St. Louis, Missouri.

Bacterial Infections

Infections of the nail folds may be either acute or chronic. Acute paronychial infections are erythematous and tender and contain pus. They are frequently caused by bacterial organisms such as *Staphylococcus aureus*. Initial treatment may require the lancing of a localized abscess. Often oral antibiotics are required. In addition, warm soaks to the area are followed by adequate drying and the application of an antibiotic such as 2 per cent mupirocin ointment.

Acute paronychial infections commonly only involve one nail. However, a subungual metastasis from a primary visceral tumor can mimic an acute paronychia of a single nail.[114] Alternative possibilities should be entertained when several nails are involved by what appears to be an acute paronychia. For example, subacute or chronic paronychial involvement of multiple nails secondary to either chronic dermatitis, psoriasis vulgaris, or Reiter's syndrome can morphologically mimic an acute paronychia.[115]

Chronic paronychial infections appear as swollen, uncomfortable (but usually not painful) nail folds. There is a clear space that results from the loss of the cuticle and the creation of a patent proximal nail groove between the proximal nail fold and the nail plate. *Candida* species and gram-negative bacteria, such as *Proteus* or *Klebsiella* species, are the causative organisms for chronic paronychial infections. In comparison with acute paronychial infections, which rarely cause a nail plate deformity, multiple transverse ridges may be present secondary to repeated acute exacerbations in chronic paronychial infection.

Treatment of chronic paronychia is often prolonged. It primarily requires keeping the nail folds and surrounding skin areas dry. To do this, a topical antifungal lotion or cream should be applied two to three times daily to these sites. In addition, a topical antiseptic agent, such as 4 per cent thymol in chloroform or alcohol, may also be helpful.[116] If chronic hypertrophy of the proximal nail fold persists and is of significant concern to the patient, surgical removal is an alternative option.

Pseudomonas aeruginosa may colonize nail plates that are onycholytic. The pyocyanin pigment that the bacteria produce provides the green discoloration of the nail plate. After the onycholytic nail plate is cut away, local therapy is often successful. For example, either an antiseptic or antibiotic such as 15 per cent sulfacetamide, gentamicin, or chloram-phenicol ophthalmic solution should be applied to the area three times a day.[116,117]

Mycobacterial and Spirochetal Infections

Painful subungual abscess, paronychia, leukonychia, disappearing lunulae, pterygium, and traumatic dystrophy with nail plate thickening and ridging secondary to digital anesthesia have been observed in patients with leprosy who have *Mycobacterium leprae* infection involving the nail.[118] Rarely, individuals with syphilis may present with nail lesions. Onychodystrophy in patients with this spirochetal infection includes clubbing, fingertip chancre, fragility and thinning of the nail plate, koilonychia, loss of the nail plate substance only in the lunula area, onycholysis, and ulcerative paronychia.[119]

Mite Infection

In elderly patients with ordinary or crusted (Norwegian) scabies, subungual hyperkeratotic debris may harbor *Sarcoptes scabiei* (Fig. 8–9). Several reports have documented organ-

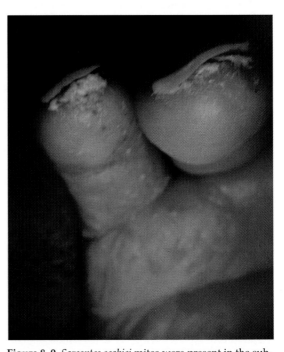

Figure 8–9. *Sarcoptes scabiei* mites were present in the subungual hyperkeratotic debris from this elderly patient living in a nursing home. Reprinted with permission from Cohen PR, Scher RK: Geriatric nail disorders: diagnosis and treatment. J Am Acad Dermatol 26:521–531, 1992. Copyright 1992, Mosby-Year Book, St. Louis, MO.

isms in this location as the cause of persistent infestations or epidemics among elderly patients and in nursing homes.[120–123] When treating elderly patients for scabies, the nail plates should be cut short and the fingertips brushed with the scabicide.

Viral Infections

Herpetic whitlow refers to a herpes simplex virus infection that involves the terminal digit and presents as a painful inflammation of the proximal and lateral nail folds. When the pustular lesion of an orf or cowpox infection occurs on the nail fold, an acute paronychia can also be mimicked. Human papillomavirus infections also involve the nail folds. Periungual warts are more common in children. However, they may be seen in elderly patients, especially those who are receiving immunosuppressive therapy. These lesions are often difficult to eradicate and may require more aggressive treatment modalities.[124–128]

Onychauxis

Localized hypertrophy of the nail plate is referred to as onychauxis. When the entire nail plate is thickened, the term *pachyonychia* is used. Onychauxis is characterized by hyperkeratotic, discolored nails and loss of translucency of the nail plate. Subungual hyperkeratosis and debris are often also present.

Subungual hyperkeratosis is the most reliable sign for distal subungual onychomycosis. It is not uncommon for elderly patients to be misdiagnosed as having tinea unguium and inappropriately treated with systemic antifungal therapy when they present with onychauxis of one or two nails, such as the great toenails. Therefore, microscopic or culture confirmation, or both, of onychomycosis should be obtained before initiating antifungal therapy in elderly patients who present with onychauxis, especially when there is accompanying subungual hyperkeratosis. A nail biopsy should be considered when mycology is persistently negative and a diagnosis of tinea is still suspected.

Idiopathic onychauxis may be associated with aging as well as with several disorders more common in the geriatric population. Distal onycholysis, increased susceptibility to acquiring onychomycosis, and pain are local complications of onychauxis. Subungual ulceration and hemorrhage may also occur in elderly patients with onychauxis as a result of constant pressure of the hypertrophic nail on the underlying and surrounding tissues.

Treatment for onychauxis involves periodic partial or total debridement of the thickened nail plate. The nail plate can be thinned using electric drills and burs. There are several potential advantages to using urea paste for partial or complete chemical avulsion of the nail in older individuals[55,56] (see Table 8–9). In addition to chemical avulsion, the hyperkeratotic nail plate can also be surgically removed. Removal of the nail plate may be followed by permanent ablation with either chemical (phenol) or surgical matricectomy when onychauxis is recurrent or associated with significant morbidity and local complications.

Onychoclavus

Onychoclavus is a hyperkeratotic process in the nail area. It has also been referred to as a subungual heloma and a subungual corn. It results from either an anatomic abnormality or a mechanical change in foot function.

The subungual heloma is most commonly located under the distal nail margin. It is caused by repeated minor trauma with accompanying localized pressure on the distal nail bed and hyponychium. For example, when the toes are contracted in a patient with a hammer toe deformity, an "end corn" may be develop beneath the pulp of the toe just below the nail plate edge.

The subungual corn typically occurs beneath the great toenail and appears as a dark spot under the nail plate. Applying pressure with a probe can elicit a circumscribed area of intense pain that corresponds to the location of the corn. In addition, the corn may cause elevation or splitting of the overlying nail plate.

The differential diagnosis of an onychoclavus includes an epidermoid cyst, a foreign body, a subungual melanoma, and a subungual exostosis (Fig. 8–10). Similar to a subungual foreign body, an onychoclavus does not blanch with pressure. In contrast to a subungual exostosis that is unchanged even after applying firm pressure, an onychoclavus will yield to slight pressure. A roentgenogram of the digit will readily identify the presence of an exostosis.[83] Subungual exostosis or chondroma may be associated with a subungual corn; therefore, a radiologic examination may be useful in the elderly patient in whom an onychoclavus is suspected. A biopsy may

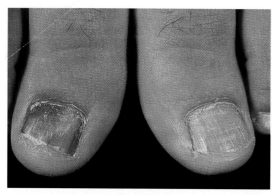

Figure 8–10. Although the distal subungual hyperkeratosis mimicked an onychoclavus, the melanocytic pigmentation of the proximal nail fold (positive Hutchinson's sign) prompted a biopsy, which revealed a subungual malignant melanoma. Reprinted with permission from Cohen PR, Scher RK: Geriatric nail disorders: diagnosis and treatment. J Am Acad Dermatol 26:521–531, 1992. Copyright 1992, Mosby-Year Book, St. Louis, MO.

be necessary when the clinical presentation suggests the possibility of a melanoma.

Lesion removal and recurrence prevention are the therapeutic cornerstones for treating onychoclavus. The subungual heloma can be enucleated by removing the corresponding section of nail plate and excising the hyperkeratotic tissue. If the corn is associated with an underlying bony abnormality, correction of the osseous lesion must also be performed. Recurrent onychoclavus can be prevented by eliminating the causative pressure. To reduce pressure to the distal toe area, modification of the footwear and use of protective pads or tube foam may be useful.

Onychocryptosis

Onychocryptosis is commonly referred to as ingrown nails. It results from the nail plate piercing the lateral nail fold. This condition can be extremely debilitating in elderly patients.

Overcurvature of the nail plate, subcutaneous ingrown toenail, and hypertrophy of the lateral nail fold are the three major types of onychocryptosis that have been described (Fig. 8–11). Inflammation, tenderness at rest, and pain on ambulation or with pressure to the digit are the clinical features of onychocryptosis. Granulation tissue at the lateral nail fold may also be present.

The most common causes of onychocryptosis are improper cutting of the nails and external pressure secondary to poorly fitting footwear.[129,130] Abnormally long toes, heredi-

tary conditions (congenital excessive convexity of the nail plate and congenital malalignment of the great toenail), hyperhidrosis, imbalance between the width of the nail plate and that of the nail bed, pointed-toe or high-heeled shoes, poor foot hygiene, and prominence of the nail folds are other etiologic factors.[131] Onychocryptosis can be a devastating problem with significant morbidity in the elderly patient with decreased sensation of the feet or toes secondary to an underlying systemic disease such as diabetes mellitus, peripheral vascular disease, or arteriosclerosis. These individuals are often unaware that a problem exists because their neuropathy results in minimal pain. Consequently, they often do not present for treatment until more serious complications such as deep infection, osteomyelitis, or gangrene have occurred.

Several therapeutic alternatives are available for the management of onychocryptosis. Correcting predisposing factors and proper nail trimming are prophylactic measures to

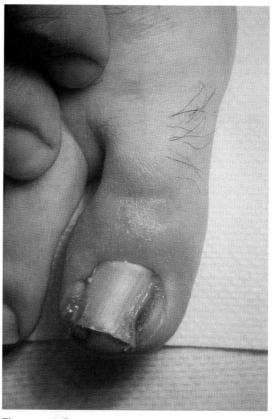

Figure 8–11. Recurrent onychocryptosis with subsequent periungual inflammation and granulation tissue. Reprinted with permission from Cohen PR, Scher RK: Geriatric nail disorders: diagnosis and treatment. J Am Acad Dermatol 26:521–531, 1992. Copyright 1992, Mosby-Year Book, St. Louis, MO.

prevent onychocryptosis. Cutting the distal nail plate straight across allows the corners of the nail plate to extend beyond the distal edge of the lateral nail folds. This decreases the opportunity for onychocryptosis to develop.

Conservative treatment of onychocryptosis involves placing a small wisp of cotton beneath the free edge of the lateral nail plate. This results in an elevation of the lateral border of the nail. As the nail subsequently grows out, its lateral edge does not penetrate into the soft tissue of the lateral nail fold.

Warm soaks and topical antibiotics are local treatment modalities that can be helpful. Microbiologic and radiographic evaluation should be performed if bacterial infection of the skin or underlying bone is suspected. Systemic antibiotics are indicated when a secondary infection is present.

More aggressive therapy is necessary for severe onychocryptosis or if the preliminary therapeutic measures have been unsuccessful. The condition may persist until the stimulus for inflammation is removed (Fig. 8–12). This usually requires complete or partial avulsion of the ingrown nail and excision of the involved adjacent tissue. Recurrence of ingrown toenails is observed in 60 to 80 per cent of onychocryptosis patients treated only with partial or complete nail plate avulsion. For these individuals, partial or total ablation of the nail matrix is often necessary.

A stainless steel wire nail brace has been used for flattening the nail plates with severe overcurvature that have caused onychocryptosis. The brace fits the overcurved nail exactly and maintains constant tension on the nail plate. Gradually, a series of adjustments are made. The nail plate is flattened painlessly within a 6-month period.[132]

Another initial treatment modality for patients with onychocryptosis is cryotherapy.[131] Liquid nitrogen is sprayed on an area that includes not only the granulomatous and infected tissue but also the adjacent nail fold. A freeze time of 20 to 30 seconds is recommended. Oral aspirin (600 mg three times daily for 3 days) and topical 0.05 per cent clobetasol propionate cream (twice daily) can minimize the immediate posttreatment inflammatory reaction.

Sonnex and Dawber[131] reported their results after treating ingrown toenails with liquid nitrogen spray cryotherapy. Twenty-four of the 44 patients treated in this manner had complete resolution without recurrence during 13 to 18 months of follow-up. Several of these individuals had previously been treated

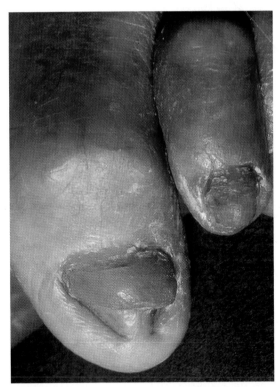

Figure 8–12. Partial regrowth of normal nail after previous nail plate avulsion for onychocryptosis secondary to severe overcurvature of the nail plate with painful constriction of the nail bed (pincer nail). Reprinted with permission from Cohen PR, Scher RK: Geriatric nail disorders: diagnosis and treatment. J Am Acad Dermatol 26:521–531, 1992. Copyright 1992, Mosby-Year Book, St. Louis, MO.

by nail avulsion or resection of the lateral nail plate and nail matrix. In the remaining 20 patients, loss of infection and granulation tissue were initially observed. However, recurrence developed within 1 to 3 months. Complete resolution, without recurrence during 14 months of follow-up, was demonstrated in 4 of 6 individuals from this latter group who were retreated with cryotherapy.

Treating onychocryptosis with cryotherapy should be considered in elderly patients with ingrown toenails. This technique is a simple, quick, and inexpensive outpatient procedure. It not only produced rapid pain relief but also an acceptable cure rate.

Onychogryphosis

Onychogryphosis is an exaggerated enlargement of the nail plate. It most often involves only the great toenails. Self-neglect or the inability of patients to perform adequate foot and nail care are primary predisposing factors for onychogryphosis. Secondary factors that influence the development of onychogryphosis include a history of nail trauma, hypertrophy of the nail bed, and biomechanical bony abnormalities such as hallux valgus. This condition is common in the elderly. It can also be observed in individuals who are homeless, have senile dementia, or are infirm.

Clinically, the shape of onychogryphotic nails appears "oyster like" or "ram's horn like." The nail plate is typically uneven, thickened, and brown to opaque. Multiple transverse striations are often present. In addition, the underlying nail bed may be hypertrophic (Fig. 8–13).

Onychogryphosis is primarily caused by the patient permitting the nail to continue to grow without treatment. The direction of the nail deformity is often determined by the pressure from the patient's footwear. In this condition, the nail plate initially grows in an upward direction. Subsequently, its growth is deviated laterally toward the other toes.[133]

Hemionychogryphosis clinically mimics onychogryphosis. It is a potential complication in patients with congenital malalignment of the great toenails, an inherited disorder in which the nail plate is deviated laterally with respect to the longitudinal axis of the distal phalanx of either one great toe or both halluces.[134–137] Hemionychogryphosis can occur in elderly patients in whom a congenital malalignment of the great toenails persists into adulthood. In contrast to onychogrypho-sis, in which the abnormal nail growth is initially upward before its lateral deviation, in hemionychogryphosis the hypertrophic nail initially grows in a lateral direction.

There are preventive, palliative, and aggressive treatments for onychogryphosis. Proper nail plate trimming and foot care will prevent the development of this condition. If elderly individuals are hampered by poor eyesight or an inability to cut their own toenails, these tasks can be done by another person.

The medical status of the patient influences the choice between a conservative and a radical treatment approach for the onychogryphotic nail. In patients with peripheral vascular disease or diabetes mellitus, the pressure on the onychogryphotic nail can result in subungual gangrene. Conservative treatment for these individuals should initially include filing of the thickened nail plate using an electric drill and bur and removal of the subungual hyperkeratosis. Subsequently, the dystrophic nail should be periodically clipped and trimmed.

More aggressive therapy is preferable for patients with a good vascular supply to the involved onychogryphotic toe. In these individuals, nail avulsion (with or without ablation of the nail matrix) should be performed. The nail can also be removed by either chemical nail destruction (using urea, potassium iodide, or salicylic acid) or surgical avulsion. When necessary, nail matrix ablation can be performed surgically (scalpel or carbon dioxide laser) or chemically (88 per cent phenol or 10 per cent sodium hydroxide).

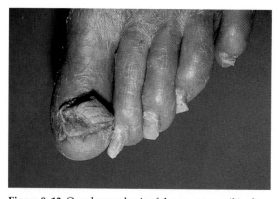

Figure 8–13. Onychogryphosis of the great toe nail is characterized by an opaque, thickened nail plate with subungual hyperkeratosis and transverse striations in which there has been exaggerated growth in an upward and lateral direction. Reprinted with permission from Cohen PR, Scher RK: Geriatric nail disorders: diagnosis and treatment. J Am Acad Dermatol 26:521–531, 1992. Copyright 1992, Mosby-Year Book, St. Louis, MO.

Onychophosis

Onychophosis refers to the localized or diffuse hyperkeratotic tissue that can develop on the lateral or proximal nail folds, in the space between the nail folds and the nail plate, and even subungually. This condition is common in elderly patients. It mainly involves the first and fifth toes and results from repeated minor trauma to the nail plate. Nail fold hypertrophy, onychocryptosis, onychomycosis, and xerosis are some of the nail plate and adjacent soft tissue deformities that predispose older individuals to the development of periungual hyperkeratotic tissue and subsequent onychophosis.

Precautionary measures to prevent the development of onychophosis include wearing comfortable shoes and relieving any pressure exerted by the nail on the surrounding soft tissue. Once onychophosis is present, the initial treatment consists of debriding the hyperkeratotic tissue. Keratolytics can be used for debridement. For this purpose, either 12 per cent ammonium lactate, 6 to 20 per cent salicylic acid preparations, or 20 per cent urea preparations may be helpful. Emollients can also be helpful to maintain hydration and lubrication. Thinning of the nail plate, packing of the nail, and surgical intervention similar to that described for onychocryptosis are additional options that may be necessary to reduce further trauma to the nail.

Splinter Hemorrhages and Subungual Hematomas

Young and Mulley[138] noted splinter hemorrhages in 35 of 220 patients older than 65 years who had been admitted to an acute geriatric ward. However, splinter hemorrhages occurred less often in elderly patients than in younger individuals. The main causative factor for these lesions in older individuals was trauma to the nails. Many of these individuals used walking aids and had fingernail splinter hemorrhages on the hand that held the walking aid.

Splinter hemorrhages have been observed in patients with various underlying systemic disorders.[139–143] In these patients, the splinter hemorrhages are usually red and are found on the proximal third of the nail plate. All of the splinter hemorrhages in Young and Mulley's elderly patients were black and were located in the middle or distal third of the fingernail.[138] Similarly, 86 of the 87 splinter hemorrhage lesions described by Robertson and Braune[144] were also situated on the distal one third of the nail plate. Therefore, the idiopathic or trauma-induced splinter hemorrhage lesions in the elderly patients are typically black, located distally, and clinically distinct from those in individuals with an associated systemic disease.

The clinical appearance and symptoms of a subungual hematoma vary with the age of the lesion. A recent hemorrhage is typically red and painful. If a fracture of the underlying phalanx is suspected, a roentgenogram of the digit may be necessary. An older lesion often appears dark blue and is usually nontender.

Idiopathic hemorrhage under the nail plate has been observed in older individuals. Trauma to the fingernail or toenail is the most common cause in these patients. Subun-gual hemorrhage has also been described in elderly individuals receiving anticoagulants. In addition, subungual hematomas have been reported in patients with bullous amyloidosis, bullous pemphigoid, chronic renal disease, dermatitis, diabetes mellitus, pemphigus vulgaris, and recent cerebrovascular accidents.[145,146]

The differential diagnosis of a subungual hematoma includes melanoma, especially when the elderly patient does not remember or associate a traumatic event with the subsequent subungual hematoma. As the nail plate grows, a pigmented lesion of the nail matrix or nail bed will persist. In contrast, a subungual hemorrhage will be replaced proximally by a normal-appearing nail plate; in some patients with a subungual hematoma, distal onycholysis and eventual autoavulsion of the nail plate occur. Microscopic evaluation of the nail plate and a biopsy specimen from the underlying nail matrix or nail bed should be considered when the diagnosis of a subungual hematoma cannot be clinically established with certainty.

Subungual Exostosis

A subungual exostosis is a benign tumor. It most commonly occurs on the medial surface of the distal great toe[147,148] (Fig. 8–14). Clinically, a subungual exostosis typically presents as a reactive hyperkeratotic nodule with secondary onychodystrophy of the overlying nail plate. Microscopically, the lesion consists of osseous bone with a fibrocartilage cap.[149–152] The patient often seeks medical attention because of symptoms related to alteration of the surrounding soft tissue such as pain, paronychia, a pyogenic granuloma, or a callus.[153]

Subungual exostoses have been described in elderly patients, the oldest being 80 years of age.[154] However, the majority of subungual exostoses occur in young adults. Less commonly, in a minimum of 51 of the 312 reported cases, these lesions appeared in children no older than 18 years.[152]

Subungual exostoses occur twice as often in women as in men. Local trauma to the involved digit was mentioned for almost two thirds of the patients.[152] In nearly all patients, especially those with solitary lesions, the subungual exostosis was an acquired lesion, and there was no family history of similar lesions.[152] However, four patients had multiple exostoses syndrome, which is an autosomal dominant condition characterized rarely by

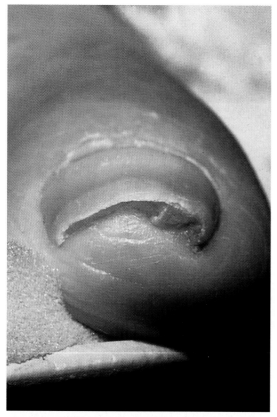

Figure 8–14. Radiographic examination confirmed that the incurvature of the medial and lateral aspects of this elderly patient's great toe nail was caused by a subungual exostosis. Reprinted with permission from Cohen PR, Scher RK: Geriatric nail disorders: diagnosis and treatment. J Am Acad Dermatol 26:521–531, 1992. Copyright 1992, Mosby-Year Book, St. Louis, MO.

subungual exostoses and more commonly by multiple exostoses that involve the endochondrally ossifying long bones of the extremities.[155–157]

The differential diagnosis of a subungual exostosis not only includes benign and malignant tumors[158] but also several other conditions.[159–162] Osteochondromas and enchondromas are additional bony lesions that can clinically mimic a subungual exostosis.[149,152,162–164] These lesions can usually be differentiated on the basis of radiologic findings. In a subungual exostosis, the radiograph often shows a broad-based lesion of trabeculated bone with an expanding distal flare[165]; the fibrocartilage cap is radiolucent, and areas of calcification are absent.[166] Distinguishing features of osteochondromas and enchondromas are a scalloped dome with a hyaline cartilage cap and a loculated medullary bone cyst with calcification, respectively.[152]

The treatment of a subungual exostosis involves removal of the excess bone aseptically after the suspected diagnosis has been confirmed radiographically.[152,157] Neither radiation nor simple cautery is effective in the management of subungual exostoses.[168] After a local anesthetic block is given, the nail plate is avulsed and the exostosis is exposed via a longitudinal incision of the overlying nail bed. With a bone rongeur, chisel, or mastoid curet, the tumor is then separated from the underlying bone. In an attempt to prevent local recurrence, the rough edges are chiseled flat and the tumor bed is saucerized by curettage to remove the lesion completely. Finally, the cutaneous wound is closed by suturing the nail bed, and an impregnated paraffin gauze dressing is applied.[168]

CONCLUSIONS

Age-associated nail changes in color, contour, histology, linear growth, surface, and thickness have been observed in elderly individuals. Age-related onychodystrophies that occur in older patients include brittle nails, faulty biomechanics, trauma, infections, onychauxis, onychoclavus, onychocryptosis, onychogryphosis, onychophosis, splinter hemorrhages and subungual hematomas, and subungual exostoses. The ability to evaluate, diagnose, and manage the onychologic needs of older individuals can be enhanced by an awareness and understanding of the clinicopathophysiology of nail changes and disorders in this patient population.

References

1. Cohen PR, Scher RK: Geriatric nail disorders: Diagnosis and treatment. J Am Acad Dermatol 26:521, 1992.
2. Cohen PR, Scher RK: Nail changes in the elderly. J Geriatr Dermatol 1:45, 1993.
3. Beauregard S, Gilchrest BA: A survey of skin problems and skin care regimens in the elderly. Arch Dermatol 123:1638, 1987.
4. Hsu JD: Foot problems in the elderly patient. J Am Geriatr Soc 19:880, 1971.
5. Finlay OE: Footwear management in the elderly care programme. Physiotherapy 72:172, 1986.
6. Zaias N: Embryology of the human nail. Arch Dermatol 87:37, 1963.
7. Scher RK: Nail surgery. Clin Dermatol 5:135, 1987.
8. Fleckman P: Basic science of the nail unit. *In* Scher RK, Daniel CR III (eds): Nails: Therapy, Diagnosis, Surgery. WB Saunders, Philadelphia, 1990, pp 36–51.

9. Fleckman P: Anatomy and physiology of the nail. Dermatol Clin 3:373, 1986.

10. Dawber R: The effect of immobilization on fingernail growth. Clin Exp Dermatol 6:533, 1981.

11. Bean WB: Nail growth: 30 years of observation. Arch Intern Med 134:497, 1974.

12. Orentreich N, Markofsky J, Vogelman JH: The effect of aging on the rate of linear nail growth. J Invest Dermatol 73:126, 1979.

13. Bean WB: Nail growth: Thirty-five years of observation. Arch Intern Med 140:73, 1980.

14. Baran R, Dawber RPR: The ageing nail. In Fry L (ed): Skin Problems in the Elderly. Churchill Livingstone, Edinburgh, 1985, pp 315–330.

15. Cohen PR: The lunula. J Am Acad Dermatol, 34: 943-953, 1996.

16. Horan MA, Puxty JA, Fox RA: The white nails of old age (neapolitan nails). J Am Geriatr Soc 30:734, 1982.

17. Lindsay PG: The half-and-half nail. Arch Intern Med 119:583, 1967.

18. Terry R: White nails in hepatic cirrhosis. Lancet 1:757, 1954.

19. Stone OJ, Maberry JD: Spoon nails and clubbing: Review and possible structural mechanisms. Tex Med 61:620, 1965.

20. Stone OJ: Spoon nails and clubbing: Significance and mechanisms. Cutis 16:235, 1975.

21. Stone OJ: Clubbing and koilonychia. Dermatol Clin 3:485, 1985.

22. Baran R: Nail care in the "golden years" of life. Curr Med Res Opinion 7(Suppl 2):95, 1982.

23. Helfand AE: Nail and hyperkeratotic problems in the elderly foot. Am Fam Physician 39:101, 1989.

24. Gilchrist AK: Common foot problems in the elderly. Geriatrics 34:67, 1979.

25. Lewis BL, Montgomery H: The senile nail. J Invest Dermatol 24:11, 1955.

26. Parker SG, Diffey BL: The transmission of optical radiation through human nails. Br J Dermatol 108:11, 1983.

27. Germann H, Barban W, Plewig G: Morphology of corneocytes from human nail plates. J Invest Dermatol 74:115, 1980.

28. Fenske NA, Lober CW: Structural and functional changes of normal aging skin. J Am Acad Dermatol 15:571, 1986.

29. Hamilton JB, Terada H, Mestler GE: Studies of growth throughout the lifespan in Japanese: Growth and size of nails and their relationship to age, sex heredity, and other factors. J Gerontol 10:401, 1955.

30. Balin AK, Pratt LA: Physiological consequences of human skin aging. Cutis 43:431, 1989.

31. Orentreich N, Scharp NJ: Keratin replacement as a ageing parameter. J Soc Cos Chem 18:537, 1967.

32. Silver H, Chiego B: Nails and nail changes: II. Modern concepts of anatomy and biochemistry of the nails. J Invest Dermatol 3:133, 1940.

33. Ronchese F: Pecular nail anomalies. Arch Dermatol 63:565, 1951.

34. Baran R, Dawber RPR: The nail in childhood and old age. In Baran R, Dawber RPR (eds): Diseases of the Nails and their Management, ed 2. Blackwell Scientific, Oxford, England, 1994, pp 81–96.

35. Daniel CR III, Sams WM Jr, Scher RK: Nails in systemic disease. In Scher RK, Daniel CR III (eds): Nails: Therapy, Diagnosis, Surgery. WB Saunders, Philadelphia, 1990, pp 167–191.

36. Chevrant-Breton J, Simon M, Bourel M, Ferrand B: Cutaneous manifestations of idiopathic hemochromatosis: Study of 100 cases. Arch Dermatol 113:161, 1977.

37. Samman PD: Principal nail symptoms. In Samman PD, Fenton DA (eds): The Nails in Disease. William Heinemann, London, 1986, pp 20–26.

38. Scher RK: Lichen planus of the nail. Dermatol Clin 3:395, 1985.

39. Basuk PJ, Scher RK, Ricci AR: Dermatologic diseases of the nail unit. In Scher RK, Daniel CR III (eds): Nails: Therapy, Diagnosis, Surgery. WB Saunders, Philadelphia, 1990, pp 127–152.

40. Pajarre R, Kero M: Nail changes as the first manifestation of the HLA-B27 inheritance: A case report. Dermatologica 154:350, 1977.

41. Samman PD: The nails in lichen planus. Br J Dermatol 73:288, 1961.

42. Urowitz MB, Gladman DD, Chalmers A, Ogryzlo MA: Nail lesions in systemic lupus erythematosus. J Rheumatol 5:441, 1978.

43. Baran R, Haneke E: Tumours of the nail apparatus and adjacent tissues. In Baran R, Dawber RPR (eds): Diseases of the Nails and Their Management, ed 2. Blackwell Scientific, Oxford, England, 1994, pp 417–497.

44. Fenton DA: Nail changes associated with general medical conditions. In Samman PD, Fenton DA (eds): The Nails in Disease. William Heinemann, London, 1986, pp 102–120.

45. Hamilton EBD: Nail studies in rheumatoid arthritis. Ann Rheum Dis 19:167, 1960.

46. Scher RK: Cosmetics and ancillary preparations for the care of nails: Composition, chemistry, and adverse reactions. J Am Acad Dermatol 6:523, 1982.

47. Engasser PG, Matsunaga J: Nail cosmetics. In Scher RK, Daniel CR III (eds): Nails: Therapy, Diagnosis, Surgery. WB Saunders, Philadelphia, 1990, pp 214–223.

48. Edelstein JE: Foot care for the aging. Phys Ther 68:1882, 1988.

49. Samman PD: Nail disorders associated with other dermatological conditions. In Samman PD, Fenton DA (eds): The Nails in Disease. William Heinemann, London, 1986, pp 66–88.

50. Baker H, Barth JH: Acanthosis nigricans (case report). Br J Dermatol 109(Suppl 1):101, 1983.

51. Edwards EA: Nail changes in functional and organic arterial disease. N Engl J Med 239:362, 1948.

52. Sonnex TS, Dawber RPR, Zachary CB, Millard PR, Griffiths AD: The nails in adult type I pityriasis rubra pilaris: A comparison with Sézary syndrome and psoriasis. J Am Acad Dermatol 15:956, 1986.

53. Sonnex TS, Dawber RPR, Zachary CB, et al: The importance of nail morphology in the differential diagnosis of pityriasis rubra pilaris, psoriasis and chronic erythroderma (abstract). Br J Dermatol (Suppl 26): 16, 1984.

54. Cohen PR, Prystowsky JH: Pityriasis rubra pilaris: A review of diagnosis and treatment. J Am Acad Dermatol 20:801, 1989.

55. Farber EM, South DA: Urea ointment in the nonsurgical avulsion of nail dystrophies. Cutis 22:689, 1978.

56. South DA, Farber EM: Urea ointment in the nonsurgical avulsion of nail dystrophies—A reappraisal. Cutis 25:609, 1980.

57. Buselmeier TJ: Combination urea and salicylic acid ointment nail avulsion in nondystrophic nails: A follow-up observation. Cutis 25:397, 1980.

58. Dorn M, Kienitz T, Ryckmanns F: Onychomycosis: Experience with nontraumatic nail avulsion. Hautarzt 31:30, 1980.

59. Hardjoko FS, Widyanto S, Singgih I, Susilo J: Treatment of onychomycosis with a bifonazole-urea combination. Mycoses 33:167, 1990.

60. Hay RJ, Roberts DT, Doherty VR, et al. The topical treatment of onychomycosis using a new combination urea/imidazole preparation. Clin Exp Dermatol 13:164, 1988.

61. Torres-Rodriguez JM, Madrenys N, Nicolas MC: Non-traumatic topical treatment of onychomycosis with urea associated with bifonazole. Mycoses 34:499, 1991.

62. Scher RK: Brittle nails. Int J Dermatol 28:515, 1989.

63. Kechijian P: Brittle fingernails. Dermatol Clin 3:421, 1985.

64. Scher RK, Bodian AB: Brittle nails. Semin Dermatol 10:21, 1991.

65. Lubach D, Cohrs W, Wurzinger R: Incidence of brittle nails. Dermatologica 172:144, 1986.

66. Baran R, Dawber RPR: Physical signs. In Baran R, Dawber RPR (eds): Diseases of the Nails and their Management, ed 2. Blackwell Scientific, Oxford, England, 1994, pp 35–80.

67. Wallis MS, Bowen WR, Guin JD: Pathogenesis of onychoschizia (lammelar dystrophy). J Am Acad Dermatol 24:44, 1991.

68. Colombo VE, Gerber F, Bronhofer M, Floersheim GL: Treatment of brittle fingernails and onychoschizia with biotin: Scanning electron microscopy. J Am Acad Dermatol 23:1127, 1990.

69. Hochman LG, Scher RK, Meyerson MS: Brittle nails: Patient response to daily biotin supplementation. Cutis 51:303, 1992.

70. Samman PD: Nail deformities due to trauma. In Samman PD, Fenton DA (eds): The Nails in Disease. William Heinemann, London, 1986, pp 135–153.

71. Gross NJ, Tall R: Clinical significance of splinter haemorrhages. BMJ 2:1496, 1963.

72. Robertson JC, Braune ML: Splinter haemorrhages, pitting, and other findings in fingernails of healthy adults. BMJ 4:279, 1974.

73. Farrington GH: Subungual haematoma—An evaluation of treatment. BMJ 1:742, 1964.

74. Baran R, Kechijian P: Longitudinal melanonychia (melanonychia striata): Diagnosis and management. J Am Acad Dermatol 21:1165, 1989.

75. Scher RK, Silvers DN: Longitudinal melanonychia striata (letter). J Am Acad Dermatol, in press.

76. Grossman M, Scher RK: Leukonychia: Review and classification. Int J Dermatol 29:535, 1990.

77. Wernick J, Gibbs RC: Pedal biomechanics and toenail disease. In Scher RK, Daniel CR III (eds): Nails: Therapy, Diagnosis, Surgery. WB Saunders, Philadelphia, 1990, pp 244–249.

78. Riccitelli ML: Foot problems of the aged and infirmed. J Am Geriatr Soc 14:1058, 1966.

79. Combes FC, Scott MJ: Onychotillomania: Case report. Arch Dermatol 63:778, 1951.

80. Samman PD: A traumatic nail dystrophy produced by a habit tic. Arch Dermatol 88:895, 1963.

81. Macaulay WL: Transverse ridging of the thumbnails: "Washboard thumbnails." Arch Dermatol 93:421, 1966.

82. van Dijk E: Dystrophia unguium mediana canaliformis. Dermatologica 156:358, 1978.

83. Cohen PR, Scher RK: Nail disease and dermatology (commentary). J Am Acad Dermatol 21:1020, 1989.

84. Haneke E: Fungal infections of the nail. Semin Dermatol 10:41, 1991.

85. English MP, Atkinson R: Onychomycosis in elderly chiropody patients. Br J Dermatol 91:67, 1974.

86. Gad ZM, Youssef N, Sherif AA, et al: An epidemiologic study of the fungal skin flora among the elderly in Alexandria. Epidemiol Infect 99:213, 1987.

87. Zaias N: Onychomycosis. Arch Dermatol 105:263, 1972.

88. Norton LA: Nail disorders: A review. J Am Acad Dermatol 2:451, 1980.

89. Hay RJ: Infections affecting the nails. In Samman PD, Fenton DA (eds): The Nails in Disease. William Heinemann, London, 1986, pp 27–50.

90. Cohen PR, Scher RK: Topical and surgical treatment of onychomycosis. J Am Acad Dermatol 31:S74, 1994.

91. Hay RJ: Onychomycosis: Agents of choice. Dermatol Clin 11:161, 1993.

92. Dompmartin D, Dompmartin A, Deluol AM, Coulaud JP: Onychomycosis and AIDS: Treatment with topical ciclopirox olamine (letter). Int J Dermatol 29:233, 1990.

93. Faergemann J, Swanbeck G: Treatment of onychomycosis with a propylene glycol-urea-lactic acid solution. Mycoses 32:536, 1989.

94. Hay RJ, Mackie RM, Clayton YM: Tioconazole nail solution—An open study of its efficacy in onychomycosis. Clin Exp Dermatol 10:111, 1985.

95. Lauharanta J: Comparative efficacy and safety of amorolfine nail lacquer 2% versus 5% once weekly. Clin Exp Dermatol 17(Suppl 1):41, 1992.

96. Zaug M, Bergstraesser M: Amorolfine in the treatment of onychomycoses and dermatomycoses (an overview). Clin Exp Dermatol 17(Suppl 1):61, 1992.

97. Reinel D: Topical treatment of onychomycosis with amorolfine 5% nail lacquer: Comparative efficacy and tolerability of once and twice weekly use. Dermatology 184(Suppl 1):21, 1992.

98. Meyerson MS, Scher RK, Hochman LG, et al: Open-label study of the safety and efficacy of fungoid tincture in patients with distal subungual onychomycosis of the toes. Cutis 49:359, 1992.

99. Meyerson MS, Scher RK, Hochman LG, et al: Open-label study of the safety and efficacy of naftifine hydrochloride 1 percent gel in patients with distal subungual onychomycosis of the fingers. Cutis 51:205, 1993.

100. Suringa DWR: Treatment of superficial onychomycosis with topically applied glutaraldehyde. Arch Dermatol 102:163, 1970.

101. Logan R, Hay RJ, Whitefield M: Antifungal efficacy of a combination of benzoic and salicylic acids in a novel aqueous vanishing cream formulation. J Am Acad Dermatol 16:136, 1987.

102. Korting HC, Schafer-Korting M: Is tinea unguium still widely incurable? A review three decades after the introduction of griseofulvin. Arch Dermatol 128:243, 1992.

103. Rollman O, Johansson S: Hendersonula toruloidea infection: Successful response of onychomycosis to nail avulsion and topical ciclopiroxolamine. Acta Derm Venereol (Stockh) 67:506, 1987.

104. Quadripur VSH, Horn G, Hohler T: On the local efficacy of cyclopyroxolamine in onychomycosis. Arzneimittelforschung 31:1369, 1981.

105. Zaias N: Management of onychomycosis with oral terbinafine. J Am Acad Dermatol 23:810, 1990.

106. Meinhof W: Kinetics and spectrum of activity of oral antifungals: The therapeutic implications. J Am Acad Dermatol 29:S37, 1993.

107. Roseeuw D, DeDenocker P: New approaches to the treatment of onychomycosis. J Am Acad Dermatol 29:S45, 1993.

108. Hettinger DF, Valinsky MS: Treatment of onychomycosis with nail avulsion and topical ketoconazole. J Am Podiatr Med Assoc 81:28, 1991.

109. Daniel CR III: Basic nail plate avulsion. J Dermatol Surg Oncol 18:685, 1992.

110. Geronemus RG: Laser surgery of the nail unit. J Dermatol Surg Oncol 18:735, 1992.

111. Rothermel E, Apfelberg DB: Carbon dioxide laser use for certain diseases of the toenails. Clin Podiatr Med Surg 4:809, 1987.

112. Apfelberg DB, Rothermel E, Widtfeldt A, et al: Preliminary report on use of carbon dioxide laser in podiatry. J Am Podiatr Med Assoc 74:509, 1984.

113. Augustine DF: CO_2 laser enhances treatment for variety of podiatric conditions. Clin Laser Monthly 5:S, 1987.

114. Cohen PR, Buzdar AU: Metastatic breast carcinoma mimicking an acute paronychia of the great toe: Case report and review of subungual metastases. Am J Clin Oncol 16:86, 1993.

115. Haneke E, Baran R (with the participation of Brauner GJ): Nail surgery and traumatic abnormalities. *In* Baran R, Dawber RPR (eds): Diseases of the Nails and Their Management, ed 2. Blackwell Scientific, Oxford, England, 1994, pp 345–416.

116. Wilson JW: Paronychia and onycholysis, etiology and therapy. Arch Dermatol 92:726, 1965.

117. Gunnoe RE: Diseases of the nails: How to recognize and treat them. Postgrad Med 74:357, 1983.

118. Patki AH, Mehta JM: Pterygium unguis in a patient with recurrent type 2 lepra reaction. Cutis 44:311, 1989.

119. Kingsbury DH, Chester EC Jr, Jansen GT: Syphilitic paronychia: An unusual complaint (letter). Arch Dermatol 105:458, 1972.

120. Witkowski JA: Scabies: Subungual areas harbor mites. JAMA 252:1318, 1984.

121. Scher RK: Subungual scabies. Am J Dermatopathol 5:187, 1983.

122. Scher RK: Subungual scabies (letter). J Am Acad Dermatol 12:577, 1985.

123. DePaoli RT, Marks VJ: Crusted (Norwegian) scabies: Treatment of nail involvement (letter). J Am Acad Dermatol 17:136, 1987.

124. Shumer SM, O'Keefe EJ: Bleomycin in the treatment of recalcitrant warts. J Am Acad Dermatol 9:91, 1983.

125. Gibson JR, Harvey SG: Interferon in the treatment of persistent viral warts. Dermatologica 169:47, 1984.

126. Halpern LK, Lane CW: Treatment of periungual warts. Missouri Med 50:765, 1953.

127. Gardner LW, Acker DW: Bone destruction of a distal phalanx caused by periungual warts. Arch Dermatol 107:275, 1973.

128. Zaias N: Benign tumors. *In* Zaias N (ed): The Nail in Health and Disease. Appleton & Lange, Norwalk, CT, 1990, pp 209–220.

129. Lloyd-Davies RW, Brill GC: The aetiology and outpatient management of ingrowing toenails. Br J Surg 50:592, 1963.

130. Mortimer PS, Dawber RPR: Trauma to the nail unit including occupational sports injuries. Dermatol Clin 3:415, 1985.

131. Sonnex TS, Dawber RPR: Treatment of ingrowing toenails with liquid nitrogen spray cryotherapy. BMJ 291:173, 1985.

132. Dawber RPR, Baran R: Nail surgery. In Samman PD, Fenton DA (eds): The Nails in Disease. William Heinemann, London, 1986, pp 194–206.

133. Baran R, Bureau H, Sayag J: Congenital malalignment of the big toe nail. Clin Exp Dermatol 4:359, 1979.

134. Baran R, Bureau H: Congenital malalignment of the big toe-nail as a cause of ingrowing toe-nail in infancy: Pathology and treatment (a study of thirty cases). Clin Exp Dermatol 8:619, 1983.

135. Dawson TAJ: An inherited nail dystrophy principally affecting the great toe nails. Clin Exp Dermatol 4:309, 1979.

136. Cohen J, Scher RK, Pappert A: Congenital malalignment of the great toenails. Pediatr Dermatol 8:40, 1991.

137. Cohen PR: Congenital malalignment of the great toe nails: Case report and literature review. Pediatr Dermatol 8:43, 1991.

138. Young J, Mulley G: Splinter haemorrhages in the elderly. Age Ageing 16:101, 1987.

139. Horder T, Libman E, Poynton FJ, et al: Discussion on the clinical significance and course of subacute bacterial endocarditis. BMJ 2:301, 1920.

140. Blum M, Aviram A: Splinter hemorrhages in patients receiving regular hemodialysis. JAMA 239:47, 1978.

141. Lang PG Jr: Keratosis lichenoides chronica: Successful treatment with psoralen-ultraviolet-A therapy. Arch Dermatol 117:105, 1981.

142. Carmel R: Hair and fingernail changes in acquired and congenital pernicious anemia. Arch Intern Med 145:484, 1985.

143. Kassis V, Kassis E, Thomsen HK: Benign cutaneous periarteritis nodosa with nail defects (letter). J Am Acad Dermatol 13:661, 1985.

144. Robertson JC, Braunne ML: Splinter haemorrhages, pitting, and other findings in fingernails of healthy adults. BMJ 4:279, 1974.

145. Baumal A, Robinson MJ: Nail bed involvement in pemphigus vulgaris. Arch Dermatol 107:751, 1973.

146. Bluhm JF, Johnson SC, Norback DH: Bullous amyloidosis: Case report with ultrastructural studies. Arch Dermatol 116:1164, 1980.

147. Salasche SJ, Garland LD: Tumors of the nail. Dermatol Clin 3:521, 1985.

148. Bendl BJ: Subungual exostosis. Cutis 26:260, 1980.

149. Dahlin DC, Unni KK: Bone tumors, ed 4. Charles C Thomas, Springfield, Ill, 1986, pp 18–30.

150. Miller-Breslow A, Dorfman HD: Dupuytren's (subungual) exostosis. Am J Surg Pathol 12:368, 1988.

151. Kato H, Nakagawa K, Tsuji T, Hamada T: Subungual exostoses—Clinicopathological and ultrastructural studies of three cases. Clin Exp Dermatol 15:429, 1990.

152. Davis DA, Cohen PR: Subungual exostosis: Case report and literature review. Pediatr Dermatol, in press.

153. Shaffer LW: Subungual exostosis. Arch Dermatol 24:371, 1931.

154. Houle RJ: Spur-shaped phalangeal exostosis. J Am Podiatr Med Assoc 57:21, 1967.

155. Hazen PG, Smith DE: Hereditary multiple exostoses: Report of a case presenting with proximal nail fold and nail swelling. J Am Acad Dermatol 22:132, 1990.

156. Baran R, Bureau H: Multiple exostosis syndrome. J Am Acad Dermatol 25:333, 1991.

157. Del Rio JM, Navarra R, Ferrando E, Mascaro J: Hereditary multiple exostoses syndrome presenting as nail malalignment and longitudinal dystrophy of fingers. Abstract presented at the 18th World Congress of Dermatology, New York City, June 12–18, 1992, p 49A.

158. Vine JE, Cohen PR: Renal cell carcinoma metastatic to the thumb: A case report and review of subungual metastases. Manuscript submitted for publication.

159. Cohen HJ, Frank SB, Minkin W: Subungual exostosis. Arch Dermatol 107:431, 1973.
160. Zimmerman EH: Subungual exostosis. Cutis 19:185, 1977.
161. Norton LA: Nail disorders. J Am Acad Dermatol 2:451, 1980.
162. Schulze KE, Hebert AA: Diagnostic features, differential diagnosis and treatment of subungual osteochondroma. Pediatr Dermatol 11:39, 1994.
163. Lemont H, Christman RA: Subungual exostosis and nail disease and radiologic aspects. *In* Scher RK, Daniel CR III (eds): Nails: Therapy, Diagnosis, Surgery. WB Saunders, Philadelphia, 1990, pp 250–257.
164. Guidici MA, Moser RP, Kransdorf MJ: Cartilaginous tumors. Radiol Clin North Am 31:244, 1993.
165. Resnick D, Niwayama G: Diagnosis of Bone and Joint Disorders, ed 2. WB Saunders, Philadelphia, 1988, pp 3701–3719.
166. Evison G, Price CHG: Subungual exostosis. Br J Radiol 39:451, 1966.
167. Landon GC, Johnson KA, Dahlin DC: Subungual exostosis. J Bone Joint Surg 61A:256, 1979.
168. Oliveira ADS, Picoto ADS, Verde SF, Martins O: Subungual exostosis: Treatment as an office procedure. J Dermatol Surg Oncol 6:555, 1980.

CHAPTER 9

Onychomycosis

Boni E. Elewski, Maria A. Charif, and C. Ralph Daniel III

Onychomycosis refers to fungal infection of one or more of the components of the nail unit and can be caused by dermatophytes, yeasts, or nondermatophyte molds. The term *tinea unguium* is generally applied to dermatophytosis of the nail unit. There are four patterns of fungal invasion into the nail unit: distal lateral subungual onychomycosis (DLSO), white superficial onychomycosis (WSO), proximal subungual onychomycosis (PSO), and *Candida* onychomycosis. Each of these varieties has distinct clinical manifestations and may be caused by a different group of fungal organisms.

The exact prevalence of onychomycosis is unknown, but it is estimated to occur in 15 to 20 per cent of persons 40 to 60 years of age[1] and up to 90 per cent in the elderly.[2] Studies in the United Kingdom,[3] Spain,[4] and Finland[5] found an overall prevalence of 3, 1.7, and 8.4 per cent, respectively. It is probably the most common nail disorder, accounting for up to 50 per cent of all nail diseases. The incidence of onychomycosis has been rising sharply in the United States and in other developed countries. Predisposing factors include increasing age, diabetes mellitus, immunosuppression, hyperhidrosis, poor peripheral circulation, trauma, and onychogryposis.

Dermatophytes cause the majority of infections. In a large study by Summerbell and others[6] of 2662 nail-invading infective agents, dermatophytes were isolated in 91 per cent of cases, *Candida albicans* in 5.5 per cent, and various nondermatophyte molds in 3 per cent. Because the clinical manifestations may be identical, a fungal culture is essential in determining the infective agent. Not all patients with dystrophic nails have onychomycosis, and a thorough understanding of the disease process is needed to establish the proper diagnosis and make informed decisions regarding therapy.

TINEA UNGUIUM

It is not surprising that dermatophyte fungi are the most common cause of onychomycosis because they are keratinolytic pathogens and invade normal keratin of the skin, hair, and nail. Few other fungi have the ability to decompose native keratin. The most common dermatophyte nail pathogens are *Trichophyton rubrum* and *T. mentagrophytes,* which are also the most common causes of tinea pedis. *Epidermophyton floccosum, T. violaceum,* and miscellaneous *Microsporum* species account for a small percentage of cases. The various causative agents of tinea unguium are listed in Table 9–1.

The one hand, two feet syndrome is not uncommon. One of the authors (CRD) has

Table 9–1. MAJOR CAUSES OF ONYCHOMYCOSIS

Dermatophyte Fungi
Trichophyton rubrum
Trichophyton mentagrophytes
Epidermophyton floccosum
Nondermatophyte Fungi
Acremonium
Aspergillus species
Fusarium species
Onycochola canadensis
Scopulariopsis brevicaulis
Scytalidium dimidiatum
Scytalidium hyalinum
Yeasts
Candida albicans

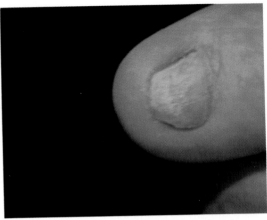

Figure 9–1. Distal subungual onychomycosis, *Trichophyton rubrum*, chronic; note keratinization of distal nail bed.

recently done a retrospective study of 80 patients with this disorder.[32] The age at which symptoms first developed on the feet was 37.1 ± 2.4 years and 45.7 ± 2.2 years for the hands. A traumatic event often preceded the appearance of the fungus in the nails. The hand involved was usually the one used to scratch the feet or pick the toenails. *Trichophyton rubrum* was the usual causative organism.

Toenails are four times more likely than fingernails to be infected. The longest toe, either the first or the second, which bears the brunt of pressure and trauma from footwear, is particularly susceptible to invasion. Some authors believe that eliminating the instigating factor may often result in spontaneous resolution.[7] Approximately 30 per cent of patients who have dermatophyte infections elsewhere on their bodies also acquire tinea unguium. Premenopausal females with no predisposing factors are less frequently affected than men of the same age group,[8] suggesting that estrogen may offer a protective effect. Prepubertal children are rarely affected, possibly because of the protective element of faster nail growth in this age group.[9] Numerous patients associate onset of disease with military service, especially those stationed for prolonged periods in hot, humid areas wearing heavy, occlusive footwear. Years of repeated trauma and impaired peripheral vascular supply are believed to account for an increased prevalence in the elderly.

Distal Subungual Infection

The most common variety of distal subungual infection (Fig. 9–1), DLSO, starts as an infection of the cornified layer of the hyponychium and distal or lateral nail bed and is generally associated with tinea pedis. It is best described as "nail bed dermatophytosis." Proximal invasion of the nail bed and ventral invasion of the nail plate then occur. The first clinical sign of infection is a discrete, distal, or lateral focus of onycholysis, yellow-brown discoloration, and hyperkeratosis of the nail bed. A mild inflammatory reaction occurs in the hyponychium and nail bed, resulting in hyperkeratosis with accumulation of subungual debris, discoloration, and onycholysis. The nail bed becomes cornified, and normal nail contour is lost. According to Zaias,[1] most cases begin with tinea pedis with subsequent invasion of the nail unit. This disorder may be autosomal dominant with incomplete penetration.[10,11]

DLSO may progress to total dystrophic onychomycosis in which the entire nail plate and bed are involved. The dystrophic nail plate is retained as a residual stump at the proximal nail fold or is traumatically lost.

White Superficial Onychomycosis (Leukonychia Trichophytica)

WSO (Fig. 9–2), a less common variety, is a distinctive pattern in which the nail plate is the primary site of invasion. The infection then proceeds to include the nail bed and hyponychium. It is most frequently seen in toenails and is primarily caused by *T. mentagrophytes*, which possesses enzymes that allow it to digest and invade the nail plate directly. *Microsporum persicolor* is an occasional etiologic agent as is *C. albicans* in infants. WSO may also be caused by nondermatophyte molds, *Aspergillus terreus*, *Fusarium oxysporum*, and *Acremonium* species.

The infection manifests as speckled or punctate porcelain-white lesions randomly distributed along the surface of the nail plate, gradu-

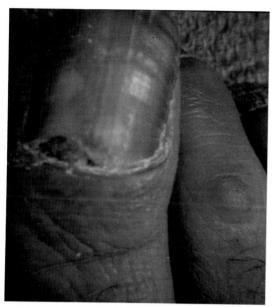

Figure 9–2. Proximal subungual onychomycosis, *Trichophyton rubrum.*

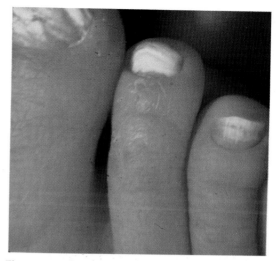

Figure 9–3. White superficial onychomycosis, *Trichophyton mentagrophytes.*

ally coalescing to involve the whole surface.[2] The nail plate becomes white and crumbly, with the consistence of plaster. The crumbled appearance can be used as a differentiating point from leukonychia. Older lesions may acquire a yellow hue. The morphology of the fungus in WSO is typically that of a saprophyte with modified hyphal elements (eroding fronds) as opposed to the usual parasitic hyphal forms seen in stratum corneum invasion.[1]

Proximal Subungual Onychomycosis

PSO (Fig. 9–3), a rarely seen pattern that affects fingernails and toenails equally, is primarily caused by *T. rubrum. T. megninii, T. mentagrophytes, T. schoenleinii,* and *T. tonsurans* have also been reported to cause the condition.[12] It starts with invasion of the stratum corneum of the proximal nail fold and subsequently penetrates the newly formed nail plate. The clinical result is a white discoloration under the proximal nail plate in the area of the lunula; the distal nail unit remains normal. As opposed to WSO, the nail plate is intact. Subungual hyperkeratosis, onychomadesis, and eventual destruction and shedding of the entire nail plate may occur in advanced disease. Because it is infrequent, some authors believe that a preceding episode of trauma is a

prerequisite for it to occur in immunocompetent patients.[7]

Proximal white subungual onychomycosis (PWSO) has been described with increasing frequency in patients with acquired immunodeficiency syndrome (AIDS). In fact, this rare form of onychomycosis was seldom encountered before AIDS became prevalent.[12] Toenail rather than fingernail involvement is more common, and, unlike other instances of onychomycosis, concurrent tinea pedis is rare. In one study of 61 human immunodeficiency virus (HIV)–infected individuals with onychomycosis, 54 (87.1 per cent) had PWSO.[12] *T. rubrum* is the most common pathogen. The explanation for the increased prevalence in this patient population remains unclear. PWSO may be the presenting sign of HIV infection and should prompt health care providers to obtain serologic tests for HIV infection in individuals at risk.

CANDIDA INFECTIONS

C. albicans is the etiologic agent in 70 per cent of cases of onychomycosis caused by yeast. *C. parapsilosis, C. tropicalis,* and *C. krusei* account for the remainder of cases.[13,24] Recently onychocola canadensis has been associated with onychomycosis.[31]

Candida onychomycosis refers to a rare syndrome limited to patients afflicted with chronic mucocutaneous candidiasis. In this type of onychomycosis, the organism invades the nail plate directly. Both toenails and fingernails may be involved, and the full thickness of the nail can be affected. Nail bed thickening occurs as does swelling of the proximal and lateral nail folds, resulting in the characteristic "drumstick" appearance of the digits.

Candida can also be a secondary pathogen in nails previously damaged by dermatophytes, trauma, or other skin diseases or in a setting of chronic paronychia. *Candida* infection is two to three times more common in women.[14] Seventy per cent of cases affect the hands, especially the middle finger, which may be infected from an intestinal or vaginal reservoir.[13] Recurrent infection of the nail matrix may result in transverse striations (Beau's lines) and nail plate dystrophy. Onycholysis and subungual hyperkeratosis may also occur, resulting in a clinical picture similar to that of distal subungual onychomycosis.

A third type of *Candida* infection, primary *Candida* onycholysis, may also occur. Whether this represents a distinct entity is open to debate. Some argue that *Candida* merely colonized onycholytic nails, whereas others believe *Candida* infection is the primary process.

Factors that predispose to *Candida* infection include diabetes mellitus, hypoparathyroidism, thyroid disease, Addison's disease, malabsorption, malnutrition, malignancies, and intake of steroids, antibiotics, and antimitotic medications. Local factors include chemical or mechanical damage to the cuticle, frequent exposure to water, frequent contact with sugar-containing food items, hyperhidrosis, chilblains, and psoriatic onycholysis.

OTHER FUNGAL INFECTIONS

Molds cause 1.5 to 6 per cent of onychomycosis.[13,15] In Summerbell and colleagues'[6] study, molds constituted up to 3.3 per cent of the organisms cultured from nail infections. Only *Scytalidium dimidiatum*[30] and *S. hyalinum* have demonstrated ability of keratinolysis, and there is presumptive evidence that *Scopulariopsis brevicaulis* also has an ability to invade keratin directly. Other nondermatophyte molds only invade nails that have altered keratin, secondary either to trauma or disease. An exception are the molds that cause WSO. Onychomycosis secondary to nondermatophyte molds is seen most frequently in the elderly, in patients with skin diseases that affect the nails, and in immunocompromised patients. It is more frequent in toes than in fingers. Only one nail may be affected. Confinement in tight shoes, trauma from repeated pressure, and

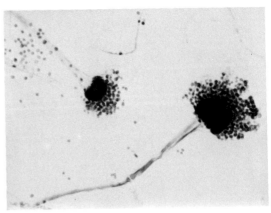

Figure 9–4. A teased preparation of *Aspergillus fumigatus*.

close contact between digits are believed to account for this.

Although several nondermatophyte molds have been reported to cause onychomycosis, *Scopulariopsis brevicaulis* is the most common.[6] Other pathogens include *Alternaria, Aspergillus, Acremonium, Fusarium, Scytalidium dimidiatum, Scytalidium hyalinum,* and *Cladosporium carrionii*.[6] *Fusarium oxysporon, Aspergillus terreus,* and *Acremonium roseogriseum* cause WSO, which may progress to total dystrophic onychomycosis. *Scytalidium dimidiatum*, a dematiaceous mold that occurs commonly in West Africa, the West Indies, and Southeast Asia, is distinctive in its ability to cause paronychia as well as infections that resemble classic tinea manuum and tinea pedis.[16] *Scytalidium hyalinum* may also cause a classic "one hand–two feet" pattern of skin infection (Figs. 9–4 to 9–7).

Aspergillus (Fig. 9–8) is frequently cultured from the nails. In most instances, it is a saprophytic inhabitant rather than a pathogen and

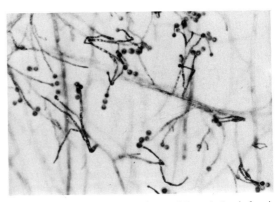

Figure 9–5. A teased preparation of *Scopulariopsis brevicaulis*.

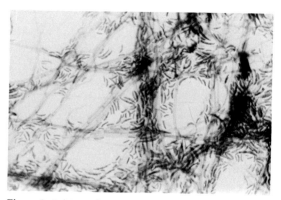

Figure 9–6. A teased preparation of a *Fusarium* species.

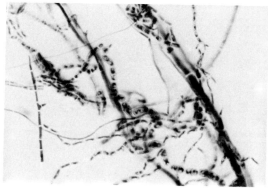

Figure 9–7. A teased preparation of *Scytalidium* species.

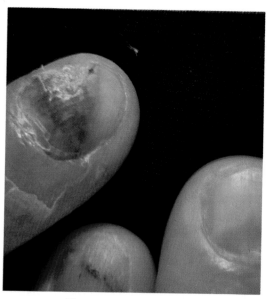

Figure 9–8. *Aspergillus niger.*

may impart a bluish-green tint to the involved nail structure, reminiscent of the discoloration caused by *Pseudomonas*.

Many of these fungi are highly sensitive to cycloheximide and may be missed if the specimen is not also inoculated on a cycloheximide-free medium, such as Sabdex or Littman's Oxgall agar. Clinical clues that a nondermatophyte mold is the causative pathogen include the absence of tinea pedis, only one or two infected toenails, a history of trauma before nail dystrophy, and a history of nonresponsiveness to the new systemic antimycotics (fluconazole, itraconazole, and terbinafine).

LABORATORY DIAGNOSIS

Collection of Specimens[24]

A stepwise approach to diagnosis is outlined in Figure 9–9. The first step in diagnosis is obtaining an adequate specimen. In patients with distal subungual onychomycosis, the specimen should be obtained from the nail bed, which is the primary site of infection, ideally with a small curet and as proximal to the cuticle as possible. Care must be taken to avoid penetration of the nail bed and bleeding. Scrapings from the undersurface of the nail should also be collected. It is important to obtain nail material from the advancing infected edge most proximal to the cuticle, where the likelihood of viable hyphae is the greatest. If nail bed debris is unavailable or insufficient, the affected nail plate can be sampled with special nail clippers. Nail clippings and portions of nails that have been avulsed are the least desirable specimens because they have a very low yield of viable hyphae and require special processing.[25,26]

In WSO, the fungi directly invade the nail plate surface. This infected nail debris can be removed with a no. 15 blade or sharp curet.

In PSO, the fungus invades under the cuticle and then settles in the proximal nail bed. The overlying nail plate is intact. To obtain culture material, the overlying healthy nail plate should be gently pared away with a no. 15 blade scalpel, and material from the proximal nail bed should be collected with a sharp curet. A nail drill may yield a more satisfactory specimen when the infection is deep and difficult to reach.

The sampled material can be divided in two portions: one for direct microscopy and the remainder for culture. If nail material is to be

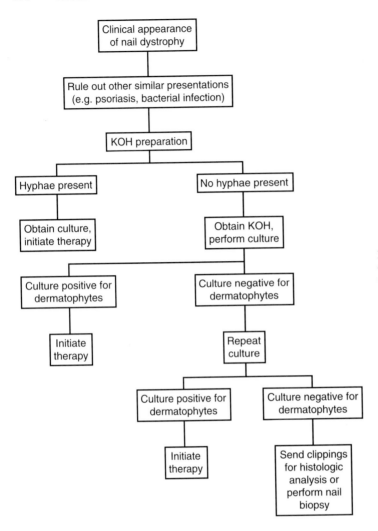

Figure 9–9. Stepwise approach to diagnosis. (KOH = potassium hydroxide.)

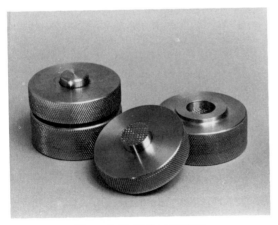

Figure 9–10. Nail micronizer.

used, fine shavings or minute clippings are preferred to large pieces. It is also helpful to pulverize thick clippings in a nail micronizer (Fig. 9–10)[24,25] or manually by placing the clippings between two pieces of cardboard and crushing them with a hammer before using them for a potassium hydroxide (KOH) preparation or culture.

Direct Microscopy

Direct microscopy of KOH preparations (Fig. 9–11) is only a screening test for the presence or absence of fungi; it cannot identify among pathogens. KOH dissolves keratin in nail material, leaving fungal elements intact. However, because large pieces of debris are often obtained in nail specimens, this procedure can be time consuming. The use of 15 to

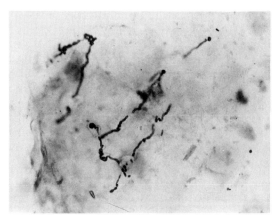

Figure 9–11. Hyphal elements in a potassium hydroxide preparation of nail scrapings.

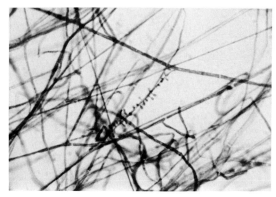

Figure 9–13. A teased preparation of *Trichophyton rubrum*.

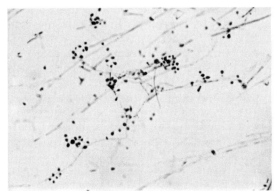

Figure 9–12. A teased preparation of *Trichophyton mentagrophytes*.

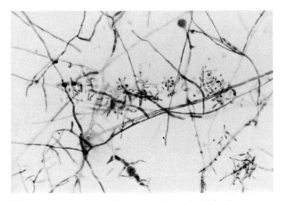

Figure 9–14. A teased preparation of *Trichophyton tonsurans*.

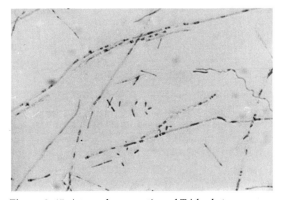

Figure 9–15. A teased preparation of *Trichophyton verrucosum*.

20 per cent KOH in dimethyl sulfoxide will hasten the process. The counterstain, chlorazol black E, which is highly specific for chitin, will selectively accentuate hyphae and is, therefore, particularly useful for nail specimens because fungal elements are scarce. Furthermore, it will not stain potential contaminants such as cotton or elastic fibers, which eliminates many false-positive findings.[17] Another counterstain is Parker's blue-black ink, but it is not chitin specific. For best results, the microscope should be set on low power (using the × 10 objective), and the light should be reduced. If direct microscopy is negative, and the KOH reagent used contains glycerol, the preparation may be left standing on the workbench overnight and re-examined the next day.[8] A teased preparation directly from the culture plate may also be utilized (Figs. 9–12 to 9–15).

Culture Techniques

Fungal culture is the only method that can identify the genus and species of the causative pathogen. Although most cases of onychomycosis are caused by dermatophytes, the occasional nondermatophyte fungus that is generally resistant to oral agents needs to be ruled out before selecting appropriate treatment. Two types of media are needed for culturing nail specimens. One medium should contain cycloheximide, an antifungal agent that is added to agar to isolate selectively many pathogenic fungi but inhibits many nondermatophyte molds that can be pathogens. Examples of media containing cycloheximide are dermatophyte test media, Mycosel (BBL), and Mycobiotic (DIFCO).[18] Sabouraud's glucose agar and Littman's Oxgall medium have no added cycloheximide and serve as the other media to ensure isolation of nail pathogens sensitive to cycloheximide, such as *Scopulariopsis brevicaulis*, *Scytalidium dimidiatum*, and *Scytalidium hyalinum*.[16] The addition of antibiotics such as chloramphenicol and gentamicin to Sabouraud's glucose agar, referred to as inhibitory mold agar, is an additional precaution to eliminate bacterial pathogens and may be used in lieu of Sabouraud's glucose medium.[18]

Ideally, the specimen should be cultured when the patient has been off both topical and systemic antifungal drugs for 2 to 4 weeks.[18] If the specimen is shipped to an outside laboratory, a sterile container (i.e., urine cup), a pill packet, a clean sheet of white paper, which is then folded and sealed with tape,[8] or a specially designed mailer such as a Dermapack can be used. Specimens should not be placed in sealed containers or in broth, saline, or other moist media. Bacteria and fungal spores that may be contaminants can multiply quickly under such conditions, making it difficult to recover any pathogenic fungus. Ideally, nail specimens should be processed within a week, but infective fungal elements can remain viable for years after specimen collection.

Although some dermatophytes may be recognized by their characteristic colonies, microscopic examination of isolates is usually required for precise identification. Nondermatophyte molds do not have characteristic colonies and, therefore, require morphologic studies. Molds are studied by obtaining teased or Scotch tape preparations in lactophenol cotton blur.[8] *Trichophyton* agars, urea testing, and hair perforation tests can also be useful in differentiating among various dermatophytes.

Histopathology

If KOH preparation and fungal culture fail to yield a diagnosis, a large nail plate fragment can be sent in a 10 per cent buffered formalin container for histologic analysis. Because special techniques may be required in processing specimens, it is helpful to inform the pathologist that nail material is enclosed and to request fungal stains, such as periodic acid–Schiff. The finding of hyphae in a nail plate may permit differentiation from psoriasis, lichen planus, and other causes of nail dystrophy, but, like KOH, this preparation does not identify the particular pathogen. Nail biopsy is the last resort.

STRATEGIES OF THERAPY

Onychomycosis is a medical, not a surgical, problem; however, for decades, because there was no effective therapy, nail avulsion was commonly used for palliative purposes. Today, choosing which of the available antifungal agents to use can be difficult. In most instances, initial therapy consists of a systemic agent because topical antimycotics are generally ineffective as sole therapy. The various systemic drugs overlap in their range of effectiveness, and there are no comparative studies to date. Factors to consider in choosing therapy include the causative pathogen (Table 9–2), potential adverse events and drug interactions, cost of treatment (Table 9–3), dosage schedule, and patient compliance. Determining the minimum inhibitory concentration of the cultured pathogen may also help narrow the choice, although that test is not routinely performed. Should patients not improve, consider incorrect dosage, poor patient compliance, drug interaction, and wrong diagnosis.

Remember to review the patient's needs and prospective compliance. The dosage schedule would be relatively important to a patient taking multiple medications, for example, who might prefer the convenience of a once-a-week dose of fluconazole. Others might prefer to select the one-week-a-month regimen of itraconazole or a fixed 3-month course of either terbinafine or itraconazole.

Table 9–2. **FACTORS TO CONSIDER WHEN SELECTING THERAPY**

Causative pathogen
Potential adverse events
Potential drug interactions
Dosage schedule
Compliance of patient
Cost of treatment regimen
Age and health of patient

Table 9–3. **COST OF TREATMENT**

Antifungal Agent	Unit (mg)[a]	Cost/Unit[b]	Dose Range(mg)	Dose/Mo	Duration (Mo)	Cost/Regimen
Griseofulvin	250	$1.38	1000	30	12	$1987
	330	$0.96	990	30	12	$1037
Ketoconazole	200	$2.35	200	30	12	$846
Itraconazole	100	$4.58	200	30	3	$824
			400	7	4	$513
			400	7	3	$385
Fluconazole	100	$5.82	150	4	9	$314
	200	$9.45	300	4	9	$550
Terbinafine	250	Unknown	250	30	3	Unknown

[a]Ultra–micro-size.
[b]Cost to patient in retail chain pharmacy in Cleveland, Ohio, as of July 15, 1994.

Additionally, cost may be a significant factor; griseofulvin and ketoconazole are the most expensive therapies, and fluconazole and itraconazole are somewhat less costly, depending on the regimen chosen (see Table 9–3). The cost of terbinafine is comparable tablet-for-tablet to that of itraconazole.

Dermatophyte Onychomycosis

Systemic Antifungals

Possible drug interactions should be kept in mind with all oral antifungals.

Griseofulvin. Of the available oral antimycotics, griseofulvin is the least effective in onychomycosis. Its spectrum of action includes only dermatophyte fungi, with no activity on *Candida* or other nondermatophyte fungi. Griseofulvin must be administered daily until the infected nail plate grows out, which is generally 6 to 9 months for fingernails and 12 to 18 months for toenails.

Griseofulvin is delivered to the nail plate via the matrix, but the pharmacokinetics of the drug have not been well studied. This fungistatic medication does not persist in the nail plate more than 1 to 2 weeks, which explains the long duration of therapy.[19] The ultra–micro-size form is best suited for onychomycosis, and most patients require 750 to 1000 mg daily in divided doses to eradicate the infection. Both underdosing and patient compliance are common reasons for failure (Table 9–4).

Laboratory monitoring during griseofulvin therapy is controversial, but periodic monitoring of hematopoietic and hepatic functions is reasonable, especially when long-term therapy is planned. Griseofulvin is contraindicated in pregnancy, lupus erythematosus, and acute intermittent porphyria. Additionally, the drug may interfere with oral contraceptives and cause fetal abnormalities. Appropriate precautions are, therefore, necessary in women of childbearing potential. Long-term regimens are frequently accompanied by minor annoyances such as gastrointestinal disturbances and headaches, causing patients to discontinue therapy prematurely and resulting in treatment failure. Cure rates are low and recurrence rates are high.

Table 9–4. **POTENTIAL ADVERSE EVENTS**

Griseofulvin

Nausea, gastrointestinal disturbance
Headache
Thrombocytopenia, anemia, leukopenia, hepatotoxicity, proteinuria
Photosensitivity
Precipitates SCLE
Interferes with oral contraceptives

Itraconazole

Nausea, GI disturbance
Rash
Pruritus
Hypokalemia
Reversible telogen effluvium
Hepatotoxicity

Fluconazole

Nausea, GI disturbance
Rash
Pruritus
Thrombocytopenia
Hepatotoxicity
Reversible telogen effluvium

Terbinafine

Nausea, GI disturbance
Taste disturbance, reversible upon discontinuation of therapy
Hepatic toxicity
Leukopenia
Rash

SCLE, Subacute lupus erythematosus; GI, gastrointestinal.

Ketoconazole. The first broad-spectrum oral antifungal and first oral azole, ketoconazole has activity not only against dermatophyte fungi but also *Candida* and some nondermatophytes. It is fungistatic and has no persistent binding to the nail plate.[19] Daily dosages of 200 mg are generally sufficient, but they need to be continued until the nail plate has grown out. Cure rates in onychomycosis are comparable or only slightly higher than those with griseofulvin.

The potential risk of hepatotoxicity has limited the use of ketoconazole in onychomycosis (see Table 9–4). The published risk is 1 in 10,000 to 15,000 patients, but it may be more common in those with onychomycosis. Ketoconazole may be useful in patients who are allergic or resistant to griseofulvin, in patients who are intolerant to griseofulvin, and in cases of *Candida* onychomycosis. An acid environment enhances absorption, and ketoconazole should be administered 2 hours before antacids or H_2 blockers. A baseline liver profile followed by monitoring of hepatic parameters in 2 weeks and, then at monthly intervals is recommended. Those at highest risk for hepatotoxicity are women, persons older than 40 years, and those with a history of drug allergies or hepatotoxicity. Additionally, ketoconazole is contraindicated in patients taking terfenadine or astemizole.

Fluconazole. This is a member of the azole family and has activity against dermatophytes, *Candida,* and some nondermatophyte fungi. Fluconazole has only recently been studied as a potential therapy for onychomycosis. The pharmacokinetics of fluconazole in the nail have not been well studied, but the drug reaches the nail plate via the nail bed, and there is evidence it persists in the nail for several months. Dosages of 50 to 100 mg either daily or on alternate days until the normal nail has grown out are often effective.[29] A new "pulse" or intermittent regimen also reported to be effective is 150 mg administered once a week until the nail has grown out. The use of chemical urea nail avulsion improves cure rates. In those patients not responding, the dose can be increased to 300 to 450 mg once per week. Patients on multiple medications may enjoy the freedom of the 1 day per week dosage. Assaf and Elewski[20] evaluated 11 patients with onychomycosis of the fingernail or toenail, with a total of 43 infected nails. *T. rubrum* was the predominant organism cultured, although 2 patients with fingernail infections had *C. albicans.* Eight patients re-

ceived fluconazole 300 mg once weekly, 1 patient received 200 mg once weekly (a child), and 2 patients received an alternate-day dosage of 100 to 200 mg. Eight of the patients also used an adjunctive topical antimycotic preparation. All 6 patients, with 32 toenails involved, were clinically cured after a mean duration of 6 months, and 5 patients, with 11 fingernails involved, were cured after 3.7 months. No clinical or laboratory adverse events were recorded. One of these patients had previously experienced a morbilliform eruption while on itraconazole but was successfully treated with fluconazole without a similar problem.

Fluconazole can be administered with or without food and without regard to gastric acidity. The drug is well tolerated, and instances of hepatotoxicity are rare. Laboratory monitoring is controversial, but periodic testing of hepatic and hematopoietic functions may be indicated for those on long-term therapy (see Table 9–4). In a recent study by Scher and coworkers, treatment of toenail onychomycosis with fluconazole yielded greater than 86 percent clinical success with a low relapse rate at a dose schedule of 300 mg once weekly for a mean period of 6–7 months.[34]

Itraconazole. This is the newest member of the azole family. Effective against dermatophytes, *Candida,* and some nondermatophyte molds, itraconazole probably has the broadest spectrum of all oral antifungal drugs. Additionally, the pharmacokinetics in the nail have been thoroughly investigated. Itraconazole is detected in the nail plate within 7 days of administration.[19] It penetrates from the nail bed and matrix and persists in the nail plate for 6 to 9 months after therapy is discontinued.[19] This is probably related to its lipophilic property, causing the drug to adhere to the lipophilic cytoplasm of the keratinocytes in the nail plate.

Two schedules have been investigated: the fixed (continuous)[28] and the pulse or intermittent. The fixed dosage is 200 mg daily for 12 weeks in pedal onychomycosis or for 6 weeks in fingernail disease. The U.S. study results for toenail onychomycosis showed a mycologic cure rate of 54 per cent, a clinical success rate of 65 per cent, and an overall success rate of 35 per cent (clinical success and mycologic cure). It is important to emphasize to the patient that when therapy is discontinued the nail is not normal. Because of the persistence of itraconazole in the nail plate, however, the nail grows out fungus free. The pulse or intermittent regimen is based on the rationale that the drug reaches the nail within 7 days of therapy and persists in the nail for 6 to 9 months, whereas serum levels are not detectable 1 week after discontinuation. Recently two pulse doses have been FDA approved for fingernail tinea.[33] Intermittent cycles of 400 mg daily for 1 week per month can be continued for 2 months when treating fingernails and for 3 months for toenail infection. Like the fixed dosage, the nail is not normal when therapy is discontinued. The U.S. data for intermittent studies are currently not available, but cure rates of almost 80 per cent have been obtained in Europe.[21] Itraconazole should be given with food. Although hepatic toxicity has been estimated to be less than 1:500,000, periodic monitoring of hepatic parameters is not unreasonable (see Table 9–4). This drug appears to be safe and effective.

Terbinafine. This is a member of the allylamine family of antifungals and is currently the only fungicidal oral antimycotic. It is broad spectrum and is effective against dermatophyte fungi, some nondermatophytes, and some species of *Candida*. Terbinafine is lipophilic and persists in the nail plate for several months after discontinuation. It is detected in the nail plate in 1 week, apparently delivered via the nail bed and matrix.

On the basis of pharmacokinetics, a 12-week course of 250 mg every day is generally effective in toenail disease; a 6-week course of the same dose is effective in fingernail disease. The U.S. study had clinical success rates of 71 per cent at 12 weeks and 77 per cent at 24 weeks and an overall clinical success rate of 74 per cent.[22] As anticipated, the nail is not clinically normal when the drug is discontinued. Although hepatotoxic reactions are rare, periodic monitoring of hepatic and hematopoietic parameters is reasonable (see Table 9–4). This drug also appears to be safe and effective and has few if any significant drug interactions.

Miscellaneous Therapies. Two topical antifungals currently under investigation in the United States, amorolfine and tioconazole, are available in other countries. Topical therapy has the greatest potential as primary therapy in mild infections and as a prophylactic agent. Avulsion of the nail combined with topical 2 per cent ketoconazole cream under occlusion may be effective in select patients. However, because of the inherent problems of nail avulsion, this is best limited to those with only one or two dystrophic nails. Topical therapy is messy and cumbersome.

Nondermatophyte Mold Onychomycosis

Nondermatophyte molds seldom cause onychomycosis (see Table 9–1). In general, when a nondermatophyte mold is determined to be the pathogen, there is no effective oral treatment. Surgical treatment or debridement followed by application of a topical antifungal may benefit some select patients. *Scytalidium dimidiatum* and *Scytalidium hyalinum* have not responded to fluconazole, itraconazole, or terbinafine. When *Scopulariopsis* species are cultured, they are frequently contaminants. However, they also can function as a pathogen, and some infections have responded to itraconazole.

Fusarium and *Acremonium* species and *Aspergillus terreus* can cause WSO. The treatment of WSO is curettage or debridement of the dystrophic superficial nail plate followed by application of a topical antifungal. However, when the infection has progressed to total dystrophic onychomycosis, no systemic antimycotic is uniformly effective. In these instances, surgical debridement or avulsion may be beneficial in some select patients. A trial of itraconazole, terbinafine, or possibly fluconazole may also result in improvement in some patients.

Candida "Onychomycosis"

C. albicans is the most common species of *Candida* that can secondarily cause or exacerbate nail disease. When other species of *Candida* are isolated, they are generally saprophytes and not pathogenic. If *C. albicans* is determined to be the pathogen,[23] an oral azole would be appropriate. Griseofulvin is ineffective, and terbinafine is only of borderline effectiveness. *Candida* has also been implicated in onycholysis and paronychia infections.[24] Topical antifungal therapy is appropriate.

References

1. Zaias N: Onychomycosis. Dermatol Clin 3:445, 1985.
2. Norton LA: Disorders of the nail. *In* Moschella SL, Hurley HJ (eds): Dermatology. WB Saunders, Philadelphia, 1992, pp 1563–1585.
3. Roberts DT: Prevalence of dermatophyte onychomycosis in the United Kingdom: Results of an omnibus survey. Br J Dermatol 126(Suppl 39):23, 1992.
4. Sais G, Juggla A, Peyri J: Prevalence of dermatophyte onychomycosis in Spain: A cross-sectional study. Br J Dermatol 132:758, 1995.

5. Heikkila H, Stubb S: The prevalence of onychomycosis in Finland. Br J Dermatol 133:699, 1995.
6. Summerbell RC, Kane J, Kradjden S: Onychomycosis, tinea pedis and tinea mannum caused by non-dermatophyte filamentous fungi. Mycoses 32:609, 1989.
7. Cohen JL, Scher RK, Pappert AS. The nail and fungus infections. *In* Elewski BE (ed): Cutaneous Fungal Infections. Igaku-Shoin, New York, 1992, pp 106–123.
8. Haley L, Daniel RC III: Fungal infections. *In* Scher RK, Daniel CR III (eds): Nails: Therapy, Diagnosis, Surgery. WB Saunders, Philadelphia, 1990, pp 106–119.
9. Martin AG, Kobayashi GS. Fungal diseases with cutaneous involvement. *In* Fitzpatrick TB, Eisen AZ, Wolff K, et al (eds): Dermatology in General Medicine, vol 2. New York, McGraw-Hill, 1993, pp 2421–2451.
10. Zias N, Tosti A, Rebell G, et al: Autosomal dominant pattern of distal subungual onychomycosis caused by *Trichophyton rubrum.* J Am Acad Dermatol 34:302, 1996.
11. Daniel CM, Daniel MP, Daniel CR: Onychomycosis update. J Miss State Med Assoc 36:37, 1995.
12. Elewski BE: Clinical pearl: Proximal white subungual onychomycosis in AIDS. J Am Acad Dermatol 29:631, 1993.
13. Andre J, Achten G: Onychomycosis. Int J Dermatol 26:481, 1987.
14. Achten G, Wanet-Rouard J: Onychomycosis in the laboratory. Mykosen 14 (suppl):125, 1978.
15. Greer DL: Evolving role of nondermatophytes in onychomycosis. Int J Dermatol 34:521, 1995.
16. Elewski BE, Greer DL: *Hendersonulea toruloidea* and *Scytalidium hyalinum.* Arch Dermatol 127:1041, 1991.
17. Burke WA, Jones BE: A simple stain for rapid office diagnosis of fungal infections of the skin. Arch Dermatol 120:1519, 1984.
18. Elewski BE: Clinical pearl: Diagnosis of onychomycosis. J Am Acad Dermatol 32:500, 1995.
19. Elewski BE: Mechanism of action of systemic antifungal agents. J Am Acad Dermatol 28S:28, 1993.
20. Assaf RR, Elewski BE. Intermittent fluconazole dosing in patients with onychomycosis: Results of a pilot study. J Am Acad Dermatol, 35:216, 1996.
21. DeDoncker P, Decroix J, Pierard GE, et al: Antifungal therapy for onychomycosis. A pharmacokinetic and pharmacodynamic investigation of monthly cycles of 1-week pulse therapy with itraconazole. Arch Dermatol 132:34, 1996.
22. Gupta AK, Sauder DN, Shear NH. Antifungal agents: An overview. Part II. J Am Acad Dermatol 30:911, 1994.
23. Daniel CR, Elewski BE: *Candida* as a nail pathogen in healthy patients. J Miss State Med Assoc 36:379, 1995.
24. Daniel CR III: The diagnosis of nail fungal infection. Arch Dermatol 127:1566, 1991.
25. Daniel CR: Nail micronizer. Cutis 36:118, 1985.
26. Daniel CR, Elewski BE, Gupta AK: Surgical pearl: Nail micronizer. J Am Acad Dermatol 34:278, 1996.
27. Daniel CR: Traditional management of onychomycosis. J Am Acad Dermatol 35:S21, 1996.
28. Odom R, Daniel CR, Aly R: A double-blind, randomized comparison of itraconazole capsules and placebo in the treatment of onychomycosis of the toenail. J Am Acad Dermatol 35:110, 1996.
29. Montero-Gei F, Robles-Soto M, Schlager H: Fluconazole in the treatment of severe onchomycosis. Int J Dermatol 35:587, 1996.
30. Elewski BE: Onchomycosis caused by *Scytalidium dimidiatum.* J Am Acad Dermatol 35:336, 1996.
31. Gupta AK, Horgen-Bell J, Summerbell R: Onychocola canadensis: Two cases with toenail onychomycosis and a review of the literature. Poster presentation, International Summit on Cutaneous Antifungal Therapy, Vancouver, British Columbia, May 26-May 28, 1996.
32. Daniel CR, Gupta AK, Daniel MP, Daniel CM: Two feet–one hand syndrome—A retrospective multicentre serving. Int J Dermatol, accepted for publication; 1997.
33. Odom RB, Devillez R, Daniel CR, et al: A multicentre placebo-controlled double blind study of intermittent therapy with itraconazole capsules for the treatment of onychomycosis of the fingernail. J Am Acad Dermatol 35:110, 1996.
34. Scher RK, et al: A placebo-controlled randomized, double-blind trial of once weekly fluconazole (150 mg, 300 mg, or 450 mg) in the treatment of distal subungual onychomycosis of the toenail. J Am Acad Dermatol, in press.

CHAPTER 10

Nonfungal Infections and Paronychia

C. Ralph Daniel III, Melissa P. Daniel, and Aditya K. Gupta

INFECTIONS RESULTING FROM HIGHER ORGANISMS

Some parasitic organisms must be included in the differential diagnosis of ungual diseases. For the most part, the disorders discussed next are rare. Several causative organisms are mentioned.

Scabies

Sarcoptes scabiei is the most common higher organism to cause nail disease. Significant nail damage most often occurs in individuals with Norwegian (or crusted) scabies. The person is usually debilitated and in some way immunologically compromised. Mental institutions have been breeding grounds for this disorder. The nail plate is usually dystrophic and brittle, with subungual hyperkeratosis.[1] With this disorder, keratotic areas may be present in the scalp, the face (rare in regular scabies), the palms, and the soles.[2] It is well known that large numbers of organisms may be involved. Nail changes similar to those in nail scabies may be seen in chronic granulomatous disease of childhood[2] or in other disorders producing dystrophic, crumbling nails with subungual hyperkeratosis.

The nail may also be instrumental in perpetuating recurrent scabies by harboring the organism and protecting it from topical scabicides.[3,4]

Diagnosis and Treatment. Simple microscopic examination after placing the specimen in mineral oil is all that is usually needed to diagnose the organism. A biopsy also readily shows the organism.

Chemical or surgical avulsion of the involved nail plates may sometimes be necessary to allow scabicides to reach the diseased tissue. Urea may be used to avulse the nail.[5] Removing patients from a predisposing environment or improving their immunologic status, if possible, may also be necessary.

Various treatment regimens have been used in the past including lindane 1 per cent, permethrin 5 per cent, precipitated sulfa, and so on.

Gamma benzene hexachloride (GBH) has been used according to the following procedure[6]:

1. Isolate the patient.
2. Provide weekly total body treatment with daily trimming of nails and scrubbing the nails with GBH, and daily application of GBH to hyperkeratotic crusts.
3. Treat fomites with acaricide.

163

A 10-month-old infant was treated with 10 per cent water-soap suspension of benzyl benzoate, which cleared the skin and nail plates.[7]

Oral ivermectin has been discussed as a possible therapy. No controlled studies have been done to date.[79]

Trichinosis

The organism *Trichinella spiralis* is hematogenously spread before it becomes encysted in muscle. It may find its way into the small vessels of the nail bed. Splinter hemorrhages may result, and if they undergo biopsy, the organism can be found.[8] It has been said that transverse splinter hemorrhages may be seen.[9] Because the nail bed vessels are oriented longitudinally, the mechanism for this is at best unclear. Splinter hemorrhages caused by systemic disorders as well as trichinosis tend to occur simultaneously in multiple nails and begin in the more proximal portions of the nail bed.

Tungiasis (Jigger Flea)

Dermatitis caused by *Tunga penetrans*, a sand flea, has been described in the United States by citizens traveling abroad.[10,11] *T. penetrans* may initially present with an asymptomatic, noninflammatory, translucent nodule with a central dark spot.[10] Complications include severe itching, pain, inflammatory reaction that may lead to autoamputation of the digits, cellulitis, and tetanus.[10] Periungual involvement may occur.[10–12] The periungual central black pit is typical.[13]

Treatment. Treatment consists of removing the flea.[10,11] Left untreated, the condition may progress to include the just-mentioned complications, which require appropriate therapy. More advanced cases may be treated by niridazole.[14]

Subungual Myiasis

Myiasis, an infestation by maggots or larvae or *Musca domestica*, the common housefly, is uncommon in the United States.[15] A subungual hematoma associated with trauma was found to be teeming with these larvae.[15]

Treatment. The larvae may be physically removed, antibiotics given, and predisposing conditions alleviated.

Cutaneous Larva Migrans

The larvae of the nematode *Ancylostoma braziliense* are most often the cause of cutaneous larva migrans.[16] Secondary nail dystrophy, probably caused by the migration of the organism near the matrix, occurred on the thumbnail of one individual.[16]

Treatment. Topical or systemic thiabendazole is administered.

Pediculosis[17,18]

Diemer reported pediculosis involving the toenails. Débridement of a great toenail manifested 10 to 12 body lice.

Post–Kala-Azar Dermal Leishmaniasis[19]

A verrucous eruption has been reported at the base of the nails.

VIRUS INFECTIONS

Herpes Simplex

Herpes simplex type 1 or type 2[20] may affect the nail apparatus. The condition is usually described as herpetic whitlow or herpetic paronychia. Medical and dental personnel are most commonly affected because of their direct contact with patients harboring the infection. Infection follows minor local trauma, even though patients often deny this.[20] Individuals with oral infection may inoculate themselves if they are nail biters or finger suckers.[21,22] One finger is usually involved, usually the forefinger or thumb.[20] Involvement of the toes has been reported but is rare.[21] Any cut or compromise in the periungual tissue allows the infection to penetrate more easily.

As with other herpetic infections, after inoculation there is a latency period of about 3 to 10 days. Local tenderness appears first, followed by erythema, vesicle formation, and pain.[20] The vesicles may coalesce, and a yellowish, honeycomb appearance may be evident.[20] Sometimes vesicles are less apparent and ulcerations are seen. Gradual healing takes place over 2 to 3 weeks. Superinfection with Staphylococcus aureus and streptococci as well as other bacteria may occur. Periodic recurrences occur in a small minority of persons.[23] Diagnosis is based on the clinical picture plus Tzanck smear, culture, or rapid immunofluorescence. A fourfold rise in viral antibody titer is diagnostic but is usually used as a confirmatory measure after treatment is initiated because of the time lag. Herpes simplex may secondarily affect the nails by triggering erythema multiforme.

Treatment. The infection may be highly contagious. Medical and dental personnel as well as others should be aware of this fact. Contact with infants and immunosuppressed individuals should especially be avoided. The wearing of heavy vinyl gloves may decrease transmission, but the safest option is avoidance of direct contact while the infection is active. We tell patients that they may still be contagious up to 7 days or longer after the vesicles completely heal. This is erring on the side of safety. Appropriate patient education, treatment of secondary bacterial infection, and close follow-up are often all that is indicated in minor cases.[22] Elevation, analgesics, immobilization of the involved extremity, and hospitalization may be necessary in more severe infections.[22] Intravenous or oral acyclovir may be used and is now readily available. Foscarnet is available and is indicated for severe herpes infection. Famciclovir and other agents are being tested as treatment for herpes simplex.

As a general rule, surgical drainage should be avoided because it does not usually provide added comfort, and it exposes the patient to the risk of superinfection.[23] Large or tense vesicles may be carefully opened to ease discomfort. This is especially true in the area of the nail matrix because permanent nail deformity may occur if this structure is damaged. Upon incising and draining a lesion, we use prophylactic penicillinase-resistant antibiotics for about 7 days. Idoxuridine has been given by cathodic iontophoresis. Rapid relief of symptoms and rapid healing were reported in two patients.[24]

Herpes Zoster

Shingles may coincidentally affect the nail apparatus if that particular dermatome is involved. This is rare. Treatment is the same as for herpes zoster elsewhere on the body.

Oral acyclovir or oral famciclovir may be instituted.

Verruca Vulgaris

Verruca vulgaris, or the common wart, is discussed under benign tumors in the chapter on neoplasms and under "Treatment" in the appendices. More recent information has been published on intralesional bleomycin,[25,26] infrared coagulation,[27] and the carbon dioxide laser.[28]

Human Immunodeficiency Virus

See the discussion of the nails in patients with human immunodeficiency virus in Chapter 13.

Miscellaneous Infections

Orf virus can affect the nail unit, often the dorsum of the right index finger.[29] Milker's nodules, caused by paravaccinia virus, affect mainly agricultural workers and veterinarians.[29] Leprosy may affect the nails by a number of mechanisms, including neuropathy, vascular deficit, and infection.[30] Some of the clinical manifestations include Beau's lines,[31] pterygium inversum unguis,[31] pseudomacrolunula,[32] leukonychia,[32] macronychia,[32] melanonychia,[30] subungual bleeding,[30] and hapalonychia.[32]

Bacterial Infection

Bacteria are ubiquitous. Our hands provide much of our physical contact with our environment; therefore, we are constantly coming in contact with bacteria. Nails are known to harbor bacteria.[33] Artificial nails may provide an additional home for these organisms.[34] Bacterial infections may manifest themselves in a number of ways in the vicinity of the nail apparatus, including bacterial felon, which requires aggressive systemic antibiotic therapy, blistering distal dactylitis,[35] and acute paronychia.

Paronychia

The word paronychia means inflammation of the nail folds. Paronychia may be infectious or noninfectious.

Acute Paronychia

Allergic contact, contact irritant, fixed drug eruption,[36] methotrexate,[37] and dyshidrotic eczema are among the entities that may cause acute periungual inflammation (Fig. 10–1A) not associated with infections. This section focuses on bacterial causes.

Trauma to the nail folds, as may occur with overaggressive manicuring or pulling a hangnail, can allow pathologic bacteria to invade the nail apparatus. Once a primary, active infection has occurred in a nail fold, the seal between the fold and nail is broken, which often predisposes to chronic paronychia (see Fig. 10–1B). This is true for several reasons. First, the alignment and integrity of the nail folds may be chronically or permanently disrupted. Irritants such as detergents, bath soaps, or nail cosmetics may disrupt the healing structure. The patient's increased personal attempts to heal the area may cause further damage. *S. aureus,* streptococci, and *Pseudomonas* are the most common offenders. Usually only one nail is involved. When several nails are involved, one should suspect subacute or chronic paronychia secondary to either chronic dermatitis or psoriasis vulgaris.[38] Acute paronychia has been reported to be caused by *Candida albicans*[39] and *Trichosporon cutaneum.*[40]

Treatment. One must try to eliminate predisposing factors. For mild cases, the following regimen should be implemented:

1. Warm saline or aluminum acetate (1:80 Domeboro) for 10 to 15 minutes two to four times a day continued for 1 to 2 days after the infection has clinically disappeared.[22]

2. Two per cent mupirocin ointment or polymyxin B–bacitracin ointment should be applied after each soak.

3. Erythromycin (bacteriostatic), 250 to 500 mg, should be taken by mouth with food four times a day for 5 to 14 days. (Continue the treatment for several days after the infection has clinically disappeared.)

For more severe cases, the following protocol should be followed:

1. Painful bulging nail folds should be carefully drained, especially if the nail matrix area is involved, because permanent damage to the nail matrix may occur. An 18-gauge needle or a no. 11 scalpel blade may be used to gently "tease" an opening to release purulent material. Cephalosporin (bacteriocidal), 250 to 500 mg by mouth four times a day, is the initial drug of choice until Gram's stain results or culture and sensitivity studies have returned. Continue antibiotics for at least 5 to 7 days after the infection has resolved clinically. Soaking is begun as previously discussed. The hand should be elevated if much swelling is apparent.[36] Nonadherent gauze[37] or Telfa pads may help drainage.

Chronic Paronychia

Inflammation of the periungual soft tissues over a period of time of 6 weeks or longer may cause chronic paronychia. Some common noninfectious causes include frequent water con-

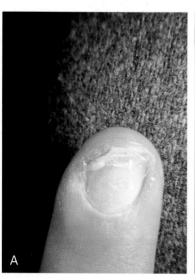
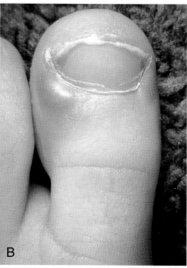

Figure 10–1. *A,* Acute paronychia fingernail. *B,* Acute paronychia toenail.

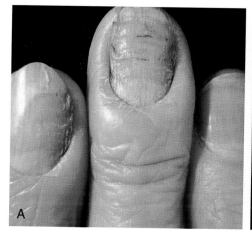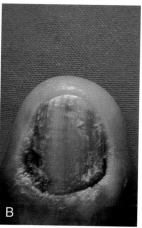

Figure 10–2. *A* and *B,* Chronic paronychia.

tact and contact irritants,[41–43] psoriasis,[41,42,44] and atopic eczema.[41,42] Certain occupations[45] (e.g., bakers) (see Chapter 17) may predispose to paronychia.[46] Immediate hypersensitivity to food can be responsible for some cases of chronic paronychia in food handlers.[46]

Paronychia has often been associated with psoriasis. Ganor found that 38 per cent of his adult female dermatology patients with chronic paronychia and 10 per cent of adult female control dermatology patients suffered from psoriasis.[47] He explained this as follows:

1. Psoriasis injures nails and allows *Candida* to proliferate.
2. In patients with psoriasis, increased rate of turnover of skin enhances growth of *Candida*. (Fig. 10–2*A* and *B*.)
3. Impairment of peripheral blood flow contributes to chronic paronychia (disturbance of microvesiculation of skin in psoriasis).

Trauma and contact irritants are usually the primary cause of inflammation of the nail folds. Once the seal is broken between the nail folds and nail plate, various organisms can secondarily populate the area and cause further inflammation and retard the "resealing" of the nail apparatus. We conducted a retrospective study showing that *Candida* is commonly cultured from these patients about 70% of the time.[80] We believe it is an important secondary factor.[82]

One of the first requirements for proper care is to ascertain an etiologic agent and proceed from there. In adults, infectious paronychia is usually caused by a combination of *Candida* and low-grade bacterial infection. In adults, such gram-negative organisms as *E. coli, Proteus*,[38] and *Klebsiella*[38] may be involved. In studies of adult Israeli women,[48] infected fingers are usually on the dominant hand, and the same holds true in our practice. Ganor and Pumpiansky further found that the number of fingers affected is associated with chronicity.[48] In their study of patients and families, the mouth and bowel, but not the vagina, were sources of *C. albicans* in chronic paronychia.[48] A pathognomonic sign of severe infection by *Candida* may sometimes be seen: fine transverse splits that are only a few millimeters wide and never involve the whole width of the nail.[1] This is seen primarily in mucocutaneous candidiasis, in severe candidal paronychia with onycholysis, and in acrodermatitis enteropathica.[1] Maceration of the posterior nail folds allows passage of foreign material from organisms into the dermis and nail folds, inciting a chronic inflammatory reaction.[1] Splinting of the finger in children has also been suggested as a treatment.[49]

The chief predisposing factor in children is probably finger sucking.[51,52] Poor skin hygiene also plays an important role.[53] Bacteria involved are usually mixed aerobic and anaerobic, with 18 per cent of cultures growing *Candida*.[53] The aerobic bacteria are usually group A streptococcus, *S. aureus*, or *Eikenella corrodens*.[53] Anaerobic bacteria are usually *Bacteroides*, gram-positive anaerobic cocci, and *Fusobacterium nucleatum*.[52,53,54] Brook[54] found that anaerobic infections are more common than aerobic infections, in a ratio of 3:2, because of organisms residing in the mouth. He furthermore stated that *Eikenella corrodens* is susceptible to ampicillin and penicillin but often resistant to methicillin, nafcillin, and clindamycin. There have been many associations in the literature with paronychia (Table 10–1).

Table 10–1. **DISEASES, FACTORS, OCCUPATIONS, AND CONDITIONS ASSOCIATED WITH PARONYCHIA**

Entity	Comment
Diseases	
Subungual epidermoid inclusions[57]	
Psoriasis (also sometimes sterile paronychia-like lesions)[43,44,47]	
Retinoids (sometimes painful paronychia)[58,59]	
5-Fluorouracil[58,60]	Usually from direct contact
Reiter's syndrome[61]	
Histiocytosis X[62,63]	Sometimes granulating
Rubinstein-Taybi syndrome[64]	Chronic, fingernails and toenails
Enchondroma[65]	May first present as paronychia
Verrucous nevus and nevus unius lateris[66]	Recurrent inflammatory changes possible
Multicentric reticulohistiocytosis[50]	Paronychial nodules, "like coral beads"[18]
Pemphigus[67]	May herald exacerbation[68]
Stevens-Johnson syndrome[69]	
Systemic lupus erythematosus[70]	
Progressive systemic sclerosis[71]	Periungual vesiculation, chronic paronychia[45]
Factors	
Sarcoid[72]	Painful paronychia
Tunga penetrans[11]	
Bazex's paraneoplastic syndrome[72]	
Chilblain (and a distinctive variant of chilblain)[47,73]	
Vasculitis[73]	
Traumatic injury[73]	
Ionizing radiation[29]	Chronic relapsing paronychia
Leukemia cutis (chronic lymphocytic leukemia)[74]	
Vascular thrombosis,[73] thrombophlebitis[47]	
Frostbite[73]	
Leprosy[30]	
Zinc deficiency,[75] pustular paronychia	
Erysipeloid[75]	
Tulip bulbs[72]	Periungual eruption
Hypoparathyroidism[72]	Chronic paronychia
Acrodermatitis enteropathica	
Celiac disease[72]	
Cold hands[72]	
Varicose veins[47]	
Diabetes mellitus	
Dyskeratosis congenita[72]	
Cosmetics around nails[41]	
Occupations	
Bartenders	
Janitorial and domestic workers	
Oil rig workers[56]	
Barbers and hairdressers	
Waitresses and waiters[43]	
Homemakers	
Gardeners	
Grounds keepers	
Secretaries (clerical)	Upon filing
Florists	
Dentists	
Dental hygienists	
Cosmetologists	
Cooks	
Carpenters, builders	
Fishermen	
Photographic and x-ray developers	
Meat (and other raw food) handlers	
Mechanics	
Engravers[29]	
Etchers[29]	
Glaziers[29]	
Painters[29]	

Table 10–1. **DISEASES, FACTORS, OCCUPATIONS, AND CONDITIONS ASSOCIATED WITH PARONYCHIA**
Continued

Entity	Comment
Radio workers[29]	
Shoemakers[29]	
Pianists[29]	
Legume shellers[29]	
Conditions	
Hydrocarbon exposure	
Transplants (renal)[76]	
Granulomatous disease (chronic)[77]	
Yellow nail syndrome	
Bandages around the nail[78]	

Treatment. The following is a list of points to consider in the treatment of chronic paronychia:

1. Avoid or treat the previously mentioned predisposing conditions. Avoid moisture and contact irritants.
2. Educate the patient as to proper nail care.[51]
3. The patient should be instructed to do the following:
   a. Wear light cotton gloves under heavy-duty vinyl gloves for wet work. Heavy-duty vinyl gloves are available at paint stores and pharmacies.
   b. Wear the cotton and vinyl gloves when peeling or squeezing citrus fruits, handling tomatoes, and peeling potatoes or other raw food.
   c. Avoid direct contact with paints, metal polish, paint thinner, turpentine, other solvents, and polish, and wear the cotton and vinyl gloves when using them.
   d. Use lukewarm water and very little mild soap when washing hands; be sure to rinse the soap off and dry gently.
   e. Protect hands from chapping and drying in windy or cold weather by wearing unlined leather gloves.
   f. Push cuticles back as little as possible and do not use fingernails, a metal file, or orange stick to do this. Cuticle removers are not good for people with paronychia and those predisposed to acquiring paronychia.
   g. If necessary, cuticles can be pushed back gently at the end of a shower or bath using a wet washcloth or the end of a finger.
   h. Avoid nail cosmetics of all kinds while the disorder is healing. Frequent application and removal of nail cosmetics are harmful. Commercial cuticle treatments are often harmful.
   i. Treatment of the bacterial component is usually not necessary. Short courses of erythromycin, cephalosporin, or ciprofloxacin may be used, especially for an acute exacerbation of chronic paronychia.
   j. Topical broad-spectrum antifungal solutions are helpful as drying and anti-yeast agents. Haloprogin (now hard to find), clotrimazole, and sulconazole solutions are available and should be applied two to three times daily. Ketoconazole or other creams may also be tried.
   k. Oral ketoconazole, itraconazole, or fluconazole may be used as anti-yeast agents in more resistant cases. Pulse dosing with itraconazole has some success.[83] At the time of this printing, these are not approved by the Food and Drug Administration for this indication. Terbinafine is also being studied in these patients.
   l. Topical steroids are useful for 1 to 2 weeks. Pulse therapy with systemic steroids should be reserved for particularly recalcitrant cases. Intralesional steroids are used less commonly.
   m. Marsupialization or excision of the proximal nail fold has been advocated by Baran[56] for resistant cases.
   n. Some older therapies used in the past include the following:
      1) Tetracycline with amphotericin V (Mysteclin-F) and nystatin with tetracycline (Achrostatin V).[22]
      2) Four per cent thymol in 95 per cent ethanol or in chloroform.
      3) Sulfacetamide, 15 per cent, in 50 per cent alcohol topically three to four times a day.[9]

4) Paronychia occurring among children who suck their fingers may be considered as bite wounds with respect to their microbiology, because the normal oral flora often are involved.[81]

References

1. Runne U, Offanos CE: The human nail. Curr Probl Dermatol 9:102, 1981.
2. Zais N: The Nail in Health and Disease. SP Medical and Scientific Books, New York, 1980.
3. Scher RK: Subungual scabies. Am J Dermatopathol 5:87, 1983.
4. Koesard E: The dystrophic nail of keratotic scabies. Am J Dermatopathol 6:308, 1984.
5. De Paoli RT, Marks VJ: Crusted (Norwegian) scabies: Treatment of nail involvement. J Am Acad Dermatol 17:136, 1987.
6. O'Donnell BF, O'Loughlin S, Powell FC: Management of crusted scabies. Int J Dermatol 29:258, 1990.
7. Sokolova TV, Sizov IE: Involvement of fingernails in scabies in an infant. Vestn Dermatol Venerol 2:68, 1989.
8. Farah FS: Protozoan and helminth infections. In Fitzpatrick TB, Eisen AZ, Wolf K, et al (eds): Dermatology in General Medicine, ed 2. McGraw-Hill, New York, 1979.
9. Samman PD: The Nails in Disease, ed 3. William Heinemann, London, 1978.
10. Brothers WS, Heckman RA: Tungiasis in North America. Cutis 25:636, 1980.
11. Zalar GL, Walther RR: Infestation by Tunga penetrans. Arch Dermatol 116:80, 1980.
12. Baran R: Onychia and paronychia. In Pierre M (ed): The Nail. Churchill Livingstone, New York, 1981.
13. Wentzell JM, Schwartz BK: Tunga penegrans. J Am Acad Dermatol 15:117, 1986.
14. Sanusi ID, Brown EB, Shepard TG, Grafton WD: Tungiasis: Report of one case and review of the 14 reported cases in the US. J Am Acad Dermatol 20:941, 1989.
15. Munyon TG, Urbanc AN: Subungual myiasis: A case report and literature. J Assoc Military Dermatol 4:60, 1978.
16. Edelglass JW, Douglass MC, Steifler R, et al: Cutaneous larva migrans in northern climates. J Am Acad Dermatol 7:353, 1982.
17. Diemer JT: Isolated pediculosis. J Am Podiatr Med Assoc 75:99, 1985.
18. Hay RJ, Baran R, Haneke E: Fungal and other infections involving the nail apparatus. In Baran R, Dawber RPR (eds): Diseases of the Nails and Their Management, ed 2. Blackwell Scientific, Oxford, England, 1994, pp 97–134.
19. Moschella SL: Benign reticuloendothelial diseases. In Moschella SL, Pillsbury DM, Hurly HJ (eds): Dermatology, vol 1. WB Saunders, Philadelphia, 1975, pp 751–836.
20. Giacobetti R: Herpetic whitlow. Int J Dermatol 18:55, 1979.
21. Muller SA, Hermann EC Jr: Association of stomatitis and paronychias due to herpes simplex. Arch Dermatol 101:396, 1970.
22. Daniel CR III: Diseases of the nail. In Conn HF (ed): Current Therapy. WB Saunders, Philadelphia, 1983, p 656.
23. Andiaman WA: Questions and answers, herpetic whitlow in a nursing student. JAMA 245:2531, 1981.
24. Gangarosa LP, Payne LJ, Hayakawa K, et al: Iontophoretic treatment of herpetic whitlow. Arch Phys Med Rehabil 70:336, 1989.
25. Epstein E: Intralesional bleomycin and Raynaud's phenomenon. J Am Acad Dermatol 24:785, 1991.
26. Shelley WB, Shelley D: Intralesional bleomycin sulfate therapy for warts: A novel bifurcated needle puncture technique. Arch Dermatol 127:234, 1991.
27. Halasz CLG: Treatment of common warts using the infrared coagulator. J Derm Surg Oncol 20:252, 1994.
28. Street ML, Roenigk RK: Recalcitrant periungual verrucae: The role of carbon dioxide laser vaporization. J Am Acad Dermatol 23:115, 1990.
29. Baran RJ, Dawber RPR: Diseases of the Nails and Their Management. Blackwell Scientific, Oxford, England, 1984.
30. Kikuchi I: Some observations on the nail changes in patients with leprosy. In Burgdorf WHC, Katz SI (eds): Dermatology Progress and Perspectives. The Proceedings of the 18th World Congress of Dermatology, Parthenon, New York, 1993.
31. Patki AH: Pterygium inversum unguius in a patient with leprosy. Arch Dermatol 126:1110, 1990.
32. Patki AH, Baran R: Significance of nail changes in leprosy: A clinical review of 357 cases. Semin Dermatol 10:77, 1991.
33. Leyden JJ, McGinley KJ, Kates SG, Myung KB: Subungual bacteria of the hand: Contribution to the glove juice test; efficacy of antimicrobial detergents. Infect Control Hosp Epidemiol 10:451, 1989.
34. Senay H: Acrylic nails and transmission of infection. Can J Infect Control 6:52, 1991.
35. Telfer NR, Barth JH, Dawber RP: Recurrent blistering distal dactylitis of the great toe associated with an ingrowing toenail. Clin Exp Dermatol 14:380, 1989.
36. Baran R, Perrin C: Fixed drug eruption presenting as acute paronychia. Br J Dermatol 125:592, 1991.
37. Wantzig GL, Thomsen K: Acute paronychia after high dose methotrexate therapy. Arch Dermatol 119:623, 1983.
38. Cohen PR, Scher RK: Geriatric nail disorders: Diagnosis and treatment. J Am Acad Dermatol 26:521, 1992.
39. Fisher BK, Warner LC: Cutaneous manifestations of the acquired immunodeficiency syndrome. Int J Dermatol 26:615, 1987.
40. Zaias N: Paronychia. In The Nail in Health and Disease, ed 2. Appleton & Lange, East Norwalk, CT, 1990, pp 131–135.
41. Daniel CR: Paronychia (CME section). J Am Acad Dermatol 31:515, 1994.
42. Daniel CR: The nail. In Sams WM, Lynch PJ (eds): Principles and Practice of Dermatology. Churchill Livingstone, New York, 1990, pp 743–760.
43. Daniel CR III: Paronychia. In Greer KE (ed): Common Problems in Dermatology. Year Book, Chicago, 1988, pp 249–255.
44. Daniel CR: Paronychia. In Daniel CR (ed): The Nail, Dermatologic Clinics. WB Saunders, Philadelphia, 1985, pp 461–464.
45. Farm G: Paronychia: An occupational disease? Contact Dermatitis 22:116, 1990.

46. Tosti A, Guerra L, Morelli R, et al: Role of foods in pathogenesis of chronic paronychia. J Am Acad Dermatol 27:706, 1992.
47. Ganor S: Chronic paronychia and psoriasis. Br J Dermatol 92:685, 1975.
48. Ganor S, Pumpianski R: Chronic *Candida albicans* in adult Israeli women. Br J Dermatol 90:77, 1974.
49. Rayan GM, Turner WT: Hand complications in children from digital sucking. J Hand Surg 14:933, 1989.
50. Masahiro T, Hork K, Nakanishi T, et al: Multicentric reticulohistiocytosis. Arch Dermatol 117:495, 1981.
51. Daniel CR: Non fungal infections. *In* Scher RK, Daniel CR (ed): Nails: Therapy, Diagnosis, Surgery. WB Saunders, Philadelphia, 1990, pp 120–126.
52. Stone OJ, Mullins JF: Chronic paronychia in children. Clin Pediatr 7:104, 1968.
53. Stone OJ, Mullins JF: Experimental studies in chronic paronychia. Arch Dermatol 89:455, 1964.
54. Brook K: Bacteriologic study of paronychia in children. Am J Surg 141:703, 1981.
55. Roberts DT, Richardson MD, Dwyer PK, Donegan R: Terbenifine in paronychia. *In* Burgdorf WHC, Katz SI (eds): Dermatology, Progress and Perspectives. The Proceedings of the 18th World Congress of Dermatology. Parthenon, New York, 1993, pp 474–476.
56. Baran R: Paronychia. Presented at the annual meeting of the American Academy of Dermatology, Las Vegas, December 8, 1985.
57. Lewin K: Subungual epidermoid inclusion. Br J Dermatol 81:671, 1969.
58. Daniel CR III, Scher RK: Nail changes secondary to systemic drugs or ingestants. J Am Acad Dermatol 10:250, 1984.
59. Voorhees JJ, Organos CE: Oral retinoids. Arch Dermatol 117:418, 1981.
60. Norton L: Nail disorders. J Am Acad Dermatol 2:451, 1980.
61. Lovy MR, Bluhm GB, Morales A: The occurrence of nail pitting in Reiter's syndrome. J Am Acad Dermatol 2:66, 1980.
62. Kahn G: Nail involvement in histiocytosis X. Arch Dermatol 100:699, 1969.
63. Timpatanapong P, Hathirat P, Isarangkura P: Nail involvement in histiocytosis X. Arch Dermatol 120:1052, 1984.
64. Selmanowitz VJ, Stiller MJ: Rubinstein-Taybi syndrome. Arch Dermatol 117:504, 1981.
65. Shelley WB, Ralson EL: Paronychia due to an enchondroma. Arch Dermatol 90:412, 1964.
66. Rook A: Naevi and other developmental defects. *In* Rook A, Wilkinson DS, Ebling FJG (eds): Textbook of Dermatology, ed 3. Blackwell Scientific, Oxford, England, 1979.
67. Baumal A, Robinson MJ: Nail bed involvement in pemphigus vulgaris. Arch Dermatol 107:151, 1973.
68. Kiyama C, Sou K, Furuya T, et al: Paronychia: A sign heralding an exacerbation of pemphigus vulgaris. J Am Acad Dermatol 29:494, 1993.
69. Chanda JJ, Callen JP: Stevens-Johnson syndrome. Arch Dermatol 114:626, 1978.
70. Mackie RM: Lupus erythematosus in association with finger clubbing. Br J Dermatol 89:533, 1973.
71. Patterson JW: Pterygium-inversum-unguius-like changes in scleroderma. Arch Dermatol 113:1429, 1977.
72. Baran R: Nail changes in general pathology. *In* Pierre M (ed): The Nail. Churchill Livingstone, New York, 1981.
73. Herman EW, Kezis JS, Silvers CN: A distinctive variant of pernio. Arch Dermatol 117:26, 1981.
74. High DA, Luscombe HA, Hauh YC: Leukemia cutis masquerading as chronic paronychia. Int J Dermatol 24:595, 1985.
75. Miller SJ: Nutritional deficiency and the skin. J Am Acad Dermatol 21:1, 1989.
76. Lugo-Janer G, Sanchez JL, Santiago-Delpin E: Prevalence and clinical spectrum of skin diseases in kidney transplant recipients. J Am Acad Dermatol 24:410, 1991.
77. Dahl MV, MacCarthy KG: Immunodeficiency and graft-versus-host syndromes. *In* Sams WM, Lynch PJ (eds): Principles and Practice of Dermatology. Churchill Livingstone, New York, 1990, pp 599–607.
78. Stone OJ: Bandage-induced nail disorders. Cutis 36:259, 1985.
79. Elston DM; Lice, mites, and bug bites. Dialogues Dermatol: 39:4, 1997.
80. Daniel CR, Daniel MP, Daniel CM, et al: Chronic paronychia and onycholysis: A 13 year experience. Cutis 58:397, 1996.
81. Griego RD, Rosen T, Orengo IF, Wolf JE: Dog, cat, and human bites; A review. J Am Acad Dermatol 33:1019, 1995.
82. Daniel CR, Elewski BE: *Candida* as a nail pathogen in healthy patients, J Miss State Med Assoc 36:379, 1995.
83. Rashid A, De Doncker P: Pulse dose regimen of oral itraconazile in the therapy of *Candida* paronychia. Poster presentation. International Summit on Cutaneous antifungal Therapy May 26-28, 1996, Vancouver, British Columbia, Canada.

CHAPTER 11

Dermatologic Diseases of the Nail Unit

James Q. Del Rosso, Pamela J. Basuk,
Richard K. Scher, and Anthony R. Ricci

Alterations in the structure and appearance of the nail unit may be seen in association with a variety of dermatologic disorders. Because of the limited number of reaction patterns associated with the nail unit, many of the changes that are seen, such as onycholysis, pitting, and subungual hyperkeratosis, are not specific. However, certain findings, especially when present in combination, may be highly suggestive of a specific diagnosis or may assist in limiting the differential diagnosis.

The following chapter reviews nail changes associated with dermatologic diseases, exclusive of infections and neoplasms, which are reviewed elsewhere in other chapters of this text. The most commonly encountered noninfectious cutaneous diseases affecting the nail are inflammatory disorders, such as psoriasis, lichen planus, and eczematous dermatoses. Nail findings associated with genodermatoses that involve the skin are also reviewed in more detail elsewhere in this text.

PSORIASIS AND PSORIATIC ARTHRITIS

Current estimates indicate that psoriasis affects approximately 2 to 3 per cent of the American population, or more than 5 million people. Studies abroad have found prevalence rates approaching 5 per cent for adults living in Scandinavia and rates exceeding 2 per cent in other regions of Europe.[1] Prevalence increases with the age of the population studied.

Familial aggregation and genetic determinants of psoriasis have long been recognized. Among siblings, 8 per cent are affected if neither parent has psoriasis. This increases to 16 to 25 per cent if one parent or a sibling has the disease and up 75 per cent if both parents are affected. If one twin has psoriasis, the other is afflicted in 25 per cent of cases involving fraternal twins and 65 per cent involving identical twins.[2,3] In a questionnaire study of more than 21,000 psoriatic patients, 36 per cent reported the presence of psoriasis in at least one relative.[4] Newer data have associated psoriasis with certain human leukocyte antigen (HLA) subtypes, such as Cw6, B13, Bw57, Cw2, Cw11, and B27. In addition to HLA associations, there is evidence that a variation at a locus of chromosome 17q is linked to the development of psoriasis.[1] As with many other genetic disorders, only a limited number of genetically predisposed individuals phenotypically express the disease. Other factors such as environmental exposures may play a causative role or exacerbate existing disease. Such factors include smoking, stress, alcohol consumption, and human immunodeficiency virus infection.[1,5]

Involvement of the nails in patients with psoriasis ranges from 10 to 50 per cent.[6,7] In most cases, nail involvement coexists with cutaneous psoriasis, although psoriasis of the skin surrounding affected nails need not be present. It is not uncommon for psoriatic nail involvement to be present in patients with limited cutaneous psoriasis. Psoriatic nail disease without overt cutaneous disease occurs in 1 to 5 per cent of patients. This latter scenario is typically associated with a more formidable diagnostic challenge.

In children with psoriasis, associated nail changes have been found in up to 39 per cent of patients, usually presenting as pitting.[7,8] Parakeratosis pustulosa is a distinct entity that typically affects children, especially girls younger than 5 years. This disorder simulates localized digital psoriasis, usually involving one fingernail, and fortunately resolves spontaneously.[9]

The prevalence of arthritis in association with psoriasis has not been clearly defined. On the basis of older studies, the incidence is believed to range between 5 and 8 per cent. Other studies indicate that arthritis or other rheumatic manifestations develop in 20 to 50 per cent of patients with psoriasis.[1] The risk appears to be higher in patients with severe cutaneous psoriasis, especially pustular psoriasis.

The presence of nail disease in patients with psoriatic arthritis has been noted in 53 to 86 per cent of patients.[10–14] Psoriatic nail disease may be seen in association with all subtypes of psoriatic arthritis. Psoriatic arthritis has also been noted during childhood. Often presenting as pauciarticular disease, progression to polyarticular disease is not uncommon.[15] The diagnosis is often delayed because the onset of arthritis commonly precedes the onset of cutaneous psoriasis. In children without psoriatic skin lesions, especially when asymmetric arthritis and dactylitis are present, a family history of psoriasis or the presence of psoriatic nail changes such as pitting are important diagnostic clues suggestive of psoriatic arthritis.[16]

CLINICAL FINDINGS

The clinical findings associated with psoriatic nail disease correlate with the anatomic locations of the nail unit that are affected by

Table 11–1. PSORIATIC SIGNS OF THE NAIL UNIT

Proximal	Clinical Sign
Proximal matrix	Pitting, onychorrhexis, Beau's lines
Intermediate matrix	Leukonychia
Distal matrix	Focal onycholysis, thinned nail plate, erythema of the lunula
Bed	"Oil drop" sign or "salmon patch," subungual hyperkeratosis, onycholysis, splinter hemorrhages
Hyponychium	Subungual hyperkeratosis, onycholysis
Nail plate	Crumbling and destruction plus other changes secondary to the specific site
Proximal and lateral nail folds	Cutaneous psoriasis
Phalanx	Psoriatic arthritis with nail changes over 80 per cent of the time

psoriasis (Table 11–1). When psoriasis involves more than one segment of the nail apparatus, a combination of nail changes may become part of the clinical presentation. The presentation is ultimately affected by the severity and progression of underlying inflammation as well as the segments of the nail unit that are involved.

Because the proximal nail matrix forms the superficial portion of the nail plate, involvement of this matrix segment results in pitting of the nail plate (Fig. 11–1). Pitting is due to the loss of parakeratotic foci as the newly growing psoriatic nail plate extends distally beyond the proximal nail fold, leaving behind a random array of small, pitted indentations. Psoriatic nail pits may be shallow but often extend deeply into the plate surface. Although nail pitting is the most common nail finding asso-

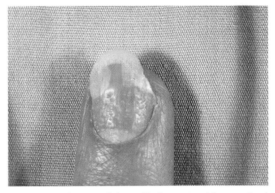

Figure 11–1. Pitting of the nail plate caused by proximal matrix disease associated with distal onycholysis.

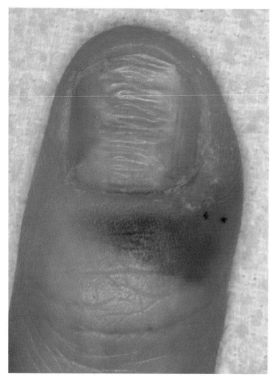

Figure 11–2. Multiple Beau's lines caused by intermittent inflammation of the proximal nail fold with resultant injury to the underlying proximal nail matrix.

ciated with psoriasis, it is not specific for this disease. Nail pitting is also seen in some patients with alopecia areata.[17,18] Unlike psoriasis, nail pitting associated with alopecia areata is usually not random, presenting as orderly rows of shallow indentations. Pitting of the nail plate has also been observed periodically in association with other conditions as described throughout this chapter. Examples include idiopathic trachyonychia[19] and punctate keratoderma.[20] In two reported cases of punctate keratoderma, several features suggestive of ungual psoriasis were noted, including subungual hyperkeratosis, onycholysis, splinter hemorrhages, and pitting.

Patchy psoriatic involvement of the nail matrix may result in a variety of nail plate changes that are less suggestive of psoriasis than pitting and not as common. Intermittent longitudinal matrix involvement produces linear variations in nail plate thickness and subsequent longitudinal ridging, resulting in onychorrhexis. Increased severity of matrix inflammation may result in full-thickness linear loss of nail plate formation, producing splitting. When transverse involvement occurs rather than longitudinal involvement,

solitary or multiple "growth arrest" lines (Beau's lines) may occur. Repeated transverse inflammation may produce a "stepladder" effect, resulting in multiple Beau's lines (Fig. 11–2). Occasionally, these changes may be severe enough to produce deep splits or crumbling of the nail plate.

Psoriatic involvement of the intermediate portion of the nail matrix leads to foci of parakeratosis within the body of the nail plate. This translates clinically to leukonychia; the extent of clinical involvement is dependent on whether psoriasis of the intermediate matrix is focal or diffuse (Fig. 11–3). Severe disease results in diminished nail plate integrity.

Involvement of the distal matrix or lunula region is typically subtle in its clinical appearance because the distal matrix produces the undersurface (inferior portion) of the nail plate. An erythematous or spotted lunula may be the only evident change (Fig. 11–4). Focal onycholysis or barely discernible nail plate thinning may result.

Nail bed psoriasis is common, resulting in proximal or distal involvement. The extent of involvement may be focal or diffuse. Focal nail bed disease at any point proximal to the hyponychium produces localized early onycholysis resulting from parakeratosis and collections of neutrophils within the nail bed stratum corneum. These foci seen through the body of the nail plate often appear like a drop of oil on a piece of paper, called the "oil drop sign."[7,21] Psoriasiform hyperplasia, exaggerated mi-

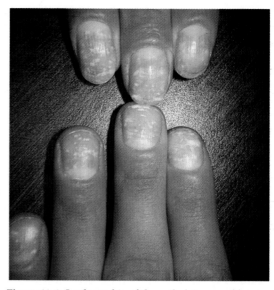

Figure 11–3. Leukonychia of the nail plate caused by psoriasis of the intermediate portion of the nail matrix.

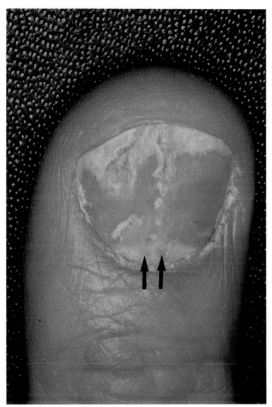

Figure 11–4. Spotted lunula (distal matrix disease) in addition to pitting, distal onycholysis, and discoloration of the nail bed.

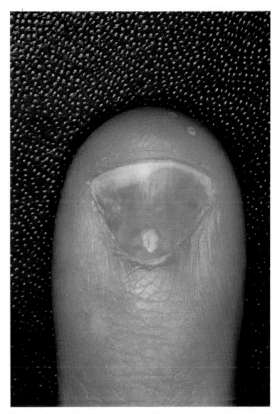

Figure 11–5. Reddish-brown discoloration of the nail bed—"oil drop" sign or salmon patch—caused by bed psoriasis.

crovascular changes of psoriasis characterized microscopically by dermal vascular dilatation and tortuosity and subungual accumulation of glycoprotein, may produce visible reddish-brown foci beneath the nail plate, called the "salmon patch sign."[7] Both of these signs are highly suggestive of psoriasis (Fig. 11–5).

When the psoriatic process occurs at the hyponychium, the initial onset of subungual hyperkeratosis and distal onycholysis develops. Continued diffuse nail bed disease produces subungual hyperkeratosis, which varies from mild to severe (Fig. 11–6). Advanced subungual hyperkeratosis leads to nail plate thickening and progression of onycholysis (Fig. 11–7). Psoriatic onycholysis represents functional separation of the plate from its underlying attachment to the nail bed, believed to be due to an intracorneal cell layer split[17] (Fig. 11–8). Trauma accentuates this process by physically enhancing the separation. In many cases, onycholysis starts distally and progresses proximally as a result of advancing psoriasis, traumatic uplifting of the distal plate, or both. Distal onycholysis enhances the develop-

ment of secondary microbial colonization. Greenish-blue discoloration of accumulated subungual debris suggests the presence of *Candida* or *Pseudomonas* organisms (Fig. 11–9).

Nail crumbling may develop as a consequence of psoriasis of the nail bed or nail matrix. Extensive involvement of the nail bed may

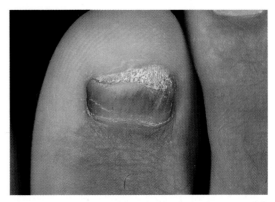

Figure 11–6. Subungual hyperkeratosis resulting in uplifting of the nail plate with distal nail bed and hyponychial psoriasis.

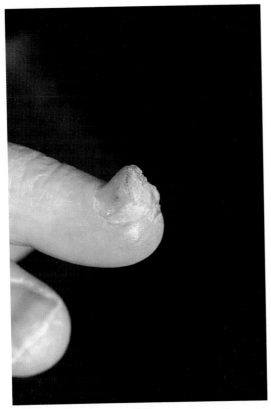

Figure 11–7. Massive subungual hyperkeratosis causing uplifting of the nail plate.

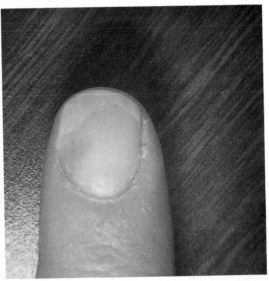

Figure 11–8. Distal onycholysis caused by distal nail bed and hyponychial psoriasis with nail bed discoloration.

lead to decreased integrity of the overlying plate and subsequent crumbling (Fig. 11–10). With diffuse matrix involvement, actual destruction of the nail plate occurs because a fully intact, discernible nail plate is not formed by the diseased matrix. A crumbled nail often presents with yellowish or grayish discoloration.

Splinter hemorrhages of the nail bed are a common finding caused by foci of capillary bleeding below the thin suprapapillary plate of the psoriatic nail bed (Figs. 11–11, 11–12). The dermal vascular dilatation and tortuosity associated with psoriasis further contribute to this phenomenon. Extravasated blood becomes trapped between the longitudinal troughs of the nail bed and the overlying nail plate, growing out distally along with the plate. The splinter hemorrhages of the psoriatic nail are analogous to the superficial foci of pinpoint bleeding seen below the surface scales of cutaneous psoriatic plaques (Auspitz sign).

Psoriasis of the proximal and lateral nail folds is equivalent to psoriasis occurring at other skin sites. When periungual skin is af-

fected, secondary nail changes may develop. If proximal nail fold inflammation is severe, injury to the underlying matrix may occur, leading to subsequent nail plate abnormalities (Fig. 11–13).

Microvascular changes of the nail folds seen in patients with psoriasis may contribute to the development of nail changes. Specific findings associated with psoriasis have been determined using nail fold capillary image analysis.[22] Changes associated with psoriasis could be differentiated from normal controls in 79 per cent of cases. A significant correlation was seen with periungual psoriasis, nail pitting, and onycholysis.

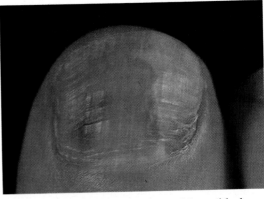

Figure 11–9. Distal onycholysis caused by nail bed psoriasis with rippling of the surface of the nail plate and early greenish-blue discoloration secondary to *Pseudomonas/Candida* infection.

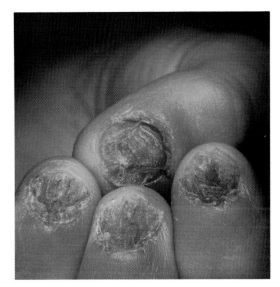

Figure 11–10. Crumbling of the nail plate from total matrix involvement.

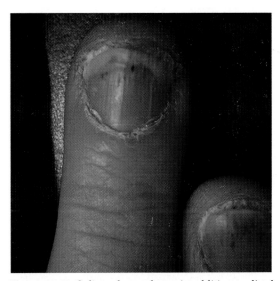

Figure 11–12. Splinter hemorrhages in addition to distal onycholysis.

Most psoriatic nail changes are potentially reversible because scarring of the affected nail segments typically does not occur. An exception to this may develop in severe cases of generalized pustular psoriasis, also referred to as pustular psoriasis of von Zumbusch. The extent of reversibility and scarring is dependent on disease progression and the effectiveness of therapy. The availability of systemic retinoid therapy has been a major advance in the treatment of pustular psoriasis; early intervention is most likely to prevent chronic sequelae.

The presence of inflammatory arthritis, seronegativity, and cutaneous or nail psoriasis suggests the diagnosis of psoriatic arthritis. Psoriatic nail disease is found more commonly at the onset of arthritis than is psoriasis of the skin. The extent of cutaneous psoriasis, when present, may be widespread or minimal.

Nail abnormalities of psoriatic arthritis are varied and include onycholysis, pitting, horizontal or longitudinal ridging, and subungual hyperkeratosis[10,23] (Fig. 11–14). In one study of 52 patients, pitting was the most common fingernail finding and subungual hyperkeratosis the most common toenail alteration.[13] The presence of ungual changes does not necessarily correlate with the subtype of psori-

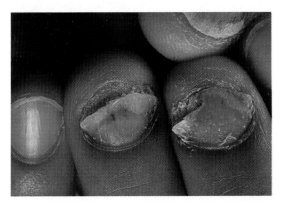

Figure 11–11. Splinter hemorrhages of the nail bed in addition to onycholysis, subungual hyperkeratosis, and pitting.

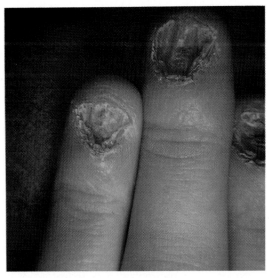

Figure 11–13. Inflammatory paronychia of the proximal nail fold resulting in injury to the total nail matrix with consequent complete onychodystrophy.

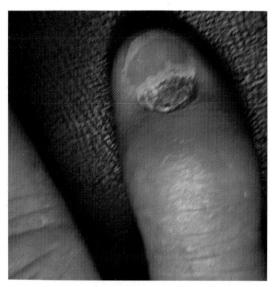

Figure 11–14. Sausage digit characteristic of distal interphalangeal joint psoriatic arthritis with proximal nail unit involvement.

Table 11–2. PSORIATIC ARTHRITIS

Type	Description
I	Classic distal interphalangeal joint involvement; about 5%
II	Arthritis mutilans, caused by osteolysis of bone; about 5%
III	Symmetric polyarthritis, similar to rheumatoid arthritis but seronegative; about 15%
IV	Asymmetric oligoarthritis, the most common type; 70%
V	Ankylosing spondylitis associated with psoriatic arthritis; about 5%

outlines the classically accepted classification of subtypes of psoriatic arthritis. Other classification systems have been suggested. One includes the three subgroups of peripheral arthritis, spondyloarthropathy, and extrarticular osseous disease.[27] An extended classification system that includes the more recently described associations between psoriasis and skeletal disease[28] is described in Table 11–3.

atic arthritis or the overall distribution of joint involvement; however, it has been suggested that nail disease may be seen more frequently in patients with distal interphalangeal joint arthritis[12,24] (Fig. 11–15). In some patients, involvement of the terminal interphalangeal joints is not associated with severe nail changes and may present only as mild pitting.[10] The severity of skin and nail psoriasis does not appear to correlate with the subgroup of psoriatic arthritis or with the severity of joint inflammation or functional impairment.[12,25]

The generally accepted definition of psoriatic arthritis defines the disorder as inflammatory arthritis associated with psoriasis, usually with rheumatoid factor seronegativity. The arthritis includes peripheral arthritis and spondylitis. Serology is not exclusively negative because occasional patients with definitive clinical and radiologic features of psoriatic arthritis test positive for rheumatoid factor. Because up to 5 per cent of normal individuals will also have positive serology, an overlap phenomenon is the most likely explanation for rheumatoid factor positivity in a small percentage of patients with psoriatic arthritis.

The classic description of psoriatic arthritis includes five subtypes of presentation. The most common form, occurring in 70 per cent of patients, is asymmetric oligoarthritis.[11,26] In this subgroup of patients, one or a few joints of the fingers or toes are involved. Table 11–2

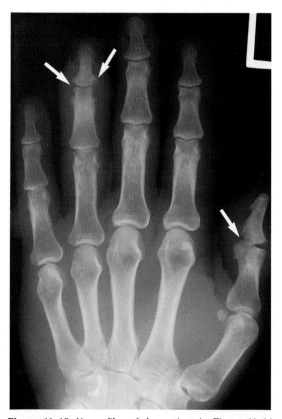

Figure 11–15. X-ray film of the patient in Figure 11–14 demonstrating distal interphalangeal joint arthritis of the left thumb with blurring of the joint space and sausage digit of the fourth finger.

Table 11–3. **PSORIATIC ARTHRITIS: EXTENDED CLASSIFICATION (1996)**

Asymmetric oligoarticular arthritis
Distal interphalangeal arthritis
Mutilating psoriatic arthritis
Spinal form of psoriatic arthritis
Pustulosis palmoplantaris with osteoarthritis sternoclavicularis
Psoriatic onychopachydermoperiostitis

The presence of onycho-osteoperiostitis of the distal phalanx appears to be more common in psoriatic arthritis than in other patient groups, suggesting that this finding may be a valuable diagnostic clue.[29] Psoriatic onychopachydermoperiostitis (POPP) is a painful variant of psoriatic arthritis first described in 1989 that includes psoriatic nail changes, soft tissue thickening above the terminal phalanx, and periosteal involvement of the terminal phalanx with bone erosions.[24,28] The large toenails are involved in most cases, although other toes and fingers may be affected. Spondyloarthropathy and peripheral arthritis, including distal interphalangeal joint disease, are usually absent. Unlike osteoarthritis of the hands, which may be associated with longitudinal nail plate ridging, the main ungual sign of POPP is onycholysis accompanied by longitudinal ridging.[24]

Interestingly, nail changes may be seen in association with osteoarthritis, especially of the hands, occurring in 13.7 per cent of patients.[30,31] Leukonychia, longitudinal lines, and ridges may occur. Distal interphalangeal joint disease and inflammation of Heberden's nodes are often present.[31] The use of nonsteroidal anti-inflammatory agents may reverse the secondary nail changes.

The diagnosis of nail psoriasis is usually straightforward when characteristic nail findings coexist with cutaneous psoriasis. Diagnostic difficulty arises when nail disease occurs as an isolated finding. Ungual psoriasis and onychomycosis, especially distal subungual onychomycosis, are often indistinguishable by clinical examination alone. Mycologic studies, including potassium hydroxide (KOH) preparation and fungal culture, are recommended. It may be necessary to repeat these mycologic studies if the first test results are negative and fungal infection remains a strong clinical suspicion. Nail biopsy processed for routine microscopy (hematoxylin & eosin stain) and fungal staining (periodic acid–Schiff [PAS] stain) may also be helpful when mycologic studies are negative. Whenever possible, treatment should be withheld until a specific diagnosis is confirmed. It should be noted that psoriasis and onychomycosis may occur concomitantly.

Psoriatic nail disease is often persistent and frequently refractory to treatment.[7] The mainstay of therapy is intralesional corticosteroid injection infiltrated into the proximal nail fold region. Depending on the response, the procedure is repeated monthly for a total of 4 to 6 months. Subsequent injections are dependent on response and the frequency and extent of recurrences. The most common agent used is triamcinolone acetonide administered at a concentration of 2.5 to 5 mg/mL. Normal saline or an anesthetic solution that does not contain epinephrine, such as plain lidocaine, may be used as a diluent. Other corticosteroid injectable preparations are available such as triamcinolone diacetate and betamethasone. Injection pain may be minimized by precooling the injection site with application of ice or a refrigerant spray and injecting with a sharply beveled 25-gauge needle. Some clinicians prefer the use of a pressure injector, such as a Dermo-Jet; however, instrument sterilization may be difficult.[7]

Intralesional corticosteroid injection is most effective in reversing nail abnormalities resulting from matrix psoriasis, such as pitting, ridging, and leukonychia. Injection into the proximal nail fold allows access to the underlying matrix (Fig. 11–16). Nail bed disease, including subungual hyperkeratosis, distal onycholysis, and "oil drop" changes, responds less favorably to proximal nail fold injection. This may be partially overcome by injecting the lateral nail folds close to the nail bed. Some absorption of steroid into the bed may occur, producing mild to moderate improvement. Unfortunately, direct injection into the nail bed is obviated by the presence of the overlying plate, and injection into the bed via the hyponychial region is too painful. Atrophy and formation of a subungual hematoma[6] (Fig. 11–17) are potential complications of nail fold injection.

Debridement of the onycholytic or dystrophic nail plate followed by application of high-potency topical corticosteroid therapy, with or without occlusion, affords minimal benefit in most patients. However, a trial of this approach may benefit some patients. Careful monitoring is indicated, especially with prolonged treatment or occlusive

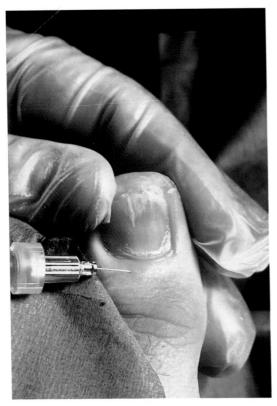

Figure 11–16. Injection of corticosteroid to the proximal nail fold in a patient with psoriatic nail changes.

therapy. Inadvertent application of the corticosteroid onto periungual skin increases the likelihood of nail fold atrophy and telangiectasia associated with prolonged use. If a beneficial response is noted, a reduction in the frequency of application or the use of a less potent agent may be warranted to reduce the risk of local side effects, such as atrophy.

Careful application of a mid- to high-potency corticosteroid solution under the free edge of the distal nail plate may slow the progression of distal onycholysis. A few drops of solution are applied from the nozzle tip of the bottle and allowed to advance proximally under the onycholytic nail plate by "capillary action." Penetration into the nail bed is enhanced by gentle massage, applying downward pressure on the overlying plate. The patient must be instructed not to physically force the solution under the plate because mechanical trauma increases uplifting of the plate.

As with topical corticosteroid therapy for cutaneous psoriasis, a beneficial response is often partial or short lived. It may be necessary to discontinue therapy intermittently or change the type of corticosteroid to avoid tachyphylaxis.

The mixture of 1 per cent 5-fluorouracil cream and 20 per cent urea is more effective in reducing subungual hyperkeratosis and may produce better overall results than the solution vehicle.[32] Usage should be limited to patients with matrix disease (i.e., pitting, leukonychia) or nail bed disease proximal to the onychodermal band (i.e., subungual hyperkeratosis). For distal onycholysis, this regimen is to be avoided because worsening may occur. The solution is gently massaged into the nail folds twice daily without occlusion for 4 to 6 months. Local side effects include irritation, hyperpigmentation, persistent telangiectasia, and suspected activation of herpes labialis caused by inadvertent transfer from the fingers.[33,34]

Psoralen plus long-wave ultraviolet light (PUVA) is very effective for the treatment of cutaneous psoriasis and may slowly improve nail changes in some patients.[35–37] Fingernail psoriasis may be responsive; however, toenail disease is refractory. Improvement requires at least 3 to 4 months of therapy, and recurrence is likely without maintenance therapy. There is no evidence that ultraviolet B (UVB) phototherapy improves nail psoriasis. Psoriatic arthritis does not appear to improve with either PUVA or UVB phototherapy.

Both oral and topical PUVA therapies have been reported to be of benefit. Local PUVA using methoxsalen application to the proximal nail fold was used to treat five patients with onycholysis and pitting.[36] Two patients cleared completely, with relapse developing after 4 and 8 months, respectively. Systemic PUVA with oral methoxsalen administered two or three times a week resulted in improvement of both skin and nail psoriasis.[35] Once patients achieved a 95 per cent clearance of skin involvement, treatments were tapered to a

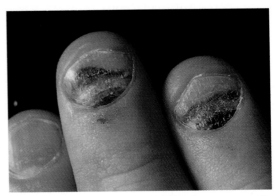

Figure 11–17. Subungual hematoma secondary to intralesional steroid injections.

maintenance schedule of once a week or less. Unfortunately, nail pitting failed to respond to PUVA. Others have reported improvement in nail pitting in 50 per cent of patients.[37] Response of nail disease lags behind improvement of skin lesions, and in some cases improvement of nail changes may not occur until after months of maintenance therapy.

Potential adverse nail changes associated with PUVA therapy include subungual photohemolysis (Fig. 11–18), pain, melanonychia,[38] and onycholysis.[39]

Oral etretinate has been found to be helpful for nail psoriasis, although improvement tends to be slow. In one study, a dose of 0.5 to 1 mg/kg/day provided a good response.[40] In another study of patients with moderate to severe chronic plaque psoriasis, etretinate, 0.5 to 0.75 mg/kg/day for 10 weeks, provided significant alleviation of nail involvement and joint disease.[41]

Oral cyclosporine has gained acceptance in the treatment of extensive moderate to severe chronic plaque psoriasis, especially in patients refractory to conventional therapy. Skin disease responds favorably in many patients, and early studies with high-dose cyclosporine demonstrated efficacy for psoriatic arthritis.[28] In another study using lower dose therapy, a mean cyclosporine dosage of 3 mg/kg/day resulted in significant improvement of skin lesions, nail changes, and joint symptomatology.[41] Remissions are better preserved if the cyclosporine dose is tapered over several weeks. Potential nephrotoxicity and numerous significant drug interactions warrant careful monitoring, even with low-dose therapy.

Oral methotrexate is known to be very effective in the treatment of moderate to severe chronic plaque psoriasis and is considered by some to be the most effective agent for psoriasis of the nails.[7] The use of methotrexate for severe, incapacitating nail disease associated with limited or no skin involvement should be initiated only after careful consideration of the risks versus benefits of treatment and after thorough informed consent. The potential hematologic and hepatic toxicity associated with methotrexate warrants strict compliance with patient monitoring guidelines. Once nail disease improves, an attempt should be made to maintain remission with other forms of therapy, such as intralesional therapy or topical PUVA.

Psoriatic nail disease that responds to systemic retinoid therapy, cyclosporine, or methotrexate recurs after discontinuation of treatment. In most cases, continued treatment

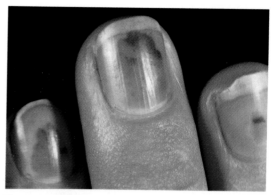

Figure 11–18. Photohemolysis secondary to psoralen and long-wave ultraviolet light.

based on the presence of psoriatic nail disease alone is difficult to justify because of potential toxicity. An exception may be severe, incapacitating nail involvement that produces discomfort, limits function, and significantly reduces the quality of life both physically and psychologically. Prolonged drug use in such cases mandates thorough patient education, informed consent, close supervision, and appropriate patient monitoring for adverse reactions. When psoriatic arthritis coexists with nail disease, improvement in joint symptomatology and function provides further support for the use of a systemic agent.

Although experience and availability are limited, superficial forms of radiotherapy have been used with some success in the treatment of psoriatic nails. In one study of three fractionated doses of superficial radiotherapy for psoriatic fingernails, treated nails demonstrated improvement for up to 15 weeks.[42] Nail thickness decreased significantly with treatment. Others have reported good responses, with remissions lasting months to years in some cases.[43] Radiotherapy is associated with both short-term and long-term dosage limitations. Sequential grenz ray therapy for psoriatic fingernails provides some improvement; however, overall results are modest.[44] Best results are achieved when nails are of normal thickness. Thick psoriatic nails are not improved. This reflects the limited penetration of grenz rays.

ACRODERMATITIS CONTINUA OF HALLOPEAU (LOCALIZED DIGITAL PUSTULAR PSORIASIS)

Acrodermatitis continua of Hallopeau is a localized form of pustular psoriasis limited to

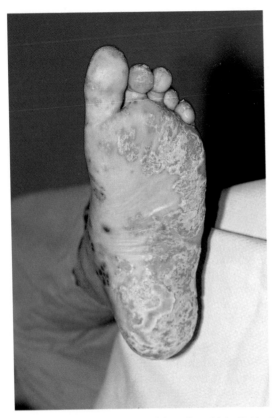

Figure 11–19. Hyperkeratoses of the soles with individual pustular and inflammatory lesions in Reiter's syndrome.

the fingers and toes. This disorder usually begins at the periungual region and extends proximally. Misdiagnosis as a bacterial pyoderma, herpetic whitlow, or a form of eczema is not uncommon. The disease usually affects a single digit and follows a relapsing course with frequent acute recurrences and absent or short-lived remissions.[45] Continued disease of the matrix may lead to dystrophic nail plate changes and in some cases anonychia. Pustular involvement of the nail bed produces onycholysis and pain. Atrophic thinning of the distal digit and bone resorption of the distal phalanx, findings not characteristic of chronic plaque psoriasis, may occur.

High-potency topical corticosteroid therapy, especially with occlusion, and oral nonsteroidal anti-inflammatory agents may reduce inflammation and symptomatology. The physician must be careful of digital atrophy, which may result from prolonged topical corticosteroid therapy. Low-dose cyclosporine therapy has been shown to be effective in one study.[46]

Generalized pustular psoriasis involving the digits may affect the nail unit, resulting in changes mentioned previously. Systemic ther-

apy with etretinate or methotrexate may prevent long-term nail complications, especially when initiated early.

REITER'S SYNDROME

Reiter's syndrome consists of a complex of arthritis and mucocutaneous manifestations. The latter include conjunctivitis, urethritis, oral erosions, balanitis circinata, and pustular or hyperkeratotic psoriasiform skin lesions. Cutaneous lesions may be clinically and histologically indistinguishable from psoriasis (Figs. 11–19, 11–20). Keratoderma blennorrhagicum refers to hyperkeratotic papules and plaques involving the palms, soles, and periungual region. The spectrum of psoriatic nail changes may occur. The presence of periungual and subungual pustules simulates generalized pustular psoriasis. Unlike chronic plaque psoriasis, Reiter's syndrome is associated with an increased prevalence of HLA-B27.

Cutaneous and ungual manifestations of Reiter's syndrome are generally refractory to therapy. Management is similar to psoriasis; however, the response to therapy is less favorable. Systemic nonsteroidal anti-inflammatory agents and topical corticosteroids are used initially, especially when disease is only mild to moderate in severity.[47] Reversal of severe nail involvement was reported in one patient with Reiter's syndrome treated with 1 g of tetracycline daily for 5 weeks.[48] A second patient with extensive nail involvement and severe arthritis was treated with intramuscular methotrexate 10 mg weekly, with resolution of skin manifestations after 1 month of therapy.[49] Methotrexate has been used in several other cases, especially those refractory to conven-

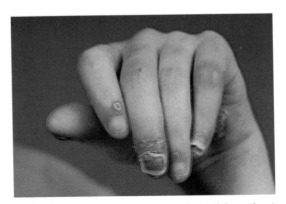

Figure 11–20. Psoriasiform acropustulosis of the nail unit characteristic of Reiter's syndrome with arthritis.

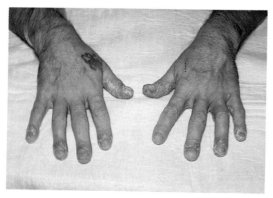

Figure 11–21. Paraneoplastic acrokeratosis (Bazex's syndrome).

tional therapy.[47] The use of chemotherapeutic agents such as methotrexate and azathioprine is usually reserved for patients with prolonged or severe episodes of articular or mucocutaneous inflammation. Improvement of joint disease usually lags behind improvement of skin disease. PUVA and systemic retinoid therapy may improve skin and nail disease.[50]

PARANEOPLASTIC ACROKERATOSIS (BAZEX'S SYNDROME)

Acral psoriasiform dermatitis associated with internal malignancy is a well-defined paraneoplastic syndrome. Paraneoplastic acrokeratosis, also known as Bazex's syndrome, presents as symmetric erythematous or violaceous psoriasiform plaques that may involve the ears, nose, cheeks, hands, knees, and feet[51–53] (Fig. 11–21). As the condition progresses, more extensive involvement may occur. The most commonly associated neoplasms include squamous cell carcinoma of the upper aerodigestive tract and unknown primary squamous cell carcinoma with cervical lymph node metastasis.[54–56] In many cases, skin and nail involvement precede the initial manifestations or diagnosis of the underlying malignancy by several months.[56,57] The astute clinician is in an excellent position to suspect the syndrome, initiate evaluation and early diagnosis of the underlying malignancy, and ensure treatment that may be lifesaving.

Nail manifestations include onycholysis, scaly white surface irregularity of the nail plate, grooving of the plate, subungual hyperkeratosis, tenderness, and erythema of the nail folds. Total nail loss or soft, thin, fragile nail plates that are prone to crumbling may also occur. Toenail changes tend be worse than fingernail changes.

Histopathologic changes of the nails are not diagnostic. However, amino acid analysis of abnormal nails has demonstrated an increased proportion of lysine, methionine, and glycine and a decrease in arginine, threonine, proline, and cystine compared with psoriatic and normal nails.[58]

The skin and nail changes associated with this syndrome are refractory to topical therapy. In greater than 90 per cent of cases, the skin eruption either improved significantly after treatment of the underlying malignancy or did not improve in the presence of persistent tumor. Even with clearance of the cutaneous eruption, nail dystrophy often persists.[56]

PITYRIASIS RUBRA PILARIS

Nails are involved in a significant number of cases of pityriasis rubra pilaris. Although the ungual changes are similar to those of psoriasis, there are distinctions that separate the two dermatoses.[59]

When the palms and soles are affected in adult patients, nails are frequently involved. In an evaluation of 24 patients with classic adult type 1 pityriasis rubra pilaris with nail abnormalities, 79 per cent demonstrated yellow-brown plate discoloration (Fig. 11–22); 75 per cent, subungual hyperkeratosis

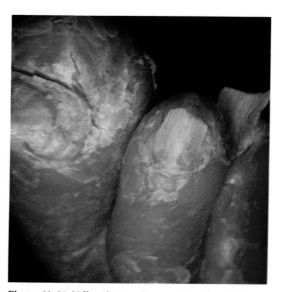

Figure 11–22. Yellow-brown discoloration of the nail plate with subungual hyperkeratosis and cutaneous involvement of the perionychium in pityriasis rubra pilaris.

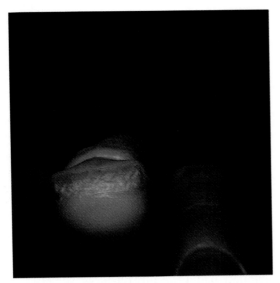

Figure 11–23. Frontal view of massive subungual hyperkeratosis seen in pityriasis rubra pilaris.

(Fig. 11–23); 71 per cent, nail thickening; 71 per cent, splinter hemorrhages; and 37 per cent, central onycholysis at the distal nail plate.[60] When nail changes of pityriasis rubra pilaris are compared with those of psoriatic nails, the latter demonstrated significantly more small pits, large and irregular indentations, salmon patches, and onycholysis. It is believed that, unlike that of psoriasis, involvement of the nail matrix is minimal or absent in pityriasis rubra pilaris.

Before the availability of systemic retinoids, pityriasis rubra pilaris was treated with high-dose vitamin A or methotrexate. Isotretinoin and etretinate are currently favored and may be combined with PUVA (RePUVA) when necessary.[50] Limited data are available regarding the response of affected nails to treatment.

LICHEN PLANUS

Nail changes of lichen planus occur in approximately 1 to 10 per cent of cases.[61] Abnormalities of the nails may be present with or without skin or mucous membrane involvement.[62–68] Onset may occur at any age in childhood or adulthood, with many cases appearing during the fifth or sixth decade of life.[67] Fingernails and toenails may be affected. Idiopathic atrophy of the nails represents a rare variant of lichen planus.[67]

Lichen planus limited to the nails is relatively uncommon and may present a formida-ble diagnostic challenge. This scenario may occur in both children and adults. Atrophic nails secondary to lichen planus without concomitant cutaneous lesions have been reported in children.[65] A case of lichen planus confined to the nails in a patient with primary biliary cirrhosis has also been reported.[69]

Ungual lichen planus may be reversible when secondary to active inflammation or permanent when secondary to matrix scarring. Fortunately, many cases do not develop early or severe permanent matrix destruction.[67] Unless matrix destruction or scarring have occurred, the disease remains amenable to treatment or spontaneous resolution.

Characteristic nail changes of lichen planus may also occur in association with lichen planopilaris, a variant associated with scarring alopecia. In one study of this disorder, approximately half of the patients had experienced glabrous skin lesions, nail changes, or mucosal lesions of lichen planus.[69a] Lichenplanus–like skin lesions and ungual changes have also been reported in a patient with graft-versus-host disease.[70]

As with psoriasis, the nail abnormalities of lichen planus are dependent on the parts of the nail unit that are affected. Matrix disease may vary in extent and severity, presenting as small atrophic foci or extensive destruction with potential for subsequent scarring. Focal disease of the proximal matrix produces onychorrhexis, with longitudinal grooves alternating with normal nail plate (Fig. 11–24). More extensive

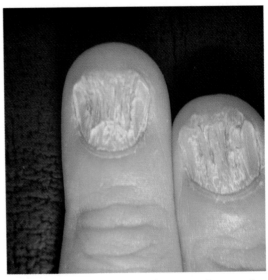

Figure 11–24. Longitudinal ridging creating onychorrhexis of the nail plate.

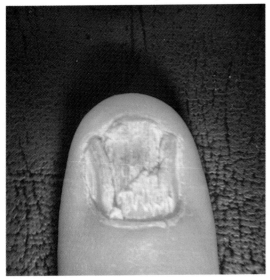

Figure 11–25. Onychorrhexis with thinning of the nail plate at both sides, giving rise to the "angel wing" deformity.

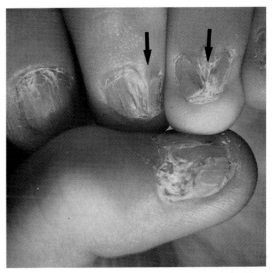

Figure 11–27. Onychorrhexis, partial nail plate destruction, and pterygia of two nails.

disease may produce splitting because the full length of the matrix is affected.

Diffuse matrix atrophy resulting in functional shortening of matrix produces thinning of the plate. This tends to predominate centrally, producing the "angel wing" deformity, a change that is often permanent (Fig. 11–25).

Matrix scarring, a late sequela that develops in some cases, produces permanent nail deformity.[67] Pterygium is the result of matrix scarring that is relatively specific for lichen planus (Fig. 11–26). This change may also occur secondary to trauma or peripheral vascular compromise, as is seen with scleroderma. Nail plate formation ceases when a large focus of matrix is replaced by cicatrix. Nail plate is no longer present to separate the proximal surface of the nail bed from the proximal nail fold. This allows the epithelial undersurface of the proximal nail fold to attach directly to the underlying nail bed. As both grow out distally, a winglike band of tissue develops (Fig. 11–27). A pterygium (from the Greek word *pterygion* meaning wing) may form centrally, laterally, or both. Total matrix scarring results in anonychia (Fig. 11–28).

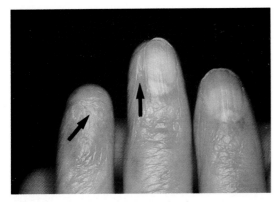

Figure 11–26. Middle nail shows a focal pterygium on one side, and nail unit on the left reveals a centrally located large triangular pterygium.

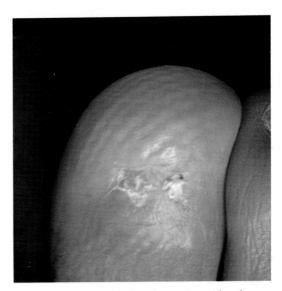

Figure 11–28. Total nail plate destruction with only remnant spicules remaining (anonychia).

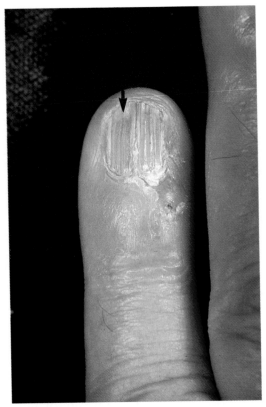

Figure 11–29. Onycholysis in lichen planus with concurrent onychorrhexis.

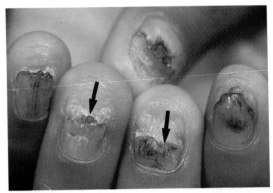

Figure 11–31. Subungual hyperkeratosis with uplifting of the nail plate and atrophy in the hyponychium area.

Lichen planus of the nail bed manifests as lichenoid papules when the disease is mild or may progress to permanent atrophy when it is more severe. Distal onycholysis may occur with involvement of the hyponychium (Fig. 11–29). If the nail bed is involved more proximally, the inflammatory process may interfere with plate-bed adhesion, resulting in more extensive onycholysis (Fig. 11–30). Involvement of the nail bed or hyponychium may also produce subungual hyperkeratosis, a change that is reflective of the hypertrophic variety of lichen planus. When extensive, marked nail plate uplifting may develop as subungual debris pushes up the nail plate in a manner similar to that seen in psoriasis or tinea unguium (Fig. 11–31).

Postinflammatory hyperpigmentation is a commonly encountered sequela of lichen planus, most prominent in blacks and Asians (Fig. 11–32). Foci of hyper- or hypopigmentation may be seen in the nail bed or matrix (Fig. 11–33). Melanonychia may be seen as the nail

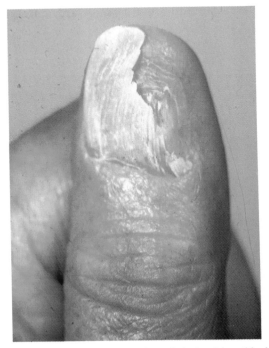

Figure 11–30. Severe degree of onycholysis with nail bed scarring.

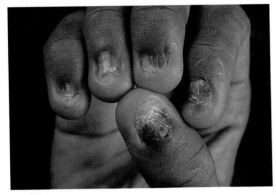

Figure 11–32. Hyperpigmentation of the nail plate and nail folds with multiple pterygia.

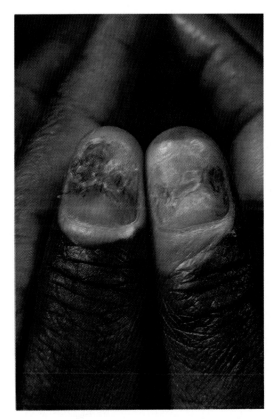

Figure 11–33. Hypopigmentation of nail bed and proximal nail fold with atrophy of the nail bed.

plate is formed, including the development of longitudinal streaks.[71] Hyperpigmentation of the nail folds may also be seen at sites preceded by cutaneous lichen planus. Although less common, hypopigmentation may also follow resolution of lichen planus and is most likely to manifest in the nail bed or nail folds.

A case of bullous lichen planus simulating yellow nail syndrome was described and confirmed histologically. The marked compact subungual hyperkeratosis was believed to cause the yellow color.[72]

Twenty-nail dystrophy was first described in 1977, affecting children between the ages of 3 and 12 years. The nail abnormality was limited to the nail plate, indicating matrix disease.[73] The plate was described as dull, opalescent, thin, and fragile, with prominent, closely arranged longitudinal ridges, distal notching, and layered splitting. Although lichen planus was considered in the differential diagnosis, a distinct entity was believed to be present because of the lack of cutaneous lesions and the absence of pterygium formation. Subsequently, biopsies of nail disease that resem-

bled this scenario demonstrated lichen planus, supporting the concept that 20-nail dystrophy is lichen planus limited to the nails.[62,64] In another case occurring in a 9-year old girl, careful examination revealed "lacy" plaques on the buccal and sublingual mucosa believed to be lichen planus.[74]

Further evaluation has revealed that 20-nail dystrophy may occur in adults[75] and may be seen in association with alopecia areata,[76] psoriasis, eczema, onychomycosis,[77] ichythyosis vulgaris,[78] and immunoglobulin (Ig) A deficiency.[79] The disorder has also been described in two siblings without other cutaneous symptoms.[80] Failure to histologically confirm lichen planus has been demonstrated in multiple studies of patients with 20-nail dystrophy.[19,71–83] This clinical pattern appears to be associated with a variety of distinct entities, with lichen planus being only one of them. The term 20-nail dystrophy simply implies that all 20 nails are involved and describes a reaction pattern rather than a specific disease. Whenever possible, the underlying diagnosis should be determined by appropriate diagnostic testing because prognostic and therapeutic implications relate directly to the underlying cause.

In a study of 20-nail dystrophy presenting as idiopathic trachyonychia, biopsies were performed in 23 patients.[19] Nineteen demonstrated spongiotic changes, lichen planus was confirmed in one patient, and three patients demonstrated psoriasiform features. The majority presented clinically with rough, lusterless nail plates with a sandpaper appearance. Some patients demonstrated less textural change characterized by a shiny appearance with numerous small superficial pits. During a mean follow-up of 2 years, none of the patients experienced alopecia areata, other cutaneous disorders, or mucosal changes. In another study of five patients with 20-nail dystrophy presenting with longitudinal ridging and loss of luster, histologic evaluation demonstrated spongiotic inflammation in all cases.[83] The underlying cause of these changes was not clear. An "eczematous process" was confirmed by biopsy in another reported case.[82] An autoimmune mechanism has been suggested in some cases because 20-nail dystrophy has been described in association with alopecia areata,[76] IgA deficiency,[79] and autoimmune hematologic abnormalities.[84]

On the basis of available clinical and histologic evidence, it may be concluded that 20-nail dystrophy is a reaction pattern associated

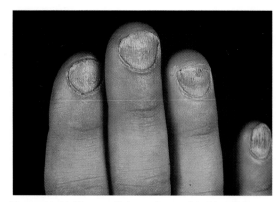

Figure 11–34. Fingernails in trachyonychia 20-nail dystrophy associated with lichen planus. There are dull-surfaced, ridged nails frayed at the edges.

with a variety of potential causes as described previously (Figs. 11–34, 11–35). Fortunately, most cases of idiopathic 20-nail dystrophy that develop during childhood resolve spontaneously.

The diagnosis of lichen planus of the nails is usually straightforward when the disorder coexists with cutaneous or mucosal involvement. Isolated nail disease is more difficult to confirm, especially when changes that are less specific for lichen planus are present. A definitive diagnosis should be obtained so that appropriate therapy can be initiated. Mycologic studies should be performed to exclude a diagnosis of onychomycosis. If mycologic studies are negative, a nail biopsy will likely be needed to confirm the diagnosis. Examination should include routine microscopy and fungal staining (PAS stain).

The cornerstone of therapy for ungual lichen planus is intralesional corticosteroid

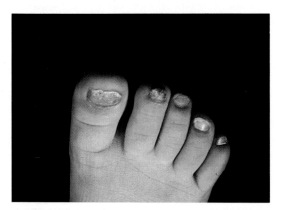

Figure 11–35. Toenails in a patient with trachyonychia 20-nail dystrophy—idiopathic. Subungual hyperkeratosis of the second toe is seen.

therapy as described in the discussion of psoriasis. If this regimen fails, oral prednisone therapy is often needed to arrest inflammation and prevent scarring. For adults, an initial dosage of prednisone 60 mg daily may be required, with treatment often continued for several weeks. Slow tapering is carried out as clinical improvement occurs. Once significant benefit is observed, changing to alternate-day therapy is preferable. Treatment failures occur even with aggressive systemic corticosteroid treatment. In one case report, no improvement was noted until after 6 weeks of systemic prednisone therapy.[85]

Other potential treatment options exist. Oral etretinate was found to be effective in a patient with lichen planus limited to all fingernails and four toenails.[86] Although oral griseofulvin has been reported to be effective for lichen planus, experience with griseofulvin has been disappointing. Grafting has been recommended as therapy for severe ulcerative lichen planus of the foot that also caused atrophic scarring of the nails.[87] Topical PUVA was used successfully for the treatment of fingernails in a patient with 20-nail dystrophy; a good response was noted after 7 months of treatment. Maintenance treatment was needed to prevent recurrence.[88]

LICHEN STRIATUS

Lichen striatus is a linear skin eruption of unknown cause that most often affects children and is frequently self-limited. Cutaneous involvement presents as discrete and confluent pinpoint lichenoid papules that most commonly occur on an extremity but may involve the neck or trunk.[3] Nail involvement is very uncommon; a total of 14 cases have been reported.[89–92] The nail changes may precede or coexist with skin involvement or may present as an isolated finding. Because of the linearity of the cutaneous eruption, the differential diagnosis includes linear lichen planus and inflammatory linear verrucous epidermal nevus, both of which may also involve nails.

Several nail changes of lichen striatus have been described. These include longitudinal splitting or ridging, nail thinning, punctate or transverse striate leukonychia, onycholysis, total nail loss, intermittent nail shedding, nail thickening, nail crumbling, hyperpigmentation, and longitudinal melanonychia.[50,89,91,93] Unlike lichen planus, scarring does not appear to occur. Although skin involvement generally resolves spontaneously within 2 years, nail abnormalities may also be self-limited or may persist for several months or years, even when the skin changes resolve.[89,91,94]

Five cases of self-limiting ungual lichen striatus were reported. The patients ranged in age from 8 to 28 years.[89] Fingers were involved in four cases and the large toe was involved in one case, with usually only one digit affected in a given patient. In three cases, the disorder affected the nail exclusively. In two patients with coexistent cutaneous lichen striatus, resolution of the nail changes occurred before the skin lesions; however, the opposite scenario has been reported. The duration of nail dystrophy ranged from 2 months to 3 years. The noted changes tended to involve the medial or lateral aspect of the nail plate.

Limited data are available on treatment of ungual lichen striatus. Because most patients are children or young adults, matrix scarring does not appear to occur, and many cases resolve spontaneously, a conservative approach to therapy is generally recommended. The response to topical corticosteroid therapy, with or without occlusion, is unsatisfactory.

LICHEN NITIDUS

Lichen nitidus is a relatively uncommon dermatosis that is seen most commonly in children but may also afffect adults. This skin disorder presents as discrete pinhead-sized, flesh-colored, or hypopigmented flat papules usually affecting the forearms, trunk, or penis.[3] The papules are typically hypopigmented in black patients. Coexistence with lichen planus has been noted; some authors believe that lichen nitidus is a variant of lichen planus. Lichen nitidus may clear spontaneously over several weeks to months, but it often persists for several years. Response of the skin eruption to topical corticosteroid therapy is poor.

Nail changes associated with lichen nitidus are uncommon and consist of nail plate thickening, deep ridging, pitting, and a roughened plate texture with associated brittleness. Some authors hypothesize that idiopathic nail pitting may be lichen nitidus in which skin changes were overlooked.[95] One patient presented with linear nail striations and ridging without pitting and was later found to have lichen nitidus on the arms, thighs, and trunk.[96] Lichen nitidus presenting as palmoplantar hyperkeratosis and nail dystrophy has been described in three patients.[97]

Because of the limited number of cases, the natural course and response to treatment of ungual lichen nitidus have not been clearly defined.

ECZEMATOUS DERMATITIS

Nail changes may be associated with all forms of eczematous dermatitis and generally result from paronychial and matrix inflammation. Atopic dermatitis, because of its high prevalence and chronicity, is the most common form of eczema associated with nail unit abnormalities. Ungual changes secondary to contact dermatitis of the hands is also common. A thorough history and careful skin examination usually allows the clinician to distinguish between the many types of eczema.

Eczematous dermatitis may produce a wide variety of nail alterations. The nail plate and nail folds are the most commonly affected sites. Changes include roughness, thickening, coarse and irregular plate pitting or grooving, transverse ridging, furrowing, nail shedding, onycholysis, and subungual hemorrhages. Acute or chronic paronychial inflammation may secondarily affect the matrix, leading to nail plate dystrophy. Onycholysis may be distal, proximal, or both, depending on the site and extent of spongiotic inflammation. Self-manipulation can induce secondary nail findings. Examples include smooth, shiny "polished" nails resulting from skin rubbing or changes secondary to nail picking. The varied ungual changes associated with eczema may simulate other nail diseases, such as paronychia or onychomycosis. Clinical confusion is most likely when findings suggestive of a specific form of eczema are limited or absent.

Specific contactants have been associated with nail unit abnormalities. Koilonychia has been produced by organic solvents and motor oils,[98] acute onycholysis by detergents, and chromonychia by well water high in iron.[99] Nail cosmetics are the fourth leading cause of contact dermatitis to cosmetics, comprising 8 to 13 per cent of cosmetic allergic reactions in studies completed in North America and The Netherlands.[100] Reactions may be either allergic or irritant in origin. Resultant inflammation can involve the matrix, bed, plate, hyponychium, and nail folds, producing a variable spectrum of clinical findings. Paronychia, yellow discoloration of the nail plate, transverse leukonychia, brittle nails, subungual hyperkeratosis, onycholysis, splinter hemorrhages, chromonychia, and permanent nail destruction have been described in relation to nail cosmetics.[98,100,101] Most reactions are secondary to toluene sulfonamide-formaldehyde resin found in most nail polishes, ethyl cyanoacrylate glue used to mend broken nails or paste on preformed nails, and methacrylates used to produce artificial nail plates.[100,101] Other components of nail cosmetics may also serve as sensitizers or irritants on rare occasions.

Diagnosis can usually be made on clinical grounds, obviating the need for biopsy. Mycologic studies may be warranted in some cases. Treatment of the underlying eczema should improve nail changes. It must be kept in mind that the rate of reversal of nail plate abnormalities depends on the extent of plate involvement and the rate of nail growth. As long as inflammation ceases and the matrix is preserved, newly formed normal nail plate should replace the distal abnormal plate. Chronic paronychia, if present, may require treatment independent of the eczema.

KERATOSIS FOLLICULARIS (DARIER'S DISEASE)

Keratosis follicularis, more commonly referred to as Darier's disease, is a genodermatosis classified as a disorder of keratinization. The nails are affected in the majority of patients (Fig. 11–36). In a study of 75 cases, nail lesions were present in 99 per cent of patients older than 20 years. Palmar pits and keratoses were found in 95 per cent and acrokeratosis verruciformis was noted in 73 per cent of patients. In 15 patients between the ages of 5 and 18 years, nail lesions were present in 60 per cent, whereas the characteristic skin eruption was present in only 27 per cent and palmar pits in 53 per cent.[102] In another study, hand involvement, primarily nail dystrophy, occurred in 96 per cent of patients.[103]

Nail abnormalities may prove to be an early diagnostic sign in many patients with Darier's disease. In some patients with less common patterns of Darier's disease, such as the flexural, nevoid, and localized hand forms, ungual changes may be the most suggestive findings.[103,104]

As with other dermatoses, the clinical features reflect the anatomic sites of the nail unit that are affected. Matrix disease leads to alter-

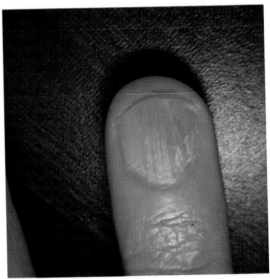

Figure 11–36. Red and white streaks of the nail bed in early Darier's disease.

ations of the nail plate. Focal matrix lesions lead to spotty leukonychia. Longitudinal white streaks may also develop from persistent matrix disease. These may look similar to the white streaks that are formed from the nail bed. The nail plate may become fragile, thickened, split, or longitudinally splintered, especially at the distal edge. Secondary microbial invasion with *Pseudomonas aeruginosa, Candida albicans,* or dermatophytes is not uncommon.

Nail bed disease may produce longitudinal red streaks, which over time change in color to white streaks.[105] A "sandwich" appearance of red and white lines is highly characteristic if not pathognomonic, of Darier's disease.[103] It should be noted that multiple long, white longitudinal streaks may be seen in patients with benign familial pemphigus (Hailey-Hailey disease).[106]

Hyponychial involvement produces a unique manifestation that appears to be specific for Darier's disease. A wedge-shaped, often triangular fragment, of subungual hyperkeratosis is formed (Fig. 11–37). A V-shaped notching of the free edge of the nail plate may be seen in fingernails and toenails.[103] The flat keratotic papules seen in this disorder may affect the nail folds.

An excellent discussion of the clinicopathologic correlations of affected nails in patients with Darier's disease appears in the literature.[105] Histologically, all segments of the nail unit may be involved, but the findings are different from those seen in the skin. There is ab-

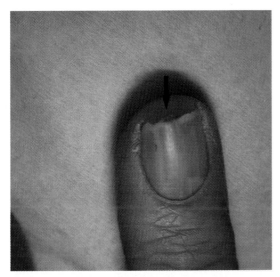

Figure 11–37. Distal wedge-shaped subungual hyperkeratosis characteristic of Darier's disease with white streaks of the nail bed.

sence of suprabasilar clefts, near absence of an inflammatory infiltrate, and presence of multinucleated epithelial giant cells.

The associated cutaneous and ungual manifestations of Darier's disease are phenotypic expressions of a genetic predisposition. Therefore, skin and nail changes are chronic and difficult to treat. As with the cutaneous lesions, treatment of nail abnormalities has met with limited success. High-dose oral vitamin A therapy, the common form of treatment before the availability of oral retinoids, has been used with inconsistent results for both skin and nail lesions, even after several months of treatment. Skin changes have responded more favorably to oral retinoids, including isotretinoin, etretinate, and acitretin in many patients[107]; however, recurrence after discontinuation of treatment is to be expected. Long-term therapy requires recognition and treatment of secondary infection, careful monitoring for adverse reactions, emotional support, and genetic counseling. Unfortunately, nail changes did not improve in a study of 18 patients treated with etretinate despite improvement or disappearance of skin lesions.[108]

ALOPECIA AREATA

Overall, alopecia areata is accompanied by nail changes in approximately 10 per cent of patients, with frequency figures ranging from 4 to 66 per cent. In a study of 272 children with alopecia areata, nail abnormalities were noted in 46 per cent of patients.[18] Fingernail pitting was the most frequent finding.

A variety of nail findings have been associated with alopecia areata, with most changes related to matrix disease. The most common finding, nail plate pitting, is often characteristic. Although not true in all cases, the nail pitting of psoriasis is often deeper and randomly arranged compared with alopecia areata. Nail pitting of alopecia areata is commonly uniform with a neatly arranged cross-hatched pattern of intermittent transverse pitting referred to as the "glen plaid design." Multiple nails are usually affected, although isolated nail involvement can occur.

In the study of 272 children with alopecia areata referred to previously, nail pitting was found in 34 per cent of children; mild disease of only a few nails was present in 21 per cent of the total population studied.[18] Only fingernails were involved with pitting. Forty per cent of children with nail pitting had alopecia totalis or universalis, and 7 per cent demonstrated lunula erythema.

Progressive matrix disease may produce diffuse roughening of the nail surface, with loss of luster and increased plate fragility. Beau's lines, transverse splitting, plate thinning, and koilonychia are seen in some patients. Punctate leukonychia may also occur and may precede the formation of nail pits by several years.[109] Greater distortion of the nail plate occurs when pits are produced rapidly, reflecting a greater intensity of active inflammation (Fig. 11–38). Alterations of the nail plate, such as trachyonychia, may involve all 20 nails, resulting in the clinical presentation of 20-nail dystrophy.[76,110] In a study of children, plate thinning and surface texture alteration consistent with trachyonychia or 20-nail

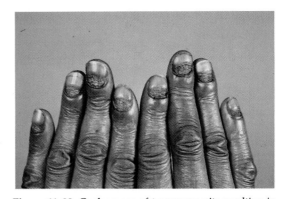

Figure 11–38. Coalescence of transverse pits resulting in surface nail plate crumbling in alopecia areata.

dystrophy occurred in 12 per cent of the patients.[18] Nail changes preceded the onset of alopecia areata by 12 to 36 months in 3 of 32 children, accompanied hair loss in 28, and followed hair loss by 18 months in 1. Progression of ungual changes did not correlate with alopecia in 23 children with trachyonychia who were monitored for 4 to 7 years. In most of these patients, nail changes resolved spontaneously.

Another study of 1095 patients with alopecia areata indicated that 3.6 per cent of patients experienced nail changes diagnosed as trachyonychia.[111] Twelve patients underwent nail biopsy. In 11 patients, the histologic findings revealed a mildly to moderately dense lymphohistiocytic infiltrate associated with exocytosis and spongiosis found in the proximal nail fold, matrix, bed, and hyponychium. The remaining biopsy indicated the histologic changes of lichen planus. Cutaneous lichen planus developed in this patient 6 months later, indicating that two distinct entities may sometimes be present.

A reversible lunula erythema[18,112,113] or a spotted effect[114] is sometimes apparent in patients with alopecia areata (Fig. 11–39). This spotting presents with a mottled appearance as small lacunae or plaques develop, resulting in loss of white color. Two patients with alopecia areata acquired red lunula within a few weeks of the acute onset of hair loss. A slow disappearance of the red lunula occurred followed by Beau's lines.[113]

Total or near-total onychodystrophy, onychomadesis (proximal nail plate shedding), longitudinal ridging with onychorrhexis, onycholysis, and a variety of color changes, including yellow, green, brown or opaque with or without leukonychia, are occasionally seen.

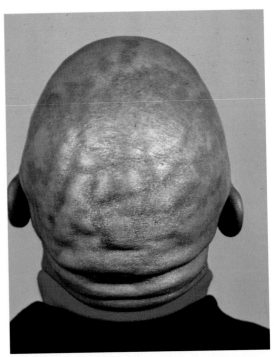

Figure 11–40. Scalp of patient in Figure 11–39 who has alopecia areata universalis.

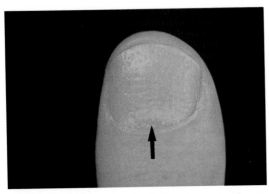

Figure 11–39. Spotted lunula of alopecia areata plus orderly linear transverse pitting.

Onychomadesis of all 20 nails has occurred during the onset of alopecia universalis.[18]

When nail changes of alopecia areata precede the onset of hair loss, the diagnosis may be difficult. As described previously, histologic examination reveals an inflammatory process that does not specifically confirm the diagnosis. Fortunately, most patients with alopecia areata experience nail changes along with or close to the onset of hair loss, resulting in a straightforward diagnosis in most cases.

It is generally believed that the nail changes associated with alopecia areata are most likely to occur in patients with severe alopecia (Fig. 11–40). The relationship between the presence of nail changes and the prognosis for hair regrowth is not clear. No relationship is likely in some cases; however, some studies have described nail changes as an adverse prognostic sign. An evaluation of 139 patients treated with diphenylcyclopropenone for alopecia areata suggested that the type and duration of alopecia areata and the presence of nail findings had prognostic significance.[115] A retrospective study of 209 patients with alopecia areata indicated that early age of onset, an atopic history in the patient or in a first-degree relative, an ophiasis pattern of hair loss, and onychodystrophy were unfavorable prognostic indicators.[116] Further study is needed to determine whether or not nail changes of alopecia areata in general, or any specific nail findings, correlate with prognosis.

Alopecia areata has been associated with other disorders, including vitiligo, psoriasis, and thyroid disease, including Hashimoto's thyroiditis, Graves' disease, and simple goiter. It has been theorized that nail pitting seen in alopecia areata is actually an expression of psoriasis.[117] In an age- and sex-matched controlled study of 152 consecutive patients with alopecia areata between the ages of 10 and 59 years, a thyroid evaluation was completed, including history and physical examination, thyroid hormone levels, thryroid stimulating hormone, and microsomal antibody testing.[118] The prevalence of positive microsomal antibodies was similar in both patient groups; no statistically significant difference was noted. None of the seven patients with positive microsomal antibody tests and alopecia areata had signs or symptoms of thyroid disease. A small, simple goiter was detected in four patients with alopecia areata. The authors concluded that routine thyroid testing in patients with alopecia areata is not recommended unless signs or symptoms suggestive of thyroid disease are observed.

Therapy with intralesional corticosteroids as described in the psoriasis section reverses nail changes in most patients, at least temporarily. Oral corticosteroid therapy is also effective but should be used only in special situations because of the high dosage and duration of therapy that are required. Temporary improvement of nail changes has been seen when dinitrochlorobenzene or squaric dibutyl ester treatment has been used to treat hair loss on the scalp.

SCABIES

Scabies, an intensely pruritic ectoparasitic infestation of the skin caused by the mite *Sarcoptes scabiei* var *hominis,* commonly affects the web spaces of the hands, wrists, elbows, axillae, waistline, buttocks, breasts in women, and genitalia in men. Mites gain access to the skin and harbor themselves within small, linear burrows that are usually scant in number. Pruritus begins within a few weeks of infestation as secondary hypersensitivity develops. At this point, patients manifest secondary urticarial papules that vary in number and extent. These skin lesions often affect the "clas-

sic" sites mentioned previously; however, the clinical presentation is highly variable. The severity of pruritus is often "out of step" with the extent of visible skin involvement. Scratching results in excoriation, which alters the clinical and histologic features of skin lesions. The onset of pruritus occurs much earlier with reinfestation.

The nail unit is usually not affected in patients with scabies. However, lodging of mites subungually secondary to excoriation of burrows may be a source of reinfestation if the subungual region is not treated during scabicide application. This mechanism has been demonstrated in a nursing home epidemic.[119] In most cases, the examining physician must carefully examine the patient for intact burrows on the skin that harbor the mite because scratching alters their appearance and may actually reduce the total number of mites on the skin.[120] Scabietic skin lesions other than burrows, such as excoriations and urticarial papules, do not contain scabies mites. Therefore, samples obtained for a scabies preparation should be obtained from intact burrows and subungual debris to achieve the highest diagnostic yield. Although dystrophic nail changes do not develop in most cases of scabies, the nails play an important role in altering the appearance of the disease and may provide assistance in obtaining the diagnosis via microscopic examination of subungual debris.

Keratotic scabies, also referred to as Norwegian or crusted scabies, is a distinct clinical presentation that occurs when scabies mites are allowed to proliferate continually without therapeutic intervention. Diffuse involvement with numerous mites produces hyperkeratotic and crusted skin lesions and extensive subungual debris. This form of scabies develops in patients with diminished cellular immunity who do not manifest the hypersensitivity reaction that produces pruritus. Many of these patients are immunocompromised by medications or disease or are mentally deficient and unable to communicate symptomatology when present. By the time an observer notes cutaneous changes, skin lesions are advanced and are teeming with scabies mites and eggs. The nail changes associated with keratotic scabies include dystrophic nail plates and extensive subungual hyperkeratosis (Figs. 11–41, 11–42). Complete destruction of the nail plate can occur as the plate becomes infested.[93] Treatment consists of proper scabicide application and trimming back of the nail plates,

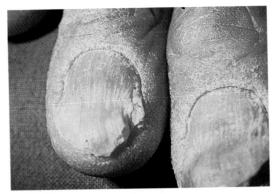

Figure 11–41. Keratotic scabies of the nail unit.

which may serve as a source for reinfestation. Additional treatment of the nails may be necessary, especially in patients with Norwegian scabies. This involves careful manual removal of subungual debris and brushing of the fingertips, especially under the free edge of the nails, with a scabicide on several consecutive days.[119] In resistant cases, segregation of the scabetic patient until healthy nail plates are produced and total destruction of the nail plate, including the matrix, have been mentioned as theoretical approaches but are not practical.[121] A combination of chemical reduction of the nail plate with topical 40 per cent urea, partial nail avulsion, and topical lindane applied under occlusion cured a patient with crusted scabies.[122]

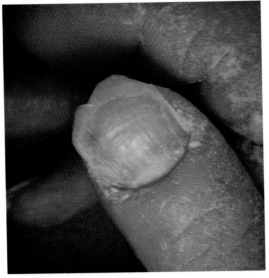

Figure 11–42. Peri- and subungual scabies associated with splinter hemorrhages with cutaneous involvement.

BULLOUS DISEASES

Pemphigus vulgaris results from the deposition of intercellular IgG within the epidermis, leading to acantholysis and bullae formation. Skin and oral mucosal involvement predominate, but the nail unit may be affected. In some cases, nail abnormalities may serve as the source of initial diagnosis. Two patients with pemphigus vulgaris were found to have dystrophic nail changes that preceded the onset of skin and mucosal lesions by many years.[123] The diagnosis of ungual involvement was confirmed by direct immunofluorescent testing of matrix epithelium.

Pemphigus vulgaris usually affects the periungual region, resulting in acute paronychia, which may become chronic as the disease persists.[124] Misdiagnosis as paronychia resulting from *Candida albicans* may occur when secondary colonization produces a positive culture. This is more likely to occur with fingernail involvement. Secondary nail plate changes can develop such as cross-ridging, Beau's lines, discoloration of the nail plate, pitting, and subungual hemorrhage. Severe microvesiculation of the matrix can produce onychomadesis.[125] Rarely, nail shedding can develop as a result of subungual involvement.[126]

Less common forms of pemphigus may also produce nail abnormalities. Pemphigus foliaceus may lead to yellowish or dark discoloration of the nails, onychorrhexis, onycholysis, pterygium formation, and subungual hyperkeratosis.[127] Pemphigus vegetans may cause onycholysis.[128]

Biopsy for routine histopathology and immunofluorescence is diagnostic. Therapy should be directed toward the treatment of cutaneous and mucosal disease. Most cases are treated with systemic corticosteroids and immunosuppressive agents. Nail symptoms may improve with treatment.

Dystrophic nail disease has been described in patients with bullous pemphigoid and in cicatricial pemphigoid.[129–131] The association was determined on the basis of clinical grounds because nail biopsies were not performed. Histopathologic and immunofluorescent studies were performed in a patient with pemphigoid, ulcerative colitis, and cicatricial nail dystrophy consisting of longitudinal nail splitting and pterygium formation. Involved adjacent skin was diagnostic for bullous pemphigoid, and direct immunofluorescence of the nail bed revealed linear deposition of C3 and IgM. Initiation of therapy before the development of scarring is necessary to prevent permanent nail abnormalities.

On the basis of studies of the basement membrane zone of the nail unit, it is not surprising that nail changes occur in association with immunobullous skin disorders. A study of three human accessory digits amputated for other purposes evaluated by immunofluorescence a battery of antibodies that react with normal basement membrane zone antigens.[132] The proximal nail fold, matrix, bed, and hyponychium expressed all the target antigens found in normal nonappendageal basement membrane. Dermal components were also normally expressed. Another study using tissue specimens from eight patients with ingrown toenails and one fetus with Herlitz junctional epidermolysis bullosa confirmed that the antigenic expression of basement membrane zone components in normal nail matrix is similar to that of normal skin.[133]

Hailey-Hailey disease, also known as benign familial pemphigus, usually presents in the second to fourth decade of life and most frequently involves the axillae and groin regions. Because intertriginous sites are typically involved, the disorder usually presents as macerated erythematous plaques. Rubbing and irritation often obscure the blistering component; however, fine surface slits may be seen and are highly suggestive of this disease. Pain and tenderness are common associated complaints.

In a study of 38 cases of Hailey-Hailey disease, asymptomatic longitudinal white bands of the nail bed were present in the fingernails of 71 per cent of patients examined.[106] Because the histologic features of this disorder are similar to those of Darier's disease, and because both disorders may be associated with longitudinal white bands, the diagnosis is based on clinical criteria and careful evaluation of the histologic features that distinguish between the two entities.

Epidermolysis bullosa refers to a family of inherited disorders characterized by blistering of the skin and mucous membranes after minor trauma that results from the separation of the epidermis from the dermis along the basement membrane zone. More than 20 genetic and clinical subtypes have been described in the literature.[134] The major disease categories include epidermolysis bullosa simplex (EBS), junctional epidermolysis bullosa (EBJ), and epidermolysis bullosa dystrophica (EBD). The site of detachment varies among these three main forms of the disorder. In EBS, cytolysis and separation occur within the basal keratinocyte layer, in EBJ the separation occurs along the lamina lucida, and in EBD the level of detachment occurs in the upper segment of the dermis immediately below the basement membrane. More recent studies have defined gene-coding defects for basement membrane proteins in some subtypes and abnormal structural protein expression in others. Mutations of keratin genes have also been discovered.[135]

Nail changes are commonly observed in some forms of epidermolysis bullosa. Some changes that are secondary to the effects of the primary disease on the nail matrix and nail bed are highly suggestive. However, chronic inflammation and secondary traumatic alterations appear to play a major role, producing nail abnormalities that are not always consistent with cutaneous changes. In general, the nail changes are the least discriminatory sign that can help in differentiating these entities and are not usually characteristic of specific subtypes of epidermolysis bullosa.[136] Some nail findings may also be seen in other skin disorders, such as onychogryphosis, hyperkeratosis, and change of longitudinal growth direction. Exceptions do exist. Nail abnormalities are often very typical in the EBJ-Herlitz subtype and may be the first sign of disease in the EBJ-progressiva subtype.[135]

The nails remain normal in most common subtypes of EBS.[135] In many rare subtypes, onychodystrophy with or without onychogryphosis may be seen. Changes in toenails are not uncommon and likely represent a response to repeated trauma and persistent inflammation.[135] Matrix and nail bed injury results, and scarring can develop. In the dominant EBS varieties, curved, thick, and dystrophic nails, including large toe onychogryphosis, have been described.[134,137] Large toe onychogryphosis is also a significant finding in the EBS-Ogna subtype. In the EBS–mottled hyperpigmentation variety, the nails may be thickened, curved, and onycholytic.[134] Frequent loss of nails with normal regrowth of fingernails and toenail dystrophy occur in the EBS–mottled with punctate keratoderma variety of the disease.[134] In the EBS-herpetiformis subtype, nail dystrophy or anonychia may result secondary to continual subungual blister formation. Nail loss after blistering with normal regrowth has been seen in association with the Dowling-Meara subtype.

Dystrophic nail changes, including subungual debris formation or anonychia, may be found in all junctional forms of epidermolysis bullosa and in some varieties of dystrophic epidermolysis bullosa.[134,138] Although EBJ is a nonscarring form, dystrophic nail changes are seen with most EBJ subtypes.[135] In the EBJ–Herlitz lethalis type, the most severe form of EBJ, paronychia-like periungual changes develop early and are followed by severe blistering with loss of the nail and large granulation tissue plaques that cover the dorsal fingertip.[135] EBJ subtypes are not associated with scarring unless induced by secondary traumatic factors. Therefore, initial normal nail regrowth follows subungual blistering and loss of the plate. Regrown nails subsequently become thickened and dome shaped.[135] Onychogryphosis may also develop. Dystrophic nail changes are even more likely to occur after repeated cycles of loss and regrowth and as sequelae secondary to repeated trauma and chronic inflammation.

Dystrophic nail changes and nail loss may be the presenting feature of EBJ-progressiva, a rare subtype. This develops without any signs of cutaneous disease between the ages of 5 to 15 years.[135] Nail changes are followed by blistering of the palms and soles.

Loss of nails is a consistent feature of EBD-mutilans and generalized EBD-nonmutilans, the most severe forms of recessive dystrophic epidermolysis bullosa.[135] Repeated blistering at the upper dermal (sub-basement membrane) cleavage plane leads to scarring and nail matrix obliteration. As a result, the ability to regrow nail plate is permanently lost. Nail dystrophy and loss of some nails is commonly seen in the generalized dominant and localized recessive forms of EBD, developing secondary to nail bed scarring and atrophy, hyperkeratosis or scarring of the nail matrix.[135] The DEB–Cockayne-Touraine subtype is associated with nails that are variably involved with dystrophic nail changes and onychogryphosis, which at times are the only sign of the disease.[136] Extensive nail alterations have been noted in the Pasini (albopapuloid) subtype, with changes often predominant on the feet.[134] The EBD–Hallopeau-Siemens subtype has also been reported to be associated with nail dystrophy and anonychia.

"Mitten hands" is a designation describing a classic late stage of development seen in patients with the EBD-mutilans subtype.[135] The fingers and toes fuse together secondary to destruction of the digits with scarring. The skin is then covered by a thin atrophic skin surface, resulting in the mitten-like appearance.

In some forms of EBD, some or all of the nails remain normal, or nail changes may be the only clinical sign of the disorder. Most of these patients are affected by milder localized EBD subtypes.[135] Nail abnormalities have not been described in patients with the EBD-pretibial variety, are minimal to absent in the EBD-inversa form, and at times are the only residual adulthood manifestation in patients affected by EBD-minimus.

Treatment should be directed toward avoidance of trauma, meticulous skin and wound care, and rapid detection and treatment of secondary skin infection. Adjunctive therapy directed toward maximal maintenance of function is also very important.

ERYTHEMA MULTIFORME–TOXIC EPIDERMAL NECROLYSIS

Erythema multiforme is a mucocutaneous reaction pattern that has been related to many potential stimuli. Certain drugs and recurrent herpes simplex infection have been the most clearly defined underlying associations. The characteristic "iris lesion" is targetoid and may develop bullae. The clinical expression of the disease may be mild (minor form) or severe, and extensive mucocutaneous involvement may develop (major form). The latter is commonly referred to as Stevens-Johnson syndrome.

Bullous lesions of erythema multiforme may affect the nail matrix, resulting in nail sloughing with regrowth or cicatricial anonychia.[139] Pterygium formation[140] and leukonychia striata[141] have also been reported. The latter finding may be due to nutritional deficiency that occurred during the acute phase of erythema multiforme, especially when oral mucosal erosions interfere with eating and drinking.

No definitive conclusions can be stated about treatment of the nails in both the minor and major forms of erythema multiforme. When severe nail unit inflammation raises concern that anonychia may ensue, intralesional corticosteroid injection may be of benefit in preventing permanent matrix destruction. Although controversial, systemic corticosteroids are sometimes used for the treatment of severe cases with extensive skin and mucosal involvement. Systemic corticosteroid therapy may improve the nail changes.

Toxic epidermal necrolysis is sometimes followed by failure of nail regrowth, corneal scarring, and cutaneous scarring. Pterygium formation affecting most of the digits and nail shedding followed by absent nail formation has been described in a patient with toxic epidermal necrolysis.[142]

ACANTHOSIS NIGRICANS

Acanthosis nigricans, which can be a marker of internal malignancy or an underlying endocrinopathy, usually affects the skin alone but may also involve the nail unit. The clinical features include thickened, discolored nails that exhibit interrupted leukonychia or are dull gray and friable. Diffusely white and thickened nails have also been reported. Successful therapy of the underlying causative disease may reverse the cutaneous and ungual changes.

INFLAMMATORY LINEAR VERRUCOUS EPIDERMAL NEVUS

Extension of an inflammatory linear epidermal nevus to the nail fold may produce longitudinal and transverse depressions of the nail plate.[143] Other reported changes include periungual psoriasiform plaques, loss of the cuticle, and onycholysis.[144] There is no known adequate treatment.

SARCOIDOSIS

Although skin involvement is present in approximately 30 per cent of cases, nail involvement is rare in patients with sarcoidosis. In a study of 400 patients with sarcoidosis, only 1 patient had nail involvement that could not be attributed to another entity.[145] The nail may exhibit thickening, longitudinal ridging, increased fragility, anonychia,[146] pterygium formation,[147] subungual papules,[93] brownish discoloration of the nail bed with scaling and fissuring of the surrounding skin,[146] convex nails with layering and splinter hemorrhages,[50] pitting, and cracking.[145] The ungual changes may occur in the absence of other cutaneous signs of sarcoidosis. A biopsy of the nail unit should demonstrate the specific histologic changes of sarcoidosis, thus excluding other causes. Treatment of the underlying disorder with oral corticosteroids or antimalarial agents may also reverse the nail abnormalities.

HISTIOCYTOSIS X

Histiocytosis X includes Letterer-Siwe disease, Hand-Schüller Christian disease, and eosinophilic granuloma. Nail involvement associated with histiocytosis X is rare but may involve the proximal nail fold, matrix, and nail bed. Ungual changes have not been reported in patients with eosinophilic granuloma. In one study of histiocytosis X, 3 of 15 patients were found to have nail involvement.[148] Two presented with fingernail and toenail dystrophy, onycholysis, subungual hyperkeratosis, and paronychial erythema with subungual pustules, and the third patient exhibited subungual purpura of all nails with slight thickening of some fingernails. A case of Langerhans' cell histiocytosis presenting initially with skin findings during infancy was reported. At 9 months of age, nail changes became prominent as the systemic features of the disease evolved. Nail findings included paronychia, nail fold destruction, onycholysis with subungual expansion, and nail plate loss.[149] Other nail changes reportedly included longitudinal grooving, distal nail plate notching,[150] and pitting.[148] It has been suggested that nail abnormalities are a poor prognostic sign, paralleling the course of the disease; however, this remains controversial.

A longitudinal nail biopsy reveals diagnostic histologic changes in the nail bed, proximal nail fold, and matrix. Electron microscopy demonstrates an increase in epidermal Langerhans' cells.[151] Therapy of the underlying disorder may result in clearing of the associated nail findings.

References

1. Stern RS: Epidermiology of psoriasis. Dermatol Clin 13:717, 1995.
2. Watson W, Cann HM, Farber EM, et al: The genetics of psoriasis. Arch Dermatol 105:197, 1972.
3. Hurwitz S: Clinical Pediatric Dermatology, ed 2. WB Saunders, Philadelphia, 1993.
4. Farber EM, Bright RD, Nall ML: Psoriasis: A questionnaire survey of 2,144 patients. Arch Dermatol 98:248, 1968.
5. Baughman RD: Psoriasis and cigarettes: Another nail in the coffin. Arch Dermatol 129:1329, 1993.
6. Scher RK: Psoriasis of the nail. Dermatol Clin 3:387, 1985.
7. Farber EM, Nall L: Nail psoriasis. Cutis 50:174, 1992.
8. al-Fouzan AS, Nanda A: A survey of childhood psoriasis in Kuwait. Pediatr Dermatol 11:116, 1994.
9. Daniel CR, Diagnosis of Onychomycosis and Other Nail Disorders—A Pictorial Atlas. Springer, New York, 1996.

10. Baker H, Golding DN, Thompson M: The nails in psoriatic arthritis. Br J Dermatol 76:549, 1964.
11. Wright V: Psoriatic arthritis. *In* Kelly WN, Harris ED Jr, Ruddy S, et al (eds): Textbook of Rheumatology, ed 2. WB Saunders, Philadelphia, 1985.
12. Jones SM, Armas JB, Cohen MG, et al: Psoriatic arthritis: Outcome of disease subsets and relationships of joint disease to nail and skin disease. Br J Rheumatol 33:834, 1994.
13. Lavaroni G, Kokelj F, Pauluzzi P, et al: The nails in psoriatic arthritis. Acta Derm Venereol Suppl (Stockh) 186:113, 1994.
14. Torre-Alonso JC, Rodriguez-Perez A, Arribas-Castrillo JM, et al: Psoriatic arthritis (PA): A clinical, immunological and radiological study of 180 patients. Br J Rheumatol 30:245, 1991.
15. Southwood TR, Petty RE, Malleson PN, et al: Psoriatic arthritis in children. Arthritis Rheum 32:1007, 1989.
16. Truckenbrodt H, Hafner R: Psoriatic arthritis in childhood: A comparison with subgroups of chronic juvenile arthritis. Rheumatol 49:88, 1990.
17. Robins TO, Kouskoukis LE, Ackerman AB: Onycholysis in psoriatic nails. Am J Dermatopathol 5:39, 1983.
18. Tosti A, Morelli R, Bardazzi F, et al: Prevalence of the nail abnormalities in children with alopecia areata. Pediatr Dermatol 11:112, 1994.
19. Tosti A, Bardazzi F, Piraccini BM, et al: Idiopathic trachyonychia (twenty-nail dystrophy): A pathological study of 23 patients. Br J Dermatol 131:866, 1994.
20. Tosti A, Morelli R, Fanti PA, et al: Nail changes of punctate keratoderma: A clinical and pathological study of two patients. Acta Derm Venereol 73:66, 1993.
21. Kouskoukis CE, Scher RK, Ackerman AB: The "oil drop" sign of psoriatic nails. Am J Dermatopathol 5:259, 1983.
22. Ohtsuka T, Yamakage A, Miyachi Y: Statistical definition of nailfold capillary pattern in patients with psoriasis. Int J Dermatol 33:779, 1994.
23. Eastmond CJ, Wright V: The nail dystrophy in psoriatic arthritis. Ann Rheum Dis 38:226, 1979.
24. Boisseau-Garsaud AM, Beylot-Barry M, Marie-Sylvia D, et al: Psoriatic onycho-pachydermo-periostitis. Arch Dermatol 132:176, 1996.
25. Golfieri R, Giampalma E, Tosti A, et al: Psoriasis arthropathica: A review of the literature, general considerations and the authors' personal experience. Radiol Med (Torino) 84:228, 1992.
26. Moll JMH, Wright V: Psoriatic arthritis. Semin Arthritis Rheum 3:55, 1973.
27. Helliwell P, Marchesoni A, Peters M, et al: A reevaluation of the osteoarticular manifestations of psoriasis. Br J Dermatol 30:339, 1991.
28. Ruzicka T: Psoriatic arthritis—New types, new treatments. Arch Dermatol 132:215, 1996.
29. Goupille P, Laulan J, Vedere V, et al: Psoriatic onycho-periostitis: Report of three cases. Scand J Rheumatol 24:53, 1995.
30. Cimmino MA, Seriolo B, Accardo S: Prevalence of nail involvement in nodal osteoarthritis. Clin Rheumatol 13:203, 1994.
31. Cutolo M, Cimmino MA, Accardo S: Nail involvement in osteoarthritis. Clin Rheumatol 9:242, 1990.
32. Fritz K: Psoriasis of the nail: Successful topical treatment with 5-fluorouracil. Z Hautkr 64:1083, 1989.
33. Burnett JW: Two unusual complications of topical fluorouracil therapy. Arch Dermatol 111:398, 1975.
34. Burnett JW: Further observations on two unusual complications of topical fluorouracil therapy. Arch Dermatol 188:74, 1982.
35. Marx JL, Scher RK: Response of psoriatic nails to oral photochemotherapy. Arch Dermatol 116:1023, 1980.
36. Handfield-Jones SE, Boyle J, Harman RRM: Local PUVA treatment for nail psoriasis. Br J Dermatol 116:280, 1987.
37. Morrison WL, Fitzpatrick TB: Phototherapy and photochemotherapy of skin disease, ed 2. Raven, New York, 1991.
38. Hann SK, Hwan SY, Park YK: Melanonychia induced by systemic photochemotherapy. Photodermatol 6:98, 1989.
39. Morgan JM, Weller R, Adams SJ: Onycholysis in a case of atopic eczema treated with PUVA photochemotherapy. Clin Exp Dermatol 17:65, 1992.
40. Rabinowitz HS, Scher RK, Shupack JT: Response of psoriatic nails to the aromatic retinoid etretinate. Arch Dermatol 119:627, 1983.
41. Mahrle G, Schulze HJ, Farber L, et al: Low-dose short-term cyclosporine versus etretinate in psoriasis: Improvement of skin, nail, and joint involvement. J Am Acad Dermatol 32:78, 1995.
42. Yu RC, King CM: A double-blind study of superficial radiotherapy in psoriatic nail dystrophy. Acta Derm Venereol 72:134, 1992.
43. Goldschmidt H, Panizzon RG: Modern Dermatologic Radiation Therapy. Springer-Verlag, New York, 1991.
44. Lindelof B: Psoriasis of the nails treated with grenz rays: A double-blind bilateral trial. Acta Derm Venereol 69:80, 1989.
45. Piraccini BM, Fanti PA, Morelli R, et al: Hallopeau's acrodermatitis continua of the nail apparatus: A clinical and pathological study of 20 patients. Acta Derm Venereol 74:65, 1994.
46. Peter RU, Ruzicka T, Donhauser G, et al: Acrodermatitis continua-type of pustular psoriasis responds to low dose cyclosporine. J Am Acad Dermatol 23:515, 1990.
47. Lally EV, Ho G: A review of methotrexate therapy in Reiter syndrome. Semin Arthritis Rheum 15:139, 1985.
48. Dijkstra JWE: Nail involvement in Reiter's disease. Br J Dermatol 102:480, 1980.
49. Ingram GJ, Scher RK: Reiter's syndrome with nail involvement: Is it psoriasis? Cutis 36:37, 1985.
50. Baran R, Dawber RPR: Diseases of the Nails and their Management. Blackwell Scientific Publications, Oxford, England, 1984.
51. Braverman IM: Skin Signs of Systemic Disease, ed 2. WB Saunders, Philadelphia, 1981.
52. Handfield-Jones SE, Matthews CN, Ellis JP, et al: Acrokeratosis paraneoplastica of Bazex. J R Soc Med 85:548, 1992.
53. Douglas WS, Bilsland DJ, Howatson R: Acrokeratosis paraneoplastica of Bazex—A case in the UK. Clin Exp Dermatol 16:297, 1991.
54. Arregui MA, Raton JA, Landa N, et al: Bazex's syndrome (acrokeratosis paraneoplastica)—First case report of association with a bladder carcinoma. Clin Exp Dermatol 18:445, 1993.
55. Mounsey R, Brown DH: Bazex syndrome. Otolaryngol Head Neck Surg 107:475, 1992.
56. Bolognia JL, Brewer YP, Cooper DL: Bazex syndrome (acrokeratosis paraneoplastica): An analytic review. Medicine (Baltimore) 70:269, 1991.
57. Baran R: Paraneoplastic acrokeratosis of Bazex. Arch Dermatol 113:1613, 1977.

58. Juhlin L, Baran R: Abnormal amino acid composition of nails in Bazex's paraneoplastic acrokeratosis. Acta Derm Venereol 64:31, 1984.

59. Sonnex TS, Dawber RPR, Zachary CB, et al: The importance of nail in the differential diagnosis of pityriasis rubra pilaris, psoriasis, and chronic erythroderma. Br J Dermatol (Suppl) 111:16, 1984.

60. Sonnex TS, Dawber RPR, Zachary CB, et al: The nails in adult type I pityriasis rubra pilaris. J Am Acad Dermatol 15:956, 1986.

61. Scher RK: Lichen planus of the nail. Dermatol Clin 3:395, 1985.

62. Burgoon CF, Kostrazewa RM: Lichen planus limited to the nails. Arch Dermatol 100:371, 1969.

63. Kanwar AJ, Govil DC, Singh OP: Lichen planus limited to the nails. Cutis 32:163, 1983.

64. Scher RK, Fischbein R, Ackerman AB: Twenty-nail dystrophy: A variant of lichen planus. Arch Dermatol 114:612, 1978.

65. Colver GB, Dawber RPR: Is childhood idiopathic atrophy of the nails due to lichen planus? Br J Dermatol 116:709, 1987.

66. Tosti A, De Padova MP, Taffurelli M, et al: Lichen planus limited to the nails. Cutis 40:25, 1987.

67. Tosti A, Peluso AM, Fanti PA, et al: Nail lichen planus: Clinical and pathologic study of twenty-four patients. J Am Acad Dermatol 28:724, 1993.

68. Peluso AM, Tosti A, Piraccini BM, et al: Lichen planus limited to the nails in childhood: Case report and literature review. Pediatr Dermatol 10:36, 1993.

69. Sowden JM, Cartwright PH, Green JR, et al: Isolated lichen planus of the nails associated with primary biliary cirrhosis. Br J Dermatol 121:659, 1989.

69a. Mehregan DA, Van Hale HM, Muller SA: Lichen planopilaris: Clinical and pathologic study of forty-five patients. J Am Acad Dermatol 27:935, 1992.

70. Liddle BJ, Cowan MA: Lichen planus-like eruption and nail changes in a patient with graft-versus-host disease. Br J Dermatol 122:841, 1990.

71. Baran R, Jancovi E, Sayag J, et al: Longitudinal melanonychia in lichen planus. Br J Dermatol 113:369, 1985.

72. Haneke E: Isolated bullous lichen planus of the nails mimicking yellow nail syndrome. Clin Exp Dermatol 8:425, 1983.

73. Hazelrigg DE, Duncan C, Jarratt M: Twenty-nail dystrophy of childhood. Arch Dermatol 113:73, 1977.

74. Silverman RA, Rhodes AR: Twenty-nail dystrophy of childhood: A sign of localized lichen planus. Pediatr Dermatol 1:307, 1984.

75. Synkowski DR: Twenty-nail dystrophy. Arch Dermatol 113:1462, 1977.

76. Horn RT, Odom RB: Twenty-nail dystrophy of alopecia areata. Arch Dermatol 116:573, 1980.

77. Kechijian P: Twenty-nail dystrophy of childhood: A reappraisal. Cutis 35:38, 1985.

78. James WD, Odom RB, Horn RT: Twenty-nail dystrophy and ichthyosis vulgaris. Arch Dermatol 117:316, 1981.

79. Leong AB, Gange RW, O'Connor RD: Twenty-nail dystrophy (trachyonychia) associated with selective IgA deficiency. J Pediatr 100:418, 1982.

80. Menni S, Piccinno R, Sala F, et al: Twenty-nail dystrophy of childhood—Two cases in one family. Clin Exp Dermatol 9:604, 1984.

81. Donofrio P, Ayala F: Twenty-nail dystrophy: Report of a case and review of the literature. Acta Derm Venereol 64:180, 1984.

82. Wilkinson JD, Dawber RPR, Bowers RP, et al: Twenty-nail dystrophy of childhood. Br J Dermatol 100:217, 1979.

83. Jerasutus S, Suvanprakorn P, Kitchawengkul O: Twenty-nail dystrophy: A clinical manifestation of spongiotic inflammation of the nail matrix. Arch Dermatol 126:1068, 1990.

84. Germain-Lee EL, Zinkham WH: Twenty-nail dystrophy associated with hematologic abnormalities. Acta Pediatr Scand 80:977, 1991.

85. Zaias N: The nail in lichen planus. Arch Dermatol 101:264, 1970.

86. Kato N, Ueno H: Isolated lichen planus of the nails treated with etretinate. J Dermatol 20:577, 1993.

87. Crotty CP, Su WPD, Winkelman RK: Ulcerative lichen planus. Arch Dermatol 116:1252, 1980.

88. Halkier-Sorensen L, Cramers M, Kragballe K: Twenty-nail dystrophy treated with topical PUVA. Acta Derm Venereol 70:510, 1990.

89. Tosti A, Miseiali C, Fanti A, et al: Histologic study of lichen striatus with nail involvement. Presented as Scientific Poster Session 157 at the meeting of the American Academy of Dermatology, Washington, DC, February 1996.

90. Baran R: Onychodystrophy in lichen striatus (letter). Pediatr Dermatol 11:283, 1994.

91. Goskowicz MO, Eichenfield LF: Onychodystrophy with lichen striatus (letter). Pediatr Dermatol 11:282, 1994.

92. Karp DL, Cohen BA: Onychodystrophy in lichen striatus. Pediatr Dermatol 10:359, 1993.

93. Zaias N: The Nail in Health and Disease. Spectrum Publications, New York, 1980.

94. Niren NM, Waldaman GD, Barsky S: Lichen striatus with onychodystrophy. Cutis 27:610, 1981.

95. Kellett JK, Beck MH: Lichen nitidus associated with distinctive nail changes. Clin Exp Dermatol 9:201, 1984.

96. Natarajan S, Dick DC: Lichen nitidus associated with nail changes. Int J Dermatol 25:461, 1986.

97. Munro CS, Cox NH, Marks JM, et al: Lichen nitidus presenting as palmoplantar hyperkeratosis and nail dystrophy. Clin Exp Dermatol 18:381, 1993.

98. Fisher AA: Contact Dermatitis, ed 3. Lea & Febiger, Philadelphia, 1986.

99. Olsen TG, Jattow P: Contact exposure to elemental iron causing chromonychia. Arch Dermatol 120:120, 1984.

100. Marks JG, DeLeo VA: Contact dermatitis and occupational dermatology. Mosby-Year Book, St. Louis, 1992.

101. Scher RK: Cosmetics and ancillary preparations for the care of nails. J Am Acad Dermatol 6:523, 1982.

102. Munro CS: The phenotype of Darier's disease: Penetrance and expressivity in adults and children. Br J Dermatol 127:126, 1992.

103. Burge SM, Willeinson JD: Darier-White Disease: A review of the clinical features in 163 patients. J Am Acad Dermatol 27:40, 1992.

104. Jorda E, Revert A, Montesinos E: Unilateral Darier's Disease. Int J Dermatol 35:288, 1996.

105. Zaias N, Ackerman AB: The nail in Darier-White disease. Arch Dermatol 107:193, 1973.

106. Burge SM: Hailey-Hailey disease: The clinical features, response to treatment and prognosis. Br J Dermatol 126:275, 1992.

107. Christopher J, Geiger JM, Danneskiold-Samsoe P, et al: A double blind comparison of acitretin and etretinate in the treatment of Darier's disease. Acta Derm Venereol 72:150, 1992.

108. Burge SM, Wilkinson JD, Miller AJ, et al: The efficacy of an aromatic retinoid, Tegison (etretinate), in the treatment of Darier's disease. Br J Dermatol 104:675, 1981.

109. Dotz WI, Lieber CD, Vogt PJ: Leukonychia punctata and pitted nails in alopecia areata. Arch Dermatol 121:1452, 1985.

110. Norton SA, Demidovich CW: Down syndrome, alopecia universalis, and trachyonychia. Pediatr Dermatol 10:187, 1993.

111. Tosti A, Fanti PA, Morelli R, et al: Trachyonychia associated with alopecia areata: A clinical and pathologic study. J Am Acad Dermatol 25:266, 1991.

112. Misch KJ: Red nails associated with alopecia areata. Clin Exp Dermatol 6:561, 1981.

113. Bergner T, Donhauser G, Ruzicka T: Red lunulae in severe alopecia areata. Acta Derm Venereol 72:203, 1992.

114. Shelley WB: The spotted lunula. J Am Acad Dermatol 2:385, 1980.

115. van der Steen PH, van Baar HM, Happle R, et al: Prognostic factors in the treatment of alopecia areata with diphenylcyclopropenone. J Am Acad Dermatol 24:227, 1991.

116. De Waard van der Spek FB, Oranje AP, De Raeymaecker DM, et al: Juvenile versus maturity-onset alopecia areata—A comparative retrospective clinical study. Clin Exp Dermatol 14:429, 1989.

117. Ganor S: Diseases sometimes associated with psoriasis: II. Alopecia areata. Dermatologica 154:338, 1977.

118. Puavilai S, Puavilai G, Charuwichitrana S, et al: Prevalence of thyroid disease in patients with alopecia areata. Int J Dermatol 33:632, 1994.

119. Scher RK: Subungual scabies. Am J Dermatopathol 5:187, 1983.

120. Gurevitch AW: Scabies and lice. Pediatr Clin North Am 32:990, 1985.

121. Koscard E: The dystrophic nail of keratotic scabies. Am J Dermatopathol 6:308, 1984.

122. DePaoli RT, Marks VJ, Crusted (Norwegian) scabies: Treatment of nail involvement. J Am Acad Dermatol 17:136, 1987.

123. Berker DD, Dalziel K, Dawber RP: Pemphigus associated with nail dystrophy. Br J Dermatol 129:461, 1993.

124. Dhawan SS, Zaias N, Pena J: The nail fold in pemphigus vulgaris (letter). Arch Dermatol 126:1374, 1990.

125. Parameswara VR, Chinnappaiah Naik RP: Onychomadesis associated with pemphigus vulgaris. Arch Dermatol 117:759, 1981.

126. Mortimer PS, Dawber RPR: Dermatologic diseases of the nail unit other than psoriasis and lichen planus. Dermatol Clin 3:401, 1985.

127. Azulay RD: Brazilian pemphigus foliaceus. Int J Dermatol 21:122, 1982.

128. Kechijian P: Onycholysis of the fingernails: Evaluation and management. J Am Acad Dermatol 12:552, 1985.

129. Burge SM, Powell SM, Ryan TJ: Cicatricial pemphigoid with nail dystrophy. Clin Exp Dermatol 10:472, 1985.

130. Esterly NB, Gotoff SP, Lolekha S, et al: Bullous pemphigoid and membranous glomerulopathy in a child. J Pediatr 83:466, 1973.

131. Miyagawa S, Kiriyama Y, Shirai T, et al: Chronic bullous disease with co-existing circulating IgG and IgG anti-basement membrane zone antibodies. Arch Dermatol 117:349, 1981.

132. Sinclair RD, Wojnarowska F, Leigh IM, et al: The basement membrane zone of the nail. Br J Dermatol 131:499, 1994.

133. Cameli N, Picardo M, Pisani A: Characterization of the nail matrix basement membrane zone: An immunohistochemical study of normal nails and of the nails in Herlitz junctional epidermolysis bullosa. Br J Dermatol 134:182, 1996.

134. Pearson RW: Clinicopathologic types of epidermolysis bullosa and their nondermatological complications. Arch Dermatol 124:718, 1988.

135. Bruckner-Tuderman L, Schnyder UW, Baran R: Nail changes in epidermolysis bullosa: Clinical and pathogenetic considerations. Br J Dermatol 132:339, 1995.

136. Gedde-Dahl T: Sixteen types of epidermolysis bullosa. Acta Derm Venereol 95 (Suppl):74, 1981.

137. Nielsen PG, Sjolund E: Epidermolysis bullosa simplex localista associated with anodontia, hair and nail disorders: A new syndrome. Acta Derm Venereol 65:526, 1985.

138. Fine JD: Epidermolysis bullosa. Int J Dermatol 25:143, 1986.

139. Hansen RC: Blindness, anonychia, and oral mucosal scarring as sequelae of the Stevens-Johnson syndrome. Pediatr Dermatol 1:298, 1984.

140. Wanscher B, Thornmann J: Permanent anonychia after Stevens-Johnson syndrome. Arch Dermatol 113:90, 1977.

141. Bryer-Ash M, Kennedy C, Ridgway H: A case of leukonychia striata with severe erythema multiforme. Clin Exp Dermatol 6:565, 1981.

142. Burns DA, Sarkany I: Junctional naevi following toxic epidermal necrolysis. Clin Exp Dermatol 3:323, 1978.

143. Landwehr AJ, Starink TM: Inflammatory linear verrucous epidermal nevus. Dermatologica 166:107, 1983.

144. Cheesbrough MJ, Kilby PE: The inflammatory linear verrucous epidermal nevus—A case report. Clin Exp Dermatol 3:293, 1978.

145. Patel KB, Sharma OP: Nails in sarcoidosis: Response to treatment. Arch Dermatol 119:277, 1983.

146. Mann RJ, Allen BR: Nail dystrophy due to sarcoidosis. Br J Dermatol 105:599, 1981.

147. Kalf RE, Grossman ME: Pterygium formation due to sarcoidosis. Arch Dermatol 121:276, 1985.

148. Timpatanapong P, Hathirat P, Isarangkura P: Nail involvement in histiocytosis X. Arch Dermatol 120:1052, 1984.

149. de-Berker D, Lever LR, Windebank K: Nail features in Langerhans cell histiocytosis. Br J Dermatol 130:523, 1994.

150. Diestelmeier MR, Soden CE, Rodman OG: Histiocytosis X: A case with nail involvement. Cutis 30:483, 1982.

151. Holzberg M, Wade TR, Buchanan ID, et al: Nail pathology in histiocytosis X. J Am Acad Dermatol 13:522, 1985.

CHAPTER 12

Pigmentation Abnormalities

C. Ralph Daniel III

Color changes in the nail unit make up a significant portion of onychopathology. The ability to examine the abnormality properly is needed to pursue a cause.

One should study all 20 nails. If polish or lacquer is on the nails, it should be removed before examination. One should examine the nails with the digits relaxed and not pressed against any surface.[1,2] Failure to do so may alter nail hemodynamics and obscure subtle changes. The observer should squeeze the digit tip to see whether the color change is altered substantially. This may help to differentiate discoloration of the nail plate from that caused by a vascular alteration. The latter is often grossly changed by pressing on the distal digit. In addition, unless the digit is too thick, it is frequently possible to transilluminate a digit by shining a strong penlight upward through the pulp. This procedure may aid in pinpointing more closely the location of the color change or possibly the etiologic agent.

A thorough history may be necessary. The review of systems, occupational and recreational activities, medications, topical contactants, and a physical examination may provide valuable information.

Various causes of nail pigmentation abnormalities have been compiled and presented previously in different communications.[1–6]

Subdivision according to cause yields (1) systemic disorders and predominantly dermatologic conditions, (2) systemic drugs, and (3) local factors near the nail.[1] Also various nail pigmentation abnormalities with eponymic or specific descriptions are tabulated. The cause, discoloring agent, color description, and site of discoloration in the nail complex are given in many instances.[1,4]

Most of the nail disorders associated with systemic diseases are not diagnostic when they are considered alone.[1] Zaias appropriately stated that if nail discoloration follows the shape of the lunula, it is more likely caused by internal factors, whereas if it corresponds to the shape of the proximal nail fold, external factors predominate.[8,9] Also many of the inherent pigment abnormalities seen in nails are the result of increased melanogenesis in the matrix.[9] Other mechanisms include imperfect keratinization, infection, by-products of metabolism, ischemia, genetic abnormalities, and lack of nutrients. Table 12–1 lists some systemic disorders that may cause changes in nail pigmentation.

Tables 12–2 and 12–3 list some abnormalities resulting from predominantly dermatologic disorders and inherited or congenital disorders, respectively.

Table 12–4 lists numerous color changes caused by systemic drugs. For the most part,

Table 12–1. **ABNORMAL NAIL PIGMENTATION ATTRIBUTABLE TO SOME SYSTEMIC DISORDERS**

Disorders	Discoloring or Causal Agent	Color	Site
Adrenal insufficiency[17]	Melanin	Longitudinal brown lines or diffusely brown	Nail plate
Alkaline metabolic diseases[18]	?	Variable white	?
Anemia	Vascular	Pallor	Vascular bed
Vitamin B_{12} deficiency[19–22]	Melanin	Variable brown-black	Nail plate, nail bed
Bazex's syndrome[23]	?	Yellow	Nail plate
Breast cancer[24] (vs. postirradiation)	Melanin	Diffuse hyperpigmentation	Nail plate (?)
Bronchiectasis (with hapalonychia)[a]	?	Light blue tinge or yellowish	Nail plate
Carbon monoxide poisoning	Hemoglobin	Cherry red, especially lunula	Vascular bed
Cardiac decompensation[17]	?	Yellow	Distal nail plate
Cardiac failure[b]	Abnormal adhesion of nail bed to nail	Red lunula	Lunula
Carpal tunnel syndrome[25]	Melanin	Longitudinal brown band	Nail plate
Cirrhosis[18,26,27]	Probable vascular alteration, a vasodilator polypeptide	Distal red band, white proximal nail; red lunula alone	Vascular bed (?)
Cronkhite-Canada syndrome[28]	?	Yellowish	?
Cushing's syndrome[a]	Melanin	Black	Nail bed, matrix
Cyanotic disease	Hemoglobin	Diffuse bluish	Vascular bed
Diabetes mellitus[29]	?	Yellow	Toenails with distal accentuation
Fogo selvagem[a]	?	Yellow canalized lines	?
Fucosidosis[30]	?	Purple nail bands	?
Gangrene[31]	Necrosis	Black	Probable nail bed
Hemochromatosis[32]	Iron or melanin (?)	Diffuse gray, brown, white	Nail plate
Hyperbilirubinemia[32]	Melanin	Diffuse brownish	Nail plate
Hyperthyroidism[33,34]	Dirt (?) melanin	Variable brown	Nail plate
Hypoalbuminemia[35] (e.g., nephrotic syndrome, cirrhosis)	See Muehrcke's lines, Table 12–4		
Hypocalcemia[18]	?	Variable white	?
Hypopituitarism[18]	?	Diffuse brown	Nail plate
Impaired peripheral blood supply[36]	?	Variable brownish discoloration	?
Leprosy[37]	?	Diffuse white	Nail plate
Lichen planus[20,38]	Melanin	Variable brownish discoloration, longitudinal pigmented band[c]; bluish or reddish color (early change)[c]	Nail plate, nail bed
Lupus erythematosus (discoid)[39]	?	Red-blue longitudinal striae	Nail plate
Lymphogranuloma venereum[18]	Vascular	Red lunula	Lunula
Malabsorption[18]	?	Variable white	Lunula
Malaria[18,37]	Vascular (?)	Variable gray (?)	Vascular bed
Malnutrition[40]	Melanin	Diffuse brown or brown bands	Nail plate (?)
Melanosis (postinflammatory)[41]	Melanin	Diffuse brown-black	Nail plate
Menstruation[42]	?	Leukonychia striata	Nail plate
Multiple myeloma[43]	?	Absent lunula	Lunula
Pellagra[18]	?	Diffuse milky white	?
Pinta[21,22]	Melanin	Diffuse brown-black	Nail bed
Pregnancy[30,44]	?	Brown longitudinal pigmented bands	Nail plate
Reiter's syndrome	?	Diffuse brown	?
Renal failure (chronic)[9,45–49]	Melanin	Distal brownish portion	Nail plate
Reticulohistiocytosis (multicentric)[50]	?	Periungual red nodules, "hyperpigmented"	Periungual
Reticulosarcoma[18]	Vascular	Red lunula	Lunula

Table 12–1. **ABNORMAL NAIL PIGMENTATION ATTRIBUTABLE TO SOME SYSTEMIC DISORDERS**
Continued

Disorders	Discoloring or Causal Agent	Color	Site
Rheumatoid arthritis[18]	?	Lilac line of Milan (as in syphilis)	Nail bed or lunula area (?)
Sarcoid[51]	?	Yellowish	Nail plate
Syphilis with hypertrophic onychauxis[52]	?	Diffuse grayish brown	?
Visceral leishmaniasis[43]	?	Diffuse gray	?
Yellow nail syndrome (acquired)[22,53]	Serum	Diffuse yellow	Nail plate

See Chapter 13 for additional entries.
[a]D. Swinehart, personal communication, 1979.
[b]C.R. Daniel III, personal observation, 1982.
[c]R. Baran, personal communication, December 1982.
Data from Cutis.[1–4]

these changes are simple asymptomatic side effects of treatment. Phototoxic, photoallergic, and other allergic reactions may cause pain, nail shedding, and other symptoms. Clues of ingestion of arsenic may first appear in the nail as Mees' lines. See the chapters on nails in systemic disease and systemic drugs elsewhere in this book for further information (Chapters 13 and 14).

Table 12–5 lists numerous local agents that may affect the nails. Examples of cosmetics, medications, fungi, bacteria, neoplasms, and occupational and physical agents are listed. Numerous topical agents affect the nail plate through adsorption of the substance.[1,10] Various mechanisms are present for other categories. If the substance is impregnated more deeply into the nail or is subungual, specific diagnostic studies such as potassium hydroxide preparations, nail composition studies, a biopsy specimen examined with a light microscope, special stains, or possibly an electron microscopic study may be indicated.[1] The initial presenting symptom of melanoma of the nail complex is often a discolored nail. If one cannot rule out melanoma as a case of longitudinal nail pigmentation (Table 12–6) or if Hutchinson's sign is noted (leaching of pigment from the nail to a nail fold), a biopsy is mandatory.

Longitudinal pigmented bands (LPB) are found normally in more heavily pigmented individuals. In these individuals, it is commonly seen in multiple nails. Baran[11,12] gave

Table 12–2. **ABNORMAL NAIL PIGMENTATION ATTRIBUTABLE TO SOME PREDOMINANTLY DERMATOLOGIC CONDITIONS**

Disorder	Causal Agent	Color	Site
Acantholytic epidermolysis bullosa[17]	?	Longitudinal red and white bands	Nail plate
Acanthosis nigricans[41]	?	Variable brownish discoloration	Nail plate
Alopecia areata[23]	?	Pale yellow leukonychia[42]	Lunula
Dyshidrosis[11]	?	White	Plate
Keratosis lichenoides chronica (possible variant of lichen planus)[54]	?	Yellow-brown	Nail plate
Laugier's essential melanotic pigmentation	Melanin	Brownish	Plate
Frictional melanonychia[11]	Melanin	Longitudinal brown streaks	Plate
Pityriasis rubra pilaris (may be familial)[24]	?	Diffuse gray or brownish	?
Prurigo vulgaris[18]	?	Longitudinal yellow-brown lines	Nail plate
Psoriasis[9,43,55]	Blood glycoprotein	Brown-yellow	Nail plate
Psoriasis[a]	Green nail syndrome (?)	Greenish	?
Senile nails[18]	?	Absent lunula and opaque	Lunula
Vitiligo[9]	Lack of melanin	Variable brown	Nail bed

[a]R. Baran, personal communication, 1981.

Table 12–3. **ABNORMAL NAIL PIGMENTATION ATTRIBUTABLE TO SOME INHERITED OR CONGENITAL DISEASES**

Disorders	Discoloring or Causal Agent	Color	Site
Pili torti[4,96]	?	Leukonychia	Nail plate
Pernicious anemia[57]	?	Blue	?
Acquired immunodeficiency syndrome[58,59]	?	Yellowish	?
Vitamin B$_{12}$ deficiency[60]	?	Bluish-black	?
Acrodermatitis enteropathica[43]	?	Variable brownish discoloration	?
Amyloidosis with polyneuropathy (familial)[29]	?	Yellow	Toenails with distal accentuation
Bart-Gorlin-Anderson syndrome[42]	?	Gray-yellow	?
Coat's syndrome[30]	?	Red	Nail bed
Darier's disease[61,62]	?	Brown or white, and red streaks	Nail bed, matrix
Great toenail dystrophy[23]	?	Dark colored	Great toenails
Ectodermal defect (congenital)[41]	?	Diffuse brownish	Nail plate
Erythropoietic protoporphyria[63]	?	No lunula, grayish	Absent lunula (?)
Genetic tendency for nail pigmentation after chemotherapy?[64]	?	Brown	?
Hidrotic ectodermal defect[43]	?	Diffuse yellow	?
Hutchinson-Gilford syndrome[9]	?	Variable yellow	?
Ichthyosiform syndrome (congenital) with keratitis and deafness[65]	?	Diffuse white	?
Incontinentia pigmenti[52,66]	?	Diffuse yellowish	?
Leukonychia, knuckle pads, deafness[67]	?	Partial white	Nail plate
Leukonychia totalis (congenital)[68]	?	Diffuse white	Nail plate
Nevi (familial congenital pigmented)[69]	Melanin	Punctate or longitudinal brownish	Nail plate, matrix
Ochronosis[70]	Hemogenistic acid (?)	Diffuse grayish	Nail bed (?)
Pachyonychia congenita[9]	?	Diffuse brownish	Nail plate
Peutz-Jeghers syndrome[71,72]	Melanin	Punctate brown	Nail plate, nail bed
Phenytoin effects (congenital)[73]	?	Brown (ocher)	Nail plate
Porphyria (congenital erythropoietic)	Porphyrin	Red fluorescence with Wood's light	Nail plate
Progeria[9]	?	Yellowish	?
Racket nail (congenital)[18]	?	Diffuse white	Lunula (?)
Soft nail disease[74]	?	Absent lunula	Matrix
Telangiectasia (hereditary acrolabial)[75]	?	Diffuse blue	Nail bed
Telangiectasia (hereditary hemorrhagic)[76]	Vascular components	Punctate red	Vascular bed
Trichothiodystrophy[77]	?	Yellow	Toenails
Yellow nail syndrome (congenital)[9,53]	Thickened nail plate (?)	Diffuse yellow	Nail plate
Wilson's disease[9,78]	Copper	Blue, especially lunula	Nail plate

Data from Cutis.[1–4]

some helpful suggestions when trying to differentiate benign LPB from those associated with subungual melanoma (SM):

The clinician should be suspicious when LPB (1) begins in a single digit of a person during the sixth decade of life or later; (2) develops abruptly in a previously normal nail plate; (3) becomes suddenly darker or wider; (4) occurs in either the thumb, index finger, or great toe; (5) occurs in a person who gives a history of digital trauma; (6) occurs singly in the digit of a dark-skinned patient, particularly if the thumb or great toe is affected; (7) demonstrates blurred, rather than sharp, lateral borders; (8) occurs in a person who gives a history of malignant melanoma; (9) occurs in a person in whom the risk for melanoma is increased (e.g., dysplastic nevus syndrome); (10) is accompanied by nail dystrophy, such as partial nail destruction or disappearance.[12]

Other signs are noteworthy,[11,12] but not necessarily helpful, in establishing the likelihood of malignancy.

1. Although a melanotic SM has been reported, lightly pigmented bands are less likely

Table 12–4. **ABNORMAL NAIL PIGMENTATION CAUSED BY SOME SYSTEMIC DRUGS OR INGESTANTS**

Drug	Discoloring Agent	Color	Site
Acetanilid[52]	?	Variable purple	?
Acetylsalicylic acid[42]	?	Purpura	Nail bed
Acridine derivations[11] (acriflavine, trypaflavine)		Whitish	Distal bed
Androgen[79]	?	Half-and-half nail–like changes	?
Aniline poisoning[52]	?	Variable blue-violet	?
Antimalarials[9,21,22,79,80]	Melanin, antimalarial	Diffuse blue, brown, variable	Nail plate, nail bed
Antimony[11]	?	Leukonychia	?
Arsenic[81]	Melanin (?)	Transverse white lines, diffuse brown	Nail plate
Azidothymidine[82,83]		Dark, bluish, brownish	
Beta carotene[29,42]	Beta carotene	Yellow	Nail bed
Brome[30]	Hemorrhage	Reddish	Nail bed
Canthaxantine[11]	?	Yellow	Bed
Caustic soda[30]	?	Yellow	Nail plate
Chromium salts[11]		Yellow	Plate
Corticotropin[11]		Longitudinal diffuse brown	Plate
Dichromates[42]	?	Yellow-ocher	?
Dicyanidamide[a]	?	Brownish	?
Dinitrophenol[11]	?	Yellow or long streaks	Bed
Emetine chlorate[18]	?	Variable white	?
Fluoride (fluorosis)[40]	Melanin (?)	Brown bands	Nail plate, matrix
Gold (allergic reaction)[41]	?	Variable brown	?
Heparin[30]	Acute poisoning	Red band	Nail bed
Ibuprofen[85]	?	Longitudinal pigmented bands	Nail plate
Ketoconazole[30]	?	Longitudinal band splinter hemorrhage	Nail plate, nail bed
Lead[86]	Lead	Hyperpigmentation	?
Lithium carbonate[87]	?	Change from golden to normal	Probably nail plate
Mepacrine[23]	?	Variable brown	?
Mercury[9]	Mercury (?)	Variable brown	Nail bed[88]
Methoxsalen[84]	?	Diffuse brown	Nail plate
Minocycline[89]	?	Blue-gray	?
Mitoxantrone	?	Blue	?
Melanoyte-stimulating hormone[11]	?	Brown	Plate
Neo-Synephrine (phenylephrine)[52]	?	Nail bed purpura	Nail bed
Para-aminosalicylic acid[11]	?	Cyanosis	Bed
Picric acid[11]	?	Yellow	Bed
Phosphorus[11]	?	Hemorrhage	Bed
Polychlorinated biphenyls[30]	?	Brown to gray line	Nail plate and nail bed
D-Penicillamine[90]	?	Yellow nail syndrome	?
Penicillamine[91]	?	Absence of lunula	Lunula
Penicillamine[11]	?	Yellow	Plates
Phenindione	?	Diffuse brown-yellow,[70] orange[92]	?
Phenolphthalein[43]	?	Diffuse gray	?
Phenothiazine (photoreaction)[93]	?	Variable brown	?
Phenytoin[73]	?	Brown (ocher)	Nail plate
Pilocarpine poisoning[42]	?	Leukonychia or plate	Nail bed (?)
Practolol[7]	?	Subungual blotchy erythema	Nail bed
Santonin[29]	?	Yellow	Nail plate (?)
Silver (argyria)[22,94]	Silver	Diffuse azure, dark gray	Lunula, nail plate, matrix
Sulfonamide (allergic reaction)[18]	?	Variable brown with drug reaction	?
Sulphydrilic acid[18]	?	Variable blue	?
Tetracycline[22,56,95,96]	Photoonycholysis splinter hemorrhages	Variable brown, red	Nail plate, nail bed
Tetryl[30]	Nitramine	Yellow	Nail bed
Thallium[37]	?	Variable white	?

Table continued on following page

Table 12–4. **ABNORMAL NAIL PIGMENTATION CAUSED BY SOME SYSTEMIC DRUGS OR INGESTANTS**
Continued

Drug	Discoloring Agent	Color	Site
Timolol[97]	?	Brown	Probably nail plate
Trinitrotoluene (absorption)[52]	?	Nail bed purpura	Nail bed
Warfarin sodium[98,99]	?	Purplish	Nail bed
Cancer Chemotherapeutic Agents			
Bleomycin[100,101]	Melanin	Variable brown, blue	Nail plate
Busulfan[32]	?	Variable brown	Lunula, nail plate
Cyclophosphamide[32,102]	?	Variable black	Nail plate
Daunorubicin[88]	?	Transverse brown-black bands	Nail plate
Dinitrochlorobenzene[b]	?	Brownish	Nail plate (?)
Doxorubicin[102–105]	Melanin	Variable brown-blue	Nail plate, bed
5-Fluorouracil[79]	?	Half-and-half nail–like changes, variable brown	?
Hydroxyurea[34,103]	?	Variable brownish	Nail plate, bed
Melphalan[32]	?	Variable brown	Nail plate, bed

See Table 12–6.
[a]R. Baran, personal communication, 1980.
[b]R. Baran, personal communication, 1981.
Data from Cutis.[1–4]

to represent SM; the pathologist may have difficulty even visualizing the melanin and melanocytes that constitute light pigmented bands.

2. Darker shades of brown do not necessarily represent melanoma because nevi and melanoma may manifest identical shades of brown. In white persons, *black* bands may be an important clue to melanoma; in African-Americans, however, jet-black bands are not unusual. Theoretically, color variegation suggests melanoma; however, variegation is common in persons with multiple benign bands.

3. Theoretically, wide bands suggest melanoma; however, the critical width that signifies melanoma has yet to be established.

4. Bands that do not extend distally to the free edge of the nail are unlikely to represent melanoma because they do not take their origin from the nail matrix. However, they may represent metastatic melanoma or LPB arising from the nail bed.

The management of African-American patients with pigmented bands can be difficult. Although multiple nails demonstrate LPB, there may be substantial variability in the color and width of bands within a single nail plate and among different nails in the same patient. Whether LPB in a thumb or great toe represents melanoma or racial variation is not necessarily easily determined by history and inspection alone. *Change in the morphology of*

LPB is the most important clue to the possibility of melanoma in these patients.

Multiple bands are *usually* not neoplastic in origin, although multiple subungual melanomas have been observed. A drug history and complete system review to rule out relevant systemic disorders and a thorough examination of the skin and nails to rule out nail infection and associated cutaneous disorders will usually reveal the underlying cause of multiple LPB.[12]

A pseudo-Hutchinson's sign may be caused by drugs such as minocycline and by acquired immunodeficiency syndrome, Peutz-Jegher's syndrome, and frictional melanonychia (R. Baran, personal communication, December 4, 1993). A subungual hematoma from trauma may also cause this sign to occur.

Also in whites even multiple bands on multiple nails should be suspect, because a melanoma arose in one such case.[13]

If scraping the nail plate surface, local cleansing, or use of a solvent such as acetone removes the discoloration, a topical agent is suggested as the cause (Figs. 12–1 and 12–2).[1]

Table 12–6 lists several named nail entities with pigment changes. Much of this information may be found scattered throughout the other chapters in this book. It is helpful to have many of the causes compiled in one location for the purpose of differential diagnosis.

The term *leukonychia* has various meanings to different physicians. I evaluate a patient

Table 12–5. **ABNORMAL NAIL PIGMENTATION ATTRIBUTABLE TO SOME LOCAL AGENTS**

Cause	Discoloring Agent	Color	Site
Ammoniated mercury[106]	Mercury	Gray	Nail plate
Amphotericin B[23]	Amphotericin B	Yellow	Nail plate
Anthralin[41]	Anthralin	Variable brown	Nail plate surface
Arning's tincture[28]	Tincture	Brownish	Nail plate
Burnt sugar[52,107]	Burnt sugar	Variable brown	Nail plate surface
Chlorophyll derivations[2]	Same	Green	Plate
Chlorophyllin copper complex and sodium propionate (Prophyllin)	Sodium propionate	Variable green	Nail plate surface
Chloroxine[30]	?	Different colors	?
Chromium salts[32]	Chromium salts	Variable ocherous	Nail plate (?)
Chrysarobin[41]	Chrysarobin	Variable brown	Nail plate surface
Coffee (roasted)[52,107]	Coffee	Variable brown	Nail plate surface
Copper sulfate[a]	Copper sulfate	Greenish	Nail plate
Derifil (chlorophyllin copper complex)	Chlorophyll	Green	Nail plate
Dinitrochlorobenzene[11]	?	Yellow	Plate
Dinitroorthocresol[108]	Dinitroorthocresol	Variable yellow	Nail matrix
Dinubuton[32]	?	Variable yellow	?
Diquat[68,109]	?	Variable brown	?
Dirt	Dirt	Variable brown	Nail plate surface subungual
Dynap insecticide[b]	Insecticide	Yellow	Nail plate
Ebony workers[52]	Ebony	Dark yellow or blackish	Nail bed region
Eosin[11]	Same	Red	Plate
5-Fluorouracil[11]	?	Brown	Plate
Fluorescein[29]	Fluorescein	Yellow	Nail plate
Formaldehyde[106]	Formaldehyde	Variable brown	Nail plate surface
Fuchsin[11]	Same	Purple	Plate
Galvanizers (silver and cyanide)[107]	Silver and cyanide	Diffuse dark blue	?
Gentian violet	Gentian violet	Variable purple	Nail plate surface
Glutaraldehyde[110]	Glutaraldehyde	Golden brown	Nail plate
Hatter's chemicals[52]	?	Variable yellow	Nail plate surface
Henna[52]	?	Variable brown	?
Hydrofluoric acid[20]	Hydrofluoric acid	Yellow	Nail plate
Hydroquinone[7,c]	Hydroquinone	Orange-brown	Nail plate
Ink	Ink (variable)	Variable	Nail plate surface
Iodine	Same	Yellowish brown	Plate
Iodochlorohydroxyquin (Vioform)	Iodochlorhydroxyquin	Brownish	Nail plate
Iron (elemental)[111]	Iron	Orange-brown	Nail plate
Mahogany[112]	?	Brownish	Nail plate
Merbromin (Mercurochrome)	Same	Reddish-purple	Plate
Mercury	Same	Blackish	Plate
Mercury bichloride plus sun exposure[94]	Mercury bichloride	Gray-blue	Probable nail plate
Methylenedianiline[29a]	?	?	?
Methyl green[11]	Same	Green	Plate
Methylene blue[11]	Same	Blue	Plate
Nail enamel	?	Variable brown	Nail plate surface
Nicotine, tar	Nicotine, tar	Variable brown	Nail plate surface
Nitric acid[11]	Same	Yellow	Plate
Nitrocellulose reacting with resorcin and toluene sulfonamide[94]	?	Variable brown	Nail plate surface
Oxalic acid in radiators[106,107]	Oxalic acid	Variable blue	?
Paraquat[68,109]	?	Variable brown	?
Pecans	Pecans	Diffuse brown	Nail plate surface
Photographic developer[22,43,52]	Methol or p-methyl-aminophenol sulfate hydroquinone	Variable black	Nail plate

Table continued on following page

Table 12–5. **ABNORMAL NAIL PIGMENTATION ATTRIBUTABLE TO SOME LOCAL AGENTS** *Continued*

Cause	Discoloring Agent	Color	Site
Picric acid[43]	?	Variable brown	Nail plate surface (?)
Potassium permanganate[41]	Potassium permanganate	Variable brown or yellow	Nail plate surface
Pyrogallol[28]	Pyrogallol (?)	Brownish	Nail plate
Radiotherapy (local)[42]	Irradiation	Brown transverse or longitudinal pigmented bands	?
Resorcinol[22,41,43,95]	Resorcinol	Variable brown	Nail plate surface
Rivanol[28]	Rivanol (?)	Brownish	Nail plate
Rhus dermatitis[30]	?	Yellow	?
Shoe polish	Shoe polish	Variable	Nail plate surface
Silver nitrate	Silver	Variable black	Nail plate surface
Sodium hypochlorite[11]	Same	Whitish	Onycholysis
Sublimate[28]	Sublimate	Brownish	Nail plate
Tar	Same	Yellowish brown	Plate
Tartrazine[11]	Same	Yellow	Plate
Tetracycline (topical)[11]	Same	Yellowish	Plate
Thermal injury[a]	?	Yellow-brown	?
Triamcinolone (intradermal)[113]	Steroid	Hypopigmented	Periungual
Walnuts[52,107]	Walnuts	Variable brown	Nail plate surface
Wine (red)[107]	Wine components	Variable black	Nail plate surface

Fungi (partial listing)

Acrotherium niger[69]	Fungus	Variable brown	?
Alternaria tenuis[52]	?	Black lateral edges	?
Aspergillus flavus[52]	Fungus	Peripheral green or punctate white	Nail plate
Aspergillus terreus[11]	Same	Longitudinal pigmented brownish bands	Plate
Blastomycetes[32,52]	Fungus	Variable blue-green, black	?
Botryodiplodia theobromae[114]	Fungus	Variable brown	Nail plate
Candida albicans[115]	Fungus	Longitudinal white streaks	Nail plate
Candida species	Fungus (?)	Variable yellow	Nail plate
Cephalosporium[43]	Fungus	Punctate white	Superficial nail plate
Chaetomium perpulchrum[11]	Same	Longitudinal pigmented brownish bands	Plate
Cladosporium carrionii[11]	Same	Longitudinal pigmented brownish bands	Plate
Curvularia lunata[11]	Same	Longitudinal pigmented brownish bands	Plate
Favus (Trichophyton schoenleinii)[32]	Fungus	Variable grayish yellow	?
Fusarium oxysporum[32,116]	Fungus (?)	Variable black, whitish, or white	Superficial nail plate
Hendersonula toruloidea[117]	Fungus	Variable brown	"Nail tissue"
Homodendrum species[32]	?	Variable black	?
Microsporum persicolor[15]	Same	Longitudinal pigmented brownish bands	Plate
Scopulariopsis brevicaulis	?	Peripheral yellowish	?
Tinea imbricata[52]	Fungus	Variable ash gray	Nail plate
Numerous trichophytons (proximal subungual onychomycosis)[43]	Fungus	White areas proceeding distally from proximal nail fold	Nail plate
Pyrenochaeta unguius-hominis[11]	Same	Longitudinal pigmented brownish bands	Plate
Scytalidium dimidiatum[11]	Same	Longitudinal pigmented brownish bands	Plate
Trichophyton mentagrophytes[9]	?	Punctate white	Superficial nail plate
Trichophyton rubrum[118]	Fungus	Variable white	Nail plate
Trichophyton tonsurans[15]	Same	Longitudinal pigmented brownish bands	Plate
Wangiella dermatitidis[11]	Same	Longitudinal pigmented brownish bands	Plate

Table 12–5. **ABNORMAL NAIL PIGMENTATION ATTRIBUTABLE TO SOME LOCAL AGENTS** *Continued*

Cause	Discoloring Agent	Color	Site
Bacteria			
Concomitant with dermatophytes[32]	?	Variable brown, gray, green	?
Various other causes of paronychia[43]	Variable	Variable	Variable
Proteus mirabilis[32]	Bacteria (?)	Variable black	Nail plate
Pseudomonas[22]	Pyocyanin, fluorescein	Variable green	Nail plate
Nevi and Tumors			
Angioma	Vascular	Variable red	Vascular bed
Enchondroma	Tumor	Bluish	Subungual, nail bed[d]
Exostosis[11]	Same	Brown	Bed
Glomus tumor	Vascular	Localized red	Vascular bed
Mucous cyst[e]	?	Longitudinal brownish band	?
Nevi (junctional)[68,119,120]	Melanin	Punctate brown	Nail plate
Pigmented cutaneous horn[8]	Cutaneous horn	Pigmented	Matrix–nail bed
Subungual epidermal cysts[121]	?	Yellowish white	Nail bed
Subungual epidermoid inclusions[122]	Subungual epidermoid inclusions	Black	Nail bed
Subungual melanoma or Hutchinson's melanotic whitlow[21,22]	Melanin	Variable black	Nail plate, nail bed periungual
Physical Agents			
Hemorrhage	Blood components	Variable red-brown	Nail bed
Ionizing radiation[8]	?	Longitudinal red	Lunula–nail bed
Irradiation[22,123]	Melanin	Variable brown-black	Nail plate
Microwaves[30]	?	Whitish	Nail bed
Trauma	Variable	Variable	Variable
Vibrating power tools[30]	?	Yellow-white longitudinal bands	?
Yellow staining in molded plastic workers	4,4-methylenedianiline	Yellow	Nail plate

See further additions in Table 12–6 (longitudinal pigmented bands).
[a]R. Baran, personal communication, 1981.
[b]C.R. Daniel III, unpublished data, 1980.
[c]C.R. Daniel III, unpublished observation, 1981.
[d]D. Swinehart, personal communication, 1979.
[e]S. Salasche, personal communication, December 1982.
Data from Cutis.[1–4]

with leukonychia by asking myself the following questions.[14,15]

1. Is it congenital or acquired?
2. Is the color change caused by an aberration mainly of the nail plate (parakeratosis) or elsewhere?
3. Is it endogenously induced or idiopathic (more often multiple nails) or caused by exogenous or nonsystemic factors (more often fewer nails)?
4. What is the pattern (partial, total, striate, punctate, location, number of nails, and so forth)?

Various modifiers of the term leukonychia may be added as a result of the answers to these questions and may help the clinician describe leukonychia, so that more readers may know exactly the disease process.

As one may conclude from perusing the tables, among the causes of acquired leukonychia are trauma, drugs and ingestants, systemic disease, and other disorders. The majority of the cases of acquired partial leukonychia seem to result from trauma to the matrix. Thus, dyskeratinization often resulting in parakeratotic foci imparts a whitish color to the nail plate. The nail unit may appear white with a normal nail plate because of vascular changes, among other causes. In some cases of traumatic leukonychia, airspaces may be found instead of dyskeratosis.[16]

In various cases, a pigmentary abnormality was arbitrarily placed in one category rather

Text continued on page 214

Table 12–6. **ABNORMAL NAIL PIGMENTATION ATTRIBUTABLE TO SOME NAMED NAIL ENTITIES**

Entity	Cause or Association	Discoloring Agent	Color	Site
Arcs (brown)[32,46]	Chronic renal failure	Melanin	Distal brown arc	Nail plate
Bissell's lines[17,124]	Adrenal insufficiency	Melanin	Longitudinal brown lines	Nail plate
Crescents[46,47,125]	Systemic illness	Probable vascular alteration	Distal red band	Vascular bed
Great toenail dystrophy[23]	Inherited	?	Dark colored	?
Expedition nails[23]	Possible protein deficiency	?	Transverse white bands	Nail plate (?)
Half-and-half nails[45,46,48,49,69]	Chronic renal failure— stimulation of matrix melanocytes	Melanin	Proximal white or proximal normal brown distal nail	Nail plate
Idiopathic azure nails[26]	?	?	Diffuse azure	?
Laugier's essential melanotic pigmentation[32,64a]	?	Melanin	Diffuse brownish or patterned	Nail plate
Leukonychia (white discoloration)	Acrokeratosis verruciformis,[126] acute rejection of renal allograft[127] alkaline metabolic disease,[18] alopecia antimony,[127] areata,[42] anemia, cachectic state,[18] carbon monoxide,[128] carcinoid syndrome,[127] cirrhosis,[27] congenital leukonychia,[68] cortisone,[127] cryoglobulinemia,[128] Darier's disease,[62,68] diquat,[18] dyshidrosis,[42] emetine chlorhydrate,[18] endemic,[127] erythema multiforme,[11] exfoliative dermatitis,[8] fluorosis,[8] formaldehyde (nail hardener),[129,130] fungi,[9,43] gout,[11] half-and-half nail,[46,47] herpes zoster,[11] Hodgkin's disease,[35] hypoalbuminemia,[35] hypocalcemia,[18] Kawasaki syndrome,[127] kidney transplantation,[127] lead poisoning,[52,127] LEOPARD syndrome,[42,127] leprosy,[127] leukonychia striata semilunaris,[52] malaria,[8] manic-depressive illness,[18] Mees' lines,[37,131] Muehrcke's lines[35,132] (see previous tables), pachyonychia congenita (autosomal recessive),[127] paraquat,[18] pellagra,[18] pilitorti,[49a] pilocarpine,[127] pneumonia,[8] rickettsial infection,[127] sickle cell anemia,[8] some diseases with fever,[18] sulfonamides,[18] sympathetic symmetric punctate leukonychia[133] (syndrome of leuko᠎hia, knuckle			

Table 12–6. **ABNORMAL NAIL PIGMENTATION ATTRIBUTABLE TO SOME NAMED NAIL ENTITIES**
Continued

Entity	Cause or Association	Discoloring Agent	Color	Site
	pads, deafness),[67] syphilis,[11] tuberculosis,[11] trauma,[68,134] trichinosis,[18] ulcerative colitis,[18] zinc deficiency (see other tables as well as Chapter 13)			
Leukonychia (longitudinal)	Erythema multiforme,[30] gout,[30] herpes zoster,[30] leuko-onycholysis paradentotica,[30] microwaves,[110] nevoid matrix changes,[28] Darier's disease			
Longitudinal brownish pigmented bands	Acrodermatitis enteropathica,[135] *Acrotherium niger,*[69] adrenal insufficiency,[17] doxorubicin (Adriamycin),[12,88,136] acquired immunodeficiency syndrome,[137] *Alternaria tenuis,*[138] antimalarials,[23,135] arsenic poisoning,[18] *Blastomycetes,*[12] bleomycin,[7] *Botryodiplodia theobromae,*[135] Bowen's[16a] disease,[139] busulfan,[135] bullous primary amyloidosis,[42] *Candida,*[71] carpal tunnel syndrome,[25] cyclophosphamide,[136] daunorubicin,[135] diquat,[12] exostosis,[135] fluorosis,[40] foreign body,[12] *Fusarium,*[12] gangrene,[135] gold therapy,[18] hematoma,[12] hemosiderosis,[12] *Hendersonula toruloidea,*[12] *Homodendrum elatum,*[12] hydroxyurea,[140] hyperbilirubinemia,[137] hyptherthyroidism,[137] hypopituitarism,[135] idiopathic,[118,124,141] ketoconazole,[30] Laugier-Hunziker syndrome, lichen planus,[32] local radiotherapy,[42] gemfibrozil (Lopid),[142] malnutrition,[54] melphalan,[7] mepacrine,[12,135] mercury,[135] methotrexate,[135] minocycline,[143] mucous cyst,[a] nevi,[69] nitrogen mustard,[12] nitrosourea,[12] ochronosis,[135] onychophagia,[144] osteomyelitis,[135] Peutz-Jegher's syndrome,[71,72] phenolphthalein, phenol, regressing nevoid melanosis in childhood,[170] phthalein poisoning,[18] phenothiazine,[135] phenytoin, pinta,[12]	Variable		

Table continued on following page

Table 12–6. **ABNORMAL NAIL PIGMENTATION ATTRIBUTABLE TO SOME NAMED NAIL ENTITIES**
Continued

Entity	Cause or Association	Discoloring Agent	Color	Site
	porphyria,[145] post-inflammatory hyperpigmentation,[12] pregnancy,[30] *Proteus mirabilis*,[12] prurigo vulgaris,[18] psoralen,[12] subungual epidermal inclusions,[146] subungual fibrous histiocytoma,[12] sulfonamide,[12] syphilis (secondary),[30,135] tetracycline,[12] thermal injury,[135] 3'azidodeoxythymidine,[147] timolol,[12] trauma,[115,148] *Trichophyton soudanese*,[12] verucca vulgaris,[135] vitamin B_{12} deficiency,[94a] Bowen's disease of nail unit,[60,108] basal cell carcinoma,[111a, 149] melanoma,[6] azidothymidine,[83] ibuprofen[85] (see Chapter 13)			
Mees' lines[37]	Arsenic, cardiac insufficiency, Hodgkin's disease, leprosy, malaria, myocardial infarction, pellagra, pneumonia, psoriasis, renal failure, sickle cell anemia, thallium, other serious systemic diseases (see Chapter 13)	Variable	Single or multiple white transverse	Nail bed
Muehrcke's lines	Hypoalbuminemia	Alteration of nail bed–plate attachment (?)	Usually double white transverse	Vascular bed vs. nail bed plate attachment
Senile nails[18,41]	Age, solar, refractile (?)	?	No lunula and/or brown or opaque	Matrix or nail plate
Splinter hemorrhages	Bacterial endocarditis,[93,134] Darier's disease,[62] dialysis,[150,151] drug reaction,[93] methoxsalen,[152] fungi,[68] general illness,[150,153] mycosis fungoides,[28] Osler-Weber-Rendu disease,[18] peptic ulcer,[68] psoriasis,[93] radiodermatitis,[128] rheumatoid arthritis,[68] scurvy,[93] 10 to 20% of normal population,[70,153] tetracycline,[96] thyrotoxicosis,[93,153,154] trauma,[150,154] trichinosis,[68,93,153] vasculitis[93]			
Terry's nails[27]	Cirrhosis	Probable vascular alteration	Prominent onychodermal band, white proximal nails	Vascular bed
Yellow nail syndrome	Bronchiectasis,[155] carcinoma larynx,[155] chronic bronchitis,[155] chronic lymphedema,[155] rheumatoid arthritis,[156] sinusitis,[155] thyroid disease[155] (see Chapter 13)			

Table 12–6. **ABNORMAL NAIL PIGMENTATION ATTRIBUTABLE TO SOME NAMED NAIL ENTITIES**
Continued

Entity	Cause or Association	Discoloring Agent	Color	Site
	Miscellaneous Changes of Lunula (see also other tables)			
All pigmented individuals[18]	?	Smaller linula	Lunula change	Lunula
Blue lunulae	Argyria,[94] hereditary acrolabial telangiectasia,[30] paronychia (bacterial, probably *Pseudomonas*),[94] quinacrine,[94] topical bichloride or mercury followed by sunlight (see Wilson's disease, Table 12–1), zidovudine			
Diffusion of lunula	Ischemia[157]	?	Whitish	Lunula
Diminished or absent abnormal lunula	Acromegaly,[18] adiposogenital syndrome,[18] atherosclerosis,[171] chronic obstructive pulmonary disease,[171] chronic polyarthritis,[18] brachyonychia,[171] congenital onychodysplasia of the index fingers (ISO and Kikuchi syndrome),[160] erythropoietic protoporphyria,[171] hereditary osteoungual dysplasia,[18] hyperthyroidism,[171] hypothyroidism,[171] hypopituitarism,[18] Goltz's syndrome,[42] malnutrition,[171] lymphedema,[171] iron deficiency anemia,[171] leprosy,[18] multiple myeloma,[158] HIV,[171] pachyonychia congenita,[171] penicillamine,[91] renal failure,[171] rheumatoid arthritis,[171] porphyria cutanea tarda,[171] porphyria,[42] nail patella syndrome,[171] nerve injury,[171] soft nail disease,[171] monosomy 4p,[42] scleroderma,[159] trisomy 21[171]			
Indians (India)[18]	?	Extended lunula	Lunula	Lunula
Large lunulas	Habit tic,[42] hydrocortisone on cuticle,[161] median nail dystrophy[23]	?	Large lunulas	Lunula
Multiple myeloma[43]	?	No lunula	Lunula change	Lunula
Pseudo-Hutchinson's sign[170]	Ethnic pigmentation,[170] Laugier-Hunziker syndrome,[170] Peutz-Jeghers syndrome,[170] radiation therapy,[170] malnutrition,[170] menopause,[170] patients with AIDS,[170] trauma induced,[170] congenital vevus,[170] after biopsy of longitudinal melanonychia,[170] regressing nevoid melanosis in childhood,[170] subungual hematoma,[170]			
Punctate red spots	Alopecia areata,[28,162] psoriasis[b]	?		Lunula

Table continued on following page

Table 12–6. **ABNORMAL NAIL PIGMENTATION ATTRIBUTABLE TO SOME NAMED NAIL ENTITIES**
Continued

Entity	Cause or Association	Discoloring Agent	Color	Site
Miscellaneous Changes of Lunula (see also other tables)				
Reddish lunula (see Table 12–1 for the following: cardiac failure, cirrhosis, lymphogranuloma venereum, reticulosarcoma, rheumatoid arthritis [iliac]),[116] systemic lupus erythematosus, possibly chronic obstructive pulmonary disease,[163] carbon monoxide				
Dark red lunulae [42]	Sometimes seen in 20-nail dystrophy	?	Reddish lunula change	Lunula
Alopecia areata[164,165]	?	?	Reddish lunula	Lunula
Psoriasis[c]	?	? Serum glycoprotein	Reddish lunula often spotted	Lunula
Dermatomyositis[116]	?	?	Reddish lunula	Lunula
Soft nail disease[74]	?	No lunula	Lunula change	Lunula
Triangular lunulae[9,166]	Nail patella syndrome trauma,[171] trisomy 21,[171] idiopathic	Matrix damage (?)	Triangular white lunula	Lunula
Yellow lunulae[20] Trisomy 21[167]	Tetracycline	Tetracycline	Yellow	Lunula

[a]S. Salasche, personal communication, December 1982.
[b]C.R. Daniel III, unpublished observation, 1982.
[c]C.R. Daniel III, unpublished data, 1980.
Data from Cutis.[1–4]

than in multiple listings to refrain from repeating identical information.[1] Furthermore, some material may have been listed several times to ensure that readers can locate their objective in a short period of time without having to use too many cross-references. In some situations, personal experience was noted without the use of a reference.[1,4] In numerous instances in

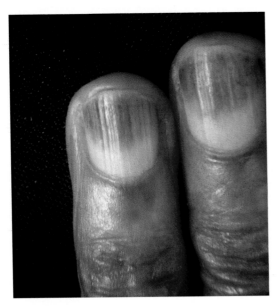

Figure 12–1. Hydroquinone pigmentation from a "fade" cream.

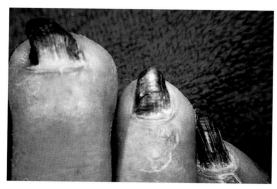

Figure 12–2. Potassium permanganate soaks.

the tables, an exact entry could not be assigned. The uncertainties are indicated by a question mark.[1,4] Nail pigmentation is an important facet of onychopathology and is worthy of further study.

References

1. Daniel CR III, Osment LS: Nail pigmentation abnormalities: Their importance and proper examination. Cutis 25:595, 1980.
2. Daniel CR III, Osment LS: Nail pigmentation abnormalities: Their importance and proper examination. Cutis 30:348, 1982.
3. Daniel CR III: Nail pigmentation abnormalities, updated entries. Cutis 30:627, 1982.
4. Daniel CR III: Nail pigmentation abnormalities, an addendum. Cutis 30:364, 1982.
5. Daniel CR III: Nail pigmentation abnormalities. Dermatol Clin 3:431, 1985.
6. Daniel CR III, Zaias N: Pigmentation abnormalities of the nails with emphasis on systemic diseases. Dermatol Clin 6:305, 1988. 313.
7. Norton LA: Nail disorders. J Am Acad Dermatol 6:451, 1980.
8. Zaias N: The Nail in Health and Disease. SP Medical Books, New York, 1980.
9. Zaias N: Disease of the nails. In Demis J, Dobson RL, Crounse RG (eds): Clinical Dermatology. Harper & Row, New York, 1974.
10. Scher RK: Cosmetics and ancillary preparations for the care of nails. J Am Acad Dermatol 6:523, 1980.
11. Baran R, Dawber RPR: Physical signs. In Diseases of the Nails and Their Management, ed 2. Blackwell Scientific, Oxford, England, 1994, pp. 35–80.
12. Baran R, Kechijian P: Longitudinal melanonychia (melanonychia striata): Diagnosis and management. J Am Acad Dermatol 21:1165, 1989.
13. Beltrani VP, Scher RK: Evaluation and management of melanonychia striata in a patient receiving phototherapy. Arch Dermatol 127:319, 1991.
14. Daniel CR III: Leukonychia (letter). J Am Acad Dermatol 13:158, 1985.
15. Zaias N: The Nail in Health and Disease, ed 2. Appleton & Lange, Norwalk, CT, 1990, p. 93.
16. Hudson JA, Cockrell CJ: Traumatic leukonychia striata: An electron microscopic and morphologic study.

Poster presented at the annual meeting of the American Academy of Dermatology, Dallas, TX, December 1991.
16a. Baran R, Simon CI: Longitudinal melanonychia: A symptom of Bowen's disease. J Am Acad Dermatol 18:1359, 1988.
17. Bissell GW, Surakomol K, Greenslit F: Longitudinal banded pigmentation of nails in primary adrenal insufficiency. JAMA 215:1666, 1971.
18. DeNicola P, Morsiana M, Zavagli G: Nail Diseases in Internal Medicine. Charles C Thomas, Springfield, IL, 1974.
19. Baker SJ, Ignatius M, Johnson S, et al: Hyper-pigmentation of skin. BMJ 1:1713, 1963.
20. Localized hyperpigmentation: Signs and symptoms of the skin. In Roche Handbook of Differential Diagnosis. Roche Laboratories, New York, 1976, p. 9.
21. Nail discoloration: Signs and symptoms of the skin. In Roche Handbook of Differential Diagnosis. Roche Laboratories, New York, 1978, pp. 3, 7, 9.
22. Zaias N, Boden HP: Disorders of nails. In Fitzpatrick TB, Arndt KA, Clark WH Jr, et al (eds): Dermatology in General Medicine. McGraw-Hill, New York, 1971.
23. Samman PD: The Nails in Disease, ed 3. William Heinemann, Chicago, 1978.
24. Krutchik AN, Toshima CK, Buzdar AU, et al: Longitudinal nail banding associated with breast carcinoma unrelated to chemotherapy. Arch Intern Med 138:1302, 1978.
25. Aratari E, Regesta G, Rebora A: Carpal tunnel syndrome appearing with prominent skin symptoms. Arch Dermatol 120:517, 1984.
26. Baran R, Gioanni T, Holla D: Nail dyschromias. Cutis 9:307, 1972.
27. Terry RB: The onychodermal band in health and disease. Lancet 1179, 1955.
28. Runne U, Orfanos CE: The human nail. Curr Probl Dermatol 9:102, 1981.
29. Hendricks AA: Yellow lunulae with fluorescence after tetracycline therapy. Arch Dermatol 116:438, 1980.
29a. Cohen SR: Yellow staining caused by 4, 4'-methylenedianiline exposure. Arch Dermatol 121:1022, 1985.
30. Baran R, Dawber RPR: Diseases of the Nails and Their Management. Blackwell Scientific, Oxford, England, 1984.
31. Klock JC: Nails may reveal first sign of many internal disorders. Dermatol Pract 9:1, 1976.
32. Baran R: Pigmentations of the nails (chromonychia). J Dermatol Surg Oncol 4:250, 1978.
33. Caravata CM, Richardson DR, Wood BT, et al: Cutaneous manifestations of hyperthyroidism. South Med J 62:1127, 1969.
34. Thomas HM Jr: Pigment in the nails during hyperthyroidism. Bull Johns Hopkins Hosp 52:315, 1933.
35. Muehrcke RC: The fingernails in chronic hypoalbuminemia. BMJ 1:1327, 1956.
36. Samman PD, Strickland B: Abnormalities of the fingernails associated with impaired peripheral blood supply. Br J Dermatol 74:165, 1962.
37. Hudson JB, Dennis AJ Jr: Transverse white lines in the fingernails after acute and chronic renal failure. Arch Intern Med 117:276, 1966.
38. Zaias N: The nail in lichen planus. Arch Dermatol 101:264, 1970.
39. Kint A, Herpe LV: Ungual anomalies in lupus erythematosus discoides. Dermatologica 153:298, 1976.

40. Bisht DB, Singh SS: Pigmented bands on nails: A new sign in malnutrition. Lancet 1:507, 1962.

41. Samman PD: The nails. *In* Rook AH, Wilkinson DS, Ebling FJG (eds): Textbook of Dermatology, ed 2. Blackwell Scientific, London, 1968.

42. Baran R: The nail. *In* Pierre M (ed): The Nail. Churchill Livingstone, Edinburgh, 1981.

43. Moschella SL, Pillsbury DM, Hurley HJ (eds): Dermatology. WB Saunders, Philadelphia, 1975.

44. Fryer JM, Werth VP: Pregnancy-associated hyperpigmentation: Longitudinal melanonychia. J Am Acad Dermatol 26:493, 1992.

45. Baran MF, Gioanni T: Half and half nail. Fitiale L'ouest Sud-Ouest-Séance 16:399, 1968.

46. Daniel CR III, Bower JD, Daniel CR Jr: The half-and-half fingernail: A clue to chronic renal failure. Proc Clin Dial Transplant Forum 5:1, 1975.

47. Daniel CR III, Bower JD, Daniel CR Jr: The half-and-half fingernail: The most significant onychopathological indicator of chronic renal failure. J Miss State Med Assoc 16:376, 1975.

48. Leyden JJ, Wood MG: The half-and-half nail. Arch Dermatol 105:591, 1972.

49. Lindsay PG: The half-and-half nail. Arch Intern Med 119:583, 1967.

49a. Giustina TA, Woo TX, Campbell JP, Ellis CN: Association of pili torti and leukonychia. Cutis 35:533, 1985.

50. Barrow MV: The nails in multicentric reticulohistiocytosis. Arch Dermatol 95:200, 1967.

51. Baran R: Nail changes in general pathology. *In* Pierre M (ed): The Nail. Churchill Livingstone, Edinburgh, 1981, pp 5–101.

52. Castello V, Pardo OA: Diseases of the Nails, ed 3. Charles C Thomas, Springfield, IL, 1960.

53. Marks R, Ellis HP: Yellow nails. Arch Dermatol 120:619, 1970.

54. Petrozzi JW, Shore RN: Keratosis lichenoides chronica, possible variant of lichen planus. Arch Dermatol 112:709, 1976.

55. Zaias N: Psoriasis of the nail. Arch Dermatol 99:567, 1969.

56. Orentreich N, Harber LC, Tromovitch TA: Photosensitivity and photo-onycholysis due to demethylchlortetracycline. Arch Dermatol 83:730, 1961.

57. Carmel R: Hair and fingernail changes in acquired and congenital pernicious anemia. Arch Intern Med 145:484, 1985.

58. Chernovsky ME, Finley VK: Yellow nail syndrome in patients with acquired immunodeficiency disease. J Am Acad Dermatol 13:731, 1985.

59. Daniel CR III: Yellow nail syndrome and acquired immunodeficiency disease. J Am Acad Dermatol 14:844, 1986.

60. Norton L: Nail disorders. Lecture presented at the annual meeting of the American Academy of Dermatology, Las Vegas, December 11, 1985.

61. Ronchyese F: The nail in Darier's disease. Arch Dermatol 91:617, 1965.

62. Zaias N, Ackerman AB: The nail in Darier-White disease. Arch Dermatol 107:193, 1973.

63. Redeker AC, Levan NE, Beake M: Erythropoietic protoporphyria with eczema solare. Arch Dermatol 86:569, 1962.

64. Sulis E, Floris C: Nail pigmentation following cancer chemotherapy: A new genetic entity? Eur J Cancer 15:1517, 1980.

64a. Koch SE, LeBoit PE, Odon RB: Laugier-Hunziker syndrome. J Am Acad Dermatol 16:431, 1987.

65. Cram DL, Resneck JS, Jackson G: A congenital ichthyosiform syndrome with deafness and keratitis. Arch Dermatol 115:467, 1979.

66. Sulzburger MB: Incontinentia pigmenti. Arch Dermatol 38:65, 1938.

67. Bart RS, Pumphrey RE: Knuckle pads, leukonychia and deafness: A dominantly inherited syndrome. N Engl J Med 276:202, 1967.

68. Samman PD: The Nails in Disease, ed 2. Charles C Thomas, Springfield, IL, 1972.

68a. Lazar P: Reactions to nail hardeners. Arch Dermatol 94:446, 1973.

69. Caron GA: Familial congenital pigmented nevi of the nails. Lancet 1:508, 1962.

70. Degowin EL, Degowin RL: Bedside Diagnostic Examination, ed 20. Macmillan, New York, 1969.

71. Achord JL, Proctor HD: Malignant degeneration and metastasis in Peutz-Jeghers syndrome. Arch Intern Med 111:498, 1963.

72. Valero A, Sherf K: Pigmented nails in Peutz-Jeghers syndrome. Am J Gastroenterol 43:56, 1965.

73. Johnson RB, Goldsmith IA: Dilantin digital defects. Am Acad Dermatol 5:191, 1981.

74. Prandi G, Caccialanza M: An unusual congenital nail dystrophy (soft nail disease). Clin Exp Dermatol 2:265, 1977.

75. Millns JL, Dicken HC: Hereditary acrolabial telangiectasia. Arch Dermatol 115:474, 1979.

76. Braverman IM: Skin Signs of Systemic Disease. WB Saunders, Philadelphia, 1970.

77. Price VH, Odon, RB, Ward WH, et al: Trichothiodystrophy. Arch Dermatol 116:1375, 1980.

78. Bearn AG, McKusick VA: Azure lunulae. JAMA 166:904, 1958.

79. Nixon DW, Pirozzi D, York RM, Black M, Lawson DH, et al: Dermatologic changes after systemic cancer therapy. Cutis 27:181, 1981.

80. Modny C, Barondess JA: Nail pigmentation secondary to quinacrine. Cutis 11:789, 1973.

81. Madorsky DD: Arsenic in dermatology. J Assoc Milit Dermatol 3:19, 1977.

82. Furth PA, Lazakis AM: Nail pigmentation changes associated with azidothymidine (zidovudine). Ann Intern Med 107:350, 1987.

83. Fisher CA, McPoland PR: Azidothymidine-induced nail pigmentation. Cutis 43:552, 1989.

84. Naik RPC, Gurmohan S: Nail pigmentation due to oral 8-methoxypsoralen. Br J Dermatol 100:229, 1979.

85. Scher R: The Nail. Lecture presented at Columbia University Nail and Hair Symposium, September, 1989.

86. Zhu WY, Xia MY, Huang SD, Du D: Hyperpigmentation of the nail from lead deposition. Int J Dermatol 28:273, 1989.

87. Hooper JF: Lithium carbonate and toenails. Am J Psychiatry 138:1519, 1981.

88. Granstein RD, Sober JA: Drug- and heavy-metal-induced hyperpigmentation. J Am Acad Dermatol 5:1, 1981.

89. Morgan DB: Blue nails from minocycline. Schoch Letter 29:2, 1979.

90. Krebs A: Drug-induced nail disorders. Praxis 70:1951, 1981.

91. Bjellerup M: Nail changes induced by penicillamine. Acta Derm Venereol (Stockh) 69:339, 1989.

92. Ross JB: Side effect of phenindione. BMJ 1:886, 1963.

93. Seckler SG: A handful of pearls. Hosp Physician 12:4, 1976.

94. Koplon BS: Azure lunulae due to argyria. Arch Dermatol 94:333, 1966.

94a. Noppakum N, Swasdikul D: Reversible hyperpigmentation of skin and nails with white hair due to vitamin B$_{12}$ deficiency. Arch Dermatol 122:896, 1986.

95. Loveman AB, Fliegelman MT: Discoloration of the nails. Arch Dermatol 72:153, 1955.

96. Sanders CV, Saenz RE, Lopez M: Splinter hemorrhages and onycholysis: Unusual reactions associated with tetracycline hydrochloride therapy. South Med J 69:1090, 1976.

97. Fieler-Ofry V, Godel V, Lagan M: Nail pigmentation following timolol maleate therapy. Ophthalmologica 182:153, 1981.

98. Feder W, Auerbach R: "Purple toes": An uncommon sequela of oral coumarin drug therapy. Ann Intern Med 55:911, 1961.

99. Lebsack CS, Weibert RT: "Purple toes" syndrome. Postgrad Med 71:81, 1982.

100. Shah PC, Rao KRP, Patel AR: Cyclophosphamide-induced nail pigmentation. Br J Dermatol 98:675, 1978.

101. Shetty MR: Case of pigmented banding of the nail caused by bleomycin. Cancer Treat Rep 61:501, 1977.

102. Morris D, Aisner J: Horizontal pigmented banding of the nails in association with Adriamycin Chemotherapy. Cancer Treat Rep 61:499, 1977.

103. Kennedy BJ, Smith LR, Goltz RW: Skin changes secondary to hydroxyurea therapy. Arch Dermatol 111:183, 1975.

104. Nixon DW: Alterations in nail pigment with cancer chemotherapy. Arch Intern Med 36:1117, 1976.

105. Pratt CV, Shanks EC: Hyperpigmentation of the nails from doxorubicin (letter). JAMA 228:460, 1974.

106. Fisher AA: Contact Dermatitis, ed 3. Lea and Febiger, Philadelphia, 1973.

107. Schwartz L, Tulipan L, Birmigham DJ: Occupational Diseases of the Skin, ed 3. Lea & Febiger, Philadelphia, 1957.

108. Baran R: Nail damage caused by weed killers and insecticides (letter). Arch Dermatol 110:467, 1974.

109. Samman PD, Johnston EN: Nail damage associated with handling of paraquat and diquat. BMJ 1:818, 1969.

110. Suringa DW: Treatment of superficial onychomycosis with topically applied glutaraldehyde. Arch Dermatol 102:153, 1970.

111. Olsen TG, Jatlav P: Contact exposure to elemental iron causing chromonychia. Arch Dermatol 120:102, 1984.

111a. Rudophy RI: Subungual basal cell carcinoma presenting as longitudinal melanonychia. J Am Acad Dermatol 16:229, 1987.

112. Harris AO, Rosen T: Nail discoloration due to mahogany. Cutis 43:55, 1989.

113. Bedi TR: Intradermal triamcinolone treatment of psoriatic onychodystrophy. Dermatologica 155:24, 1977.

114. Restrepo A, Arango M, Vedlez H, et al: The isolation of *Botryodiplodia theobromae* from a nail lesion. Sabouraudia 14:1, 1976.

115. Zaias N: Onychomycosis. Arch Dermatol 105:263, 1972.

116. Jorizzo JL, Gonzalez EB, Daniels JC: Red lunulae in a patient with rheumatoid arthritis. J Am Acad Dermatol 8:711, 1983.

117. Campbell CK, Kurwa A, Abdel-Aziz AHM, et al: Fungal infection of the skin and nails by *Hendersonula toruloides*. Br J Dermatol 89:45, 1973.

118. Reiss F: Leukonychia trichophytica caused by *Trichophyton rubrum*. Cutis 20:223, 1977.

119. Higashi N: Melanocytes and nail matrix and nail pigmentation. Arch Dermatol 97:570, 1968.

120. Higashi N, Saito T: Horizontal distribution of the dopa-positive melanocytes in the nail matrix. J Invest Dermatol 53:163, 1969.

121. Yung CW, Estes SA: Subungual epidermal cyst. J Am Acad Dermatol 3:599, 1980.

122. Lewin K: Subungual epidermoid inclusions. Br J Dermatol 81:671, 1969.

123. Shelley WB, Rawnsley HM, Pillsbury DM: Postirradiation melanonychia. Arch Dermatol 90:174, 1964.

124. Ronchese F, Kern AB: Longitudinal pigmentation of the nails (letter). JAMA 216:1352, 1971.

125. Daniel CR III, Sams WM, Scher RK: Nails in systemic disease. Dermatol Clin 3:465, 1985.

126. Rook A: Textbook of Dermatology, ed 3. Blackwell Scientific, Oxford, England, 1979.

127. Grossman M, Scher RK: Leukonychia, review and classification. Int J Dermatol 29:535, 1990.

127a. Stewart WK, Raffle EJ: Brown nail-bed arcs and chronic renal disease. BMJ 1:784, 1972.

128. Fitzpatrick TB: Dermatology in General Medicine, ed 2. McGraw-Hill, New York, 1979.

129. Jawny L, Spada F: Contact dermatitis to a new nail hardener. Arch Dermatol 5:191, 1981.

130. March CH: Allergic contact dermatitis to a new formula to strengthen nails. Arch Dermatol 93:720, 1966.

131. Held JL, Chew S, Grossman ME, Kohn SR: Transverse striate leukonychia associated with acute rejection of renal allograft. J Am Acad Dermatol 20:513, 1989.

132. Feldman SR, Gammon WR: Unilateral Muehrcke's lines following trauma. Arch Dermatol 125:133, 1989.

133. Arnold HL: Sympathetic symmetric punctate leukonychia. Arch Dermatol 115:495, 1979.

133a. Terry R: Red half-moons in cardiac failure. Lancet 2:842, 1954.

134. Leyden JJ: Chromonychia. Cutis 10:161, 1972.

135. Pappert AS, Scher RK, Cohen JL: Longitudinal pigmented nail bands. Dermatol Clin 9:703, 1991.

136. Markenson AL, Chandra M, Miller DR: Hyperpigmentation after cancer chemotherapy. Lancet 2:128, 1975.

137. Fisher BK, Warner LC: Cutaneous manifestations by the AIDS: Update 1987. Int J Dermatol 26:615, 1987.

138. Haneke E: Fungal infections of the nail. Semin Dermatol 10:41–53, 1991.

139. Saijos KT: Pigmented nail streaks associated with Bowen's disease of the nail matrix. Dermatologica 181:156, 1990.

140. VomVouras S, Pakula AS, Shaw JM: Multiple pigmented bands during hydroxyurea therapy: An uncommon finding. J Am Acad Dermatol 24:1016, 1991.

141. Leyden JJ, Spott DA, Goldschmidt H: Diffuse and banded melanin pigmentation in nails. Arch Dermatol 105:548, 1972.

142. Klein ME: Linear lateral black nail discoloration after months on Lopid. Schoch Letter 40:29, 1990.

143. Litt JZ: A dark streak in the nail. Diagnosis 4:23, 1982.

144. Baran R: Nail biting and picking as a possible cause of longitudinal melanonychia: A study of 6 cases. Dermatologica 181:126, 1990.

145. Canizares O: Chronic porphyria. Arch Dermatol Syphilol 63:269, 1951.

146. Lewin K: Subungual epidermal inclusions simulating melanoma. Br J Dermatol 81:671, 1969.

147. Tosti A, Gaddoni G, Fanti PA, et al: Longitudinal melanonychia induced by 3'azidodeoxythymidine. Dermatologica 180:217, 1990.

147a. Scheithauer W, Ludwig H, Kotz R, Depisch D: Mitoxantrone-induced discoloration of the nails. Eur J Cancer Clin Oncol 25:763, 1989.

148. Baran R: Frictional longitudinal melanonychia: A new entity. Dermatologica 174:280, 1987.

149. Baran R: Frictional longitudinal melanonychia: A new entity. Dermatologica 174:280, 1987.

150. Blum M, Avinam AL: Splinter hemorrhages in patients receiving regular hemodialysis. JAMA 1239:44, 1978.

151. Kilpatrick ZM, Greenberg PA, Sanford JP: Splinter hemorrhages—Their clinical significance. Arch Intern Med 115:730, 1965.

152. Zala L: Photo-onycholysis induced by 8-methoxypsoralen. Dermatologica 154:203, 1977.

153. Gross NJ, Tall R: Clinical significance of splinter hemorrhages. BMJ 12:1496, 1963.

154. Robertson JC, Braune ML: Splinter hemorrhages, pitting, and other findings in fingernails of healthy adults. BMJ 4:279, 1974.

155. Guin JD, Elleman JH: Yellow-nail syndrome: Possible association with malignancy. Arch Dermatol 115:734, 1979.

156. Mattingly PC, Bossingham DH: Yellow-nail syndrome in rheumatoid arthritis: Report of three cases. Ann Rheum Dis 38:475, 1979.

157. Edwards EA: Nail changes in functional and organic arterial disease. N Engl J Med 239:362, 1948.

158. Fromer JL: Multiple myeloma. In Moschella SL, Pillsbury DM, Hurley HJ (eds): Dermatology. WB Saunders, Philadelphia, 1975, pp 1420–1422.

159. Patterson JW: Pterygium-inversum-unguis-like changes in scleroderma. Arch Dermatol 113:1429, 1977.

160. Baran R, Stroud JD: Congenital onychodysplasia of the index fingers. Arch Dermatol 120:243, 1984.

161. Baran R: Nails. Lecture presented at the meeting of the American Academy of Dermatology, San Francisco, December, 1981.

162. Ringrose EJ: Alopecia symptomatica with nail base changes (society transactions). Arch Dermatol 76:263, 1957.

163. Wilkerson MG, Wilkin JK: Red lunulae revisited: A clinical and histopathologic examination. J Am Acad Dermatol 20:453, 1989.

164. Misch KJ: Red nails associated with alopecia areata. Clin Exp Dermatol 6:561, 1981.

165. Rigrose EJ, Bahcall CR: Alopecia symptomatica with nail base changes. Arch Dermatol 76:263, 1957.

166. Daniel CR III, Osment LS, Noojin RO: Triangular lunulae. Arch Dermatol 116:448, 1980.

167. Beaver DW, Brooks SE: Color Atlas of the Nail in Clinical Diagnosis. Year Book, Chicago, 1984, p. 39.

168. McGeorge BCL: Lunula change induced by psoralen plus ultraviolet A radiation. Photodermatol Photoimmunol 9:15, 1992.

169. Kose O, Baloglu H: Knuckle pads, leukonychia, and deafness. Int J Dermatol 35:728, 1996.

170. Baran R, Kechijian P: Hutchinson's sign: A reappraisal. J Am Acad Dermatol 34:87, 1996.

171. Cohen PR: The lunula. J Am Acad Dermatol 34:943, 1996.

172. Hoffman MD, Fleming MG, Pearson PW: Acantholytic epidermolysis bullosa. Arch Dermatol 131:566-589, 1995.

CHAPTER 13

Nails in Systemic Disease

C. Ralph Daniel III, W. Mitchell Sams, Jr., and Richard K. Scher

Nail abnormalities secondary to systemic disease are important to dermatologists because they are readily examined and may be the initial signal that systemic disease is present. Some abnormal nail findings represent part of a symptom complex that may or may not be useful in physical diagnosis. The knowledge of the correct onychopathologic cause may give the patient the correct nail prognosis and may prevent institution of possible incorrect lengthy and costly treatment regimens. There are no hard and fast rules concerning nails in systemic disease, but several points are worthy of mention:

1. Always examine all 20 nails because multiple nails are usually involved.
2. In general, fingernails provide more subtle information than toenails because trauma is more likely to mask or change certain manifestations in toenails.
3. Examine the rest of the skin and mucous membranes for additional abnormalities, and perform a complete physical examination if indicated.
4. A detailed history is important, including close attention to the chronologic sequence of events.
5. Obtain appropriate laboratory tests as indicated by the history and physical examination.

6. Nail pigmentation changes associated with systemic disease often arise in the area of the matrix. In this case, the leading edge of the abnormal pigmentation is often shaped similarly to the distal matrix (lunula or half-moon).[1] If this color change is transmitted to the nail plate, it will grow out with that structure. By measuring the distance from the proximal nail fold (cuticle) to the leading edge of the pigmentation change and calculating from the rate of nail growth (0.1–0.15 mm per day), one can estimate the time at which the initial insult occurred.

In the balance of this chapter, reaction patterns often associated with systemic disease and a system-by-system approach are presented and varied subheadings are used. Several diseases have arbitrarily been placed in certain categories, although they certainly could just as correctly have been grouped elsewhere.

REACTION PATTERNS (LESS SPECIFIC NAIL SIGNS)

Splinter Hemorrhages and Subungual Purpura

Splinter hemorrhages are formed by the extravasation of blood from the longitudinally oriented vessels of the nail bed. The blood attaches itself to the underlying nail plate and moves distally. The splinter hemorrhages occasionally appear to remain stationary, probably because of attachment to the nail bed rather than to the plate.

Splinter hemorrhages can be caused by physical factors, including trauma, drugs, dermatologic diseases, systemic diseases, and idiopathic conditions, among others. Trauma is by far the most common cause of splinter hemorrhages.[2,3] At times, certain presentations of splinter hemorrhages should make one consider a systemic cause, particularly bacterial endocarditis.[295] Their simultaneous appearance in multiple nails is more frequently associated with systemic disease. Also their occurrence closer to the lunula as opposed to the distal nail plate seems to be more directly correlated with systemic disease.[2,3]

Other miscellaneous facts have been noted:

1. Splinter hemorrhages occur more frequently in black patients.[4]

2. In one study, the left hand was involved greater than three times more frequently than the right hand in patients with single hemorrhages; the left thumb was the digit most frequently involved.[4]

3. In patients with multiple hemorrhages, more occurred on the left hand than the right hand, but the thumb was the most frequently involved digit, followed by the left index finger and the left thumb.[4]

4. In one study, peritoneal dialysis was the single most frequently encountered factor in patients with splinter hemorrhages.[5]

5. Splinter hemorrhages were found to occur in 10.3 per cent of patients admitted to a general medicine ward of a large city-county hospital in one study and 19.5 per cent and 19.1 per cent, respectively, in two other studies.[4]

6. Biopsy of splinter hemorrhages that are associated with trichinosis may reveal the organism.[6]

7. In trichinosis splinter hemorrhages may be oriented transversely instead of longitudinally.[7]

8. The pathologic factors of splinter hemorrhages have been described.[8]

9. Splinter hemorrhages do not blanch upon pressure to the nail plate as do some other disorders such as ataxia-telangiectasia.[9]

10. Splinter hemorrhages are less common in the elderly, are more common among blacks, and are located distally.[10]

11. When found in women, splinter hemorrhages are more likely to indicate systemic disease.[11]

12. Splinter hemorrhages and pain have been associated with subacute bacterial endocarditis,[12] trichinosis,[12] an indwelling arterial catheter,[12] and leukocytoclastic vasculitis (C.R. Daniel, personal observation).

Table 13–1 lists various diseases that have been associated with splinter hemorrhages, subungual purpura, and their many causes. Most commonly, systemic disease is not the cause but, when keeping the points just listed in mind, one may more rationally evaluate their true significance.

Beau's Lines

Beau's lines are probably one of the most common but least specific nail changes associated with systemic disease. The exact cause is unclear.[13] Temporary cessation of nail growth or decreased nail plate deposition results in a transverse depression across the nail plate. There is probably an approximate direct correlation with the degree of general body trauma sustained and the likelihood of manifesting Beau's lines. Local injury or trauma to the proximal nail fold region may also cause a similar lesion. It seems that the most useful information that this finding gives is found by measuring the distance from the proximal nail fold distally to the leading edge of the Beau's line. Then one may approximate the time the insult occurred because the fingernail grows about 0.1 mm to 0.15 mm a day.

The width of the furrow is an indicator of the duration of the disease that has affected the matrix.[14] A transverse groove such as this is the most common ischemic deformity of the nail seen by the hand surgeon after the use of the upper extremity tourniquet.[14]

Histologic studies have shown an inflammatory infiltrate consisting of lymphocytes, plasma cells, and a moderate number of polymorphonuclear leukocytes. The epidermis shows abnormal keratinization; many of the cells retain their cellular outline and granularity.[15]

DeNicola and colleagues described Rosenau's depression, which seems to be similar if not identical to Beau's lines.[16]

Table 13–1. **CONDITIONS ASSOCIATED WITH SPLINTER HEMORRHAGES AND SUBUNGUAL PURPURA**

Alopecia mucinosa[233]	Malignant neoplasms[7]
Altitude (high)[1]	Mitral stenosis[235,237]
Amyloid[10]	Multiple sclerosis[14]
Anemia[233]	Mycosis fungoides[55]
Antigen-antibody complex disease	Normals[18,235]
Antiphospholipid coagulopathy[234]	Onychomycosis
Antiphospholipid syndrome[304]	Osler-Weber-Rendu disease[16]
Behçet's syndrome[1]	Pemphigoid[10]
Blood diseases[1]	Pemphigus[47]
Buerger's disease[76]	Pen-push purpura[242]
Cirrhosis[235]	Peptic ulcer disease[7]
Cryoglobulinemia[76]	Periarteritis nodosa[243]
Cystic fibrosis[1]	Pityriasis rubra pilaris[163b]
Darier's disease[236]	Porphyria[12]
Diabetes mellitus (in about 10% of patients)[16]	Psittacosis[12]
Dialysis[5,235]	Psoriasis[26,75,237,244]
Drug reactions (in general),[237] especially phototoxic	Pterygium[12]
Arterial emboli[76]	Pulmonary disease[233]
Endocarditis[238,239]	Purpura[8]
Eczema[76]	Radial artery puncture[12]
Exfoliative dermatitis[16]	Raynaud's disease[76]
Fungal[7]	Rheumatic fever[12]
General illness[5,235]	Rheumatoid arthritis[7]
Glomerulonephritis[12]	Sarcoid[47]
Heart disease[233]	Scurvy[237]
Hemochromatosis[1]	Septicemia[12]
Hepatitis[6]	Systemic lupus erythematosus[6,75]
Histiocytosis X[205]	Tetracycline[245]
Human immunodeficiency virus[12a]	Thrombocytopenia[16]
Hypertension[7]	Thyrotoxicosis[235,237,238]
Hypoparathyroidism[76]	Transplant patients[c]
Irradiation[16,240]	Trauma[2,3,5,26,235,238,244]
Keratosis lichenoides chronica[241]	Trichinosis[6,75]
Letterer-Siwe disease[205]	Vasculitis[237a]
Leukemia[16]	Wegener's granulomatosis[246]

[a] C.R. Daniel, personal observation.
[b] H.W. Randle, personal communication, 1982.
[c] J.M. Mascaro, personal communication, December 8, 1992.

Onycholysis

Onycholysis has been discussed elsewhere (see Chapters 11 and 17). Its correlation with systemic disease is overrated, especially because it is associated much more frequently with such diverse conditions as trauma, drug reactions, psoriasis, fungus, local allergy, and irritant reactions.[17]

Onycholysis is believed by some to be correlated with thyroid disease. It has been said that separation often occurs in thyrotoxicosis,[18,19] in which the earliest stage is conversion of the curved adhesion to a straight line. This adhesion line later dips proximally into the nail bed as a jagged projection.[18] This description is that of Plummer's nails, which usually starts at the fourth and then the fifth fingers.[16] X-ray examination has been used to help differentiate between onycholysis associated with thyroid disease and that resulting from other causes.[16] Most cases of thyroid disease do not manifest onycholysis.

Table 13–2 lists several systemic diseases that have been associated with onycholysis.

Pitting

Pitting has been described earlier (see Chapter 11). Its diagnostic relationship to systemic disease is doubtful because numerous dermatitides in the vicinity of the proximal nail fold may cause parakeratotic foci in the proximal matrix and thus pitting. Once the pits are visible in the more distal nail, sufficient time has passed so that the etiologic lesion may have disappeared or the patient may not remember whether there ever was an abnormality in that area.

Table 13–2. **SYSTEMIC DISEASES ASSOCIATED WITH ONYCHOLYSIS**

Amyloid and multiple myeloma[203]
Anemia[16]
Bantu porphyria[17]
Bronchiectasis (see yellow nail syndrome)[a]
Carcinoma (lung)[247]
Circulatory disorders
Cronkhite-Canada syndrome[248]
Cutaneous T cell lymphoma (mycosis fungoides)[17]
Diabetes mellitus[17]
Drug reaction (see Chapter 14)
Erythropoietic porphyria[55]
Erythropoietic protoporphyria[17]
Histiocytosis X[206]
Ischemia (peripheral)
Leprosy[16]
Lupus erythematosus[22]
Neuritis[16]
Pellagra[1]
Pemphigus vulgaris[55]
Pleural effusion[a]
Porphyria cutanea tarda[55]
Pregnancy[17]
Pseudoporphyria of hemodialysis[249] (possible photo induced)
Psoriatic arthritis
Pustular eruption of pregnancy[250] (impetigo herpetiformis)
Raynaud's phenomenon[14]
Reiter's syndrome
Scleroderma[124]
Sézary syndrome[251]
Syphilis[16] (secondary and tertiary)
Thyroid disease[18]
Vitamin C deficiency[63]
Yellow nail syndrome[125,126]

[a]See discussion of yellow nail syndrome in text.

We find pitting occasionally helpful in building a clinical case for psoriatic arthritis in the absence of other definitive markers, especially when it is the only cutaneous manifestation of psoriasis. Lovoy[20] and Pajarre[21] and their colleagues associated pitting with human leukocyte antigen (HLA) inheritance, psoriatic arthritis, and Reiter's syndrome. Urowitz and others reported pitting in association with systemic lupus erythematosus.[22] We have seen, and Dupre and associates[23] have noted, pitting in patients with dermatomyositis. The pitting may exhibit tight longitudinal rows in HLA-B27 inheritance.[21] We have only seen the latter orientation of pits in alopecia areata. Large pitting (elkonyxis) confined to the lunula has been described in syphilis.[16] Sarcoid[24] and pemphigus vulgaris[25] have been reported to cause nail pitting.

Transverse White Bands

Transverse white bands appearing in the nail unit are common. Most are caused by trauma to the more proximal matrix in the area of the proximal nail fold, such as with overaggressive manicuring. Several important points help differentiate local trauma-induced lesions from those associated with systemic disease:

1. Mees' and Muehrcke's lines tend to occur on several nails at once (traumatically induced lines may also but less frequently).
2. These systemic disease–associated lines usually spread across the entire breadth of the nail bed or plate and tend to be more homogeneous and have smoother borders.[26]
3. It has been our experience, as well as Zaias',[1] that these lines tend to have similar contour to the distal lunula, with a rounded distal edge. Trauma-induced lines tend to be more linear and resemble the contour of the proximal nail fold[1] and often do not span the entire breadth of the nail plate.
4. One usually finds no specific history of sufficient physical trauma to the cuticle area in patients with Mees' or Muehrcke's lines (Fig. 13–1).
5. A systemic insult usually may be correlated with the onset of the lines.

Mees' lines tend to be single but may be multiple transverse white lines that occur in the nail plate and move distally as the nail grows. If one squeezes the distal digit, the line does not disappear because it is a permanent alteration of that particular focus of nail plate. Biopsy of a probable Mees' line has shown the nail plate to appear "fragmented," with the

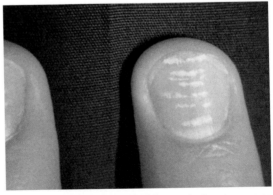

Figure 13–1. Trauma to cuticle producing transverse leukonychia, not Mees' lines.

underlying nail bed and nail matrix showing nothing of note.[15] This fragmentation probably represents a focus of abnormally formed cells exhibiting parakeratosis imparted to the nail plate by the compromised matrix.

Arsenic intoxication was classically believed to be the major cause of Mees' lines. It is now well known that many severe systemic insults may be the stimuli to initiate the abnormality (Table 13–3).[26,27] It has been said that Mees' lines that occur as a result of arsenic poisoning are due to actual deposition of arsenic in the nail plate (Fig. 13–2).[28] One may approximate the time of onset of systemic illness by measuring the distance from the Mees' line to the proximal nail fold, as one can do with Beau's lines.

In our experience, only one consistent mimic of a Mees' line exists: the situation in which only the distal aspect of the lunula is apparent. This may sometimes be caused by an erythematosus masking of the more proximal lunula. The tip-off is that this line (or lines) does not move out with the growing nail plate.

Muehrcke's Lines

Muehrcke's lines are double white transverse lines that represent an abnormality of the nail vascular bed. Squeezing the distal digit will cause the lines to disappear temporarily.[26] They are not palpable and do not indent the nail, and it has been noted that they are usually found on the second, third, and fourth fingernails.[29] They sometimes occur when chronic hypoalbuminemia persists and tend to disappear when the serum albumin is above 2.2 g/100 mL.[30] Their exact pathogenesis has not been adequately explained, but possibly a localized edematous state in the nail bed exerts pressure on the underlying vasculature, thus decreasing the normal erythema seen through the nail plate.[15] (See Fig. 13–3.)

A number of disease states causing hypoalbuminemia may be associated with Muehrcke's lines, such as the nephrotic syndrome and glomerulonephritis. Liver disease[30] and malnutrition[29] are among those that have been mentioned. A case has been reported attempting to correlate Muehrcke's lines with normal serum albumin, but this patient may have had Mees' lines (Fig. 13–3).[31] A case of Muehrcke's lines has been reported after trauma.[32]

Table 13–3. DISORDERS ASSOCIATED WITH MEES' LINES

Acute rejection of renal allograft[252]
Antimony poisoning[252]
Arsenic poisoning[27,253,254]
Cachectic state[14]
Carbon monoxide poisoning[204]
Carcinoid[255]
Cardiac failure[27]
Childbirth[a]
Chemotherapeutic drugs
Crush injury[b]
Cryotherapy (local)[14]
Endemic typhus[252]
Erythema multiforme[14]
Fluorosis[14]
Fracture[14]
Glomerulonephritis[33]
Gout[14]
Herpes zoster[14]
Hodgkin's disease[27]
Hyperalbuminemia[14]
Lead poisoning[252]
Leprosy[27]
Malaria[27]
Measles[14]
Menstrual cycle[14b]
Myocardial infarction[27]
Parathyroid insufficiency[14]
Pellagra[27]
Peripheral neuropathy[14]
Pneumonia[27]
Protein deficiency[14]
Psoriasis[27]
Renal failure[26,27,33,34]
Renal transplant[252]
Shock[14]
Sickle cell anemia[27]
Syphilis[14]
Tuberculosis[14]
Thallium poisoning[27]
Ulcerative proctitis[b]
Vitamin B_{12} deficiency[14]
Warm-reacting antibody immunohemolytic anemia[256]
Zinc deficiency[14]

[a]C.R. Daniel, unpublished observation.
[b]C.R. Daniel, personal observation.

Erythematous Crescent

The erythematous crescent represents a nail disorder that has received little attention.[26,33,34] It is defined as an abnormally prominent erythematous band that is seen at the distal portion of the nail vascular bed and is an anomaly of that structure. The proximal nail is normal. It may be thought of as a prominent onychodermal band. This band de-

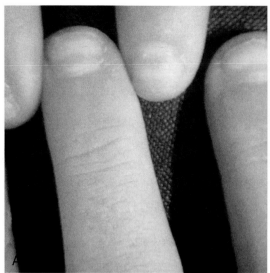

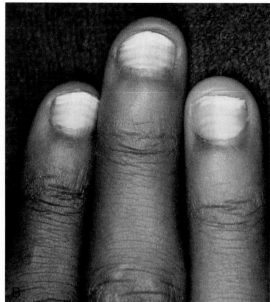

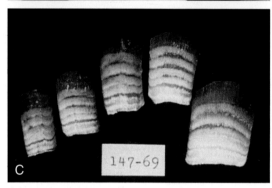

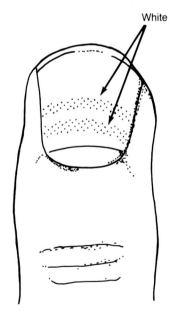

Figure 13–2. Arsenic-induced Mees' lines. *A*, Observation of nails led to discovery of criminal case of arsenic poisoning. *B*, Mees' lines caused by chemotherapy. *C*, Nails taken at autopsy of patient with arsenic poisoning. (Courtesy of Dr. N. Grannemann.)

White

Figure 13–3. Muehrcke's lines.

scribed by Terry[35] in combination with a proximal whitish portion of the nail illustrates Terry's nail associated with cirrhosis.

In our experience, the erythematous crescent may or may not be associated with an abnormally white proximal nail portion. Crescents were seen more frequently in patients with chronic medical illnesses such as renal failure[33,34,36] but may appear in healthy persons as well. Thus, the crescent is more of academic interest and not of particular diagnostic importance (Fig. 13–4).[26,33,34] It may mimic the half-and-half nail.[37]

Longitudinal Pigmented Bands

The vast majority of cases of longitudinal pigmented bands have no clear association with systemic disease. It seems that the more heavily pigmented the individual's skin, the

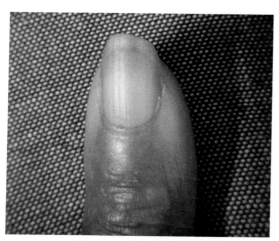

Figure 13–4. Erythematous crescent.

Table 13–5. **OTHER NAMES FOR CLUBBED FINGERS**

Acropachy
Digital hippocratism[16]
Drumstick fingers[18]
Dysacromelia[38]
Hippocratic nails (or fingers)[18]
Parrot-beak nails[18]
Serpent-head nails[18]
Trommelschlagelfinger[56]
Watch-glass nails[18]

bands associated with systemic changes are usually in multiple nails, although blacks not infrequently manifest them idiopathically (see Chapters 12 and 15).

Clubbing

Clubbing is an important physical finding that seems unique to humans.[29] Although this abnormality may be familial or idiopathic, its relationship to systemic disease is at times unquestionable. Much as been written on the subject from antiquity to the present. It has been called by many names (Table 13–5). Stone and Maberry studied clubbing extensively and rationally classified it into three major categories: idiopathic, hereditary-congenital, and acquired.[38,39] Each of these three categories is addressed later.

In our opinion, two major findings are important to classify nail changes as clubbing. First, and most important, the ungual-phalangeal angle must be increased. The normal nail proceeds from the finger at an obtuse angle of about 160°.[40] This may be visualized by placing the base of a "V" at the proximal nail fold and then pointing one of its arms toward the distal end of the nail and the other proximally toward the wrist. With gross clubbing, the angle at the base of the nail becomes greater than or equal to 180 degrees[40] (Fig. 13–5). Two common conditions may seem to mimic the increasing of the angle. Curved nails usually manifest their abnormal appearance by the distal part of the nail curving downward.[40] Paronychia[40] exhibiting inflamed proximal nail fold tissue may cause an apparent pseudoclubbing by the bulging of the cuticular area. Pseudoclubbing may be seen in osteitis fibrosa cystica[41] as well as in other conditions causing resorption of the distal phalanx. However, close measurement of the ungual-phalangeal angle will show that,

more likely it is that longitudinal pigmented bands will form in the nails. Trauma, dermatologic conditions, nevi, drugs, fungi, and other factors may cause these bands.[16,26]

Melanoma is certainly a possible cause and must be considered in any patient with these bands (see Chapter 15). Melanocyte-stimulating hormone often plays a role in the pathogenesis of longitudinal pigmented bands associated with systemic diseases. The more lightly pigmented an individual, the more likely it is that longitudinal pigmented bands are associated with melanoma or systemic disease (Table 13–4). Longitudinal pigmented

Table 13–4. **LONGITUDINAL PIGMENTED BANDS AND SYSTEMIC DISORDERS***

Acrodermatitis enteropathica[257]
Addison's disease[72]
Acquired immunodeficiency syndrome[92]
Amyloid (primary)[47]
Arsenic intoxication[16]
Carcinoma of the breast[258]
Carpal tunnel syndrome[259]
Cushing's syndrome (postadrenalectomy)[260]
Fluorosis[26,120]
Gastrointestinal diseases[16]
Hemosiderosis[257]
Hyperbilirubinemia[92]
Hyperthyroidism[92]
Hypopituitarism[257]
Irradiation[257]
Malnutrition[120]
Melanoma (metastatic)[257]
Ochronosis[257]
Peutz-Jeghers syndrome[26,261]
Porphyria[26]
Pregnancy[76]
Syphilis (secondary)[257]

*See also Chapter 12.

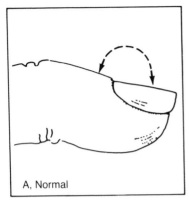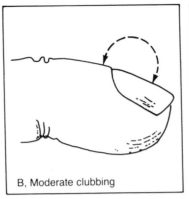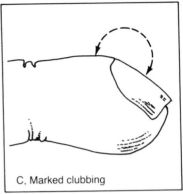

Figure 13–5. Clubbing. *A,* Normal. *B,* Moderate clubbing. *C,* Marked clubbing. From Stone OJ, Maberry JD: Spoon nails and clubbing. Tex State J Med 61:620, 1965. Used with permission.

unless the digit is truly clubbed, the angle has not been sufficiently increased to designate the digit as clubbed. Another important physical finding is the development of a spongy feel as one pushes downward on the tissue just proximal to the cuticle. This finding is probably due to fibrovascular hyperplasia of the underlying soft tissue.

Numerous hypotheses have been presented to explain clubbing. Stone and Maberry theorized that clubbing is caused by angulation of the nail matrix secondary to connective tissue changes. They believed that the distal nail matrix is relatively high compared with the proximal matrix.[38,39]

Mendlowitz[42] found, in all the cases of simple clubbing he studied, except hereditary clubbing, that the blood flow per unit surface or per volume of fingertip was abnormally high. These excessive flow rates were at least partially caused by elevated digital arterial pressure. He also concluded that abnormally high blood flow and digital arterial pressure, after release of sympathetic tone, are peculiar to ordinary clubbing and are integral forces in its development. Blood flow and pressure values were normal in hereditary clubbing. In addition, he noted that the blood flow per unit of tissue and the digital arterial pressure were within normal limits in hypertrophic osteoarthropathy.[42] Hall[43] believed that the capillary blood flow is less than in normal fingers even though overall flow is increased through dilated arteriovenous anastomoses. He indicated that this abnormal circulation was due to the presence of reduced ferritin. Hall also suggested that many intrathoracic diseases that induce clubbing manifest pulmonary arteriovenous shunts or their equivalents, which allow reduced ferritin to pass into the peripheral circulation instead of being rendered inert by oxidation in normal lung tissue.[43] (Bashour had a similar opinion and stated that reduced tissue oxygen tension secondary to blood shunting caused by a peripheral vasodilator rather than an increased oxygen supply over tissue demand was the cause of clubbing.[44]) Ginsburg and Brown found increased urinary estrogen excretion in a group of 11 men with hypertrophic pulmonary osteoarthropathy.[45]

Acquired, simple, bilateral clubbing most often is associated with cardiopulmonary disease. Approximately 80 per cent of simple clubbing is associated with respiratory ailments, and 10 to 15 per cent is associated with cardiovascular and extrathoracic diseases.[38,39] In our experience, this clubbing is most frequently bilateral. It often begins in the thumb and index finger.[45] "In chronic bronchial infections, the appearance of clubbing depends on three criteria: long duration, often more than 10 years, hypoxia, and hyperglobulinemia. If one is missing, there is little likelihood of clubbing developing."[47]

Acquired unilateral or single-digit clubbing is usually related to vascular lesions in that extremity, such as a peripheral shunt, aneurysm, or arteriovenous fistula, but Pancoast's tumors, erythromelalgia, or lymphadenitis may cause unilateral clubbing.[38,39] When a single nail is involved, the cause is usually traumatic but may be congenital.[38,39]

Acquired hypertrophic osteoarthropathy has six characteristics, according to Stone and Maberry[38,39]:

1. Simple clubbing, including the toes
2. Hypertrophy of the upper and lower extremities, with soft tissue proliferation and, at times, edema simulating elephantiasis

3. Peripheral neurovascular diseases such as local cyanosis, hyperhidrosis, paresthesia, and erythema

4. Bone pain aggravated by lowering the extremity, proliferative periostitis radiographically manifesting a laminated sheath along the shaft or a compact layer like wax dripping along a candle

5. Joint pain and swelling

6. Muscle weakness

They also emphasized that when the syndrome is complete a malignant thoracic tumor, especially bronchogenic carcinoma, is seen in at least 90 per cent of the cases.[38,39]

Several miscellaneous diseases associated with acquired clubbing and not mentioned in Stone's extensive compilation of causes of clubbing (Table 13–6) include systemic lupus erythematosus,[42,48] poisoning[14] with phosphorus, vinyl chloride, alcohol, mercury or beryllium, hyperparathyroidism,[49] Down syndrome,[50] Ayerza's syndrome (asthma in infancy),[14] amebiasis,[14] familial polyposis,[14] Gardner's syndrome,[14] chronic active hepatitis,[14] POEMS syndrome,[14] Graves' disease,[14] causalgia,[14] sarcoidosis and painful clubbing with discomfort relieved by colchicine therapy,[51] alpha heavy-chain disease (diffuse intestinal lymphoma),[52] Osler-Weber-Rendu disease,[52] laxative abuse,[53] chronic obstructive jaundice,[18] Crohn's disease,[54] and vinyl chloride disease.[55] Burgdorf stated that clubbing found in Crohn's disease may help differentiate it from ulcerative colitis,[54] but we have not found this useful. Idiopathic and hereditary clubbing may be transmitted as a simple mendelian-dominant or autosomal-dominant sex-limited trait with variable penetrance. It has an insidious onset, usually starting after puberty, and may affect both fingernails and toenails.[56] Pachydermoperiostosis is rare and is generally considered idiopathic. It is familial in more than half of the cases and consists of clubbing, pawlike or spadelike enlargement of the hands, thickening of the legs and forearms involving the bones as well as the soft tissue, thickening of the forehead and scalp (cutis verticis gyrata), and symmetric periosteal bone ossification.[38,39] It is more likely to initially affect adolescent males and be self-limited. The sella turcica is normal, distinguishing pachydermoperiostosis from classic acromegaly.[38,39] Chronic lymphedema and endocrine abnormalities have been associated with pachydermoperiostosis.[57]

Generally, there is no specific treatment for clubbing other than eliminating the predispos-

Table 13–6. CLASSIFICATION OF CLUBBING

I. Idiopathic
II. Hereditary, congenital[262]
   Citrullinemia[263]
   Other[76]
III. Acquired
  A. Pulmonary
    1. Neoplasms of lung
    2. Bronchitis, bronchiectasis, emphysema, lung abscess, cyst, tuberculosis, pulmonary fibrosis, blastomycosis, acute pneumonia, pulmonary endarteritis, chronic passive congestion
    3. Mediastinal: fibrosarcoma, mesoendothelioma, Hodgkin's disease, lymphoma, pseudotumor (dilation of esophagus)
    4. Metastatic neoplasm (fibrosarcoma, giant cell tumor)
  B. Cardiovascular
    1. Congenital heart disease (cyanotic)
    2. Subacute bacterial endocarditis
    3. Congestive heart failure
    4. Chronic myelogenous leukemia
    5. Myxoid tumor
    6. Acyanotic congenital heart diseases (rare)
  C. Hepatic
    1. Cirrhosis (cholangiolitic, malarial, hemochromatotic)
    2. Portal cirrhosis, secondary amyloidosis
  D. Gastrointestinal
    1. Chronic diarrhea, sprue
    2. Ulcerative colitis
    3. Neoplasms
    4. *Ascaris*
  E. Renal: chronic pyelonephritis (rare)
  F. Toxic: phosphorus, arsenic, alcohol, mercury, beryllium, reduced ferritin
  G. Miscellaneous (rare): syphilis, syringomyelia, Maffucci's syndrome, congenital dysplasia, angiectasis, chronic familial neutropenia, postthyroidectomy, myxedema, cretinism, primary polycythemia, leprosy, rheumatic fever, Raynaud's disease, scleroderma, acrocyanosis, chilblains, Kaposi's sarcoma, transitory physiology in newborn resulting from reversal of circulation at birth,[47] Gottron's syndrome (acrogeria)[47]
  H. Unilateral or unidigital
    1. Arterial aneurysm (aortic auxillary)
    2. Brachial arteriovenous fistula
    3. Subluxation of shoulder
    4. Pancoast's tumors
    5. Erythromelalgia
    6. Lymphangitis
    7. Median nerve injury
    8. Local trauma
    9. Felon
    10. Tophaceous gout
    11. Sarcoidosis

From Stone OJ: Spoon nails and clubbing. Cutis 16:235, 1975; Stone OJ, Maberry JD: Spoon nails and clubbing. Tex State J Med 61:620, 1965. Used with permission.

ing cause. As mentioned, colchicine has been used for the subsequent pain. Remission of clubbing has been observed after cutting the vagus nerve in the thorax, even when the associated pulmonary malignancy was not removed.[46]

The histologic picture of the tissue involved illustrates three histologic patterns corresponding to the severity of clubbing.[15]

1. Early clubbing is associated with an increase in dermal fibroblasts and connective tissue.

2. Moderate clubbing is accompanied by mucoid degeneration of the ground substances.

3. Severe clubbing is accompanied by marked interstitial edema and a mild infiltrate of plasma cells, lymphocytes, and primitive fibroblasts.

It is not clear from Lewin's article, but the prior description probably relates to simple, acquired clubbing. Interestingly, bulbous rete pegs (or keratin cysts) were noted in all cases.[15]

DeNicola and colleagues mentioned that the nail plate is thickened.[16] "It has rightly been said that clubbing is one of those phenomena with which we appear to know more about it than we really do."[40]

Koilonychia (Spoon Nails)

Spoon-shaped nails are not uncommon. Their relationship to systemic disease is at times relatively clear but most frequently nebulous. Classically, when koilonychia is mentioned, one's thoughts turn to iron deficiency anemia or Plummer-Vinson syndrome. In our experience, however, this is not one of the more common causes. A drop of water placed on a spoon nail will not roll off.[38] The spooning is best viewed from the side.

The exact cause of koilonychia is at best elusive, but several hypotheses have been given. Stone suggested that angulation of the nail matrix secondary to connective tissue changes is the cause. "Spooning of the nail occurs when the distal matrix is relatively low compared to the proximal matrix and vice-versa for clubbing."[39] Jalili and Al-Kassaf[58] found that the cystine content was somewhat low in the nails of patients with anemia and very low when koilonychia was present. They thus concluded that a deficiency of sulfur-containing amino acids played a role in the pathogenesis of koilonychia.[58] This association might be more apparent than real and could possibly reflect malnutrition. Samman believed that the cause is thinning and softening of the nail

plate.[7] Most publications categorize spoon nails into three major groups: idiopathic, hereditary, and acquired. We believe that acquired is the largest group. Trauma, dermatologic diseases such as psoriasis and fungal infection, and distal ischemia as in Raynaud's phenomenon seem to be the most common offenders. Occupational koilonychia has been reported in numerous instances and unusually in the toenails of boys who pull rickshas.[59] The authors of this article state that spoon nails caused by systemic diseases exhibit a concavity from side to side, with the edges everted and the nail plates themselves thinned. Ricksha boys tended to have the concavity from end to end, with eversion of the free margin of the nail plate associated with thickening.[59] The inertia of stopping and starting the ricksha was the probable cause. Koilonychia has also been associated with an upper gastrointestinal tract carcinoma.[1]

The petaloid nail is an early stage of koilonychia and is characterized by flattening of the nail.[47]

The idiopathic group is probably the second largest and may be the most common if the investigator does not rigorously pursue a cause. We most frequently find that children fit into this group more often than adults. One should rule out trauma from shoes and finger sucking before categorizing children as such. Serrated koilonychia syndrome has been described as a combination of koilonychia and deep longitudinal grooving of all nails.[55]

Koilonychia can be inherited in a dominant manner with a high degree of penetrance.[60] Inherited koilonychia may be seen in association with total leukonychia.[61] This group is probably the least commonly encountered.

Stone compiled an extensive list of possible diseases associated with koilonychia (Table 13–7).[38,39] Some additions include alopecia areata,[62] carpal tunnel syndrome,[14] and scurvy.[63]

NAIL CHANGES ASSOCIATED WITH SPECIFIC ORGAN INVOLVEMENT

The following is a brief system-by-system or category approach to nail changes associated with particular disorders. Emphasis is not placed on minor findings, and tables include a partial listing of associated disorders. For additional information, see the remainder of this chapter and Chapter 12 on nail pigmentation.

Table 13–7. CLASSIFICATION OF SPOON NAILS

I. Idiopathic
II. Hereditary, congenital, and associated with other ectodermal defects
  A. Spoon nails only, as a dominant
  B. Monilethrix
  C. Palmar hyperkeratoses
  D. Steatocystoma multiplex
  E. Spoon-fissured nail
  F. LEOPARD syndrome (leukokoilonychia)[47]
  G. Nail-patella syndrome[47,166]
  H. Nezelof syndrome[47]
  I. Incontinentia pigmenti[47]
  J. Gottron's syndrome (acrogeria)[47]
  K. Ectodermal dysplasia with anhydrosis[47]
  L. Chondroectodermal dysplasia (Ellis-van Creveld syndrome)[47]
  M. Palmoplantar keratoderma, maleda type[47]
  N. Focal dermal hypoplasia (Goltz's syndrome)[47]
III. Acquired
  A. Cardiovascular
    1. Anemia
      a. Hypochromic anemia (Plummer-Vinson syndrome)
      b. Epithelial iron deficiency (in our opinion a secondary phenomenon)
      c. Cystine deficiency (in our opinion a secondary phenomenon)
      d. Hemoglobinopathy SG[47]
    2. Polycythemia vera
    3. Coronary disease
  B. Infections: syphilis, fungus
  C. Metabolic
    1. Acromegaly
    2. Hypothyroidism
    3. Thyrotoxicosis
    4. Porphyria cutanea tarda[47]
    5. Malnutrition[52]
    6. Pellagra[16]
  D. Traumatic and occupational
    1. Petroleum products
    2. Alkalis and acids
    3. Homemakers, chimney sweeps
    4. Thioglycolate (hairdressers)[47]
    5. Frostbite[16]
    6. Thermal burns[16]
  E. Miscellaneous
    1. Psoriasis
    2. Lichen planus
    3. Acanthosis nigricans
    4. Banti's syndrome: nails cured with splenectomy
    5. Postgastrectomy
    6. Raynaud's disease
    7. Cachexia
    8. Scleroderma
    9. Toenails of some normal children (our experience)
    10. Hypovitaminoses (B_2 and especially C)[47]
    11. Darier's disease[47]
    12. Alopecia areata[7,47]
    13. Renal transplant[47]
    14. Polyglobulias (erythropoietin-producing tumors)[16]
    15. Primary amyloid (slight spooning)[47]
    16. Alopecia areata

From Stone OJ: Spoon nails and clubbing. Cutis 16:235, 1975; Stone OJ, Maberry JD: Spoon nails and clubbing. Tex State J Med 61:620, 1965. Used with permission.

Cardiovascular, Hematologic, and Ischemic Disorders

Reddish lunulae have been associated with heart failure,[64] even though other causes of this color change have been noted (see Chapter 12). Raynaud's phenomenon and other causes of peripheral ischemia, including koilonychia, may cause nail dystrophy.

Blood groups may be demonstrated from nail clippings and may be important if only hands and feet are obtainable for study or if mummification or putrefaction has set in.[55,65] Also a victim's blood-tinged material under an assailant's nails may be important in legal cases. Generally, few if any nail changes are pathognomonic in this group. Table 13–8 lists changes associated with cardiovascular, hematologic, and ischemic conditions (see also Tables 13–1, 13–6, and 13–7).

Samman treated his patients who have cold hands or Raynaud's phenomenon with isoni-

Table 13–8. NAIL CHANGES ASSOCIATED WITH CARDIOVASCULAR, HEMATOLOGIC, AND ISCHEMIC CONDITIONS

Disease	Nail Abnormality
Aortic insufficiency	Quincke's pulse
Anemia (general)[6]	Nail dystrophy
Endocarditis (bacterial)	Splinter hemorrhages,[7] clubbing[264]
Fabry's disease[77]	Turtle-back nail configuration
Heart failure[64]	Reddish lunulae
Hypertension[7]	Splinter hemorrhages
Ischemia	Nonspecific dystrophy; pterygium, nail thickening[265]
Leukemia[16]	Splinter hemorrhages
Marfan syndrome (aneurysm)[18]	Long and narrow nails
Mitral stenosis[26]	Splinter hemorrhages
Myocardial infarction (see Chapter 12)	Mees' lines
Osler-Weber-Rendu disease	Telangiectasia[16]
Pernicious anemia[266]	Splinter hemorrhage[1]
Porphyria (erythropoietic)[52]	Blue fingernails
Periarteritis nodosa[243]	Splinter hemorrhages
Scurvy[26]	Splinter hemorrhages
Sickle cell anemia (see Chapter 12)	Mees' lines
Thrombocytopenia[16]	Splinter hemorrhages
Thrombosis[16]	Onychomadesis
Vasculitis[26]	Splinter hemorrhages
Polyglobulias (erythropoietin-producing tumor)[16]	Koilonychia, reddish nail
Erythropoietic porphyria[55]	Onycholysis
Varicose lesions (trophic)[47]	Pachyonychogryphosis
Wegener's granulomatosis[267]	Periungual infarcts

cotinic acid hydrazide, thymoxamine hydrochloride, warm gloves, and ultraviolet B exposure of the terminal phalanges. He stated that the latter treatment may provide relief for several months.[66]

Gastrointestinal Disorders

It is our opinion that there are no specific nail findings in gastrointestinal disorders. Several onychopathies are worthy of mention, however, because they have in the past been thought to be relatively specific (Table 13–9).

Azure lunulae are associated with hepatolenticular degeneration (Wilson's disease). This discoloration is localized to the lunulae as opposed to a similar azure color in other parts of the nail bed in argyria, with antimalarials, and *Pseudomonas* infections.[26,67] A patient taking a phenolphthalein-containing laxative exhibited a similar color change localized to the lunulae; the change was especially marked in the thumbnails and was unaffected by pressure on the nail.[67] Terry's nails, supposedly indicative of cirrhosis, are described as an abnormal white appearance of the nail except for the distal portion that is just proximal to the free end of the nail. This portion, the distal pink zone, is exaggerated in this disorder and is named the onychodermal band. Its appearance does not diminish upon squeezing the digit.[35]

On the basis of their definition of Terry's nail, Holzberg and Walker found the condition in 25.2 per cent of a hospital population. They associated it with cirrhosis, chronic congestive heart failure, adult-onset diabetes mellitus, and increased age. In younger patients, it was associated with an increased risk of systemic disease. Tissue biopsy showed that the abnormality was due to distal telangiectasias.[68] Their description is very close to Daniel's description of the crescents.[26,33,34] Thyrotoxicosis, "pulmonary eosinophilia," malnutrition, or "keratoses" were found in other patients who had Terry's nails but who did not exhibit cirrhosis.[35] We have noticed numerous patients who had a similar nail appearance but who never had liver disease, and we concluded that this disorder is a reaction pattern and is not pathognomonic for cirrhosis (also see previous discussion of erythematous crescents). The white color has been said to be caused by overgrowth of connective tissue between the nail and bone, reducing the

Table 13–9. **NAIL CHANGES ASSOCIATED WITH GASTROINTESTINAL DISEASES**

Disease	Nail Finding
Acrodermatitis enteropathica	Paronychia
Basex's syndrome[248,268]	See Pulmonary System
Biliary cirrhosis[6]	Clubbing
Cirrhosis	Flat nails,[269] Terry's nails
Chylous ascites, intestinal lymphangiectasia[270]	Yellow nail syndrome
Crohn's disease[271]	Nail bed vasospasm
Cronkhite-Canada syndrome[6,272]	Ventral nail shaped like a triangle and nonspecific nail dystrophy, sometimes yellowish,[55] onychomadesis, onychoschizia,[273] and onycholysis[301]
Cystic fibrosis[1]	Periungual telangiectasia
Diabetes mellitus (pancreatic dysfunction)	Paronychia more likely
Duodenal ulcer, gallstones[274]	Hereditary leukonychia
Hepatic disease (other nonspecific changes)	Erythema at base of nails,[6] Muehrcke's lines,[30] Beau's lines, melanonychia striata[16]
Hepatitis[6] (chronic active)	Clubbing, white nails, splinter hemorrhages
Hemochromatosis[275]	Koilonychia, leukonychia, longitudinal striation, brittleness
Intestinal leiomyosarcoma[276]	Brownish nail pigmentation
Jaundice (chronic obstructive)[18]	Clubbing, nail yellowing[277]
Malabsorption[52]	Abnormal growth
Plummer-Vinson syndrome (esophageal web)	Koilonychia
Porphyria cutanea tarda	Onycholysis,[55] dystrophy, clubbing, disappearance of lunula,[47] longitudinal band[26]
Progressive systemic sclerosis (gastrointestinal manifestation)	Ischemic changes and periungual telangiectasias
Peutz-Jeghers syndrome[278]	Brownish pigmentation
Regional enteritis[264] (Crohn's disease)	Clubbing

See Table 13–6 for other gastrointestinal diseases not mentioned here.

amount of blood in the subcapillary plexus[6] (Fig. 13–6).

There is an interesting report of hand and nail contact with methacrylate causing nausea and diarrhea.[69] Because nail cosmetics may contain methacrylate, the association is worth remembering. See the pulmonary section in this text for a discussion of Basex's paraneoplastic syndrome.

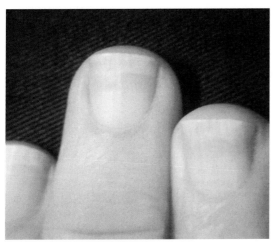

Figure 13–6. Terry's nail. Note close resemblance to what has been labeled by some as half-and-half nail.

Metabolic-Hormonal-Endocrine Condition

Almost all onychopathies associated with the endocrine system are nonspecific (Table 13–10).[70,71] Bissell and colleagues described longitudinal pigmented bands that may occur in patients with Addison's disease.[72] These have more meaning than when they occur in lightly pigmented individuals than in more heavily pigmented patients.[26] (See prior discussion of longitudinal pigmented bands and, in Chapter 12, nail pigmentation.) DeNicola and others suggested a radiologic method to distinguish onycholysis in thyroid disease from that caused by other diseases.[16] Nails in general are often brittle with hormonal disease.[73,74]

Some Infectious Diseases

Findings associated with infectious diseases are basically nonspecific. Syphilis has been associated with numerous nail changes. Some of these include elkonyxis (loss of nail plate substance in the lunula only)[16]; paronychia (sometimes ulcerative),[16] thought in the past to be a typical sign of congenital lues[75]; thinning and onychomadesis[16]; fragility with fissuring of the free margin[16]; racket nail[16]; and deep violet arch of Milan.[16] Several characteristics have been reported: reddish lunulae in lymphogranuloma venereum,[16] gray ardesia nail color during fever[16] or Mees' lines in malaria patients,[27] paronychia in tularemia,[6] nonspecific changes in typhoid fever,[6] at-

rophic nail changes in Job's syndrome,[76] and grayish discoloration in visceral leishmaniasis.[77] Leprosy may show numerous manifestations, including leukonychia and painful subungual abscess,[16] disappearing lunula,[16] lilac line of Milan,[16] and pterygium unguium.[78]

Toxoplasmosis has been associated with lichene planus verrucosus et reticularise of Kaposi and "nail dystrophy."[79] Beau's lines and nail shedding may occur with toxic shock.[80]

Accumulation of occult blood under the fingernails, especially the thumb and index finger in dentists, may be a mechanism for the spread of blood-borne infection such as hepatitis B.[81] It is recommended that dentists and others who have contact with blood and body fluids wear surgical gloves.[81] Scabies may take refuge under nails, leading to reinfection.[82,83]

Other associations[84] are listed elsewhere (also see Chapter 12).

The Nails in Patients With Human Immunodeficiency Virus

Because of the mobility of our society, human immunodeficiency virus (HIV) infection is becoming more prevalent worldwide. Whether one practices in a university setting, rural environment, or third world country, one can expect to encounter this disorder. Patients with HIV-positive disease (as well as other immunodeficiency disorders) often have numerous cutaneous manifestations.[85,86] Usually these cutaneous manifestations follow their normal patterns. Sometimes, however, the presentation of these infections may be atypical.[85,86]

Dermatophyte Infections

It is well known that dermatophyte infection is common in patients with HIV disease. The presence of onychomycosis generally correlates with helper T cell numbers less than 100 cells/mm[3].[87,88] Even though the causative organisms and clinical presentation in onychomycosis are usually similar to that in patients without HIV, there appear to be some notable differences:

1. The disorder may spread rapidly to all the fingernails and toenails.[87] In immunocompetent individuals, only the fingernails of one hand are usually involved (if at all).

Table 13–10. **HORMONAL-ENDOCRINE-METABOLIC ASSOCIATIONS**

Disease	Nail Findings
Acromegaly	Thick nails[6]; short, wide, flat nails[16]; onychoschizia[16]; absent lunulae[16]
Addison's disease	Longitudinal pigmented bands[72] of deep yellow color with brown background[16]
Adiposogenital syndrome (Frölich's syndrome)[16]	Absent lunulae, onychauxis, longitudinal striations
Alkaptonuria[12]	Pigmented nail beds
Amyloid (bullous)[279]	Subungual hematoma
Amyloid (primary)[47]	Slight spooning, longitudinal melanotic band, subungual papillomatosis, striations, crumbling of the free margin, punctated erosions, fragility, anonychia: nail changes may be the first sign[280]
Cushing's disease[12]	Onycholysis, chronic paronychia
Diabetes mellitus	Yellowish toenails,[281] proximal nail bed telangiectasia, capillary dilation or blush,[281] splinter hemorrhages,[12] periungual erythema,[12,296] paronychia, tinea unguium, onycholysis, periungual skin-colored papules[299]
Fabray's disease[77]	Turtle-back configuration of the nails
Fucosidosis[12]	Purple nail bands, onychogryphosis
Glucagonoma syndrome[91]	Brittle nails
Gout[12]	Longitudinal streaks, brittleness, onychogryphosis
Hartnup disease[282]	Nail streaks
Histidinemia[12]	Pachyonychia, onychoschizia, Beau's lines
Homocystinuria[12]	Periungual telangiectasias and longitudinal ridging
Hypercalcemia[283]	Hypergranulation of nail bed
Hyperoxaluria[12]	Ungual oxalate granulomas
Hypogonadism[12]	Onychauxis
Lipoid proteinosis[6]	Poor nail growth
Menstruation (dysmenorrhea) ?	Striate leukonychia,[47] Beau's lines[284]
Metabolic acidosis[16]	Onychoschizia
Parathyroid disease	Beau's lines,[285] nail textural changes,[6] candidal paronychia[6]
1. Hypoparathyroidism	Longitudinal striations,[16] opaque,[6] brittle,[6] splinter hemorrhages[12]
2. Hyperparathyroidism (osteitis fibrosa cystica)[41]	Chronic paronychia,[47] pseudoclubbing
Pituitary disease (hypopituitarism)	Lunula may disappear[16]; brown spots[16]; long, thin nails[18]; *Candida* infection[12]; brittleness[12]; Beau's lines[12]
Pseudohypoparathyroidism[12]	Brachydactyly
Thyroid disease	
1. Hypothyroidism	Nail plate wider than it is long,[16] hapalonychia,[16] slow growth,[16] longitudinal sulci,[16] transverse striations,[286] brittle,[16] onycholysis (dry, flat, thick, lackluster)[12]
2. Hyperthyroidism	Plummer's nail: free edge is undulated and curves upward,[6] clubbing,[52] yellow nail syndrome,[126] splinter hemorrhage,[16] increased growth rate,[16] increased nail calcium,[287] soft, shiny, onycholysis,[286,288] koilonychia[12]

2. Mycotic keratoderma of both palms may be found in HIV-positive individuals.[85,86] This would be quite rare in immunocompetent individuals.

3. A proximal white subungual onychomycosis often appears[85-87,298] (Fig. 13–7). This is unusual in the general population, especially in the fingernails. There has been a report of a patient with systemic lupus erythematosus with this presentation in the toenails.[89] Indeed, this presentation has prompted us[85] and others[90] upon seeing it to check for HIV and thus diagnose HIV in a previously unknown HIV-positive patient.

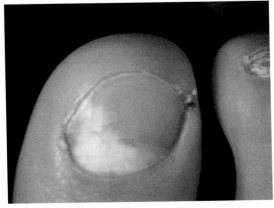

Figure 13–7. Proximal white subungual onychomycosis.

4. In immunocompetent individuals, chalky white involvement of the outer nail plate (superficial white onychomycosis) is rare in fingernails and is usually caused by *Trichophyton mentagrophytes*. In HIV-infected individuals, this presentation is not unheard of in fingernails or toenails and is usually caused by *Trichophyton rubrum*.[87]

5. The periungual region may be involved with the dermatophyte infection.[88]

6. Fingernail involvement may occur without toenail involvement (T. Berger, personal communication, February 6, 1995).

Treatment is disappointing, and relapse is the rule. Consideration of therapy is important, however, because the nails act as a reservoir of infection. We have had poor results with griseofulvin. Itraconazole and, to a lesser extent, fluconazole have shown better efficacy than griseofulvin. We have not used terbinafine in these patients.

For patients who decide against systemic therapy, the nails should be kept short and treated with topical[85] antifungal preparations as ketoconazole, terbinafine, ciclopirox, oxiconazole, econazole, or sulconazole.

Candida

It is uncommon for *Candida* to be a primary pathogen that directly invades the nail plate of a healthy individual.[95,292] *Candida* nail dystrophies are common in HIV-infected patients, especially when the helper T cell count is less than 100 cells/mm^3.[87,88] Onycholysis and paronychia may occur. As with dermatophyte infection, numerous nails are often involved.[88] A hypertrophic nail bed *Candida* infection is more typical in HIV-infected patients,[91] as it is in chronic mucocutaneous candidiasis. We have not seen this in nonimmunocompromised individuals. Acute *Candida* paronychia has been reported in one publication[92] in an HIV-positive patient. However, it has also been reported in a healthy individual.[93]

Some cases have responded to itraconazole, fluconazole, or ketoconazole, but relapse is the rule.[85]

Candida albicans is the major fungal agent in pediatric acquired immunodeficiency syndrome (AIDS).[94] In this age group, chronic *Candida* paronychia seems to occur most commonly between the ages of 2 and 6 years and is sometimes associated with severe nail dystrophy.[94]

Other Fungi

Undoubtedly, the entire spectrum of fungal infection in the general population[95] (see Chapter 11) will appear in HIV-positive individuals. *Pityrosporum ovale* was thought to cause onychomycosis in two patients with AIDS.[12,87] *Alternaria* nail infection has also been reported.[96,97] We certainly will find organisms affecting the nails that are most unusual in nonimmunosuppressed individuals. When performing fungal studies, one must do a potassium hydroxide test and culture on Sabouraud's agar, one with cycloheximide and chloramphenicol and one without chlorheximide so as not to hinder the growth of some organisms that are not ordinarily a pathogen.[90,95,98]

Viral Infection[85]

Herpetic whitlow has been reported in adults and in children with HIV.[99] Relapses are common, and recalcitrant, progressive disease may be ulcerative and scar the nail apparatus.[85] Acyclovir, famciclovir, or foscarnet may be instituted.

Papillomavirus may infect the nail unit. Biopsy should be performed on unusual or persistent lesions to rule out squamous cell carcinoma. We had a young adult patient who manifested a typical "wart" on a finger. This later developed into an invasive squamous cell carcinoma of the nail bed. The patient was then tested for HIV and found to be positive. Human papillomavirus type 16 deoxyribonucleic acid has been found in periungual squamous cell carcinoma.[100] Human papillomavirus type 35 and other strains have also been reported.[100]

Scabies[85]

Crusted scabies[101,102] may occur in patients with HIV infection. The nail bed and plate may be hypertrophic and loaded with the organisms. Proper treatment of the nail, especially in refractory cases, is important.[103,104] This may consist of nail debridement and then multiple treatments with lindane or permethrin cream.

Neoplastic Disease[85]

Squamous cell carcinoma (see discussion of viral infections), metastatic lesions, and Kaposi's sarcoma may appear in the region of the nail. Almost 100 per cent of AIDS patients with Kaposi's sarcoma have onychomycosis (T. Berger, personal communication, February 6, 1995). A nail unit lymphoma was the first manifestation in a patient with human T cell leukemia-lymphoma virus type I infection.

Inflammatory Disease[85]

Psoriasis or a psoriatic-like eruption may commonly affect patients with HIV. The typical nail manifestations of psoriasis may be present, but an eruption similar to pustular psoriasis may affect the nail. A proliferative, almost granulomatous process may permanently damage the nail. A psoriasis–Reiter's syndrome overlap process may occur.[86,87] Zidovudine may improve psoriasis in HIV-positive patients.[105] The antipsoriatic effect appears to be dose dependent and is associated with the development of erythrocyte macrocytosis, a side effect of zidovudine.[105] One psoriasis patient experienced improvement with high-dose co-trimoxazole,[106] and another did so with peptide T treatment.[107] Methotrexate should not be used because it increases the chance of encephalopathy, leukopenia, infection, and death.[92] Systemic antimicrobial agents have been effective in some instances.[108] Etretinate has improved a Reiter's syndrome diathesis.[109]

Pityriasis rubra pilaris has been reported in two patients with HIV infection.[110] One had nail "dystrophy" and one had normal nails. The disorder did not respond to etretinate.[110]

An atopic-like disease may occur with xerosis and brittle nails. Lichen spinulosus and "nail dystrophy" in an HIV-positive person have been reported.[111]

In general, nail manifestations of inflammatory disease among HIV-infected persons and among the general population are similar.[85] However, as the helper T cell counts become lower, more secondary infection is seen as is delayed healing.[85]

Systemic Disease[85,86]

Systemic disease in general can affect the nail apparatus.[112] There have been no specific nail changes associated with systemic disease (other than those mentioned previously) that suggest HIV infection. (See Table 13–11 for some nonspecific findings.) We have noticed an apparent increase in erythematous crescents[33] in HIV-infected patients (unpublished

Table 13–11. **SOME SYSTEMIC DISEASE EFFECTS ON THE NAILS**

Slow growth
Beau's lines
Splinter hemorrhages
Slow healing
Clubbing, especially with pneumocystis pneumonia[12]
Brittle nails
Leukonychia[91]
Nail plate yellowing[96,114]
Psoriatic changes (Reiter's syndrome)[289]
Smooth nails (scratching)

observation). The condition has been reported to be more frequent in "ill" patients.[33] We have not confirmed an increased frequency of yellow nail syndrome.[113–116] There may be a correlation between nail yellowing and *Pneumocystis carinii* pneumonia.[117] With wasting, slower nail growth and nail brittleness are observed.[85] Beau's lines may also occur, with exacerbation and remission of the underlying disease.[85]

Systemic Drugs[86]

Systemic drugs may affect the nails in a number of ways (see Chapter 14).[118] The incidence of drug reactions is increased in patients with HIV infection, especially with trimethoprim-sulfamethoxazole. Cancer chemotherapeutic agents used to treat developing malignancies are known to produce a wide array of pigmentary changes in patients without HIV infection,[118] and similar patterns in patients with HIV are expected. Zidovudine may produce dark brown, bluish, or blackish discoloration of the nail apparatus. However, blue nails may occur in HIV-positive disease and not be associated with zidovudine.[293] The pattern may vary and may be longitudinal, transverse, or diffuse. The color change is more commonly seen in blacks.

Miscellaneous. The lunula may be smaller than usual in HIV-positive disease.[294] Also periungual erythema was found in 2.4 per cent of one HIV study population.[296] Sometimes the erythema is painful.[297]

Nail Care in Patients With HIV Disease[86]

Nails should be kept relatively short. Longer nails are more likely to abrade the skin when scratching. Longer nails are also more likely to harbor infectious agents. Toenails should be cut straight across and not rounded at the edges to help avoid in-grown nails. Onychophagia and onychotillomania are not uncommon,[12] and these should be discouraged. Hangnails should not be pinched or pulled off but gently clipped off. A dual-action nail nipper, when used correctly, may painlessly clip onycholytic nails with less chance of nail bed damage. Power-driven drills should not be used to pare down nails in patients with HIV in-fection because they scatter many small pieces of nail debris and may release a "plume" of infectious material. Cotton gloves should be worn underneath vinyl gloves for wet work. Patients should notify their nail care professional if they are HIV positive so that appropriate precautions may be taken. All cases of nail surgery should be done as though the patient had HIV.

Summary

There are no known pathognomonic nail signs of HIV infection in nails. However, several presentations should increase the index of suspicion:

1. Proximal white subungual onychomycosis or *Trichophyton rubrum* appears to cause both most commonly in HIV-infected patients. Periungual dermatophyte involvement and involvement in all fingernails is unusual in non–HIV-infected individuals.

2. *Candida* as a primary pathogen of the nail bed and nail plate, especially if many nails are involved.

3. A destructive, almost granulomatous-like psoriatic diathesis of the nails.

4. Squamous cell carcinoma of the nail bed in a young adult.

Malnutrition

Much has been written about nails in malnutrition, but these findings seem to be nonspecific. Slow growth and fissuring,[6] koilonychia,[16] pustular paronychia with zinc deficiency,[119] spearlike nails,[120] Muehrcke's lines,[29] pellagra and koilonychia,[16] vitamin A deficiency associated with eggshell nails,[18] and brittle nails[16] have been reported. Hypocalcemia is usually not a cause of brittle nails. Chronic, severe hypocalcemia as seen in severe malnutrition probably can contribute to abnormal nails.

Central and Peripheral Nervous Systems

Probably no onychopathy is specific in this group, but one is of particular interest (Table 13–12). Several decades ago, Maricq noted that a significant correlation exists between a family history of schizophrenia and visibility of

Table 13–12. **ASSOCIATIONS WITH CENTRAL AND PERIPHERAL NERVOUS SYSTEMS**

Disorder	Nail Finding
Carpal tunnel syndrome[290]	Beau's lines, yellow-brown discoloration and transverse furrows, koilonychia[12]
Causalgia[16]	Long convex nails with vertical ridging, unilateral clubbing[12]
Central nervous system disease[16]	Splinter hemorrhages
Central and peripheral nervous system disorders[16]	Onycholysis
Epidemic encephalitis[12]	Multiple paronychia
Epilepsy[16]	Beau's lines
Hemiplegia[16]	Longitudinal striations
Lesch-Nyhan syndrome	Self-destruction of the tips of the digit
Manic-depressive disease[16]	Striated leukonychia
Morgagni-Stewart-Morel syndrome[47]	Hard, thickened nails
Multiple sclerosis	Longitudinal striations[16]
Neurofibromatosis	Pterygium inversus unguium–like changes[124]
Peripheral neuritis and hemiplegia[16]	Onychomadesis
Psychosis[16]	Double-edged nail
Reflex sympathetic dystrophy[291]	Increased nail growth, excessive transverse curvature, brittleness and periungual whitlow-like changes
Spinal cord injuries[12]	Ingrown toenails
Syringomyelia	Longitudinal striations,[16] periungual crusting[12]

the subcapillary plexus in the nail fold.[121] The duration of illness was greater in these patients, and they did not perform well academically.[121] Several years later, she added that the abnormal capillary appearance is not a permanent characteristic.[122] In a later article, she noted that, when these patients had a more clearly visible subcapillary plexus, they more frequently had smooth, glossy skin and more capillary hemorrhages in the nail fold area and tended to have longer and straighter sweat ducts.[123]

A double-edged nail in psychoses,[16] onycholysis with central and peripheral nervous system problems,[16] destruction of the tips of the digits in Lesch-Nyhan syndrome, onychomadesis with peripheral neuritis and hemiplegia,[16] splinter hemorrhages in central nervous system disease,[16] long and convex nails with vertical ridging in the causalgic syndrome,[6] Beau's lines in epilepsy,[16] striated leukonychia in manic-depressive illness,[16] longitudinal striations in hemiplegia, multiple sclerosis, syringomyelia,[16] pterygium inversus

unguium–like change in a patient with neurofibromatosis,[124] and hard, thickened nails in Morgagni-Stewart-Morel syndrome[47] have been noted.

Pulmonary System

The nails in yellow nail syndrome exhibit a greatly slowed rate of growth, yellowish discoloration of the nail plate (which may be thickened and excessively curved from side to side), absent lunulae and cuticles, swelling of the periungual tissue, and a variable degree of onycholysis[125,126] (Fig. 13–8).

Yellow nail syndrome has been found in a wide array of pulmonary diseases,[127] including tuberculosis,[124] asthma,[125] pleural effusion,[125] bronchiectasis,[126] chronic sinusitis,[126] chronic bronchitis,[128] and chronic obstructive pulmonary disease.[129] The nail manifestations may be mimicked by bullous lichen planus.[76] Biopsy of an involved nail suggests primary stromal sclerosis, which may lead to lym-

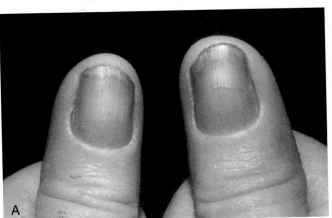

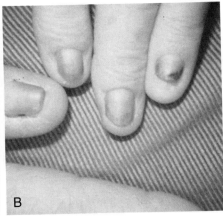

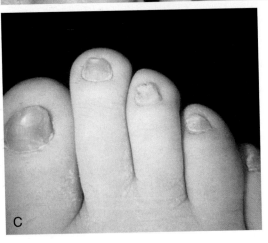

Figure 13–8. *A–C,* Yellow nail syndrome of chronic pulmonary disease.

phatic obstruction, thus possibly explaining the clinical manifestation.[130] Along with the nail and respiratory problems, lymphedema has been noted to be a third major component of the syndrome.[131]

Removal of a carcinoma of the larynx has been associated with a resolution of the yellow nails in one patient.[129] Other associated malignancies are lymphoma,[129] melanoma,[129] adenocarcinoma of the endometrium, anaplastic undifferentiated tumor, and carcinoma of the gallbladder.[132]

Some other associations include breasts of unequal size,[76] thyroid disease,[126] chronic nasal obstruction and rock-hard cerumen,[133] empyema,[134] nephrotic syndrome,[12] use of penicillamine,[135,136] psoriasis,[137] intestinal lymphangiectasia,[138] and sleep apnea.[139]

Various therapeutic regimens have been cited in the literature but with no consistent results. Guin and Elleman mentioned that gold therapy and bed rest for rheumatoid arthritis had possibly improved one case.[129] Biotin,[140] intralesional triamcinolone,[141] diethylstilbestrol,[142] zinc,[137] and management of diabetes mellitus[143] have possibly caused improvement in various patients with the abnormality. Vitamin E[137,144] given in the dosage of 400 IU two[127] to three[145] times daily has been reported to improve the nails. There is also a report of topical vitamin E solution improving the nails.[146] Oral vitamin E and itraconazole have been used in one case.[147]

Shell nail syndrome was reported to be associated with bronchiectasis. Affected nails exhibited excessive longitudinal curvature of the nail plate, dystrophic fingertips resulting from atrophy of the distal nail bed, and onycholysis.[148] This description is certainly similar to that of yellow nail syndrome, except no mention is made of abnormal color or slow rate of growth.

Clubbing has been mentioned earlier and is associated with respiratory problems. Painful clubbing in a patient with sarcoidosis was documented, and the discomfort diminished after colchicine therapy.[51] The nail in sarcoidosis may also appear dystrophic and yellowish and may manifest painful paronychia and splinter hemorrhages.[47]

Bazex's paraneoplastic syndrome[149–151] may present with psoriasis-like changes in the nails and other acral areas such as the nose and ears. Other nail changes that may be found include horizontal and vertical ridging, yellow color, thickening, onycholysis, subungual debris, softness, thinning, slow growth,

and increased glycine, lysine, and methionine.[12] These changes may occur months or years before an upper respiratory tract malignancy as well as upper gastrointestinal malignancies. Squamous cell carcinoma is most commonly found.[12] There have also been reports of associated carcinomas of the prostate or vulva.[12]

Some miscellaneous associations with pulmonary disease include interstitial pulmonary disease and dyskeratosis congenita.[152] Also nail clippings in cystic fibrosis have an elevated sodium content,[55] and splinter hemorrhages and periungual telangiectasia have been noted.[12]

Renal Disease

The half-and-half fingernail may be the most useful onychopathologic indicator of chronic renal failure.[33] The finding was originally popularized by Lindsay[153] but possibly first described by Bean.[154] Lindsay's working description reads as follows: "a nail exhibiting a red, pink, or brown transverse distal band occupying 20 to 60 per cent of the total nail length and with the remaining proximal portion exhibiting a dull whitish ground glass appearance."[153] We did not find that the proximal portion necessarily needed to be whitish. Kint and colleagues came to the same conclusion.[155] If the distal band was less than 20 per cent of the total nail length, the patient was considered to have Terry's nails.[153] Probably a more specific description of the half-and-half nail would be a nail exhibiting either a whitish or normal proximal half and a distinctly abnormal brownish distal portion. This distal portion begins proximally where the normal or whitish nail ends and terminates distally where the free end of the nail loses its attachment to the hyponychium[26,33,34] (Fig. 13–9). It has been our experience that this description most aptly describes the half-and-half nail and leaves less room for imitations. Lindsay's description, as well as crescents,[33,34,36] are seen frequently in renal failure but not infrequently otherwise.

Numerous causes of nail discoloration could mimic the half-and-half nail, but understanding how to evaluate pigment changes can remove most from the differential diagnosis.[26] Probably the most frequently encountered causes that may mimic the half-and-half nail are topical agents[26] and psoriasis. A brownish discoloration (oil-spot change) often

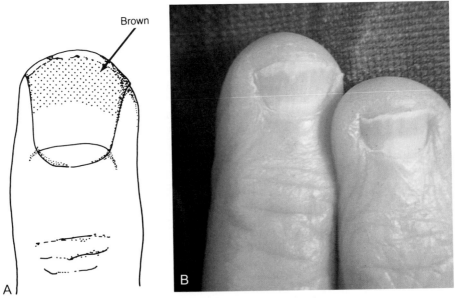

Figure 13–9. *A* and *B,* Half-and-half nail.

occurs just proximal to an area of onycholysis in a psoriatic nail, but the onycholysis as well as other nail and skin findings of psoriasis often make the diagnosis clear (Fig. 13–10). Systemic 5-fluorouracil and androgens may possibly cause a half-and-half–like nail.[156–158] Scher reported a patient with concomitant yellow nail syndrome and half-and-half nail.[159]

The exact cause of the half-and-half nail is unknown. Leyden and Wood[160] performed

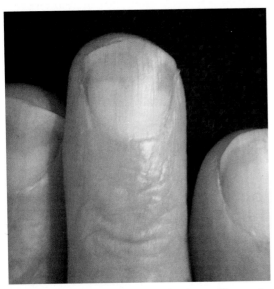

Figure 13–10. Pseudo–half-and-half nail caused by psoriasis.

a biopsy on the distal brownish area and found the pigment to be melanin. They hypothesized that renal failure stimulates matrix melanocytes and causes melanin to be deposited in the nail plate.[160] Also, because the nail grows more slowly in renal failure, pigment is more likely to accumulate.[160] Stewart and Raffle found melanin granules in the basal layer of the nail bed epidermis.[161] Kint and colleagues found increased capillaries and a distinct thickening of the walls.[155] This could be due to increased blood flow through an artificial shunt. Capillary changes that are probably reversible have been suggested as the cause.[162] Plasma melanotropic hormone has been found to be greatly increased in patients treated by maintenance dialysis for chronic renal failure.[163] This and the fact that the nails are in a sun-exposed area could possibly be responsible for the melanin deposition.[163]

An intriguing question about the half-and-half nail is why the distal brownish color is not apparent throughout the more proximal nail, considering that the melanocytes responsible are probably in the matrix and the color does not seem to migrate. The pigment apparently is more visible distally than it is proximally because of a looser attachment of the nail plate or because of a variation of the Tyndall effect. It has been noted that after a chronic hemodialysis patient received a kidney transplant the brown pigment moved distally and his half-and-half nails slowly disappeared.[34]

The half-and-half nail is not correlated with specific quantitative blood urea nitrogen or creatinine findings[153,160,161] (C.R. Daniel and J.D. Bower, unpublished data, 1975). It does seem apparent that renal disease per se is not the cause of this nail finding, but azotemia and renal failure do instigate the problem either by acting directly on the matrix melanocytes or by a melanocyte-stimulating substance released from another site. The half-and-half nail as more specifically described seems to occur in about 9[33,34] to 15[162] per cent of chronic renal failure patients sometime during the course of their disease. We described a condition called crescents that was found to occur more frequently in renal failure but also in other chronically ill patients as well as in some normal individuals. Lubach and colleagues lumped half-and-half nails, brown arcs, and possibly crescents under the term subungual erythema. Subungual erythema was found most commonly, but not exclusively, in renal failure patients.[36,164]

Levitt[165] analyzed the creatinine concentration of human fingernail and toenail clippings to determine the duration of renal failure. He concluded that patients with acute renal failure had normal nail creatinine concentration, whereas those with chronic renal failure had elevated levels that correlated with the serum creatinine concentration that had been present several months previously.[165]

Probably the only other relatively specific nail findings associated with renal failure are those seen in the nail-patella syndrome. Findings include triangular lunulae and ulnar-sided nail dystrophy, discoloration, longitudinal ridging, poorly formed lunulae, koilonychia, and absent or dystrophic nails. When triangular-shaped lunulae, alone or especially in combination with ulnar-sided nail dystrophy, are observed, nail-patella syndrome is strongly suggested and other associated abnormalities should be sought[166] (Fig. 13–11).

Mees' lines, Muehrcke's lines, splinter hemorrhages, and slow growth have been associated with renal failure, as mentioned earlier. Renal adenocarcinomas producing erythropoietin may impart a more reddish color to the nail bed.[16] Rheumatologic diseases that may produce secondary renal disease also have numerous associated nail abnormalities (see the following section). Angiokeratoma corporis diffusum (Fabry's disease) may have associated renal problems and a "turtle-back" nail configuration.[77]

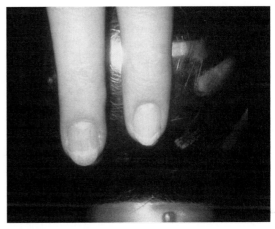

Figure 13–11. Triangular lunulae of nail-patella syndrome.

Paronychia and onychomycosis are seen with increased frequency in renal transplant patients.[167]

Rheumatologic and Other Arthritic Diseases

Numerous rheumatologic diseases[168] can either directly or indirectly affect the nail unit. The vast majority of these onychopathies represent nonspecific reaction patterns. A few are more specific, but in our opinion, none is pathognomonic of that particular rheumatologic disorder. The proximal nail fold is often the most important site of alterations.[169] Capillary changes of the nail fold may be characteristic of scleroderma, as mentioned later. Ischemia often associated with Raynaud's phenomenon probably forms the basis of most changes. Rheumatoid arthritis is often associated with nonspecific nail findings. Pronounced longitudinal ridges often having a beaded appearance, thickening, discoloration, splinter hemorrhages, and periungual vascular lesions (Bywaters' syndrome) associated with beading and longitudinal ridging have been noted.[170] "A deep violet arch like a half moon, well delimited by the adjacent plate, 0.5 to 1 mm in size, at about 4 to 5 mm from the free nail margin, to which it is parallel, can occur."[16] Milan believed that this was specific for syphilis, but it can also occur in rheumatoid arthritis, leprosy, and during the convalescence of debilitating, infectious diseases.[16]

Nail fold infarcts and yellow nail syndrome have also been associated with rheumatoid arthritis.[169] Periungual erythema is not uncommon. One case of a red lunula has been reported.[171] Nail abnormalities have been seen frequently in patients with lupus erythematosus. Erythema and fissuring of the proximal nail fold with dilated capillary loops may be seen in systemic lupus erythematosus[6] as was a case of red lunulae.[171] Clubbing,[48] paronychia,[48] pitting,[22] white nails, leukonychia striata,[22] onycholysis that may cause nail shedding,[16] and "coffin-lid" nail characterized by a flat laminar surface at the center descending steeply on both sides and penetrating the ungual sulci[16] have been noted. According to Kint and Herpe, the combination of a typical red-blue color of the crumbling nail plate and longitudinal striae should make one suspect discoid lupus erythematosus.[172] Periungual erythema and telangiectasia have been reported in coffee plantation workers without any association with lupus.[173] Their single patient's nail abnormality cleared with systemic chloroquine therapy. Also in discoid lupus a "curious atrophic spindling of the fingers sometimes with hyperextension of the terminal phalanges and nail dystrophy" has been observed.[75]

Erythema and telangiectasias of the proximal nail fold probably are the most frequently found changes in systemic lupus erythematosus. Changes secondary to Raynaud's phenomenon and distal ischemia are also common in systemic lupus erythematosus. Sclerodactyly, seen in this disease group, may also be seen in toxic oil syndrome.[174] Hyperkeratosis of the cuticle in combination with erythema and telangiectasia is probably helpful, but hyperkeratosis alone seems to be too nonspecific because xerosis alone often causes this change (Fig. 13–12). Urowitz and coworkers found that patients with systemic lupus erythematosus who had nail changes tended to have a higher incidence of Raynaud's phenomenon and mucous membrane ulceration.[22] The oil-spot change so typical of psoriasis may be seen in the nail bed of a patient with systemic lupus erythematosus.[55] Diffuse nail hyperpigmentation has been found more commonly in black patients with systemic lupus erythematosus.[175] Also nail fold capillary density has been associated with pulmonary capillary loss.[176] Periungual erythema and onychodystrophy have been noted in chilblain lupus erythematosus.[177]

Reiter's syndrome may cause nail changes that appear identical to psoriasis, but this occurs much less frequently in Reiter's syndrome. Onycholysis, yellowing, and subungual hyperkeratosis are the most frequent

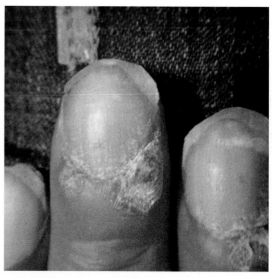

Figure 13–12. Hyperkeratosis of proximal nail fold in a patient with lupus erythematosus.

changes. Lovoy and colleagues reported a patient with nail pitting and incomplete Reiter's syndrome and suggested that this change may reflect a predisposition to the development of psoriasis or psoriasiform lesions conferred by HLA-A2 with B27 inheritance.[20] Longitudinal tight superficial nail grooving, subungual hyperkeratosis, and onycholysis have been reported as the first manifestations of HLA-B27 inheritance.[21] Small yellow pustules may develop beneath the nail, often near the lunula; they may enlarge, and erosion through the nail plate may occur.[6] Paronychia-like changes have been noted.[20]

Patients with dermatomyositis frequently have nail changes similar to those seen in systemic lupus erythematosus, including erythema and dilated capillary loops in the proximal nail folds (Fig. 13–13), bluish-red plaques around the base of the nails, hyperkeratotic cuticles, and pitting.[6,23,75,178] One case of a red lunula has been reported.[171]

Patients with scleroderma (progressive systemic sclerosis) may exhibit nail abnormalities, including telangiectasia and erythema of the proximal nail fold, tightening of the skin of the digits, and distal digital infarcts resulting from ischemia and Raynaud's phenomenon. Pterygium inversus unguium–like changes may be seen and are characterized by adherence of the distal portion of the nail bed or hyponychium to the ventral surface of the nail plate, thereby obliterating the normal distal separation of these structures[124] (Fig. 13–14). Progressive systemic sclerosis and systemic lupus erythemato-

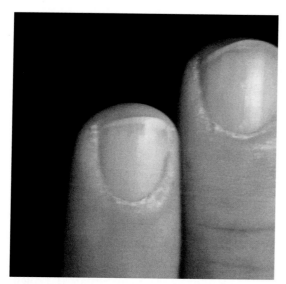

Figure 13–13. Hyperkeratosis and erythema of nail folds associated with dermatomyositis.

sus are the two most common associations.[179] Patterson noted that this finding may become symptomatic upon trauma or upon attempts to clip the nails.[124] Trauma may induce a similar disorder. A reaction to formaldehyde-containing nail cosmetics may also produce a pterygium inversus unguium–like picture.[180] Odom and colleagues described a similar finding in patients having the anomaly since birth, without apparent distal ischemia, and postulated that this change may represent an anomaly of the developing fetal nail primordia and is analogous to the claw of lower primates.[181] It has been reported that decreased manual skills and vibration exposure may be associated with systemic scleroderma and nail fold abnormalities.[305]

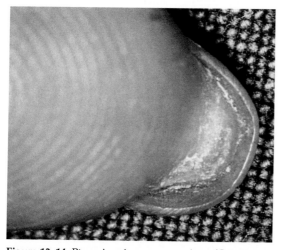

Figure 13–14. Pterygium inversus unguium. (Courtesy of Dr. R. Caputo.)

Caputo and Prandi[182] found one patient who acquired the disorder without a definite predisposing cause, an observation confirmed by others.[183] Pterygium inversus unguium of the toenails has been reported only in families.[184] Ragged cuticles,[75] widened cuticles with the proximal skinfold thin,[6] clubbing (probably secondary to pulmonary manifestations),[185] onychorrhexis,[16] vesiculation of the periungual area, absence of the lunula, deep longitudinal sulci, hapalonychia, onycholysis, and onychogryphosis have been associated with progressive systemic sclerosis.[124] Distal pulp resorption tends to occur as in other diseases with Raynaud's phenomenon, and the subsequent ulcers may be painful. Nail fold bleeding is strongly associated with anticentromere antibodies, especially in scleroderma.[186] Abnormal periungual capillaries have also been noted in morphea.[187]

Multicentric reticulohistiocytosis, with its often destructive polyarthritis, may have associated atrophy, longitudinal ridging, brittleness, and hyperpigmentation[188] of the nails in addition to papules around the nail folds,[189] onycholysis, and racket-shaped (plates wider than long) nails.[188] Barrow attributed most of these changes to a synovial reaction affecting nail growth and to the giant cell nodules producing a pressure effect on the matrix.[188]

Other rheumatologic nail associations include faster nail growth in Still's disease and acute rheumatic fever,[16] pitting with psoriatic arthritis, slow growth, and nails exhibiting decreased cystine content and absent lunulae in chronic polyarthritis.[16] In Behçets syndrome, a half-and-half–like nail diathesis was reported.[190] A peculiar nail dystrophy composed of leukonychia,[76] longitudinal striations, brittleness, and crumbling of the nail plate may be seen in patients with gout.[75] Baran and Dawber, reporting the work of others, suggested that nails in psoriatic arthritis may be differentiated from those in rheumatoid arthritis by biochemical and statistical analysis of the amino acids of the fingernails.[76,191,192] Significant nail involvement of psoriasis (e.g., advanced subungual hyperkeratosis) in children may suggest more severe psoriasis or increased chance of development of psoriatic arthritis.[193] Capillary changes of the proximal nail fold may also be found in psoriatic arthritis patients.[194]

Periungual telangiectasia is a distinctive microvascular pattern of dilated and distorted capillary loops seen in patients with connective tissue vascular diseases. Maricq and colleagues[195] proposed a simple, inexpensive, reproducible technique to predict internal multisystem involvement in scleroderma, Raynaud's phenomenon, and dermatomyositis.[195] They have not found this specific change in systemic lupus erythematosus or rheumatoid arthritis. Their method is not easily applicable to black patients.[195] Periungual telangiectasia also may be seen in schizophrenia,[121–123] cystic fibrosis,[1] graft-versus-host reaction,[76] diabetes mellitus,[1] congenital heart disease,[1] homocystinuria,[76] and mongolism.[1] Minkin and Rabhan expounded on the periungual capillary changes seen in some arthritic disorders.[196] Implementing a method described by Herd[197] and using an ophthalmoscope, they examined 130 patients with various connective tissue diseases. They placed a drop of mineral oil on each nail fold to be examined. They believed that the capillaries were best visualized in the nail fold of the fourth finger. The ophthalmoscope was set at +40, resulting in a × 10 magnification. They found the following:

1. Patients with systemic scleroderma exhibited enlarged and deformed capillaries with dilation of both limbs of the loop. This was associated with disorganization of the loop arrangement and many avascular areas. This pattern was seen in 74 per cent of the patients studied.

2. The pattern in patients with systemic lupus erythematosus consisted of widened, tortuous, "meandering" capillary loops at times resembling a renal glomerulus. There is usually some disorganization of the capillary pattern, but only rarely were avascular areas seen. These patients manifested this pattern 53 per cent of the time.

3. Of patients with dermatomyositis, 82 per cent illustrated the systemic scleroderma pattern.

4. No specific patterns were found for vasculitis, Raynaud's disease, morphea, or mixed connective tissue disease.

5. Capillary microscopy is most useful: as a prognostic factor in Raynaud's disease or mixed connective tissue disease, to differentiate "undifferentiated" connective tissue disease to distinguish cutaneous lupus from dermatomyositis, and to confirm the diagnoses of systemic scleroderma, dermatomyositis, and systemic lupus erythematosus.

6. Dark-skinned people and traumatized fields may diminish capillary visibility.

Biopsy of proximal nail folds in these patients often shows deposits positive for periodic acid–Schiff that are not specific but may help identify those patients with idiopathic Raynaud's phenomenon who are at risk for the development of a connective tissue disease.[198] Others have also confirmed the usefulness of capillary microscopy.[303]

Maricq and Maize, pioneers in the study of nail fold capillary abnormalities, added that capillary hemorrhages are more frequent in patients with scleroderma than in controls. These hemorrhages may seem to "grow out" with the cuticle.[199] Also scleroderma nail fold capillary abnormalities may be quite characteristic in early disease. Callen found that nail fold manifestations of dermatomyositis were diminished in a child he was treating with hydroxychloroquine Plaquenil Sulfate (J. Callen, personal communication, December 10, 1985).

Miscellaneous Systemic Disorders

Several more nail abnormalities that are nonspecifically associated with other systemic diseases include paronychia,[200] temporary[200] and permanent[201] nail shedding and other changes after Stevens-Johnson syndrome, canalized and yellow nails (Vieira's sign) in fogo selvagem,[202] subungual pustules in impetigo herpetiformis,[77] disappearing lunula or onycholysis in multiple myeloma,[77,203] Mees' lines and leukonychia in carbon monoxide poisoning,[204] splinter hemorrhages, paronychia onycholysis, purpura, subungual hyper-keratosis in histiocytosis X[205,206] (biopsy of the involved nail unit in histiocytosis X showed the presence of atypical histiocytes[207]), subungual purpura in Letterer-Siwe disease,[208] nail shedding in toxic shock syndrome[209] and toxic epidermal necrolysis,[1] nail dystrophy (including horizontal ridging, hemorrhage, hyperkeratosis, and shedding in bullous pemphigoid), nail dystrophy in epidermolysis bullosa simplex,[210] and onychogryphosis[211] and other bullous diseases (Fig. 13–15). Lead poisoning may manifest leukonychia, onychalgia, and onychomadesis.[28] Periodic shedding of the nails may be associated with epidermolysis bullosa[212] and leukonychia seen in cryoglobulinemia.[6] Periungual erythema may be seen in histiocytosis X, graft-versus-host disease, and Wiskott-Aldridge syndrome.[296]

In our experience, sarcoid of the nail involves a crumbling nail plate sometimes associated with pain and paronychia. Painful paronychia and splinter hemorrhages may oc-

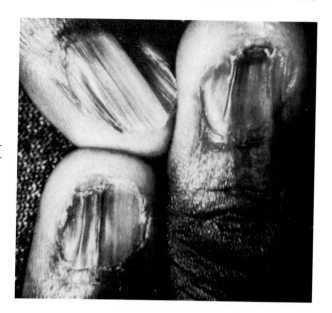

Figure 13–15. Permanently dystrophic nails secondary to matrix scarring in a patient with Stevens-Johnson syndrome.

cur,[47] as may some nail pitting.[24] Treatment with prednisone and hydroxychloroquine cleared one patient of his nail abnormalities.[24] Pterygium formation may occur.[213] Sarcoid may cause nail dystrophy with or without underlying bony involvement.[302]

Hodgkin's disease may manifest Mees' lines,[27] which may be associated with a poor prognosis.[47] Leukonychia may be seen in patients with hyperalbuminemia, zoster, and exfoliative dermatitis[76] and in Orthodox Jews who fast. Painful nails with subungual hyperkeratosis were reported in cutaneous T cell lymphoma.[214] In a child with mycosis fungoides, nail dystrophy resolved with photochemotherapy.[215] Hypertrichosis lanuginosa may be associated with nail pitting and subungual epidermal hyperplasia.[301]

Pemphigus vulgaris has been noted to exhibit numerous nail findings, as have other bullous diseases. In our experience, pemphigus, in a majority of cases, causes nail changes by contiguous effects. Onychomadesis,[216] discoloration, pitting, transverse lines, paronychia, onychoschizia,[217] and other dystrophic changes characterize the nail changes.[25] Beau's lines, pterygium, pigmentation changes, onycholysis, subungual hemorrhages, subungual hyperkeratoses, and fungal involvement may be seen.[25] Paronychia may be a sign heralding an exacerbation.[218]

An unsubstantiated report has raised the issue of whether a "radium fingernail polish" has been associated with development of cancer.[219]

"Neopolitan nails," the main features of which are loss of lunula and white appearance of the proximal half of the nail, a more normal pink band, and the opaque free edge of the nail, seems to be associated with old age, reduced bone mass, and thin skin.[220] This presentation has some of the features of the half-and-half nail,[33,153] Terry's nail,[35] and crescents,[33,34] described earlier.

Primary subungual calcification of fingers and toes may be an effect of advancing age in women. Secondary subungual calcification occurs occasionally after trauma and in psoriasis.[221] In pregnancy, nail changes occur as early as the sixth week and consist of grooving, increased brittleness and softening, distal onycholysis, and subungual keratosis[222]; longitudinal pigmented bands may occur.[76] Erythema elevatum diutinum has been reported in a periungual distribution.[223] Low nail nitrogen is found in ill neonates.[76] In graft-versus-host disease, lichen planus–like changes, including superficial ulceration of the lunula, fluting of the nails, onychatrophia,[76] onychomycosis,[224] longitudinal ridging (J.M. Mascaro, personal communication, December 8, 1992), and periungual erythema (J.M. Mascaro, personal communication, December 8, 1992) may occur.

Reversible hyperpigmentation of the nails has been reported in a patient with vitamin B_{12} deficiency.[225] Nail dystrophy has been associated with vitiligo.[226] Onycholysis, thickening, and discoloration have been reported in the Sézary syndrome.[227,228]

Other miscellaneous reports have included nail dystrophy in incontinentia pigmenti,[229] nodules under the nails in chronic lympho-cytic leukemia,[230] nail necrosis in gamma heavy-chain disease,[231] and nail shedding in Kawasaki syndrome.[217] In addition, severe psoriasis (usually with nail involvement) pa-tients have an increased incidence of autoim-mune disease in close relatives.[232]

References

1. Zaias N: The Nail in Health and Disease. Spectrum Publications, New York, 1980.
2. Daniel CR, Daniel MP: Nail signs of systemic dis-ease. Consultant 35:392, 1995.
3. Daniel CR: Nails in Systemic Disease. Audiotape presented at the meeting of the American Academy of Dermatology, New Orleans, February 7, 1995.
4. Kilpatrick ZM, Greenberg PA, Sanford JP: Splinter hemorrhages—Their clinical significance. Arch In-tern Med 115:730, 1965.
5. Blum M, Avinam AL: Splinter hemorrhages in pa-tients receiving regular hemodialysis. JAMA 239:44, 1978.
6. Fitzpatrick TB: Dermatology in General Medicine, ed 2. McGraw-Hill, New York, 1979.
7. Samman PD: The Nails in Disease, ed 3. Year Book, Chicago, 1978.
8. Zaias N: The Nail in Health and Disease. Spectrum Publications, New York, 1980, citing Alkiewicz J: Zur Histopathologie der Hamatome des Menschlichen Nagels. Arch Dermatol Syphilol 168:411, 1933.
9. Moschella SL, Hurley HJ (eds): Cutaneous Manifes-tations of Immunodeficiency in Dermatology, ed 2. WB Saunders, Philadelphia, 1985, p 218.
10. Cohen PR, Scher RK: Geriatric nail disorders: Diag-nosis and treatment. J Am Acad Dermatol 26:521, 1992.
11. Norton L: Determining if subungual bleeding signals systemic disease, trauma. Skin Allergy News 22:5, 1991.
12. Tosti A, Baran R, Dawber RPR: The nail in systemic diseases and drug-induced changes. In Diseases of the Nails and Their Management, ed 2. Blackwell Scientific, London, 1994, pp 175–261.
13. De Barber D: What do Beau's lines mean. Int J Der-matol 33:545, 1994.
14. Baran R, Dawber RPR: Physical signs. In Baran R, Dawber RPR (eds): Diseases of the Nails and Their Management, ed 2. Blackwell Scientific, Oxford, Eng-land, 1994, pp 35–80.
15. Lewin K: The fingernail in general disease. Br J Der-matol 77:431, 1965.
16. DeNicola P, Morsiani M, Zavagli G: Nail Diseases in Internal Medicine. Charles C Thomas, Springfield, IL, 1974.
17. Daniel CR: Onycholysis: An overview. Semin Der-matol 10:34, 1991.
18. Degowin EL, Degowin RL: The Nails in Bedside Di-agnostic Examination, ed 2. Macmillan, New York, 1969.
19. Luria MN, Asper SP: Onycholysis in hyperthy-roidism. Ann Intern Med 49:102, 1958.
20. Lovoy MR, Gluhm GB, Morales A: The occurrence of nail pitting in Reiter's syndrome. J Am Acad Derma-tol 2:66, 1980.
21. Pajarre R, Kemo M: Nail changes as the first manifes-tation of HLA-B27 inheritance. Dermatologica 154:350, 1977.
22. Urowitz M, Gladman DD, Chalmers A, et al: Nail le-sions in systemic lupus erythematosus. J Rheumatol 5:441, 1978.
23. Dupre A, Viraben R, Bonafe JL, et al: Zebra-like der-matomyositis. Arch Dermatol 117:63, 1981.
24. Patel KB, Sharma OP: Nail in sarcoidosis: Response to treatment. Arch Dermatol 119:277, 1983.
25. Baumal A, Robinson MJ: Nail bed involvement in pemphigus vulgaris. Arch Dermatol 107:751, 1973.
26. Daniel CR, Osment LS: Nail pigmentation abnormal-ities, their importance and proper examination. Cutis 25:595, 1980.
27. Hudson JB, Dennis AJ Jr: Transverse white lines in the fingernails after acute and chronic renal failure. Arch Intern Med 117:276, 1976.
28. Pardo-Castello V: Diseases of the Nails, ed 3. Charles C Thomas, Springfield, IL, 1960.
29. Conn RD, Smith RH: Malnutrition, myoedema Muehrcke's lines. Arch Intern Med 116:875, 1965.
30. Muehrcke RC: The fingernails in chronic hypoalbu-minemia. BMJ 1:327, 1956.
31. Schwartz RA, Vickerman CE: Muehrcke's lines of the fingernails. Arch Intern Med 139:242, 1979.
32. Feldman SR, Gummon WR: Unilateral Muehrcke's lines following trauma (letter). Arch Dermatol 125:133, 1989.
33. Daniel CR III, Bower JD, Daniel CR Jr: The half and half fingernail: The most significant onychopatho-logical indicator of chronic renal failure. J Miss State Med Assoc 16:376, 1975.
34. Daniel CR III, Bower JD, Daniel CR Jr: The half and half fingernail: A clue to chronic renal failure. Proc Clin Dial Transplant Forum 5:1, 1975.
35. Terry RB: The onychodermal band in health and dis-ease. Lancet 1:179, 1955.
36. Lubach D, Strubbe I: The frequency of subungual erythema. Z Hautkr 57:1486, 1982.
37. Daniel CR: The nail. In Sams M, Lynch P (eds): Prin-ciples and Practice of Dermatology. Churchill-Liv-ingstone, New York, 1990, pp 743–760.
38. Stone OJ: Spoon nails and clubbing. Cutis 16:235, 1975.
39. Stone OJ, Maberry JD: Spoon nails and clubbing. Tex State J Med 61:620, 1965.
40. Lovibond JL: Diagnosis of clubbed fingers. Lancet 1:363, 1938.
41. Brickman AS: Grand Rounds: Progressive shortening of the fingertips. Drug Ther 49, 1981.
42. Mendlowitz M: Measurements of blood flow and blood pressure in clubbed fingers. J Clin Invest 20:113, 1941.
43. Hall GH: The cause of digital clubbing. Lancet 1:750, 1959.
44. Bashour FA: Clubbing of the digits: Physiologic con-siderations. J Lab Clin Med 58:613, 1961.
45. Ginsberg J, Brown JB: Increased estrogen exertion in hypertrophic pulmonary osteoarthropathy. Lancet 2:1274, 1961.
46. Just-Viera JO: Clubbed digits: An enigma. Arch In-tern Med 113:122, 1964.
47. Baran R: Nail Changes in General Pathology. In Pierre M (ed): The Nail. Churchill Livingstone, New York, 1981, pp 5–105.
48. Mackie RM: Lupus erythematosus in association with finger-clubbing. Br J Dermatol 89:533, 1973.
49. Davis GM, Rubin J, Bauer JD: Digital clubbing due to secondary hyperparathyroidism. Arch Intern Med 150:452, 1990.

50. Scherbenske JM, Benson PM, Rotchford JP, James WD: Cutaneous and ocular manifestations of Down syndrome. J Am Acad Dermatol 22:933, 1990.
51. West SG, Gilbreath RE, Lawless, OJ: Painful clubbing and sarcoidosis. JAMA 246:1338, 1981.
52. Braverman IM: Skin Signs of Systemic Disease, ed 2. WB Saunders, Philadelphia, 1981.
53. Pines A, Olchovsky D, Bregman J, et al: Finger clubbing associated with laxative abuse. South Med J 76:1071, 1983.
54. Burgdorf W: Cutaneous manifestations of Crohn's disease. J Am Acad Dermatol 5:689, 1981.
55. Runne U, Orfanos CE: The human nail. In Mali WH, Karger S (eds): Current Problems in Dermatology, vol 9. S Karger, Basel, 1981, pp 102–149.
56. Demis DJ (ed): Clubbing of the Fingers in Clinical Dermatology, Vol 1. Harper & Row, New York, 1980.
57. Brenner S, Srebrnik A, Kisch ES: Pachydermoperiostosis with new clinical and endocrinologic manifestation. Int J Dermatol 31:341, 1992.
58. Jalili MA, Al-Kassaf S: Koilonychia and cystine content of nails. Lancet 1:108, 1959.
59. Bentley-Phillips B, Bayles MA: Occupational koilonychia of the toenails. Br J Dermatol 85:140, 1971.
60. Bergeron JR, Stone OJ: Koilonychia: A report of familial spooned nails. Arch Dermatol 95:351, 1967.
61. Baran R, Achten G: Les associations congenitales de koilonychia et de leuconychie totale. Arch Belges Syphiligr 25:13, 1969.
62. Hordinsky MK: Hair. In Sams M, Lynch P (eds): Principles and Practice of Dermatology. Churchill-Livingstone, New York, 1990, pp 761–780.
63. Cohen PR, Prystowsky JH: Metabolic and nutritional disorders. In Sams W, Lynch P (eds): Principles and Practice of Dermatology. Churchill-Livingstone, New York, 1990, pp 665–681.
64. Terry R: Red half-moons in cardiac failure. Lancet 2:842, 1954.
65. Garg RK: Determination of ABOCH blood group-specific substances from fingernails. Am J Forensic Med Pathol 4:143, 1983.
66. Samman PD: Management of disorders of the nails. Clin Exp Dermatol 7:189, 1982.
67. Bearn AG, McKusick VA: Azure lunulae. JAMA 166:904, 1958.
68. Holzberg M, Walker HK: Terry's nails: Revised definition and new correlations. Lancet 1:896, 1984.
69. Mathias CGT, Caldwell TM, Maibach HI: Contact dermatitis and gastrointestinal symptoms from hydroxyethylomethacrylate. Br J Dermatol 100:447, 1979.
70. Greene RA, Scher RK: Nail changes associated with diabetes mellitus. J Am Acad Dermatol 16:1015, 1987.
71. Feingold KR, Elias PM: Endocrine-skin interactions. J Am Acad Dermatol 17:921, 1987.
72. Bissell GW, Sarakomoi K, Greenslit F: Longitudinal banded pigmentation of nails in primary adrenal insufficiency. JAMA 215:1656, 1971.
73. Scher RK, Bodian AB: Brittle nails. Semin Dermatol 10:21, 1991.
74. Scher RK: Brittle nails. Int J Dermatol 28:515, 1989.
75. Rook A, Wilkinson DS, Eblins FJG, et al: Textbook of Dermatology, ed 3. Blackwell Scientific, London, 1979.
76. Baran R, Dawber RPR: Diseases of the Nails and Their Management. Blackwell Scientific, Oxford, England, 1984.
77. Moschella SL, Pillsbury DM, Hurley HJ: Dermatology. WB Saunders, Philadelphia, 1975.
78. Patki AH, Mehta JM: Pterygium unguium in a patient with recurrent type 2 lepra reaction. Cutis 44:311, 1989.
79. Menter MA, Morrison JGL: Lichen verrucosus et reticularis of Kaposi: A manifestation of acquired adult toxoplasmosis. Br J Dermatol 94:645, 1976.
80. Hirschmann JV: Cutaneous signs of systemic bacterial infection. In Sams WM, Lynch PJ (eds): Principles and Practice of Dermatology. Churchill-Livingstone, New York, 1990, pp 89–98.
81. Allen LA: Occult blood accumulation under the fingernails: A mechanism for the spread of blood-borne infection. J Am Acad Dermatol 105:455, 1982.
82. Scher RK: Subungual scabies. Am J Dermatopathol 5:187, 1983.
83. Witkowski JA, Parish LC: Scabies, subungual areas harbor mites. JAMA 252:1318, 1984.
84. Kosinski MA, Stewart D: Nail changes associated with systemic disease and vascular insufficiency. Clin Podiatr Med Surg 6:295, 1989.
85. Daniel CR, Norton LA, Scher RK: The spectrum of nail disease in patients with human immunodeficiency virus infection. J Am Acad Dermatol 27:93, 1992.
86. Daniel CR: Nail disease in patients with HIV infection. In WHC Burgdorf, SI Katz (eds): Dermatology, Progress and Perspectives: The Proceedings of the 18th World Congress of Dermatology, Parthenon, New York, 1993, 382–385.
87. Dompmartin D, Dompmartin A, Deluol AM, et al: Onychomycosis and AIDS: Clinical and laboratory findings in 62 patients. Int J Dermatol 29:337, 1990.
88. Kaplan MH, Sadick N, McNutt NS, et al: Dermatologic findings and manifestations of acquired immunodeficiency syndrome (AIDS). J Am Acad Dermatol 16:485, 1987.
89. Rongioletti F, Persi A, Tripodi S, Rebora A: Proximal white subungual onychomycosis: A sign of immunodeficiency. J Am Acad Dermatol 30;129, 1994.
90. Elewski BE: Clinical pearl: Proximal white subungual onychomycosis in AIDS. J Am Acad Dermatol 29:631, 1993.
91. Scher RK: Nail signs of systemic diseases (audiotape). Dialogues in Dermatol 28: 1991.
92. Fisher BK, Warner LC: Cutaneous manifestations of the AIDS: Update 1987. Int J Dermatol 26:615, 1987.
93. Montemarano AD, Benson PM, James WD, Croup MA: Acute paronychia apparently caused by Candida albicans in a healthy female. Arch Dermatol 129:786, 1993.
94. Prose NS: HIV infection in children. J Am Acad Dermatol 22:1223, 1990.
95. Haley L, Daniel CR: Fungal infection of the nails. In Scher RK, Daniel CR (eds): Nails: Therapy, Diagnosis, Surgery. Philadelphia, WB Saunders, 1990, pp 106–119.
96. Prose NS, Abson KG, Scher RK: Disorders of the nails and hair associated with HIV infection. Int J Dermatol 31:453, 1992.
97. Valenzano L, Giacalone B, Grillo LR, Ferraris AM: Compromissione ungueale in corso di AIDS. G Ital Dermatol Venereol 123:527, 1988.
98. Daniel CR: The diagnosis of nail fungal infection. Arch Dermatol 127:1566, 1991.
99. Straka BP, Whitaker DL, Morrison SH, et al: Cutaneous manifestations of the acquired immunodeficiency syndrome in children. J Am Acad Dermatol 18:1089, 1988.
100. Eliezri Y, Silverstein SJ, Nuoro GJ: Occurrence of hu-

man papillomavirus type 16 DNA in cutaneous squamous and basal cell carcinomas. J Am Acad Dermatol 23:836, 1990.

101. Rau RC, Baird IM: Crusted scabies in a patient with acquired immunodeficiency syndrome (letter). J Am Acad Dermatol 15:1058, 1986.

102. Drabick JJ, Lupton GP, Tompkins K: Crusted scabies in human immunodeficiency virus infection (letter). J Am Acad Dermatol 17:142, 1987.

103. Depaoli RT, Marks VJ: Crusted (Norwegian) scabies: Treatment of nail involvement (letter). J Am Acad Dermatol 17:136, 1987.

104. Scher RK: Subungual scabies (letter). Am J Dermatopathol 5:187, 1983.

105. Kaplan MH, Sadick NS, Wieder J, et al: Antipsoriatic effects of zidovudine in human immunodeficiency virus–associated psoriasis. J Am Acad Dermatol 20:76, 1989.

106. Rasokat H: Psoriasis in AIDS: Remission with high dosage cotrimoxazole. A Hautkr 61:991, 1986.

107. Marcusson JA, Wetterberg L: Peptide-T in the treatment of AIDS associated psoriasis and psoriatic arthritis. Acta Derm Venereal (Stockh) 69:86, 1989.

108. Rosenberg EW, Noah D, Skinner RB: AIDS and psoriasis. Int J Dermatol 30:449, 1991.

109. Belz J, Breneman DL, Nordlund JJ, Solinger A: Successful treatment of a patient with Reiter's syndrome and acquired immunodeficiency syndrome using etretinate. J Am Acad Dermatol 20:898, 1989.

110. Bluvelt A, Nahass GT, Pardo RJ, et al: Pityriasis rubra pilaris and HIV infection. J Am Acad Dermatol 24:703, 1991.

111. Cohen S, Dicken CH: Generalized lichen spinulosus in an HIV-positive man. J Am Acad Dermatol 25:116, 1991.

112. Daniel CR, Sams WM, Scher RK: Nails in systemic disease. In Scher RK, Daniel CR (eds): Nails: Therapy, Diagnosis, Surgery. Philadelphia, WB Saunders, 1990, pp 167–191.

113. Chernosky ME, Finley VK: Yellow nail syndrome in patients with acquired immunodeficiency disease. J Am Acad Dermatol 13:731, 1985.

114. Daniel CR: Yellow nail syndrome and acquired immunodeficiency disease. J Am Acad Dermatol 14:844, 1986.

115. Norton AL: Yellow nail syndrome controlled by vitamin E therapy (letter). J Am Acad Dermatol 15:715, 1986.

116. Scher RK: Acquired immunodeficiency syndrome and yellow nails (letter). J Am Acad Dermatol 18:758, 1988.

117. Goodman DS, Teplitz E, Wishner A, et al: Prevalence of cutaneous disease in patients with acquired immunodeficiency syndrome (AIDS) or AIDS-related complex. J Am Acad Dermatol 17:210, 1987.

118. Daniel CR, Scher RK: Nail changes secondary to systemic drugs or ingestants. In Scher RK, Daniel CR (eds): Nails: Therapy, Diagnosis, Surgery. Philadelphia, WB Saunders, 1990, pp 192–201.

119. Miller SJ: Nutritional deficiency and the skin. J Am Acad Dermatol 21:1, 1989.

120. Gisht DB, Singh SS: Pigmented bands on nails: A new sign in malnutrition. Lancet 1:507, 1962.

121. Maricq HR: Familiar schizophrenia as defined by nail fold capillary pattern and selected psychiatric traits. J Nerv Ment Dis 136:216, 1963.

122. Maricq HR: Capillary morphology and the course of illness in schizophrenic patients. J Nerv Ment Dis 142:63, 1966.

123. Maricq HR: Association of a clearly visible subpapillary plexus with other peculiarities of the nail fold skin in some schizophrenic patients. Dermatologica 138:148, 1969.

124. Patterson JW: Pterygium inversum unguius-like changes in scleroderma. Arch Dermatol 113:1429, 1977.

125. Marks G, Ellis JP: Yellow nails. Arch Dermatol 102:619, 1970.

126. Kandil E: Yellow nail syndrome. Int J Dermatol 12:236, 1973.

127. Pavlidakey GP, Hashimoto K, Blum D: Yellow nail syndrome. J Am Acad Dermatol 11:509, 1984.

128. Ayres S, Michan R: Yellow nail syndrome, response to vitamin E. Arch Dermatol 108:267, 1973.

129. Guin JD, Elleman JH: Yellow nail syndrome possible association with malignancy. Arch Dermatol 115:734, 1979.

130. Decosta SD, Imber MJ, Baden HP: Yellow nail syndrome. J Am Acad Dermatol 22:608, 1990.

131. Samman PD, White WF: The "yellow nail" syndrome. Br J Dermatol 76:153, 1964.

132. Burrows NP, Jones RR: Yellow nail syndrome in association with carcinoma of the gall bladder. Clin Exp Dermatol 16:471, 1991.

133. Moran MF: Upper respiratory problems in the yellow nail syndrome. Clin Otolaryngol 1:333, 1976.

134. Lodge JP, Hunter AM, Saunders NR: Yellow nail syndrome associated with empyema. Clin Exp Dermatol 14:328, 1989.

135. Krebs A: Drug-induced nail disorders. Praxis 70:1951, 1981.

136. Lubach D, Marghescu S: Yellou-nail syndrom durch D-enizillamin. Hautzt 30:547, 1979.

137. Mautner G, Scher RK: Yellow nail syndrome. J Geriatr Dermatol 1:106, 1993.

138. Ocana I, Bejarno E, Ruiz I, et al: Intestinal lymphangiectasia and the yellow nail syndrome (letter). Gastroenterology 94:858, 1988.

139. Knuckles MLF, Hodge SJ, Roy TM, Snider HL: Yellow nail syndrome in association with sleep apnea. Int J Dermatol 25:588, 1986.

140. Meirs HG, Gruel H, Perschmann Y, et al: Yellow nail syndrome. Dtsch Med Wochenschr 98:1529, 1973.

141. Abell E, Samman PD: Yellow nail syndrome treated by intralesional triamcinolone acetomide. Br J Dermatol 88:200, 1973.

142. Lebioda J: Yellow nail syndrome. Przegl Dermatol 59:523, 1972.

143. Nelson LM: Yellow nail syndrome. Arch Dermatol 100:499, 1969.

144. Norton L: Further observations on the yellow nail syndrome with therapeutic effects of oral alphatocopherol. Cutis 36:457, 1985.

145. Hazebrigg DE, McElroy RJ: The yellow nail syndrome. J Assoc Milit Dermatol 6:14, 1980.

146. Williams HC, Buffham R, Vivier A: Successful use of topical vitamin E solution in the treatment of nail changes in yellow nail syndrome. Arch Dermatol 127:1023, 1991.

147. Andre J, Walraevens C, DeDoncker P: Yellow nail syndrome infected by dermatophyte SPP: Experience with itraconazole pulse treatment combined with vitamin E. Poster exhibit at the annual meeting of the American Academy of Dermatology, New Orleans, February, 1995.

148. Cornelius CE, Shelley WB: Shell nail syndrome associated with bronchiectasis. Arch Dermatol 96:694, 1967.

149. Baran R: Paraneoplastic acrokeratosis of Bazex. Arch Dermatol 113:1613, 1977.
150. Pecora AL, Landsman L, Imgrund SP, et al: Acrokeratoses paraneoplastics (Bazex' syndrome). Arch Dermatol 119:820, 1983.
151. Bazex A, Salvador R, Dupre A: Syndrome paraneoplasique a type d'hyperkeratose des extremities: Guerison apres le traitement de Peoithelioma larynge. Bull Soc Fr Dermatol Syphiligr 72:182, 1965.
152. Paul SR, Perez-Atayde A, Williams DA: Interstitial pulmonary disease associated with dyskeratosis congenita. Am J Pediatr Hematol Oncol 14:89, 1992.
153. Lindsay PG: The half and half nail. Arch Intern Med 119:583, 1967.
154. Bean WB: A discourse on nail growth and unusual fingernails. Trans Am Clin Climatol Assoc 74:152, 1963.
155. Kint A, Bussels L, Fernandes M. et al: Skin and nail disorders in relation to chronic renal failure. Acta Derm Venereal (Stockh) 54:137, 1974.
156. Nixon DW, Pirozzi D, York RM, et al: Dermatological changes after systemic cancer therapy. Cutis 27:181, 1981.
157. Daniel CR III: Nail pigmentation abnormalities: An addendum. Cutis 30:364, 1982.
158. Daniel CR III, Scher RK: Nail changes secondary to systemic drugs and ingestants. J Am Acad Dermatol 10:250, 1984.
159. Scher RK: Yellow nail syndrome and half-and-half nail. Arch Dermatol 123:710, 1987.
160. Leyden JJ, Wood MG: The half and half nail. Arch Dermatol 105:591, 1972.
161. Stewart WK, Raffle EJ: Brown nail bed arcs and chronic renal disease. BMJ 1:784, 1972.
162. Bussels L, Kint A, Fernandes M, et al: Lesions cutaneous et unqueales dans l'insuffisance renale chronique. Arch Belg Dermatol Syphiligr 28:363, 1972.
163. Gilkes JJH, Eady RAJ, Rees LH, et al: Plasma immunoreactive melanotrophic hormones in patients on maintenance haemodialysis. BMJ 1:656, 1975.
164. Lubach D, Strubbe J, Schmidt J: The half and half nail phenomenon in chronic hemodialysis patients. Dermatologica 164:350, 1982.
165. Levitt JI: Creatine concentration of human fingernail and toenail clippings. Ann Intern Med 64:312, 1966.
166. Daniel CR, Osment LS, Noojin RO: Triangular lunulae: A clue to nail patella syndrome. Arch Dermatol 116:448, 1980.
167. Lugo-Janer G, Sanchez JL, Santiago-Delpin E: Prevalence and clinical spectrum of skin disease in kidney transplant recipients. J Am Acad Dermatol 24:410, 1991.
168. Sarnow MR, Plotkin EL, Spinosa FA, Cohen R: Nail changes in the seropositive and seronegative arthritides. Clin Podiatr Med Surg 6:389, 1989.
169. Tosti A: The nail apparatus in collagen disorders. Semin Dermatol 10:71, 1991.
170. Hamilton EBD: Nail studies in rheumatoid arthritis. Ann Rheum Dis 19:167, 1960.
171. Jaizzo JL, Gonzalez EB, Daniels JC: Red lunulae in a patient with rheumatoid arthritis. J Am Acad Dermatol 8:711, 1983.
172. Kint A, Herpe LV: Ungual anomalies in lupus erythematosus discoids. Dermatologica 153:298, 1976.
173. Narehari SR, Srinivas CR, Kelkar SK: LE-like erythema and periungual telangiectasia among coffee plantation workers. Contact Dermatitis 22:296, 1990.
174. Phelps RG, Fleischmajer R: Clinical, pathologic, and immunopathologic manifestations of the toxic oil syndrome. J Am Acad Dermatol 18:313, 1988.
175. Vaughn RY, Bailey JP, Field RS, et al: Diffuse nail dyschromia in black patients with SLE. J Rheumatol 17:640, 1990.
176. Pallis M, Hopkinson N, Powell R: Nailfold capillary density as a possible indicator of pulmonary capillary loss in systemic lupus erythematosus but not in MLTD. J Rheumatol 18:1532, 1991.
177. Su WPD, Perniciaro C, Robgers RS, White JW: Chilblain lupus erythematosus (lupus pernio): Clinical review of the Mayo Clinic experience and proposal of diagnostic criteria. Cutis 53:395, 1994.
178. Thiers BH, Dobson RL: Westwood Western Conference on clinical dermatology. J Am Acad Dermatol 3:651, 1980.
179. Caputo R, Cappio F, Rigorri C, et al: Pterygium inversum unguius. Arch Dermatol 129:1307, 1993.
180. Norton LA: The Nail. Lecture presented at Nail and Hair Symposium sponsored by Columbia University, September, 1989.
181. Odom RB, Stein KM, Maibach HI: Congenital painful aberrant hyponychium. Arch Dermatol 110:89, 1974.
182. Caputo R, Prandi G: Pterygium inversum unguium. Arch Dermatol 108:817, 1973.
183. Drake L, Goodman TB: Pterygium inversum unguium. Society transactions. Arch Dermatol 112:255, 1976.
184. Nogita T, Yamashita H, Kawashima M, Hidano A: Pterygium inversum unguis. J Am Acad Dermatol 24:787, 1991.
185. Fleischmajer R: Unusual Nail Findings. Lecture presented at the meeting of the American Dermatological Society of Allergy and Immunology, New Orleans, September,1980.
186. Sato S, Takehara K, Sama Y, et al: Diagnostic significance of nailfold bleeding in scleroderma spectrum disorders. J Am Acad Dermatol 28:198, 1993.
187. Maricq HR: Capillary abnormalities, Raynaud's phenomenon, and systemic sclerosis in patients with localized scleroderma. Arch Dermatol 128:630, 1992.
188. Barrow MV: The nails in multicentric reticulohistiocytosis. Arch Dermatol 95:200, 1967.
189. Tani M, Hori K, Nakanishi T, et al: Multicentric reticulohistiocytosis. Arch Dermatol 117:495, 1981.
190. Sahin AA, Kaloncu AF, Selouk ZT, et al: Behçet's disease with half and half nail and pulmonary artery aneurysm (letter). Chest 97:1277, 1990.
191. Greaves MS, Fieller NRJ, Moll JMH: Differentiation between psoriatic arthritis and rheumatoid arthritis: A biochemical and statistical analysis of fingernail amino acids. Scand J Rheum 8:33, 1979.
192. Maeda K, Kawaquchi S, Niwa T, et al: Identification of some abnormal metabolites in psoriasis nail using gas chromatography-mass spectrometry. J Chromatogr 221:199, 1980.
193. Rasmussen J: Childhood psoriasis in pediatric dermatology, Dermavision. Videotape presented at the meeting of the American Academy of Dermatology, Evanston, IL, December,1982.
194. Blockmans D, Vermylen J, Babhaers H: Nailfold capillaroscopy in connective tissue disorders in Raynaud's phenomenon. Acta Clin Belg 48:30, 1993.
195. Maricq HR, Spencer-Green C, LeRoy EC: Skin capillary abnormalities as indicators of organ involvement in scleroderma (systemic sclerosis), Raynaud's syndrome and dermatomyositis. Am J Med 61:862, 1976.
196. Minkin W, Rabhan NB: Office nail fold capillary mi-

croscopy using ophthalmoscope. J Am Acad Dermatol 7:190, 1982.

197. Herd JK: Nailfold capillary microscopy made easy. Arthritis Rheum 19:1370, 1976.

198. Scher RK, Tom DWK, Lally EV, et al: The clinical significance of PAS-positive deposits in cuticle–proximal nail fold biopsy specimens. Arch Dermatol 121:1406, 1985.

199. Maricq HR, Maize JC: Nailfold capillary abnormalities. Clin Rheum Dis 8:455, 1982.

200. Chanda JJ, Callen JP: Stevens-Johnson syndrome. Arch Dermatol 114:626, 1978.

201. Wanscher B, Thormann J: Permanent anonychia after Stevens-Johnson syndrome. Arch Dermatol 113:970, 1977.

202. Zaias H: Diseases of the nails. In Demis J, Dobson RL, Crounse RB (eds): Clinical Dermatology. Harper & Row, New York, 1974, pp 1–5.

203. Wheeler GE, Barrows GH: Alopecia universalis, a manifestation of occult amyloidosis and multiple myeloma. Arch Dermatol 117:815, 1981.

204. Leavell OW, Farley CH, McIntyre JS: Cutaneous changes in a patient with carbon monoxide poisoning. Arch Dermatol 99:429, 1969.

205. Kahn G: Nail involvement in histiocytosis X. Arch Dermatol 100:699, 1969.

206. Timpatanapong P, Hathirat P, Isarangkura P: Nail involvement in histiocytosis X. Arch Dermatol 120:1052, 1984.

207. Holzberg M, Wade TR, Buchana ID, et al: Nail pathology in histiocytosis X. J Am Acad Dermatol 13:522, 1985.

208. Harper JI, Staughton R: Histiocytosis X (letter). Cutis 31:493, 1983.

209. Chesney PJ, Davis JP, Purdy WK, et al: Clinical manifestations of toxic shock syndrome. JAMA 246:741, 1981.

210. Niemi KM, Kero M, Kanerva L, et al: Epidermolysis bullosa simplex. Arch Dermatol 119:138, 1983.

211. Haber RM, Hanna W, Ramsey CA, et al: Hereditary epidermolysis bullosa. J Am Acad Dermatol 13:252, 1985.

212. Main RA: Periodic shedding of the nails. Br J Dermatol 88:497, 1973.

213. Kalb RE, Grossman ME: Pterygium formation due to sarcoidosis. Arch Dermatol 121:276, 1985.

214. Dalziel KL, Telfer NR, Dawber RPR: Nail dystrophy in cutaneous T-cell lymphoma. Br J Dermatol 120:571, 1989.

215. Wilson AGM, Cotter FE, Lowe DG, et al: Mycosis fungoides in childhood: An unusual presentation. J Am Acad Dermatol 25:370, 1991.

216. Parameswara YR, Chinnappaiah RP: Onychomadesis associated with pemphigus vulgaris. Arch Dermatol 117:759, 1981.

217. Dhawan SS, Zaias N, Pena J: The nail fold in pemphigus vulgaris. Arch Dermatol 126:1374, 1990.

218. Akiyama C, Sou K, Furuya T, et al: Paronychia: A sign heralding an exacerbation of pemphigus vulgaris. J Am Acad Dermatol 29:494, 1993.

219. Richards B: A radium fingernail polish. Wall Street Journal, September 19, 1983, p 72.

220. Horan MA, Puxty JA, Fox RA: The white nails of old age (neopolitan nails). J Am Geriatr Soc 30:734, 1982.

221. Fischer VE: Subunguale verkalkungen. Fortschr Rontgenstr 137:580, 1982.

222. Wong RC, Ellis CN: Physiological skin changes in pregnancy. J Am Acad Dermatol 10:929, 1984.

223. Hansen U, Haersley T, Knudsen B, Jacobson GK: Erythema elevation diutinum: Case report showing an unusual distribution. Cutis 53:124, 1994.

224. Basuck PJ, Scher RK: Onychomycosis in graft versus host disease. Cutis 40:237, 1987.

225. Noppakun N, Swasdikul D: Reversible hyperpigmentation of skin and nails with white hair due to vitamin B_{12} deficiency. Arch Dermatol 122:896, 1986.

226. Barth JH, Telfer MB, Dawber RPR: Nail abnormalities and autoimmunity. J Am Acad Dermatol 18:1062, 1988.

227. Wieselthier JAS, Koh HK: Sezary syndrome: Diagnosis, prognosis, critical review of options. J Am Acad Dermatol 22:381, 1990.

228. Tosti A, Fanti PA, Varotti C: Massive lymphomatosis nail involvement in Sezary syndrome. Dermatologica 181:162, 1990.

229. Grimes PE: Diseases of hyperpigmentation. In Sams WM, Lynch PJ (eds): Principle and Practice of Dermatology, 2nd ed. Churchill-Livingstone, New York, 1996, pp 825-859.

230. Simon CA, Su WPD, Chin-Yang L: Subungual leukemia cutis. Int J Dermatol 29:636, 1990.

231. Lassoued K, Picard C, Danon F, et al: Cutaneous manifestations associated with gamma heavy chain disease. J Am Acad Dermatol 23:988, 1990.

232. Harrison PV, Khunti K, Morris JA: Psoriatic nails, joints and autoimmunity (letter). Br J Dermatol 122:569, 1990.

233. Zaias N: The Nail in Health and Disease, ed 2. Appleton and Lange, Norwalk, CT, 1990, pp 171–173.

234. Asherson RA: Subungual splinter haemorrhages: A new sign of the antiphospholipid coagulopathy (letter)? Ann Rheum Dis 49:268, 1990.

235. Gross NJ, Tall R: Clinical significance of splinter hemorrhages. BMJ 2:1496, 1963.

236. Zaias N, Ackerman AB: The nail in Darier-White disease. Arch Dermatol 107:193, 1973.

237. Seckler SG: A handful of pearls. Hosp Physician 12:4, 1976.

238. Robertson JC, Braune ML: Splinter hemorrhages, pitting and other findings in fingernails of healthy adults. BMJ 4:279, 1974.

239. Leyden JJ: Chromonychia. Cutis 10:161, 1972.

240. Peter RU, Brau-Falco O, Biricoukov A, et al: Chronic cutaneous damage after accidental exposure to ionizing radiation: The Chernobyl experience. J Am Acad Dermatol 30:719, 1994.

241. Lang PG: Keratosis lichenoides chronica. Arch Dermatol 117:105, 1981.

242. Pierson JC, Lawlor KB, Steck WD: Pen push purpura: Iatrogenic nail bed hemorrhage in the intensive care unit. Cutis 51:4221, 1993.

243. Kassis V, Kassis E, Thomsen HK: Benign cutaneous periarteritis nodosa with nail defects. J Am Acad Dermatol 13:661, 1985.

244. Scher RK, Daniel CR: Nail Basics: An Approach to Diagnosis (audiovisual teaching set). Year Book, Chicago, 1981.

245. Saunders CV, Saenz RE, Lopez M: Splinter hemorrhages and onycholysis—unusual reactions associated with tetracycline hydrochloride therapy. South Med J 69:1090, 1976.

246. Daoud MS, Gibson LE, DeRemef RA, et al: Cutaneous Wegener's granulomatosis: Clinical, histopathologic, and immunopathologic features of thirty patients. J Am Acad Dermatol 31:605, 1994.

247. Hickmann JW: Onycholysis associated with carcinoma of the lung. JAMA 238:1246, 1977.

248. Gentry WC: Paraneoplastic syndromes. In Sams M,

Lynch P (eds): Principles and Practice of Dermatology. Churchill-Livingstone, New York, 1990, pp 715–739.

249. Guilland V, Moulin G, Bennefoy M, et al: Photo-ony-cholyse bulleuse au cous o'une pseudoporphyriec des hemodialyses. Ann Dermatol Venereol 117:723, 1990.

250. Selem MME, Hegyi V: Pustular eruption of pregnancy treated with locally administered PUVA. Arch Dermatol 126:443, 1990.

251. Wieselthier JS, Koh HK: Sezary syndrome: Diagnosis, prognosis, critical review of options. J Am Acad Dermatol 22:381, 1990.

252. Zaun H: Leukonychias. Semin Dermatol 10:17, 1991.

253. Welter A, Michaux M, Blondeel A: Lignes de Mees dans un cas d'intoxication aigue a l'arsenic. Dermatologica 165:482, 1982.

254. Mees RA: Een verschijinsel by polyneuritis arsenicosa. Ned Tijdschr Geneeskd 1:391, 1919.

255. Scher RK, Grossman M: Leukonychia, review and classification. Int J Dermatol 29:535, 1990.

256. Marino MT: Mees' lines. Arch Dermatol 126:827, 1990.

257. Baran R, Kechijian P: Longitudinal melanonychia, diagnosis and management. J Am Acad Dermatol 21:1165, 1989.

258. Krutchik AN, Tashima CK, Buzdar AU, et al: Longitudinal nail banding associated with breast carcinoma unrelated to chemotherapy. Arch Intern Med 138:1302, 1978.

259. Arateri E, Regesta G, Rebora A: Carpal tunnel syndrome appearing with prominent skin symptoms. Arch Dermatol 120:517, 1984.

260. Bondy PK, Harwick HJ: Longitudinal banded pigmentation of nails following adrenalectomy for Cushing syndrome. N Engl J Med 281:1056, 1969.

261. Valero A, Sherf K: Pigmented nails in Peutz-Jeghers syndrome. Am J Gastroenterol 43:56, 1965.

262. Kitano K, Matsunaga E, Morimoto T, et al: A syndrome with nodular erythema, elongated and thickened fingers, and emaciation. Arch Dermatol 121:1053, 1985.

263. Bonafe JL, Pieraggi MT, Abravanel M, et al: Skin, hair and nail changes in a case of citrullinemia with late manifestation. Dermatologica 168:213, 1984.

264. Winetrobe MW, Thorne GW, Adams RD, et al: Harrison's Principles of Internal Medicine, ed 7. McGraw-Hill, New York, 1974.

265. Edwards EA: Nail changes in functional and organic arterial disease. N Engl J Med 239:362, 1948.

266. Carmel R: Hair and fingernail changes in acquired and congenital pernicious anemia. Arch Intern Med 145:484, 1985.

267. Spigel GT, Krall RA, Hilal A: Limited Wegener's granulomatosis. Cutis 32:41, 1983.

268. Bolognia JL, Brewer YP, Cooper DL: Bazex syndrome: An analytic review. Medicine 70:269, 1991.

269. Kleeberg J: Flat fingernails in cirrhosis of the liver. Lancet 261:248, 1951.

270. Duhra PM, Quigley EM, Marsh MN: Chylous ascites, intestinal lymphangiectasia and the "yellow-nail" syndrome. Gut 26:1266, 1985.

271. Gasser P, Affstter H, Schuppisser JP: The role of nailbed vasospasm in Crohn's disease. Int J Colorectal Dis 6:147, 1991.

272. Cronkhite LS, Canada WJ: Generalized gastrointestinal polyposis. N Engl J Med 252:1011, 1955.

273. Gregory B, Ho VC: Cutaneous manifestations of GI disorders: Part 1. J Am Acad Dermatol 26:153, 1992.

274. Ingregno AP, Yatto RP: Hereditary white nails (leukonychia totalis), duodenal ulcer, and gallstones. N Y State J Med 13:1797, 1982.

275. Chevrant-Breton J, Simon M, Bourel M, et al: Cutaneous manifestations of idiopathic hemochromatosis. Arch Dermatol 113:161, 1977.

276. Suda M, Ishii H, Kashiwazaki K, et al: Hyperpigmentation of skin and nails in a patient with intestinal leiomyosarcoma. Dig Dis Sci 30:1108, 1985.

277. Rudlinger R, Grob R, Yu YX, et al: Human papillomavirus 35-positive bowenoid papulosis of the onogenital area and concurrent human papillomavirus-35 positive verruca with bowenoid dysplasia of the periungual area. Arch Dermatol 125:655, 1989.

278. Valero A, Sherf K: Pigmented nails in Peutz-Jeghers syndrome. Am J Gastroenterol 43:56, 1965.

279. Bluhm JF, Johnson SC, Norback DH: Bullous amyloidosis. Arch Dermatol 116:1164, 1980.

280. Fanti PA, Tosti A, Morelli R, Galbaiti G: Nail changes as the first sign of systemic amyloidosis. Dermatologica 183:44, 1991.

281. Huntley AC: The cutaneous manifestations of diabetes mellitus. J Am Acad Dermatol 7:427, 1982.

282. Williams ML, Packman S, Cowan MJ: Alopecia and periorificial dermatitis in biotin-responsive multiple carboxylase deficiency. J Am Acad Dermatol 9:97, 1983.

283. Handley J, Walsh M, Path MRC, et al: Laryngo-ony-cho-cutaneous syndrome associated with benign hypercalcemia. J Am Acad Dermatol 29:906, 1993.

284. Colver GB, Dawber RPR: Multiple Beau's lines due to dysmenorrhea? Br J Dermatol 111:111, 1984.

285. Lang PG: The clinical spectrum of parathyroid disease. J Am Acad Dermatol 5:733, 1981.

286. Truhan AP, Roenigk HH: The cutaneous mucinoses. J Am Acad Dermatol 14:1, 1986.

287. Cheah JS, Jacob E, Yeo PPB, et al: Nail calcium, phosphate and magnesium in hyperthyroidism. Singapore Med J 23:273, 1982.

288. Heymann WR: Cutaneous manifestations of thyroid disease. J Am Acad Dermatol 26:885, 1992.

289. Duvic M: HIV associated psoriasis and Reiter's syndrome. Prog Dermatol 24:1, 1990.

290. Tosti A, Morelli R, D'Alessandro R, Bassi F: Carpal tunnel syndrome presenting with ischemic skin lesions, acrosteolysis, and nail changes. J Am Acad Dermatol 29:287, 1993.

291. Tosti A, Baran R, Peluso AM, et al: Reflex sympathetic dystrophy with prominent involvement of the nail apparatus. J Am Acad Dermatol 29:865, 1993.

292. Daniel CR, Elewski BE: Candida as a nail pathogen in healthy patients. J MS State Med Assn 36:379–381, 1995.

293. Glaser DA, Remlinger K: Blue nails and acquired immunodeficiency syndrome: Not always associated with azidothymidine use. Cutis 57:243, 1996.

294. Cohen PR: The lunula. J Am Acad Dermatol 34:943, 1996.

295. Daniel CR, Scher RK: The Nail. In Sams WM, Lynch PJ (eds): Principles and Practice of Dermatology, 2nd ed. Churchill-Livingstone, New York, 1996, pp 763–777.

296. Itin PH, Gilli L, Nuesch R, et al: Erythema of the proximal nailfold in HIV-infected patients. J Am Acad Dermatol 35:631, 1996.

297. Ruiz-Avila P, Villen A, Rodenas JM: Painful periungual telangiectasia in a patient with acquired immunodeficiency syndrome. Int J Dermatol 34:199, 1995.

298. Lizama E, Logemann H: Proximal white subungual onychomycosis in AIDS. Int J Dermatol 35:290, 1996.

299. Hordinsky MK: Hair. *In* Sams WM, Lynch PJ (eds): Principles and Practice of Dermatology, 2nd ed. Churchill-Livingstone, New York, 1996, pp 763–777.

300. Cohen PR, Prystowsky: Metabolic and nutritional disorders. *In* Sams WM, Lynch PJ (eds): Principles and Practice of Dermatology. Churchill-Livingstone, New York, 1996, pp 693–712.

301. Lynch PJ: Cutaneous signs of systemic malignancy. *In* Sams WM, Lynch PJ (eds): Principles and Practice of Dermatology. Churchill-Livingstone, New York, 1996, pp 739–746.

302. Wakelin SH, James MP: Sarcoidosis: Nail dystrophy with or without underlying bone changes. Cutis 55:344, 1995.

303. Ohtsuka T, Yamakage A, Tamura T: Image analysis of nail fold capillaries in patients with Raynaud's phenomenon. Cutis 56:215, 1995.

304. Nahass GT: Antiphospholipid antibodies and the antiphospholipid syndrome. J Am Acad Dermatol 36:149, 1997.

305. Shikano Y, Mori S, Kitajima Y: Detection of scleroderma with capillaroscopic abnormalities of nailfolds. Int J Dermatol 35:857, 1996.

CHAPTER 14

Nail Changes Secondary to Systemic Drugs and Ingestants

C. Ralph Daniel III and Richard K. Scher

Systemic drugs and ingestants may affect the nails. Changes vary from asymptomatic growth rate changes and pigmentation abnormalities to nail shedding and permanent deformity. The former two changes are most common.

The abnormalities that occur are frequently part of a symptom complex, including other cutaneous changes, especially affecting hair. Not infrequently, nail manifestations are the only apparent finding.

It is important for the practitioner to be aware of these changes or at least to have a reference available for the following reasons:

1. Nails are often of great cosmetic importance to the patient.
2. Nail changes may be an early manifestation of possibly serious side effects.
3. Nail changes may be a signal that covert systemic problems exist.
4. Awareness can prevent improper treatment regimens from being instituted.
5. The physician will be able to reassure the patient.

Systemic drugs alter the nails by affecting different parts of the nail unit. Some affect the matrix, nail bed, periungual region, hyponychial region, or some combination of these areas. As can be discerned from the tables, the clinical manifestation is usually related to the anatomic site affected. If the matrix is affected, growth rate changes and pigmentation abnormalities occur most frequently. The pattern of pigmentation is significant because it may give a clue to the cause. Matrix melanocyte stimulation and disturbance of cellular maturation are the probable mechanisms.[1]

When the nail bed, or hyponychium, is affected, onycholysis, subungual hyperkeratosis, splinter hemorrhages, and so forth may occur. These areas and the matrix are the most common targets in the nail apparatus. Photoactivated drugs such as tetracycline and methoxsalen may affect the nails in this region. Baran and Juhlin attempted to subdivide photo-onycholysis into three distinct subtypes by the pattern of nail plate–nail bed separation.[2] Photo-onycholysis has been said to occur spontaneously.[3] Ultraviolet light combines with by-products of the drug, and energy is released or cellular maturation is changed. Thus, the bond between the nail plate and nail bed may be broken, producing onycholysis and possibly pain and splinter hemorrhages. Periungual structures are not as commonly affected. When they are, paronychia, ingrowing nails, malalignment of the nail plate, and contiguous nail plate dystrophy may occur.

For the purpose of this discussion, drugs that affect the nails can be divided into five groups: antibiotics, cancer chemotherapeutic agents, poisons and ingestants, antimalarials, and miscellaneous drugs. See Chapter 12 also for further entries.

ANTIBIOTICS

Looking at Table 14–1, one can see that the tetracycline family of drugs has often been associated with nail changes. Demethylchlortetracycline and doxycycline are more likely to produce photosensitivity reactions than are other types of tetracycline. It is clear to us that phototoxicity, mediated by ultraviolet B light, is the cause of the vast majority of changes. Ultraviolet A light may also be involved but less commonly. Onycholysis and pain are encountered most commonly. Splinter hemorrhages, pigmentation changes, and so on are less common. Taking the medication at bedtime, using opaque nail polish, using a combination oxybenzone PABA-containing sunscreen with a sun protection factor of at least 15, judicious sun exposure, and patient education are the best safeguards one can implement.

There have been reports that tetracycline may cause onycholysis that is not photomediated.[4,5] We believe that more data must be available before this can be accepted as fact. It has also been reported that photo-onycholysis may occur spontaneously.[6]

Chloramphenicol has also been noted to cause onycholysis.[7,8] In general, other antibiotics, when they affect the nail, usually do so as part of a generalized drug eruption or hypersensitivity reaction. If a lesion, as a component of the drug eruption, is in the vicinity of the nail unit, one may see nail shedding, deformity, and so forth, depending on the part of the nail unit that is affected (Figs. 14–1 and 14–2).

CANCER CHEMOTHERAPEUTIC AGENTS

Table 14–2 lists cancer chemotherapeutic drugs that have been reported to affect the nails. For the most part, asymptomatic pigmentation changes and slower growth rate are the most common manifestations. Darkly pigmented nail changes appear more commonly in more heavily pigmented individuals. Matrix melanocyte stimulation is probably responsible. Cyclophosphamide and doxorubicin are the two agents most likely to affect the nails[9] (Fig. 14–3). Onycholysis and nail shedding, among others, have been reported. Muercke's lines have questionably been associated with chemotherapy.[10]

Dermatologists frequently prescribe methotrexate and 5-fluorouracil. Methotrexate usu-

Table 14–1. **ANTIBIOTICS**

Drug	Apparent Nail Change	Site of Change, Mechanism, Comments
Cephalexin[14]	Acute paronychia	Nail folds (fixed drug eruption)
Cephaloridine and cloxacillin[15]	Nail shedding	Probably nail bed matrix toxicity
Chloramphenicol[8,16]	Onycholysis	Nail bed: probable photosensitivity
Chlortetracycline[7]	Onycholysis	Nail bed: photosensitivity
Dapsone[17]	Beau's lines	After erythroderma, nail matrix
Demethylchlortetracycline[18,19,27a] (Declomycin)	Onycholysis, pain	Nail bed: photosensitivity
Doxycycline[20] (Vibramycin)	Onycholysis, pain	Nail bed: photosensitivity
Minocycline[21]	Onycholysis[22]; longitudinal brown band[23,24]; diffuse darkening[a]; hyperpigmentation, periungual involvement[25]	Nail bed: photosensitivity; biopsy revealed iron and calcium[26,27]
D-Penicillamine	Absence of lunula; longitudinal ridging; onychoschizia	
Sulfonamides	Partial leukonychia,[28] photoonycholysis,[29] Beau's lines,[29] paronychia[29]	Probable nail matrix toxicity
Tetracycline hydrochloride	1. Onycholysis	Nail bed: unassociated with ultraviolet light[4,5]
	2. Onycholysis: bluish residue[20,30]	Nail bed: photo-onycholysis
	3. Splinter hemorrhages,[31] pain, onycholysis	Nail bed: photo-onycholysis
	4. Yellow lunulae with fluorescence[32]	Deposition in lunulae or entire nail plate[33]

[a]R.K. Scher, unpublished data, 1983.

From Daniel CR III, Scher RK: Nail changes secondary to systemic drugs or ingestants. J Am Acad Dermatol 10:250, 1984. Used with permission.

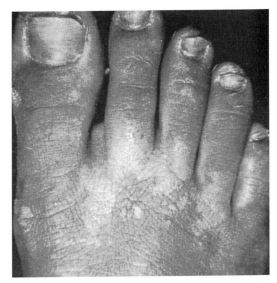

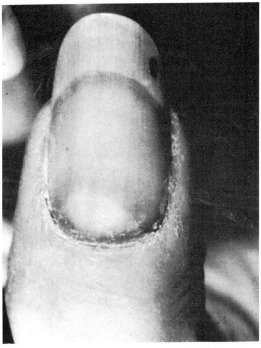

Figure 14–1. Phototoxic reaction to tetracycline hydrochloride. Opaque nails and onycholysis with nail shedding later developed. From Daniel CR III, Osment LS: Nail pigmentation abnormalities. Cutis 25:595, 1980. Used with permission.

Figure 14–2. Hyperpigmented nail, including longitudinal pigmented band, in a patient on minocycline therapy. From Daniel CR III, Scher RK: Nail changes secondary to systemic drugs or ingestants. J Am Acad Dermatol 10:250, 1984. Used with permission.

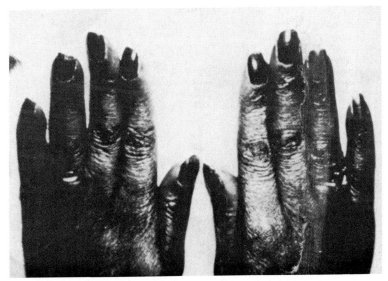

Figure 14–3. Hyperpigmented nails in a patient on doxorubicin therapy for unknown type of malignancy. From Adrian RM, Hood AF, Skarin AT: Mucocutaneous reactions to antineoplastic agents. CA 30:143, 1980. Used with permission.

Table 14–2. **CANCER CHEMOTHERAPEUTIC DRUGS**

Drug	Apparent Nail Change	Site of Change, Mechanism, Comments
Actinomycin[34]	Diffuse hyperpigmentation	? Nail matrix
Adriamycin (doxorubicin)	Onycholysis[8,35]; hyperpigmentation[9,35–38]; transverse pigmented bands[7,39,40]; longitudinal gray, brown, and black pigmented bands[40]; bluish nails[a]	Nail bed and matrix toxicity
Ametantrone[41]	Gray-blue	Unclear
Anthracycline[151]	Mees' lines	Nail plate
3-Azido-3'-deoxythymidine[42]	Longitudinal melanonychia	Matrix
Bleomycin (Blenoxane; patient also on vinblastine)[40]	Onycholysis[8,43]; dystrophy[44]; longitudinal pigmented bands[7]; shedding[45]; thickening nail bed[39]; darkening of nail cuticle[46,47]	Nail bed[40] or matrix toxicity
Bleomycin (intralesional for warts)	Dystrophy,[48] cold-sensitive distal fingers[49]; Raynaud's phenomenon[50]	
Bleomycin (intralesional)	Raynaud's phenomenon[51]	
5-Bromodeoxyuridine[52] (and radiation)	Horizontal yellow depressed bands (Beau's lines?)	? Matrix
Busulfan	Longitudinal pigmented bands[53]	? Nail matrix
Cancer chemotherapeutic drugs in general	Slow growth; sometimes Beau's lines	Matrix toxicity
	White transverse lines[54] (Mees' lines)	Combination chemotherapy (doxorubicin, cyclophosphamide, vincristine): nail plate
Cyclophosphamide (Cytoxan)	Hyperpigmentation[55]; transverse pigmented bands[7,56]; longitudinal pigmented band[56]	Nail bed and plate color change from matrix and bed toxicity[40]
Cyclosporin[57]	Faster linear growth	Matrix
Cytoxine arabinoside[57]	Periungual erythema	Nail folds
Dacarbazine (DTIC)	Hyperpigmentation[55]	Matrix toxicity
Daunorubicin	Transverse brown-black bands[40]; longitudinal pigmented bands[53]	Probable matrix toxicity
Docetaxel[152]	Onycholysis	Nail bed
Doxorubicin	Onycholysis,[58] longitudinal pigmented bands[53]	Nail bed
5-Fluorouracil (5-FU) (topical and systemic[59])	Diffuse blue superficial pigment[55]; hyperpigmentation[55]; onycholysis[7,59], other photo changes[57], diffuse brown[60], longitudinal pigmented bands[53]; dystrophy[7]; paronychial inflammation[7]; pain and thickening of nail bed[59]; transverse striations,[59] half-and-half nail–like changes[55]	Superficial blue pigment may be scraped off[55]
Ftorafur[61] (analogue of 5-FU)	Diffuse brownish	? Matrix
Genetic tendency for nail pigmentation after chemotherapy	Brownish[23,62]	Probable matrix toxicity
Hydroxyurea	Atrophic, brittle nails[45,63]; longitudinal pigmented bands[64]; diffuse pigmentation[65,155]	Nail matrix toxicity
Interferon-α[66]	Reiter's syndrome–like changes	?
Melphalan (Alkeran)	Longitudinal pigmented bands[7]	Nail bed: increase in melanin in basal melanocytes,[40] matrix toxicity
Mercaptopurine	Nail shedding[67]	Probable cytotoxic and photosensitivity effect on bed and matrix
Methotrexate	Hyperpigmentation,[55] acute paronychia,[68] increased superinfection,[69] longitudinal pigmented bands[53]	Probable matrix toxicity, periungual region
Mitozantrone[70]	Onycholysis,[70] blue,[71] black[72]	Nail bed, hyponychium
Nitrogen mustard	Hyperpigmentation,[55] longitudinal pigmented bands[53]	Probable matrix toxicity
Nitrosoureas	Hyperpigmentation,[55] longitudinal pigmented bands[53]	Probable matrix toxicity
Razoxane[73]	Beau's lines	Matrix
Tegafur[74] (analogue of 5-FU)	Longitudinal pigmented bands	? Matrix

[a]N. Esterly, personal communication, October 1982.

From Daniel CR III, Scher RK: Nail changes secondary to systemic drugs or ingestants. J Am Acad Dermatol 10:250, 1984. Used with permission.

ally causes only nail pigmentation changes and slower nail growth rate. It has more recently been reported to cause paronychial changes. As one can see from Table 14–2, 5-fluorouracil may cause numerous changes. After combination cancer chemotherapy, it is common to see subungual hemorrhage under the first and second toes as a result of trauma.[11]

POISONS AND INGESTANTS

Table 14–3 lists poisons and ingestants that cause various nail changes. Arsenic can cause a variety of nail changes, including Mees' lines. We had the opportunity to see a patient who was hospitalized for neurologic problems and incidentally had Mees' lines. Our index of suspicion was raised because of the clinical picture, and nail and hair clippings were taken and evaluated for arsenic content. It turned out that the patient as well as her father (who by then was deceased) had been poisoned with arsenic by the patient's mother. By measuring the distance from the cuticle to the leading edge of the Mees' line and knowing that the nail grows about 0.1 to 0.15 mm per day, one may ascertain approximately the tim-

Table 14–3. **POISONS AND INGESTANTS**

Drug	Apparent Nail Change	Site of Change, Mechanism, Comments
Acetylacetic acid[28]	Purpura	Nail bed–vascular damage
Aniline	Variable blue violet[75,76]	Site unclear
Arsenic	Mees' lines[23,76,154]	Matrix toxicity, probable arsenic deposition[77] in nail plate, matrix
	Onychomadesis[43]	Proximal nail bed–nail matrix toxicity
	Longitudinal brown bands[43]	Probable matrix melanocyte stimulation (matrix toxicity)
	Diffuse brown nail[78]	Probable matrix toxicity
Carbon monoxide	Cherry red nail bed and lunula[76]	Lunula, nail bed vascular changes
Diquat[81]	Leukonychia,[79] Mees' lines[80]	Probable matrix toxicity
	Transverse white bands, transverse brown bands, soft nail plate, permanent loss of one nail; hypertrophic nail plate, longitudinal pigmented bands[53]	
Fluoride[76,82] (fluorosis)	Longitudinal pigmented bands	Matrix toxicity
Fluorine[57]	Beau's lines, brittleness, onychorrhexis, transverse leukonychia	Matrix
Hydrogen selenide[83]	Transverse ridges	Matrix toxicity
Lead poisoning	Onychomadesis,[75] onychalgia,[75] hyperpigmentation[51]	Probable matrix and nail bed toxicity
	Leukonychia[28]	Probable matrix toxicity
Mercury[71,84]	Nail dystrophy (acrodynia)[67,85]; greenish-black nail discoloration, longitudinal pigmented bands[53]	Probable nail bed and matrix toxicity
	Nail shedding[79]	
Paraquat[81]	White bands, brown bands, softening nail plate, permanent loss of one nail; hypertrophic nail plate[a]	Matrix toxicity
Phosphorus[86]	Hemorrhage	Bed
Pilocarpine poisoning[28]	Leukonychia	Probable matrix toxicity
Polychlorinated biphenyls (PCBs)[1]	Flattening of nail, ingrown nail of big toe, "pigmentation"	
Selenium poisoning[87]	Horizontal white streaks, shedding of some nails	Probable matrix toxicity
Silver	Blue lunula[23,88]; bluish nail bed	Deposition of silver in sun-exposed areas[40] of matrix and bed
Sulfhydrilic acid[43]	Subungual bluish color	Vascular bed, sulfmethemoglobin
Thallium	Onychorrhexis[43]; Mees' lines[75,79]	Probable matrix toxicity
Trinitrotoluene (TNT)[76]	Purpura	Nail bed–vascular damage
Vinyl chloride[8]	Clubbing	Probably lungs with secondary nail change
	Sclerodactyly,[89] nail fold changes[89]	Nail folds,[89] distal digit[89]

[a]R. Baran, personal communication, December 1982.

From Daniel CR III, Scher RK: Nail changes secondary to systemic drugs or ingestants. J Am Acad Dermatol 10:250, 1984. Used with permission.

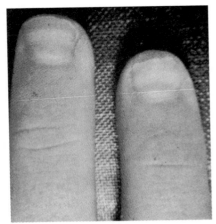

Figure 14–4. Mees' lines secondary to arsenic poisoning. From Daniel CR III, Scher RK: Nail changes secondary to systemic drugs or ingestants. J Am Acad Dermatol 10:250, 1984. Used with permission.

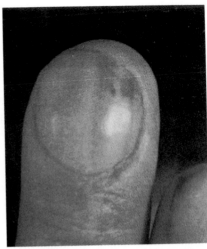

Figure 14–5. Longitudinal pigmented band appearing after antimalarial Plaquenil therapy was begun. (The patient had porphyria cutanea tarda and also mild clubbing.) From Daniel CR III, Scher RK: Nail changes secondary to systemic drugs or ingestants. J Am Acad Dermatol 10:250, 1984. Used with permission.

ing of the insult that caused the Mees' line (Fig. 14–4). Cyanide poisoning has occurred in children from the ingestion of a cosmetic nail polish remover.[12,13]

ANTIMALARIALS

Antimalarials (Table 14–4) may cause nail changes. The most common change is various kinds of pigmentation patterns. Other changes may also occur (Fig. 14–5).

MISCELLANEOUS DRUGS

Table 14–5 lists miscellaneous drugs that may cause nail changes. Of direct interest to dermatologists are methoxsalen and the vitamin A family. The former, when activated by ultraviolet A light, may cause onycholysis, splinter hemorrhages, tenderness, and nail pigmentation. The latter, especially in larger

Table 14–4. **ANTIMALARIALS**

Drug	Apparent Nail Change	Site of Change, Mechanism, Comments
Amodiaquine	Blue-brown[90] nail bed Longitudinal stripes[91] nail plate	Probable nail bed–matrix toxicity Melanin antimalarial complex[90]
Camoquin (amodiaquine)[28]	Blue-gray fluorescence in ultra-violet light	Probable nail bed–matrix toxicity,[90] melanin antimalarial complex[90]
Chloroquine	Blue-brown[90] nail bed Fluorescence in ultraviolet light[28]	Probable nail bed–matrix toxicity Melanin antimalarial combination[90]
Mepacrine	Brownish,[23] bluish color[91] Fluorescence yellow-green or white under Wood's light,[91] longitudinal pigmented bands[53]	Probable nail bed–matrix toxicity Melanin antimalarial complex[90]
Other antimalarials[29,96]	Vertical or longitudinal stripes, brownish or bluish gray	Nail bed–matrix toxicity; melanin antimalarial complex[90]
Quinacrine	Deformity, shedding[92] (may be concomitant with systemic drug reactions) Blue-gray transverse bands[93,94]; fluorescence of nails[95]; blue lunula[23,88]; longitudinal striate leukonychia[29]	Probable nail bed–matrix toxicity; melanin antimalarial complex deposition[90]
Quinine[97]	Photo-onycholysis	Nail bed

From Daniel CR III, Scher RK: Nail changes secondary to systemic drugs or ingestants. J Am Acad Dermatol 10:250, 1984. Used with permission.

Table 14–5. **MISCELLANEOUS DRUGS**

Drug	Apparent Nail Change	Site of Change, Mechanism, Comments
Acetanilid	Variable purple[75,76]	Unclear
Acetylsalicylic acid[57]	Subungual purpura	Nail bed
Acridine[98]	Whitish nail, photo-onycholysis	Nail bed
Androgen[23,55]	Half-and-half nail–like changes	Probable vascular bed
Azidothymidine[100,101]	Hyperpigmentation, slow growth,[57] diffuse pigmentation[57]	Melanin deposition[102]
Benoxaprofen	Painless onycholysis of fingernails and toenails[40a,47,56a,103–106]	Nail bed toxicity and possible matrix changes
	Possible accelerated nail growth[47]	Photosensitivity component important[107–109] but at times unclear in toenails[104]
Biotin	Accelerated nail growth[8]	Probable matrix effect
Bucillamine[153]	Yellow nail syndrome	Nail plates, nail matrix
Buspirone[110]	Thinning of nails	Nail plate
Calcium channel blockers[57]	Nail dystrophy	?
Captopril[111,112]	Onycholysis (photo)[57]	Nail bed, hyponychium
Carbamazepine[113]	Onychomadesis	Unclear
Carotene	Yellow[32,76]	Nail bed
Clofazimine[57]	Subungual hyperkeratosis, onycholysis	Nail bed
Clorazepate dipotassium[114]	Photo-onycholysis	Nail bed
Corticosteroids[57]	Mees' lines, transverse melanonychia	Nail matrix
Crack (cocaine)[38]	Acrocyanosis	Vasculature
Cystine	Accelerated nail growth[8]	Probable matrix effect
Dapsone (syndrome)[115]	Beau's lines	Matrix toxicity
Dichromates	Yellow ocher[28]	Unclear
Dicyanodiamide[23a]	Brownish appearance	Unclear
Dimercaptosuccinic acid[116]	Nail plate dystrophy	Matrix
Dinitrochlorobenzene (DNCB)[23]	Brownish appearance	Site unclear
Diphenylhydantoin[117]	Anonychia, dystrophy, hypoplasia,[118] hyperpigmentation (brown ocher),[117] longitudinal bands[53]	Congenital effect site unclear
Emetine chlorhydrate	Variable white[43,76]	Unclear
Fluoroquinolones[124]	Photo-onycholysis	Nail bed, hyponychium
Gelatin	Accelerated nail growth[8]	Probable matrix effect
Gemfibrozil (Lopid)[128]	Longitudinal pigmented bands	?
Gold (allergic reaction)[76,81]	Variable brown	Unclear
Gold salts[98]	Latent onychomadesis, longitudinal bands[53]	Nail bed
Heparin[98]	Transverse red band, slow growth[57]	Nail bed, matrix[57]
Ibuprofen[27]	Longitudinal pigmented bands	Nail plate
Ketoconazole[98]	Longitudinal brown bands; splinter hemorrhages	Nail and nail bed
L-Dopa	Accelerated nail growth[8]	Probable matrix effect
Lithium carbonate[125]	"A patient's nail changed from golden-yellow to normal color"[126] (questionable); dystrophy, psoriasis[127]	Unclear
Masoprocol (Actinex)[99]	Grayish staining	? Nail plate
Metoprolol[129]	Transverse depressions (Beau's lines)	Probable matrix toxicity
Methionine	Accelerated nail growth[8]	Probable matrix effect
Methoxsalen	Onycholysis (photo),[119] splinter hemorrhages, tenderness[120]; dark pigmentation of nail bed[121]; longitudinal melanonychia[122,123]	Nail bed and hyponychium photosensitivity
Oral contraceptive[98] (Norinyl 1[7,130] [norethindrone and mestranol])	Some reports of increased growth rate and reduced splitting and chipping; onycholysis (photo)[57]	Matrix (?), associated with porphyria cutanea tarda; probable nail bed toxicity
Parathyroid extract	Necrosis of lunulae[131]	Distal matrix toxicity
Peloprenoic acid[57]	Nail fragility	?
D-Penicillamine[99a]	Orange color (transient),[132] longitudinal ridging,[57] Beau's lines,[57] onychoschizia[57]	Unclear
Phenindione	Diffuse gray[76,133]; blue lunulae[23,88]	Unclear
Phenobarbital[134]	Hypoplasia	?
Phenolphthalein	Nail dystrophy and yellow nail syndrome[131,135]	Unclear
Phenothiazine	Variable brown[76,133]; grayish to violet,[136] photo-onycholysis,[57] longitudinal bands[53]	Nail bed,[136] especially photoexposed[29]

Table continued on following page

Table 14–5. **MISCELLANEOUS DRUGS** *Continued*

Drug	Apparent Nail Change	Site of Change, Mechanism, Comments
Phenylephrine hydrochloride (Neo-Synephrine)[23,75]	Nail bed purpura	Nail bed toxicity
Polychlorinated biphenyls (PCBs)[98]	Brown-gray lines	Nail and nail bed
Practolol[137]	Psoriasis-like onycholysis, subungual hyperkeratosis, peculiar overcurvature of nail plate with painful pincer effect (narrowing) of the distal nail bed[8,131]; ridging and subungual blotchy erythema;[7] photo-onycholysis[57]	Nail bed–hyponychial area
Propranolol	Onycholysis,[138] psoriasis-like changes[86]	Nail bed
Retinoids	Brittle nails and nail dystrophy[131]; paronychia (sometimes painful)[139,140]; friability[141]; onychorrhexis, onychoschizia, 28% acitretin patients[142]; nail shedding, granulation tissue, and ingrown nails[140,143]; Beau's lines[144]	Unclear, dose dependent[141]
Salbutamol[57]	Periungual erythema	Nail folds
Senna (chronic use) (and long-term diarrhea)[145]	Finger clubbing	Fibrovascular hyperplasia of proximal nail unit
Sodium hypochlorite	Onycholysis[146]	Nail bed, hyponychium
Thiazides[149]	Onycholysis (probably photo)	Nail bed
Timolol	Symmetric brown discoloration of fingernails and toenails,[147] longitudinal bands[53]	Unclear
Trazodone[148]	Leukonychia	Nail plate
Trypoflavine[28]	Photo-onycholysis	Nail bed
Vitamin A (large doses)	Brittle nails and nail dystrophy[131]	Unclear
Warfarin sodium[23,33,150]	Purplish appearance	Probable nail bed changes

[a]R. Baran, personal communication, December 1980.

From Daniel CR III, Scher RK: Nail changes secondary to systemic drugs or ingestants. J Am Acad Dermatol 10:250, 1984. Used with permission.

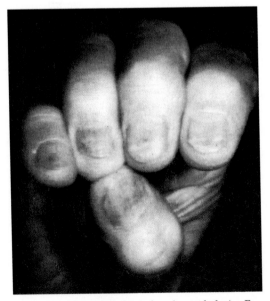

Figure 14–6. Benoxaprofen-induced onycholysis. From Daniel CR III, Scher RK: Nail changes secondary to systemic drugs or ingestants. J Am Acad Dermatol 10:250, 1984. Used with permission.

dosages, may cause brittle nails, nail "dystrophy," paronychia, ingrowing nails, and other changes (Fig. 14–6).

References

1. Urabe H, Asahi M: Past and current dermatological status of yusho patients. Am J Industr Med 5:5, 1984.
2. Baran R, Juhlin L: Drug-induced photoonycholysis. J Am Acad Dermatol 17:1012, 1987.
3. Parodi A, Guarrera M, Rebora A: Spontaneous photo-onycholysis. Photodermatology 4:160, 1987.
4. Kanwar AJ, Singh OP: Onycholysis secondary to tetracycline hydrochloride. Cutis 23:657, 1979.
5. Kestel JL: Tetracycline-induced onycholysis unassociated with photosensitivity. Arch Dermatol 106:766, 1971.
6. Hario T: Spontaneous photo-onycholysis. J Dermatol (Tokyo) 15:540, 1988.
7. Norton LA: Nail disorders. J Am Acad Dermatol 2:451, 1980.
8. Runne U, Orfanos CE: The human nail. Curr Probl Dermatol 9:102, 1981.
9. Pratt CB, Shanks EC: Hyperpigmentation of nails from doxorubicin. JAMA 228:460, 1974.
10. Schwartz RA, Vickerman CE: Muercke's lines of the fingernails. Arch Intern Med 139:242, 1979.
11. Thomsen K: Nail changes after chemotherapy. *In* Burgdorf WHC, Katz SI (eds): Dermatology Progress

and Perspectives. Parthenon Publishers, New York, 1993, p 372.

12. Geller RJ, Ekins BR, Iknoion RC: Cyanide toxicity from acetonitrile-containing false nail remover. Am J Emerg Med 9:268, 1991.

13. Losek JD, Rock AL, Boldt RR: Cyanide poisoning from a cosmetic nail remover. Pediatrics 88:337, 1991.

14. Baran R, Perrin C: Fixed drug eruptions presenting as an acute paronychia. Br J Dermatol 125:592, 1990.

15. Eastwood JB, Cutis JR, Smith EKM, et al: Shedding nails apparently induced by the administration of large amounts of cephaloridine and cloxacillin in two anephric patients. Br J Dermatol 81:750, 1969.

16. Daniel CR III, Scher RK: Nail changes secondary to systemic drugs or ingestants. J Am Acad Dermatol 10:250, 1984.

17. Patki AH, Mehta JM: Dapsone induced erythroderma with Beau's lines. Lepr Rev 60:274, 1989.

18. Carter WI: Disorders of the nails. BMJ 2:1198, 1966.

19. Orentreich N, Harber LC, Tromovitch TA: Photosensitivity and photo-onycholysis due to demethylchlortetracycline. Arch Dermatol 83:68, 1971.

20. Frank SB, Cohen HJ, Minkin W: Photoonycholysis due to tetracycline hydrochloride and doxycycline. Arch Dermatol 103:520, 1971.

21. Wolfe JD, Reichmister J: Minocycline hyperpigmentation: Skin, tooth, nail, and bone involvement. Cutis 33:457, 1984.

22. Kestel JL: Photo-onycholysis from minocycline. Cutis 28:53, 1981.

23. Daniel CR III: Nail pigmentation abnormalities: An addendum. Cutis 30:364, 1982.

24. Litt JZ: A dark streak in the nail. Diagnosis 4:23, 1982.

25. Mooney E, Bennett RG: Periungual hyperpigmentation mimicking Hutchinson's sign associated with minocycline administration. J Dermatol Surg Oncol 14:1011, 1988.

26. Gordon G, Sparans BM, Iatropoulos MJ: Hyperpigmentation of the skin associated with minocycline therapy. Arch Dermatol 121:618, 1985.

27. Scher R: Nail changes with drugs and systemic disease. Lecture presented at the Nail and Hair Symposium sponsored by Columbia University, September, 1989.

27a. Douglas AC: The deposition of tetracycline in human nails and teeth: A complication of long-term treatment. Br J Dis Chest 57:44, 1963.

28. Baran R: Modifications of colour: Chromonychias and dyschromias. In Pierre M (ed): The Nail. Churchill Livingstone, New York, 1981, pp 30–38.

29. Baran R, Temime P: Les onychodystrophies toximedicamenteuses et les onycholyses. Concours Med 95:1007, 1973.

30. Smith ZS, Scheen SR, Allen JD, et al: Argyria. Arch Dermatol 117:595, 1981.

31. Sanders CV, Rolando ES, Lopez M: Splinter hemorrhages and onycholysis: Unusual reactions associated with tetracycline hydrochloride therapy. South Med J 69:1090, 1976.

32. Hendricks AA: Yellow lunulae with fluorescence after tetracycline therapy. Arch Dermatol 116:438, 1980.

33. Feder W, Auerbach R: "Purple toes": An uncommon sequela of oral coumarin drug therapy. Ann Intern Med 55:911, 1961.

34. Vaughn RY, Bailey JP, Field RS, et al: Diffuse nail dyschromia in black patients with systemic lupus erythematosus. J Rheumatol 17:640, 1990.

35. Runne U, Mitrenga D, Pfeiff B: Braunes Nagelbett, Onycholyse und Hautveranderungen durch Adriamycin und Bleomycin. Z Hautkr 55:1590, 1980.

36. Adrian RM, Hood AF, Skarin AT: Mucocutaneous reactions to antineoplastic agents. CA Cancer J Clin 30:143, 1980.

37. Alagaratnam TT, Choi TK, Ong GB: Doxorubicin and hyperpigmentation. Aust N Z J Surg 52:531, 1982.

38. Rojas AR: Pigmentacion de unas por doxorrubicina. Dermatol Esp 3:37, 1978.

39. Giacobetti R, Esterly NB, Morgan ER: Nail hyperpigmentation secondary to therapy with doxorubicin. Am J Dis Child 135:317, 1981.

40. Granstein RD, Sober AJ: Drug and heavy metal-induced hyperpigmentation. J Am Acad Dermatol 5:1, 1981.

40a. Griest MC, Norins AL: Benoxaprofen: A new arthritis medication that causes phototoxicity (letter). J Am Acad Dermatol 5:689, 1982.

41. Hendrix JD, Greer KE: Cutaneous hyperpigmentation caused by systemic drugs. Int J Dermatol 31:458, 1992.

42. Tosti A, Gaddoni G, Fanti PA, et al: Longitudinal melanonychia induced by 3'azidodeoxythymidine. Dermatologica 180:217, 1990.

43. DeNicola P, Morsiari M, Zavagli G: Nail Diseases in Internal Medicine. Charles C Thomas, Springfield, IL, 1974.

44. Yagoda A, Mukherji B, Young C, et al: Bleomycin: An antitumor antibiotic. Ann Intern Med 77:861, 1972.

45. Dunagin WG: Clinical toxicity of chemotherapeutic agents: Dermatologic toxicity. Semin Oncol 9:14, 1982.

46. Bronner AK, Hood AF: Cutaneous complications of chemotherapeutic agents. J Am Acad Dermatol 9:645, 1983.

47. Fenton DA, English JS, Wilkinson JD: Reversal of male-pattern baldness, hypertrichosis and accelerated hair and nail growth in patients receiving benoxaprofen. BMJ 284:1228, 1982.

48. Miller RAW: Nail dystrophy following intralesional injections of bleomycin for a periungual wart. Arch Dermatol 120:963, 1984.

49. Bovednmyer DA: Cold-sensitive fingers from bleomycin. Schoch Lett 34:31, 1984.

50. Epstein E: Persisting Raynaud's phenomenon following intralesional bleomycin treatment of finger warts. J Am Acad Dermatol 13:468, 1985.

51. Zhu WY, Xia MY, Huang SD, Du D: Hyperpigmentation of the nail from lead deposition. Int J Dermatol 28:273, 1989.

52. McCuaig, Ellis CN, Greenberg HS, et al: Mucocutaneous complications of intraarterial 5-bromodeoxyuridine and radiation. J Am Acad Dermatol 21:1235, 1989.

53. Baran R, Keshijian P: Longitudinal melanocytes: Diagnosis and management. J Am Acad Dermatol 21:1165, 1989.

54. James WD, Odom RB: Chemotherapy-induced transverse white lines in the fingernails. Arch Dermatol 119:334, 1983.

55. Nixon DW, Pirozzi D, York RM, et al: Dermatologic changes after systemic cancer therapy. Cutis 27:181, 1981.

55a. Kirkham N, Holt S: Nail dystrophy after practolol. Lancet 2:1137, 1976.

56. Markenson AL, Chandra M, Miller DR: Hyperpigmentation after cancer chemotherapy. Lancet 2:128, 1975.

56a. Kligman AM, Kaidbey KH: Photosensitivity to benoxaprofen. Eur J Rheumatol Inflamm 5:124, 1982.

57. Tosti A, Baran R, Dawber RPR: The nail in systemic diseases and drug-induced changes. In Baran R,

Dawber RPR (eds): Diseases of the Nails and their Management, ed 2. Blackwell Scientific, Oxford, England, 1994, pp 175–261.

58. Curran CF: Onycholysis in doxorubicin-treated patients (letter). Arch Dermatol 126:1244, 1990.

59. Katz ME, Hansen TW: Nail plate-nail bed separation: An unusual side effect of systemic fluorouracil administration. Arch Dermatol 115:860, 1979.

60. Perlin E, Ahlgren JD: Pigmentary effects from the protracted infusion of 5-fluorouracil. Int J Dermatol 30:43, 1991.

61. Del-Pozo LJ, Vilalla J, Jimeno M, et al: Skin and ungual pigmentation caused by Ftorafur. Med Cutan Ibero Lat Am 18:78, 1990.

62. Sulis E, Floris G: Nail pigmentation following cancer chemotherapy: A new genetic entity? Eur J Cancer 15:1517, 1980.

63. Kennedy RJ, Smith LR, Goltz RW: Skin changes secondary to hydroxyurea therapy. Arch Dermatol 111:183, 1975.

64. Vomvouras S, Pakula AS, Shaw JM: Multiple pigmented bands during hydroxyurea therapy: An uncommon finding. J Am Acad Dermatol 24:1016, 1991.

65. Gropper CA, Don PC, Sadjadi MM: Nail and skin hyperpigmentation associated with hydroxyurea for polycythemia vera. Int J Dermatol 32:731, 1993.

66. Cleveland MG, Mallory SB: Incomplete Reiter's syndrome induced by systemic interferon alpha treatment. J Am Acad Dermatol 29:788, 1993.

67. Baker H: Drug reactions. In Rook A, Wilkinson DS, Ebling FJG (eds): Textbook of Dermatology, ed 3. Blackwell Scientific, Oxford, England, 1979, pp 1111–1140.

68. Wantzin GL, Thomsen K: Acute paronychia after high-dose methotrexate therapy. Arch Dermatol 119:623, 1983.

69. Delaunay M: Effets cutanes indesirable de la chemiotherapie antitumorale. Ann Dermatol Venereol 116:347, 1989.

70. Speechly-Dick ME, Owen ERTC: Mitozantrone-induced onycholysis. Lancet 1:113, 1988.

71. Scheithauer W, Ludwig H, Kotz R, Depisch D: Mitoxantrone-induced discoloration of the nails. Eur J Cancer Clin Oncol 25:763, 1989.

72. Kumar L, Kochipillai A: Mitoxantrone induced hyperpigmentation (letter). N Z Med J 103:55, 1990.

73. Tucker WFG, Church RE, Hallam R: Beau's lines after razoxane therapy for psoriasis. Arch Dermatol 120:1140, 1984.

74. Llistosella E, Codina A, Alvarez R, et al: Tegafur-induced acral hyperpigmentation. Cutis 48:205, 1991.

75. Castello VP, Pardo OA: Diseases of the Nails, ed 3. Charles C Thomas, Springfield, IL, 1960.

76. Daniel CR III, Osment LS: Nail pigmentation abnormalities: Their importance and proper examination. Cutis 25:595, 1980.

77. Althause TL, Gunther L: Acute arsenic poisoning. JAMA 92:2002, 1929.

78. Madorsky DD: Arsenic in dermatology. J Assoc Milit Dermatol 3:19, 1977.

79. Birmingham DJ: Cutaneous reactions to chemicals in dermatology. In Fitzpatrick TB, Eisen AZ, Wolf K, et al (eds): Dermatology in General Medicine, ed 2. McGraw-Hill, New York, 1979, pp 995–1006.

80. Leavell UW, Farley CH, McIntyre JS: Cutaneous changes in a patient with carbon monoxide poisoning. Arch Dermatol 99:429, 1969.

81. Samman PD: The Nails in Disease, ed 2. Charles C Thomas, Springfield, IL, 1972.

82. Bisht DB, Singh SS: Pigmented bands on nails: A new sign of malnutrition. Lancet 1:507, 1962.

83. Alderman LC, Bergin JJ: Hydrogen selenide poisoning: An illustrative case with review of the literature. Arch Environ Health 41:354, 1986.

84. Bockers M, Wagner R, Oster O: Nail dyschromia as the leading symptom in chronic mercury poisoning caused by a cosmetic bleaching preparation. Z Hautkr 15:821, 1985.

85. Wustner H, Orfanos CE: Nail changes and hair loss: Cardinal signs of mercury poisoning from hair bleaches. Dtsch Med Wochenschr 100:1694, 1975, cited by Samman PD: The Nails in Disease, ed 3. William Heinemann, London, 1978.

86. Baran R, Dawber RPR: Physical signs. In Baran R, Dawber RPR (eds): Diseases of the Nails and Their Management, ed 2. Blackwell Scientific, Oxford, England, 1994, pp 35–80.

87. Centers for Disease Control: Morbidity and mortality report. JAMA 251:1938, 1984.

88. Koplon BS: Azure lunulae due to argyria. Arch Dermatol 94:333, 1966.

89. Rycroft RJG, Baran R: Occupational abnormalities and contact dermatitis. In Baran R, Dawber RPR (eds): Diseases of the Nails and their Management, ed 2. Blackwell Scientific, Oxford, England, 1994, pp 35–80.

90. Zaias N, Baden HP: Disorders of nails. In Fitzpatrick TB, Eisen AZ, Wolf K, et al (eds): Dermatology in General Medicine, ed 2. McGraw-Hill, New York, 1979, pp 418–436.

91. Samman PD: The Nails in Disease, ed 3. William Heinemann, London, 1978.

92. Bauer F: Quinacrine hydrochloride drug eruption (tropical lichenoid dermatitis). J Am Acad Dermatol 4:239, 1981.

93. Barr JF: Subungual pigmentation following prolonged atabrine therapy. US Navy Med Bull 43:924, 1944.

94. Modny C, Barondess JA: Nail pigmentation secondary to quinacrine. Cutis 11:789, 1973.

95. Kierland RR, Sheard C, Mason HL, et al: Fluorescence of nails from quinacrine hydrochloride. JAMA 13:809, 1946.

96. Bailin PL, Matkaluk RM: Cutaneous reactions to rheumatological drugs. Clin Rheum Dis 8:493, 1982.

97. Tan SV, Berth-Jones J, Burns DA: Lichen planus and photo-onycholysis induced by quinine (letter). Clin Exp Dermatol 14:335, 1989.

98. Baran R, Dawber RPR: Diseases of the Nail and Their Management. Blackwell Scientific, Oxford, England 1984.

98a. Zamora-Quezeda JC: Muscle and skin infarction after free-basing cocaine (crack). Ann Intern Med 108:564, 1988.

99. Hart M: Grey staining of fingernails and flat wear with Actinex. Schoch Letter 43:34, 1993.

99a. Bjellerup M: Nail changes induced by penicillamine. Acta Derm Venereol (Stockh) 69:339, 1989.

100. Antoni AM, Mallolas J, Gatell J, et al: Zidovudine-induced nail pigmentation. Arch Dermatol 124:1570, 1988.

101. Furth PA, Kazakis AM: Nail pigmentation changes associated with azidothymidine (zidovudine). Ann Intern Med 107:350, 1987.

102. Valencia ME, Pikntado V, Lavilla P, Aguado A: Ungual blue striae, HIV and zidovudine: What is their etiology? (letter). Rev Clin Esp 185:167, 1989.

103. Fenton D: Side effects of benoxaprofen. BMJ 284:1631, 1982.

104. Hindson C, Daymond T, Diffey B, et al: Side effects of benoxaprofen. BMJ 284:1368, 1982.
105. Mikulaschek WM: Long-term safety of benoxaprofen. J Rheumatol 7:100, 1984.
106. Shedden WIH: Side effects of benoxaprofen. BMJ 284:1630, 1982.
107. Griest MC, Ozois II, Ridolfo AS, et al: The phototoxic effects of benoxaprofen and their management and prevention. Eur J Rheumatol Inflamm 5:138, 1982.
108. McCormack LS, Elgart ML, Turner ML: Benoxaprofen-induced photo-onycholysis. J Am Acad Dermatol 7:678, 1982.
109. Mikulaschek WM: An update on long-term efficacy and safety with benoxaprofen. Eur J Rheumatol Inflamm 5:206, 1982.
110. Barnhart ER: Physicians' Desk Reference. Medical Economics Inc, Oradell, NJ, 1989.
111. Borfders JV: Captopril and onycholysis. Ann Intern Med 105:305, 1986.
112. Brueggemeyer CD, Ramirez G: Onycholysis associated with captopril. Lancet 1:1352, 1984.
113. Mishra D, Singh G, Pandey SS: Possible carbamazepine-induced reversible onychomadesis. Int J Dermatol 28:460, 1989.
114. Torras H, Mascaro JM Jr, Mascaro JM: Photo-onycholysis caused by clorazepate dipotassium. J Am Acad Dermatol 21:1304, 1989.
115. Kromann NP, Vilhelmsen R, Stahl D: The dapsone syndrome. Arch Dermatol 118:531, 1982.
116. Thomas G, Fournier L, Garnier R, et al: Nail dystrophy and dimercaptosuccinic acid. J Toxicol Clin Exp 7:285, 1987.
117. Johnson RB, Goldsmith LA: Dilantin digital defects. J Am Acad Dermatol 5:191, 1982.
118. Hanson JW, Smith DW: The fetal hydantoin syndrome. J Pediatr 87:285, 1975.
119. Baran R, Barthelemy H: Photo-onycholysis caused by 5-MCP (Psoraderm) and the imputation method of drug effects. Ann Dermatol Venereol 112:367, 1990.
120. Zala L: Photo-onycholysis induced by 8-methoxypsoralen. Dermatologica 154:203, 1977.
121. Naik RPC, Singh G: Nail pigmentation due to oral 8-methoxypsoralen. Br J Dermatol 100:229, 1979.
122. MacDonald KJ, Ead RD: Longitudinal melanonychia during photochemotherapy. Br J Dermatol 114:395, 1986.
123. Weiss E, Sayegh-Carreno: Purva induced pigmented nails. Int J Dermatol 28:188, 1989.
124. Baran R, Brun P: Photoonycholysis induced by the fluoroquinolones pefloxacine and ofloxacine. Dermatologica 173:185, 1986.
125. Don PC, Silverman RA: Nail dystrophy caused by lithium carbonate. Cutis 41:19, 1988.
126. Hooper JF: Lithium carbonate and toenails. Am J Psychiatr 138:1519, 1981.
127. Rudolph RI: Lithium-induced psoriasis of the fingernails. J Am Acad Dermatol 26:135, 1992.
128. Klein ME: Linear lateral black nail discoloration after months on Lopid. Schach Lett 40:29, 1990.
129. Graeber CW, Lapkin RA: Metoprolol and alopecia. Cutis 28:633, 1981.
130. Bryden JP: Contraceptive pill-induced porphyria cutanea tarda presenting with onycholysis of fingernails. Postgrad Med J 52:535, 1976.
131. Krebs A: Drug-induced nail disorders. Praxis 70:1951, 1981.
132. Degowin EL, Degowin RL: The nails. In Degowin EL, Degowin RL (eds): Bedside Diagnostic Examination, ed 2. Macmillan, New York, 1969, pp 644–653.
133. Norton LA: Disorders of the nails. In Degowin EL, Degowin RL (eds): Moschella SL, Pillsbury DM, Hurley HJ (eds): Dermatology. WB Saunders, Philadelphia, 1975, pp 1222–1235.
134. Holder M, Mijewski F, Lenard HG: Hypoplasie der Nagel und Endphalangen als Folge Pranataler Barbiturat Exposition. Monatsschr Kinderheilkd 138:34, 1990.
135. Lubach D, Marghescu S: Yellow-nail syndrome durch D-penizillamin. Hautzart 30:547, 1979.
136. Santanove A: Pigmentation due to phenothiazines in high and prolonged doses. JAMA 191:263, 1965, cited by Granstein RD, Sober AJ: Drug- and heavy-metal-induced hyperpigmentation. J Am Acad Dermatol 6:1, 1981.
137. Pines A, Olchousky D, Bregman J, et al: Finger clubbing associated with laxative abuse. J South Med Assoc 76:1071, 1983.
138. Zaias N: The Nail in Health and Disease, ed 2. Appleton & Lange, Norwalk, CT, 1990, p 169.
139. Voorhees JJ, Orfanos CE: Oral retinoids. Arch dermatol 117:418, 1981.
140. Baran R: Action therapeutique et complications du retinoide aromatique sur l'appareil ungueal. Ann Dermatol Venereol (Paris) 109:367, 1982.
141. Kaplan RP, Russell DH, Lowell NJ: Etretinate therapy for psoriasis: Clinical response, remission times, epidermal DNA and polyamine responses. J Am Acad Dermatol 8:95, 1983.
142. Saurat JH, Lefranca H, Geiger JM: European experience with acitretin in psoriasis and various disorders of keratinization. Poster presented at the annual meeting of the American Academy of Dermatology San Francisco, December 8, 1993.
143. Campbell JP, Grekin RC, Ellis CN, et al: Retinoid therapy is associated with excess granulation tissue responses. J Am Acad Dermatol 9:708, 1983.
144. Ferguson MM, Simpson NB, Hammersley N: Severe nail dystrophy associated with retinoid therapy. Lancet 2:974, 1983.
145. Levine D, Goode AW, Wingate DL: Purgative abuse associated with reversible cachexia, hypogammaglobulinemia and finger clubbing. Lancet 1:919, 1981, cited by Editors: Finger clubbing associated with purgative abuse. Modern Medicine 153, 1981.
146. Coskey RJ: Onycholysis from sodium hypochloride. Arch Dermatol 109:96, 1974.
147. Feiler-Ofry V, Godel V, Lazar M: Nail pigmentation following timolol maleate therapy. Ophthalmologica 182:153, 1981.
148. Longstreth GF, Herhman J: Trazodone-induced hepatotoxicity and leukonychia. J Am Acad Dermatol 13:149, 1985.
149. Krull E: Cited by Baran R, Dawber RPR: Diseases of the Nail and Their Management. Blackwell Scientific, Oxford, England, 1984, pp 441–445. Malignant melanoma.
150. Lebsack CA, Weilbert RT: "Purple toes" syndrome. Postgrad Med 71:81, 1982.
151. Eagle K: Images in clinical medicine: Transverse leukonychia. N Engl J Med 333:98, 1995.
152. Von Hoff DD, McCullough ML, Kuhn J, et al: Acute cutaneous reactions to docetaxel, a new chemotherapeutic agent. Arch Dermatol 131:202, 1995.
153. Ishizaki C, Sueki H, Kohsokabe S: Yellow nail indiced by bucillamine. Int J Dermatol 34:493, 1995.
154. Quecedo E, San Martin O, Febrer MI, et al: Mees' lines. Arch Dermatol 132:350, 1996.
155. Kuong YL: Hydroxyurea-induced nail pigmentation. J Am Acad Dermatol 35:275, 1996.

CHAPTER 15

Tumors

Lawrence A. Norton

Tumors of the nail may be categorized as benign, premalignant or transitional, and malignant. Any portion of the nail unit may be the primary site of these tumors, except for the nail plate. The nail plate, however, will often become deformed or destroyed by the tumor growth, and in a similar fashion adjacent bone may show alterations. No tumor is unique to the nail, but neoplasms in this area may have very different clinical courses, biologic behavior, and histologic features from the same tumors located elsewhere in the body.

Diagnosis of both benign and malignant tumors of the nail tends to be delayed because of altered or indistinct morphology. In the case of nail bed tumors, the nail plate obscures morphology. Elevation of the nail plate by the tumor (onycholysis) may allow for secondary invasion of pigment-producing bacteria or fungi, further clouding the clinical picture. Nail fold infection is often present and may be mistakenly diagnosed as primary rather than secondary. Finally, because of the location of nails, they are subject to repeated trauma, and alterations in physical appearance are all too often attributed by the patient to an injury that ultimately proves to be insignificant.

A high index of suspicion is necessary to shorten delay in diagnosis. All presumptive tumors, treatment failures, and persistent infections should have x-ray studies to rule out

bone origin or involvement. Adequate biopsy of diseased tissue is necessary and should be accompanied by a differential diagnosis and request for special stains to be sent to the pathologist.

Table 15–1 lists the most common tumors of the nail unit and neighboring tissues. Some of these tumors have a clinical appearance that is reliable enough to justify treatment before tissue diagnosis is obtained. This does not pertain to nail bed tumors in which a nonspecific appearance usually requires histologic diagnosis before treatment is decided on. The recent advance of magnetic resonance imaging (MRI) allows for differential diagnosis and localization of some nail bed tumors before invasive biopsy. This is particularly helpful when bone changes are not visible on conventional x-ray film.[1,2]

BENIGN TUMORS

Warts

Warts that involve the proximal or lateral nail folds and that do not extend into the corresponding groove represent no particular treatment problem. However, warts involving the subungual region or extending into the lateral or proximal nail grooves are the most dif-

Table 15–1. **TUMORS OF THE NAIL UNIT**

Benign Warts Molluscum contagiosum Mucous cyst Eccrine poroma Giant cell tumor of tendon sheath Glomus tumor Pyogenic granuloma Periungual fibroma Recurrent digital fibrous tumor of childhood Dermatofibroma[115] Histiocytoid hemangioma[116] Onychomatrixoma[117] **Premalignant or Transitional** Actinic keratosis Bowen's disease Keratoacanthoma Arsenical keratosis Radiodermatitis **Malignant** Basal cell epithelioma Squamous cell epithelioma Melanoma Fibrosarcoma Metastatic	Acquired digital fibrokeratoma Supernumerary digit Exostosis Enchondroma Osteochondroma Epidermoid cyst Epidermal cyst Neuroma Neurofibroma Epithelioma cuniculatum[118] Porocarcinoma (malignant eccrine poroma)[119] Chondrosarcoma Epithelioid leiomyosarcoma[120] Lymphomas[121,122]

ficult warts to eliminate on the body (Fig. 15–1). If the patient is a nail biter with multiple digits involved, the number of treatments and time before cure increase geometrically. With small warts (2 to 3 mm) in either location, simple destruction by electrodesiccation or

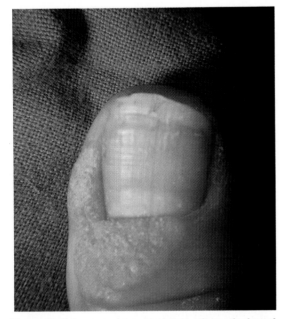

Figure 15–1. Large periungual wart involving the lateral and proximal nail grooves. It is unusually difficult to cure.

cryosurgery may be all that is required. In the subungual location, the nail plate should be cut back to reveal the most proximal portion of the wart. More extensive warts in these two locations have a high incidence of recurrence. A simple treatment that usually reduces the size of the warts and may eliminate them is occlusion of the warts with tape for 6 days a week.[3] Salicylic acid plaster may be added for part of the occlusion time. In the author's experience, the most successful treatment approach in resistant cases is the combination of intralesional bleomycin sulfate (Blenoxane) and cryotherapy.[4] Specifically, 0.1 to 0.2 mL of a 0.01 per cent solution of bleomycin is injected intralesionally into the wart with or without prior local anesthesia, followed by 10 seconds of liquid nitrogen application. Several series have reported success in using intralesional bleomycin alone with a cure rate of up to 71.4 per cent.[5–8] The patient should be informed that this is not a Food and Drug Administration–approved use of the drug, and potential side effects should be explained. The lesion turns black in 4 to 5 days, and the necrotic material is dissected away 10 to 14 days later. Alternative treatments for these difficult warts are carbon dioxide laser vaporization,[9] immunotherapy with dinitrochlorobenzene, or squaric acid dibutyl ester[10] and intralesional recombinant interferon alfa-2.[11]

Molluscum Contagiosum

Molluscum contagiosum, a viral growth, occurs less often than warts around the nail and in general responds to treatment by simple local destruction. The author has never encountered this tumor in the subungual location.

Mucous Cysts (Myxoid, Mucoid, Myxomatous Cyst, Focal Mucinosis)

Next to warts, mucous cysts are the most common ungual tumor. They may be either peri- or subungual, but the most common location is the dorsum of the distal digit between the distal interphalangeal joint and the proximal nail fold. The tumor presents as a smooth, flesh-colored to pink nodule that is semitranslucent and compressible. A high percentage of them are associated with some evidence of osteoarthritis in the joint. This lesion represents a localized degenerative tissue reaction that results in the production of a clear, viscous fluid. This mass usually impinges on the nail matrix, producing a longitudinal groove and thinning of the nail plate (Fig. 15–2). Some connect to the joint space and others do not. The nonconnecting variety are most likely to respond to simpler treatments,

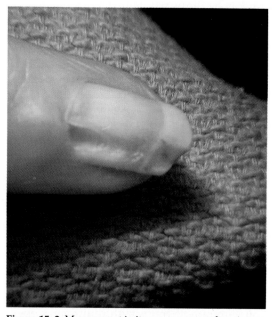

Figure 15–2. Mucous cyst in its most common location exerting pressure on the matrix, resulting in a grooved nail plate.

which include repeated evacuation of the contents with a needle,[12] injection of corticosteroids intralesionally,[13] curettage and electrodesiccation, or cryosurgery.[14,15] A newer technique is the use of an intralesional sclerosing solution such as sodium tetradecyl sulfate.[16] If they connect to the joint, complete excision will probably be required, usually followed by a graft or rotation flap to close the defect. An alternate approach is the marsupialization technique,[17] which involves excision of the entire proximal nail fold and allowance of wound healing by secondary intention. With the steroid injection procedure, the mucinous material is first evacuated and then the cavity and base are injected with triamcinolone acetonide, 5 mg/mL, the volume depending on the size of the cyst, but usually 0.1 to 0.2 mL. With cryotherapy, a 15- to 20-second application is recommended, creating an ice front 2 to 3 mm beyond the margins of the cyst with a thaw time of about 60 seconds. Again, the cyst should be emptied first. Sclerosants such as sodium tetradecyl sulfate have been used successfully by intralesional technique.[16]

Glomus Tumor

Encapsulated glomus tumors of the arteriovenous anastomosis of the digital dermis occur most often in the nail bed. These hamartomatous growths are the result of hyperplasia of the normal neuromyoarterial glomus body.[18] They are usually solitary but may be multiple and hereditary sometimes associated with von Recklinghausen's neurofibromatosis.[19,20] The clinical picture is quite characteristic, with a bluish-red discoloration visible through the nail plate (Fig. 15–3) plus pain and tenderness aggravated by direct pressure, heat, and cold exposure.[21] Warmth can sometimes relieve the pain. The pain is very sharply localized and Love's pin test using pressure with the head of a straight pin can be used to differentiate other causes of pain from pressure.[18,22,23] Sometimes application of a tourniquet to the involved extremity will relieve pain (Hildreth test).[22,24] Finally, avulsion of the nail has been advocated as a diagnostic test.[25] The differential diagnosis includes neuroma, causalgia, mucous cyst, Raynaud's phenomenon, neurofibroma, gout, and other forms of arthritis.[18]

In spite of symptomatology, signs, and clinical tests, localization of the tumor may often be difficult. Standard x-ray films are fre-

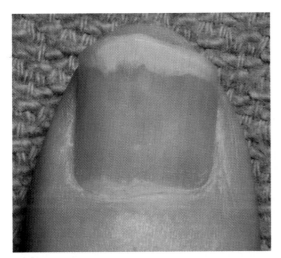

Figure 15–3. Glomus tumor. Note bluish hue in the distal nail bed.

quently negative, and, although ultrasonography has been successful in digital tumors away from the nail unit, it is less helpful in the subungual location. The diagnostic test of choice at this time appears to be MRI. This not only is capable of localizing tumors as small as 1 mm but also can differentiate other subungual tumors by their different MRI characteristics.[26–29] This increased diagnostic accuracy will lower the incidence of misdirected surgery, unnecessary psychotherapy, and delayed diagnosis and may also help the surgeon in determining the margins of the tumor and the presence of recurrence if it has been incompletely removed.[22]

Treatment consists of complete surgical removal, sparing as much normal tissue as possible. Laser has been used successfully in multiple glomus tumors.[30]

Pyogenic Granuloma

Pyogenic granuloma is probably the third most common tumor of the nail. It represents an overgrowth of vascular tissue usually secondary to trauma or infection, most often a pulled hangnail or an ingrown nail. It is reddish black and friable, and it bleeds easily (Figs. 15–4 and 15–5). In spite of a very typical appearance, a tissue specimen should be obtained before destruction because melanoma may sometimes mimic this tumor. Because of this, the author prefers curettage and electrodesiccation instead of cryotherapy. Silver nitrate application alone is apt to be inadequate treatment and leaves unsightly stains.

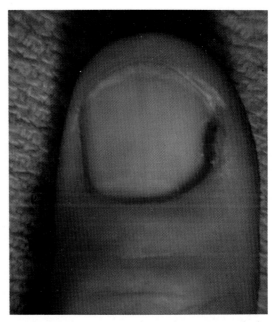

Figure 15–4. Pyogenic granuloma after trauma to the lateral nail fold.

Fibromas

A number of fibromatous tumors have been described in the nail region, including acquired digital fibrokeratomas (Fig. 15–6),[31,32] periungual fibromas, recurrent digital fibrous tumor of childhood,[33,34] garlic clove fibroma,

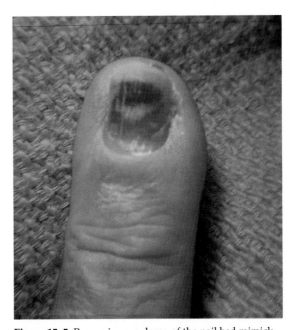

Figure 15–5. Pyogenic granuloma of the nail bed mimicking hematoma or melanoma.

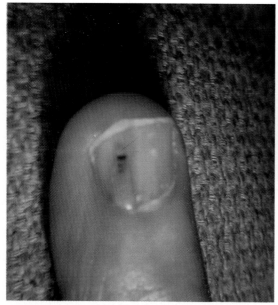

A

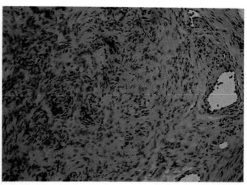

B

Figure 15–6. *A,* Acquired digital fibrokeratoma emerging from the proximal nail fold. *B,* Histology of *A* showing coarse collagen bundles and numerous connective tissue cells. The acanthotic epidermal covering is not visible in this section.

and dermatofibromas.[35] It is important to recognize periungual fibromas as a frequent marker of tuberous sclerosis and to be aware that the histology of recurrent digital fibrous tumor of childhood usually shows intracytoplasmic inclusion bodies.[33,34] Trauma appears to play a role in some of these. Treatment represents very little difficulty, and simple excision is very successful. The clinical differential diagnosis should include supernumerary digit, which can usually be distinguished histologically.

Giant cell tumors of the tendon sheath are usually on the ventral or dorsal surface of the digit but may present in the region of the lateral nail fold (Fig. 15–7). In this location, periodic inflammation and drainage may occur.

Exostosis, Enchondroma, Osteochondroma, and Epidermoid Cyst

Exostosis, enchondroma, osteochondroma, and epidermoid cyst are four benign tumors of the subungual region that involve the bone first and the nail plate secondarily. X-ray films of these lesions should be taken before biopsy, because the appearance may be characteristic enough to allow for definitive surgery initially. Table 15–2 lists the most common x-ray findings as well as some of the clinical features that aid in the differential diagnosis.[36–39] In early lesions of exostosis before the tumor is ossified, x-rays may be negative.[40] Exostosis is rare in the upper extremities, occurring mainly on the great toe.[41–47] All of these tumors produce pain with or without a visible

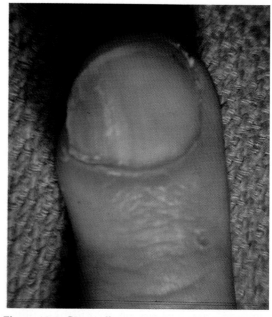

Figure 15–7. Giant cell tumor of the tendon sheath presenting lateral to the usual location on the dorsum of the digit.

Table 15–2. **DIFFERENTIAL DIAGNOSIS OF EXOSTOSIS, OSTEOCHONDROMA, ENCHONDROMA, AND EPIDERMOID CYST**

Tumor	Sex	Rate of Growth	X-Ray Findings
Exostosis	Female > male 2:1	Slow	Trabeculated bony growth with expanded distal portion covered with radiolucent fibrocartilage
Osteochondroma	Male > female 2:1	Slow	Broad-based sessile bony growth
Enchondroma	Male = female	Rapid	Loculated radiolucent cyst with flecks of calcification and surrounding bone expansion
Epidermoid cyst	Male > female 2:1	Rapid	Lucent cyst; no calcification

From Norton LA: Nail disorders. J Am Acad Dermatol 2:457, 1980. Used with permission.

mass. Epidermoid cyst (traumatic cyst, epithelial implantation cyst)[48] arising from the distal phalanx following trauma should not be confused with subungual epidermal cysts,[49] otherwise referred to as epidermal buds.[50] The latter arise in the dermis, are usually microscopic in size, and are asymptomatic. Although exostoses have been excised successfully as an office procedure,[44] I believe all four of the just-mentioned tumors should be excised under operating room conditions, and in some cases a bone graft is needed. (For further discussion, illustrations and classification of subungual exostosis, see Chapter 20.)

PREMALIGNANT AND TRANSITIONAL TUMORS

Actinic keratoses occur on the dorsum of the fingers and probably are present in the nail bed, but little reference to this is made in the literature. In contradistinction, numerous cases of Bowen's disease and squamous cell cancer of the nail bed have been reported. Furthermore, actinic alterations have been noted in the nail bed elastic tissue,[51] suggesting that the nail plate does not serve as an effective sunscreen. Studies by Parker and Diffey[52] disagree with this hypothesis. These researchers measured the transmission of radiation through toenails with a monochrometer and showed 0 to 25 per cent transmission in the sunburn spectrum, depending on thickness of the nail. Transmission in the longer wavelengths is considerably greater, probably accounting for the photo-onycholysis associated with light exposure plus tetracycline, psoralens, and more recently benoxaprophen. It may be that relatively small amounts of transmission are all that is necessary for photodamage and phototoxicity. Baran and Gormley,[53] in discussing three cases of polydactylous Bowen's disease of the nail, theorized that radiation effects probably begin in the nail folds and extend subungually. This in fact is the usual clinical picture.

Other factors that may contribute to premalignant and superficial malignant nail bed lesions are x-ray exposure,[54,55] chronic infection, trauma, and human papillomavirus.[56] It appears that papillomavirus is more likely to induce Bowen's disease or frank squamous cell cancer in patients with acquired immunodeficiency syndrome.[57,58] The finding of either of these conditions in a young person should suggest the possibility of human immunodeficiency virus.[59]

There has been an increased incidence of case reports of Bowen's disease in the nail bed over the past decade. The clinical picture is usually very nonspecific, looking like a wart or chronic irritation most frequently along the

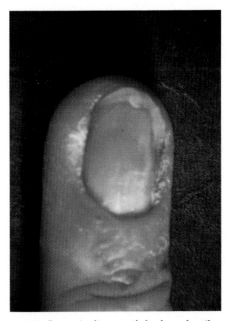

Figure 15–8. Bowen's disease of the lateral nail groove with minimal clinical changes for 2 years.

lateral nail fold, followed by onycholysis and nail plate deformity.[60–63] A helpful finding in differentiating Bowen's disease from common verrucae is the presence of scaling and onycholysis out of proportion to the verrucous changes.[64] Later changes include ulceration and nail plate destruction. The condition is more common in fingernails and in male patients. Numerous case reports have demonstrated the association of human papillomavirus 16 with the presence of Bowen's disease or squamous cell cancer of the nail bed by deoxyribonucleic acid (DNA) hybridization.[65] Ashinoff and colleagues found the polymerase chain reaction technique more sensitive in demonstrating this association.[66] Figure 15–8 shows the clinical picture and Figure 15–9 the histology of a 48-year-old woman with nail fold changes of 3 years duration before diagnosis. Figure 15–10 shows a 52-year-old woman's fingernail with subungual hyperkeratosis and pigmentation misdiagnosed clinically by the author as melanoma prior to biopsy. Both Bowen's disease[67] and basal cell skin cancer[68,69] have been reported to present as melanonychia. Although Bowen's disease by definition is superficial and noninvasive, clinical experience has shown that in the nail bed these lesions have a frequent recurrence rate if treated by desiccation and curettage, cryotherapy, or topical 5-fluorouracil. In these lesions there seems to be a higher incidence of local areas of invasion that may be missed on partial biopsy. This is probably because of relatively late diagnosis following the initial horizontal growth phase of the tumor. The treatment of choice is excision either with estimated margins and primary or graft closure or preferably by microscopically controlled surgery as in Mohs' technique. The latter allows for maximum retention of very important function, particularly with the thumb. Again, an x-ray film of the distal phalanx is mandatory before surgery.

Keratoacanthoma of the nail bed or matrix is a rapidly growing tumor that is difficult to classify as either benign or malignant.[73] The rate of growth and confinement under the nail lead to early pain and bone erosion, demonstrable on x-ray film. This biologic behavior helps dis-

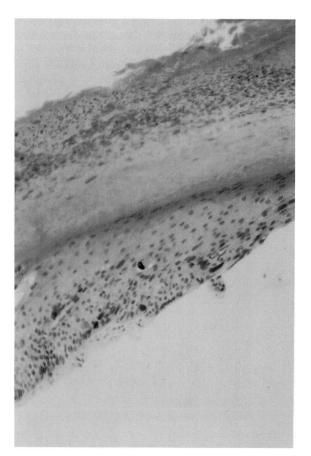

Figure 15–9. Histology of lesion in Figure 15–8 showing cellular atypia, mitoses, and individual cell keratinization. The nail plate intervenes between the nail fold on top and the nail bed on the bottom in this tangential cut.

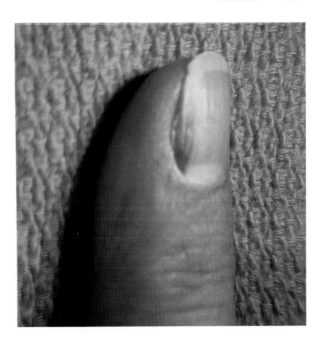

Figure 15–10. Bowen's disease masking as a pigmented streak along the lateral nail groove, clinically suspected of being a melanoma.

tinguish it from slow-growing, asymptomatic squamous cell cancer. Histologically, the mean cell diameter in squamous cell cancer is larger when compared with that of keratoacanthoma.[70] Transforming growth factor-α expression may help differentiate these two tumors.[71]

There are two reasons why keratoacanthomas of the nail bed undergo spontaneous resolution less often than do the same tumors located elsewhere on the skin. First, the pain produced by the lesion forces the patient to demand early treatment before there is time for self-healing. Second, a higher proportion of the tumors in this area are of the multiple variety, which by their biologic behavior are less likely to go away.[72]

Biopsy of the nail bed should be performed after cutting back or avulsing the nail plate and should be of adequate diameter (3.5 to 4 mm) and depth (down to the phalanx) to aid the pathologist in differentiating squamous cell cancer. In solitary lesions, local excision is usually curative[73] and as long as the matrix is not disturbed, spontaneous regrowth of a normal nail plate may be expected. In multiple keratoacanthomas, treatment with systemic methotrexate,[74] intralesional or topical fluorouracil,[75–77] or intralesional bleomycin is possible. If topical fluorouracil is used, the 5 per cent cream should be applied, with occlusion and response expected within 3 to 5 weeks. Careful follow-up is required.

MALIGNANT TUMORS

Squamous cell cancer is by far the most frequent malignant tumor of the nail unit. This is also true of the entire digit on both upper and lower extremities. Fortunately, this tumor metastasizes late and very infrequently. Of the cases described in the literature, there are few documented cases of metastasis.[78–81] In view of this, amputation appears to be too radical a surgical approach for this tumor unless there is bone invasion. Bear in mind that the thumb is the most frequent digit involved, and its loss markedly reduces the function of the entire hand. For this reason, the treatment of choice for squamous cell cancer of the nail bed without bone metastasis is microscopically controlled surgery by Mohs' technique.[82] This leaves the patient with maximum function and as high a cure rate as any other technique. Long-term follow-up is necessary, not only for possible recurrence but because of the real possibility of a second primary. In Attiyeh and colleagues' series, three of five radiation-exposed patients acquired second primaries.[83]

There have been very few reports of basal cell cancer involving the nail bed.[84–86] Because these cases failed to respond to local destruction techniques and went on to amputation, microscopically controlled surgery again appears to be the treatment of choice.

MELANOMA

Although not as rare as basal cell cancer of the nail unit, malignant melanoma in the subungual location is very uncommon, accounting for only 1 to 4 per cent of melanomas in most series.[87,88] Although it may be said of any malignant tumor that early diagnosis is essential, this is particularly true of subungual melanoma. Several series indicate that the prognosis depends a great deal more on duration, level, and thickness of the tumor than on whatever subsequent treatment is administered.[87–89] In spite of the general awareness of the seriousness of this tumor, published series still show late diagnosis averaging 2 years after the initial sign of changes and a 5-year survival in the range of 50 per cent or less. To improve this unsatisfactory situation, the clinician should

1. Be aware that approximately 20 per cent of subungual melanomas are amelanotic.
2. Consider the differential diagnosis of pigmentation of the nail bed.
3. Perform an adequate biopsy.
4. Follow up on persistent pigmentation even if the initial biopsy report is benign.

As in any subungual tumor, the early diagnosis of amelanotic melanoma in this area is dependent on early biopsy of any

1. Inflammatory process that fails to resolve in a reasonable time
2. Treatment failure of apparently benign tumors
3. Slow disappearance of signs and symptoms following injury

Prior injury to the involved digit has been reported in numerous cases, and it is interesting that the thumb on the dominant hand and the great toenails are the more common sites for these tumors.[90–92]

Table 15–3 lists a differential diagnosis of pigmentation of the nail bed.[93–96] Melanocytes are normally present in the matrix and nail bed[97,98] but usually do not produce visible darkening in Caucasians. In African-Americans and some Asians, pigmented bands are frequent and appear to increase in incidence with age.[99] Any noticeable change of these bands, particularly if they occur in the thumb or great toenail, is significant in African-Americans as well as Caucasians. Although only about 1 per cent of melanomas in the United States are in African-Americans, when they do occur, up to 25 per cent are in the subungual location, and the vast majority of these involve

Table 15–3. **CAUSES OF HYPERPIGMENTATION OF THE NAIL BED AND NAIL PLATE**

Hematoma
Chlorpromazine
Antimalarial drugs
Cancer chemotherapy
X-ray therapy
Trauma
Heavy metal exposure
Peutz-Jeghers syndrome[93]
Laugier-Hunziker syndrome[94,95]
Cushing's syndrome (postsurgical)
Idiopathic benign melanocytic hyperplasia
Lentigo
Nevus
Atypical melanocytic hyperplasia
Melanoma (acral lentiginous, lentigo maligna, superficial spreading, and nodular varieties)
Frictional longitudinal melanonychia

the thumb or great toenail.[100] In Caucasians, the significance of a pigmented band still remains uncertain once the benign conditions listed in Table 15–3 are ruled out or considered unlikely. The majority of pigmented bands seen clinically in Caucasians are in the younger adult age group, whereas the peak incidence of subungual melanoma occurs between the ages of 50 and 80 years.[101] Retrospective history in patients with proven subungual melanoma seldom discloses the recollection of any long-standing pigmentation. The onset of a pigmented band after the age of 40 years would appear to have a graver prognosis. In a publication from Japan, three of four melanoma in situ cases involved children.[102] At present, it appears best to perform a biopsy on all idiopathic pigmented nail bands in Caucasians, particularly if there are progressive color or size changes (Fig. 15–11).

The reader is referred to Chapter 20 for a discussion of biopsy techniques for nails. A few important points must be made about the biopsy of this disorder. If pigmentation is in the nail bed, hematoma is much more common than a melanocytic lesion. Time should be allowed to see whether the pigmentation migrates with nail growth (i.e., 6 weeks). If there is no outward movement, biopsy may be achieved by cutting back or avulsing the nail, followed by a longitudinal or punch biopsy. If pigmentation is in the nail plate, the origin of the pigment is in the nail matrix. To visualize the site of pigment origin, a flap must be made in the proximal nail fold. The area of matrix involvement may be very small and must be observed carefully to obtain the correct tissue for

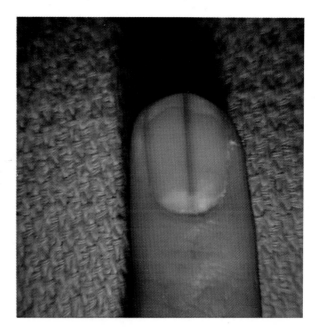

Figure 15–11. Pigmented band originating from benign melanocytic hyperplasia in the nail matrix.

biopsy. Some prefer to avulse the nail prior to a nail fold flap, whereas others prefer to leave the nail plate on and take a biopsy specimen through the plate after a flap is formed.[103] The biopsy must be repeated if the lesion is missed or if pigmentation persists and increases in spite of a benign tissue report on the initial biopsy. The tissue report of a benign lesion is more likely to reveal benign melanocytic hyperplasia rather than pigmented nevus.

Melanoma in this location may be classified as lentigo maligna, superficial spreading, nodular, or acral lentiginous. Whether these are variations of the same malignancy, depending on host resistance factors, is not certain. In any event, subungual melanomas have biologic and histologic features similar to the changes seen in melanomas of the palms, soles, and mucous membranes but different from those seen in melanomas elsewhere. These changes were described by Clark[100] and Arrington[104] and their colleagues and named acral lentiginous melanoma. Clinically, there is nothing unique in the appearance of this tumor other than its location and the fact that pigmentation of the proximal or lateral nail fold (Hutchinson's sign) may be present. Biologically, the tumor has a radial growth phase of variable duration during which the nail plate is intact. Following that, a vertical growth phase ensues, accompanied clinically by increased size and irregularity of pigmentation, nodule development, and nail plate alteration and destruction (Fig. 15–12).

Histologically, acral lentiginous melanoma shows giant melanocytes in the basal layer, uniform morphology of malignant cells, single cell invasion into the dermis, and a marked lymphocytic inflammatory response at the dermal–epidermal junction[100] (Fig. 15–13). Regardless of the histologic type of melanoma, the prognosis is worse once the vertical phase is reached, and progressively more so with lower level and increased thickness of invasion. Presence of ulceration or bone invasion has a significant effect on survival rate. In one series, the survival was significantly better in females than in males.[89]

Clark and colleagues[100] pointed out that levels are sometimes difficult to determine in subungual lesions because the interface of papillary and reticular dermis is difficult to see. For this reason, thickness by measurement is more reliable. Controversy exists as to how much local surgery should be performed and whether lymph node dissection is indicated.[88] There is general agreement that the minimum of treatment should be amputation of part or all of the involved digit, but some additionally favor removal of part or all of the corresponding metatarsal or metacarpal bone.[105] Comparative data on the results of these two degrees of surgery are not available, but particularly with the thumb, argument can be made for the much greater maintenance of function with the less radical surgery. Two studies concluded that the level of amputation did not have a significant effect on survival or local recurrence.[106,107] The

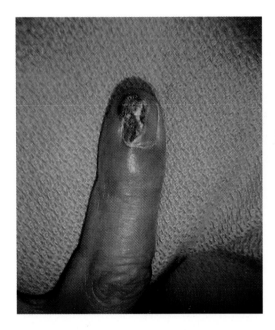

Figure 15–12. Melanoma of nail bed in vertical growth phase showing nodule formation, nail plate destruction, and very faint Hutchinson's sign of the proximal nail fold.

authors recommended amputation at the proximal interphalangeal or metacarpophalangeal-metatarsophalangeal joint provided that clear margins can be obtained.

Clark and associates believed that tumors still in their radial growth phase, level II, of thickness less than 0.76 mm have an excellent prognosis. Those still in radial growth phase but 0.76 to 1.50 mm thick have a more guarded prognosis, with an expected recurrence rate of 10 to 30 per cent.[108] They recommended axillary or inguinal lymph node dissection for any clinical stage 2 disease, all tumors greater than 1.50 mm in thickness, and any level IV or V tumor regardless of thickness. Those who advocate more liberal use of lymphadenectomy point out that a significant percentage of lymph nodes may be involved without giving clinical evidence. In the M.D. Anderson series[107] survival did not differ between patients who had amputation alone or in combination with lymph node dissection. These authors also studied the merits of chemotherapeutic limb perfusion and concluded that it did not reduce survival rate, although it did reduce the incidence of local recurrence. The relative rarity of this tumor dictates that more data will have to be obtained

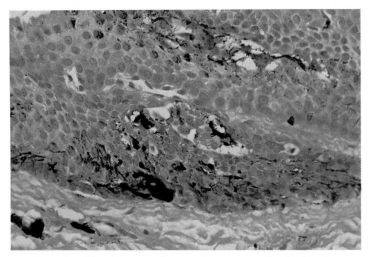

Figure 15–13. Histology of acral lentiginous melanoma showing giant dendritic melanocytes with atypia.

before these disagreements are settled. For widespread disease, radical surgery appears unwarranted, and the relative merits of chemotherapy and immunotherapy are still being evaluated. In spite of these various therapeutic efforts, it still remains clear that the single most important factor in lowering the current high mortality of subungual melanoma is earlier diagnosis.[108]

METASTATIC CANCER

The possibility of metastatic cancer should not be overlooked in the differential diagnosis of subungual and periungual tumors, particularly if there is a proven or suspected primary malignancy. The clinical picture may mimic acute or chronic infection rather than obvious tumor.[109] Clinical impressions in reported cases include cellulitis, paronychia, felon, whitlow, and osteomyelitis.[110] Lung cancer is the most common cause of metastases to the hand,[111–113] whereas foot metastases more often come from genitourinary tumors.[114] Bronchogenic carcinoma has accounted for 43 per cent of the cases of metastases to the terminal phalanges, with breast and kidney each producing 10 per cent of reported cases.[109,114] Discovery of metastatic tumor here calls for careful study in looking for other evidence of spread, identification of the primary tumor, and maximum palliative treatment.

References

1. Goettmann S, Drapé JL, Idy-Peretti I: Magnetic resonance imaging: A new tool in the diagnosis of nail tumors. Br J Dermatol 130:701, 1994.
2. Zemstov A, Lorig R: Magnetic resonance imaging of cutaneous neoplasms. J Dermatol Surg Oncol 17:416, 1991.
3. Litt JZ: Don't excise—Exorcise. Treatment for subungual and periungual warts. Cutis 22:673, 1978.
4. Cordero AA, Goglielmi HA, Woskoff A: The common wart: Intralesional treatment with bleomycin sulfate. Cutis 26:319, 1980.
5. Amer M, Diab N, Aly R, et al: Therapeutic evaluation for intralesional injection of bleomycin sulfate in 143 resistant warts. J Am Acad Dermatol 18:1313, 1988.
6. Hayes ME, O'Keefe EJ: Reduced dose of bleomycin sulfate in treatment of recalcitrant warts. J Am Acad Dermatol 15:1002, 1986.
7. Shumer SM, O'Keefe EJ: Bleomycin in treatment of recalcitrant warts. J Am Acad Dermatol 9:91, 1983.
8. Shelley WB, Shelley ED: Intralesional bleomycin sulfate therapy for warts: A novel bifurcated needle puncture technique. Arch Dermatol 127:234, 1991.
9. Street M, Roenigk R: Recalcitrant periungual verrucae: The role of carbon dioxide vaporization. J Am Acad Dermatol 23:115, 1990.
10. Naylor MF, Neldner KH, Yarbrough GK: Contact immunotherapy of resistant warts. J Am Acad Dermatol 19:679, 1988.
11. Vance JC, Bart BJ, Hansen RC, et al: Intralesional recombinant alpha-2 interferon for the treatment of patients with condyloma acuminatum or verruca plantaris. Arch Dermatol 122:272, 1986.
12. Epstein E: A simple technique for managing digital mucous cyst. Arch Dermatol 115:1315, 1979.
13. Zaias N: In the Nail. Spectrum Publications, New York, 1980, p 223.
14. Bardach HG: Managing digital mucoid cysts by cryosurgery with liquid nitrogen: Preliminary report. J Dermatol Surg Oncol 9:455, 1983.
15. Kuflik EG: Specific indications for cryosurgery of the nail unit: Myxoid cysts and periungual verrucae. J Dermatol Surg Oncol 18:702, 1992.
16. Audebert C: Treatment of mucoid cysts of fingers and toes by injection of a sclerosant. Dermatol Clin 7:179, 1989.
17. Salasche SJ: Myxoid cyst of the proximal nail fold: A surgical approach. J Dermatol Surg Oncol 10:1, 1984.
18. Rohrich RJ, Hochstein LM, Millwee RH: Subungual glomus tumors: An algorithmic approach. Ann Plast Surg 33:300, 1994.
19. Sawada S, Honda M, Kamide R, Niimura M: Three cases of subungual glomus tumor with von Recklinghausen neurofibromatosis. Arch Dermatol 32:277, 1995.
20. Kouskoukis CE: Subungual glomus tumor: A clinicopathological study. J Dermatol Surg Oncol 9:294, 1983.
21. Schneider LH: The glomus tumor. Am Fam Physician 12:140, 1975.
22. Drapé JL, Idy-Peretti I, Goettmann S, et al: Subungual glomus tumors: Evaluation with MR imaging. Radiology 195:507, 1995.
23. Carroll RE, Berman AT: Glomus tumors of the hand. J Bone Joint Surg Am 54:691, 1972.
24. Hildreth DH: The ischemia for glomus tumors: A new diagnostic test. Rev Surg 27:147, 1970.
25. Shelley ED, Shelley WB: Exploratory nail plate removal as a diagnostic aid in painful subungual tumors: Glomus tumor, neurofibroma, and squamous cell carcinoma. Cutis 38:310, 1986.
26. Goettman S, Drapé JL, Idy-Peretti I, et al: Magnetic resonance imaging: A new tool in the diagnosis of nail tumours. Br J Dermatol 130:701, 1994.
27. Holzberg M: Glomus tumor of the nail. A "red herring" clarified by magnetic resonance imaging. Arch Dermatol 128:160, 1992.
28. Idy-Peretti I, Cermakova E, Dion E: Subungual glomus tumor: Diagnosis based on high-resolution MR images (letter). AJR Am J Roentgenol 159:1351, 1992.
29. Jablon M, Horowitz A, Bernstein DA: Magnetic resonance imaging of a glomus tumor of the finger tip. J Hand Surg [Am] 15:507, 1990.
30. Barnes L, Estes SA: Laser treatment of hereditary multiple glomus tumors. J Dermatol Surg Oncol 12:912, 1986.
31. Bart RS, Andrade R, Kopf AW, et al: Acquired digital fibrokeratomas. Arch Dermatol 97:120, 1968.
32. Cahn RL: Acquired periungual fibrokeratoma: A rare benign tumor previously described as garlic-clove fibroma. Arch Dermatol 113:1564, 1977.

33. Shapiro HL: Infantile digital fibromatosis and aponeurotic fibroma. Acta Dermatol 99:37, 1969.
34. Coskey RJ, Nabai H, Rabari H: Recurring digital fibrous tumor of childhood. Cutis 23:359, 1979.
35. Baran R, Perrin C, Baudet J, et al: Clinical and histological patterns of dermatofibromas of the nail apparatus. Clin Exp Dermatol 19:31, 1994.
36. Zimmerman EH: Subungual exostoses. Cutis 19:185, 1977.
37. Apfelberg DB, Drucker D, Maser M, et al: Subungual osteochondroma. Arch Dermatol 115:472, 1979.
38. Yaffee H: Peculiar nail dystrophy caused by an enchondroma. Arch Dermatol 91:361, 1965.
39. Schulze KE, Herbert AA: Diagnostic features, differential diagnosis and treatment of subungual osteochondroma. Pediatr Dermatol 11:39, 1994.
40. Bendl BJ: Subungual exostosis. Cutis 26:260. 1980.
41. Cohen HJ, Frank SB, Minkin W, et al: Subungual exostosis. Arch Dermatol 107:431, 1973.
42. Lebovitz SS, Miller OF, Dickey RF: Subungual exostosis. Cutis 13:426, 1974.
43. Matthewson MH: Subungual exostosis of the fingers: Are they really uncommon? Br J Dermatol 98:187, 1978.
44. Oliviera ADS, Picoto ADS, Verde SF, et al: Subungual exostosis: Treatment as an office procedure. J Dermatol Surg Oncol 6:555, 1980.
45. Brenner MA, Montgomery RM, Kalish SR: Subungual exostosis. Cutis 25:518, 1980.
46. Kato H, Nakagawa T, Suj T, et al: Subungual exostosis: Clinicopathological and ultrastructural studies of 3 cases. Clin Exp Dermatol 15:429, 1990.
47. Carroll RE, Chance JT, Inan Y: Subungual exostosis of the hand. J Hand Surg [Br] 17:569, 1992.
48. St. Onge RA, Jackson IT: An uncommon sequel to thumb trauma: Epidermoid cyst. Hand 9:52, 1977.
49. Yung CW, Estes SA: Subungual epidermal cyst. J Am Acad Dermatol 3:599, 1980.
50. Samman PD: The human toenail: Its genesis and blood supply. Br J Dermatol 71:296, 1952.
51. Lewis BL, Montgomery H: The senile nail. J Invest Dermatol 24:11, 1955.
52. Parker SG, Diffey BL: The transmission of optical radiation through human nails. Br J Dermatol 108:11, 1983.
53. Baran RL, Gormley DE: Polydactylous Bowen's disease of the nail. J Am Acad Dermatol 17:201, 1987.
54. Carroll RE: Squamous cell carcinoma of the nail bed. J Hand Surg 1:92, 1976.
55. Albom MJ: Squamous cell carcinoma of the finger and nail bed. J Dermatol Surg Oncol 1:43, 1975.
56. Moy RL, Eliezri YD, Nuovo GJ, et al: Human papilloma virus type 16 DNA in periungual squamous cell carcinomas. JAMA 261:2669, 1989.
57. Tosti A, LaPlaca M, Fanti PA, et al: Human papilloma virus type 16 associated periungual squamous cell cancer in a patient with acquired immunodeficiency syndrome (letter). Acta Derm Venereol 74:178, 1994.
58. McGrae JD, Greer CE, Manos MM: Multiple Bowen's disease of the fingers associated with human papilloma virus type 16. Int J Dermatol 32:104, 1993.
59. Daniel CR, Norton LA, Scher RK: The spectrum of nail disease in patients with human immunodeficiency virus infection. J Am Acad Dermatol 27:93, 1992.
60. Coskey RJ, Mehregan A, Fosnaugh R: Bowen's disease of the nail bed. Arch Dermatol 106:79, 1972.
61. Dietman DF: Bowen disease of the nail bed. Arch Dermatol 108:577, 1973.
62. Mikhail GR: Bowen disease and squamous cell cancer of the nail bed. Arch Dermatol 110:267, 1974.
63. Baran R: Bowen disease of the nail apparatus: Report of 5 cases and review of the 20 cases of the literatures. Ann Dermatol Venereol 106:227, 1979.
64. Sau P, McMarlin SL, Sperling LC, et al: Bowen's disease of the nail bed and periungual area: A clinicopathologic analysis of seven cases. Arch Dermatol 130:204, 1994.
65. Guitart J, Bergfeld WF, Tuthill RJ, et al: Squamous cell carcinoma of the nail bed: A clinicopathological study of 12 cases. Br J Dermatol 123:215, 1990.
66. Ashinoff R, Li JJ, Jacobson M, et al: Detection of human papilloma virus DNA in squamous cell carcinoma of the nail bed and finger determined by polymerase chain reaction. Arch Dermatol 127:1813, 1991.
67. Baran RL, Simon C: Longitudinal melanonychia: A symptom of Bowen's disease. J Am Acad Dermatol 18:1359, 1988.
68. Baran R, Perrin C: Pseudo-fibrokeratoma of the nail apparatus with melanocytic pigmentation: A clue for diagnosing Bowen's disease. Acta Dermatol Venereol 74:449, 1994.
69. Rudolph RI: Subungual basal call carcinoma presenting as longitudinal melanonychia. J Am Acad Dermatol 16(Pt 2):229, 1987.
70. Allen CA, Stephens M, Steel WM: Subungual keratoacanthoma. Histopathology 25:181, 1994.
71. Ho T, Horn T, Finzi E: Transforming growth factor α expression helps to distinguish keratoacanthomas from squamous cell carcinomas. Arch Dermatol 127:1167, 1991.
72. Shapiro L, Baraf CS: Subungual epithelial carcinoma and keratoacanthoma. Cancer 25:141, 1970.
73. Pellegrini VD Jr, Tompkins A: Management of subungual keratoacanthoma. J Hand Surg [Am] 11:718, 1986.
74. Plewig G: Mutilating subungual warts: Healing through methotrexate. Hautarzt 24:338, 1973.
75. Goette DK, Odom RB, Arrott JW, et al: Treatment of keratoacanthoma with topical application of fluorouracil. Arch Dermatol 118:309, 1982.
76. Goette DK, Odom RB: Successful treatment of keratoacanthoma with intralesional fluorouracil. J Am Acad Dermatol 2:212, 1980.
77. Grupper C: Treatment of keratoacanthomas by local applications of 5-fluorouracil. Dermatologica 140:127, 1970.
78. Nelson LM, Hamilton CF: Primary carcinoma of the nail bed. Arch Dermatol 101:63, 1970.
79. Campbell CJ, Klokarn T: Squamous-cell carcinoma of the nail bed in epidermal dysplasia. J Bone Joint Surg 48:92, 1966.
80. Haber MH, Alter AH, Wheelock MC: Tumors of the hand. Surg Gynecol Obstet 121:1073, 1965.
81. Mauro JA, Maslyn R, Stein AA: Squamous-cell carcinoma of the nail bed in hereditary ectodermal dysplasia. N Y State J Med 72:1065, 1972.
82. Kouskoukis CE, Scher RK, Kopf AW: Squamous-cell carcinoma of the nail bed. J Dermatol Surg Oncol 8:853, 1982.
83. Attiyeh FF, Shah J, Booher RJ, et al: Subungual squamous-cell carcinoma. JAMA 241:262, 1979.
84. Alpert LI, Zak FG, Werthamer S: Subungual basal cell epithelioma. Arch Dermatol 106:599, 1972.
85. Hoffman S: Basal cell carcinoma of the nail bed. Arch Dermatol 108:828, 1973.
86. Guana AL, Kolbusz R, Goldberg LH: Basal cell carcinoma on the nailfold of the right thumb. Int J Dermatol 33:204, 1994.

87. Klausner JM, Inbar M, Gutman M, et al: Nail-bed melanoma. J Surg Oncol 34:208, 1987.

88. Daly JM, Berlin R, Urmacher C: Subungual melanoma: A 25-year review of cases. J Surg Oncol 35:107, 1987.

89. Patterson RH, Helwig, EB: Subungual malignant melanoma: A clinicopathologic study. Cancer 46:2074, 1980.

90. O'Toole EA, Stephens R, Young MM, et al: Subungual melanoma: A relation to direct injury? J Am Acad Dermatol 33:525, 1995.

91. Roberts AHN: Subungual melanoma following a single injury. J Hand Surg 9:328, 1984.

92. Blessing K, Kernohan NM, Park KG: Subungual malignant melanoma: Clinicopathological features of 100 cases. Histopathology 19:425, 1991.

93. Valero A, Sherf K: Pigmented nails in Peutz-Jeghers syndrome. Am J Gastroenterol 43:56, 1965.

94. Baran R: Longitudinal melanotic streaks as a clue to Laugier-Hunziker syndrome. Arch Dermatol 115:1448, 1979.

95. Laugier P, Hunziker N, Olmos L: Pigmentation melanique lenticulaire essentielle de la mugeuse jugale et des leures. Ann Dermatol Venereol 104:181, 1977.

96. Baran R: Frictional longitudinal melanonychia: A new entity. Dermatologica 174:280, 1987.

97. Higashi N: Melanocytes of nail matrix and nail pigmentation. Arch Dermatol 97:570, 1968.

98. Hashimoto K: Ultrastructure of the human toenail: Proximal nail matrix. J Invest Dermatol 56:235, 1971.

99. Monash S: Normal pigmentation of the nail in the Negro. Arch Dermatol Syphilol 25:876, 1932.

100. Clark WH Jr, Bernardino EA, Reed NJ, et al: Acral lentiginous melanomas including melanomas of mucous membranes. In Clark WH, Mastrangelo MF, Goldman AB (eds): Human Melanoma: The Benign and Malignant Lesions and their Precursors. Grune and Stratton, New York, 1978, pp 109–124.

101. Feibleman CE: Melanomas of the palm, sole, and nail bed: A clinicopathologic study. Cancer 46:2492, 1980.

102. Kato T, Usuba Y, Takematsu H: A rapidly growing pigmented nail streak resulting in diffuse melanosis of the nail: A possible sign of subungual melanoma in situ. Cancer 64:2191, 1989.

103. Kopf AW, Albom M, Ackerman AB: Biopsy technique for longitudinal streaks of pigmentation in nails. Am J Dermatopathol 6(Suppl):309, 1984.

104. Arrington JH, Reed RJ, Ichinose H: Acral lentiginous melanoma: A distinctive variant of human cutaneous malignant melanoma. Am J Surg Pathol 1:131, 1977.

105. Kopf AW, Bart RS, Rodriguez-Sains RS, et al: Subungual malignant melanoma. In Kopf AW, Bart RS, Rodriguez-Sains RS, et al (eds): Melanoma. Masson Publishing, New York, 1979, pp 159–161.

106. Finlay RK, Driscoll DL, Blumenson LE, et al: Subungual melanoma: An eighteen-year review. Surgery 116:96, 1994.

107. Heaton KM, el-Naggar A, Ensign LG, et al: Surgical management and prognostic factors in patients with subungual melanoma. Ann Surg 219:197, 1994.

108. Dawber RP, Colver GB: The spectrum of malignant melanoma of the nail apparatus. Semin Dermatol 10:82, 1991.

109. Baran R, Tosti A: Metastatic carcinoma to the terminal phalanx of the big toe: Report of two cases and review of the literature. J Am Acad Dermatol 31:259, 1994.

110. Cohen PR, Buzdar AU: Metastatic breast carcinoma mimicking an acute paronychia of the great toe: Case report and review of subungual metastasis. Am J Clin Oncol 16:86, 1993.

111. Kerin R: Metastatic tumors of the hand. J Bone Joint Surg Am 40:263, 1958.

112. Zaias N: Premalignant and malignant nail lesions. In The Nail in Health and Disease. Appleton & Lange, East Norwalk, CT, 1990, pp 221–227.

113. Kumar PP: Metastases to the bones of the hand. J Nat Med Assoc 67:275, 1975.

114. Zindrick MR, Young MP, Daley RS, et al: Metastatic tumors of the foot. Clin Orthop Rel Res 170:219, 1982.

115. Baran R, Perrin CH, Baudet J, et al: Clinical and histological patterns of dermatofibromas of the nail apparatus. Clin Exp Dermatol 19:31, 1994.

116. Tosti A, Peluso AM, Fanti PA, et al: Histiocytoid hemangioma with prominent fingernail involvement. Dermatology 189:87, 1994.

117. Baran R, Kint A: Onychomatrixoma. Br J Dermatol 126:510, 1992.

118. Tosti A, Morelli R, Fanti PA, et al: Carcinoma cuniculatum of the nail apparatus: Report of 3 cases. Dermatology 186:217, 1993.

119. Raquena L, Sanchez M, Aguilar A, et al: Periungual porocarcinoma. Dermatologica 180:177, 1990.

120. Bryant J: Subungual epithelioid leiomyosarcoma. South Med J 85:560, 1992.

121. Tosti A, Fanti PA, Varotti C: Massive lymphomatous nail involvement in Sézary syndrome. Dermatologica 181:162, 1990.

122. Pedersen LM, Nordin H, Nielsen H, et al: Non-Hodgkin malignant lymphoma in the nails in the course of a chronic lymphocytic leukemia. Acta Derm Venereol (Stockh) 72:277, 1992.

CHAPTER 16

Nail Cosmetics

Patricia G. Engasser

Patients frequently complain to dermatologists about their nails; with aging, nails grow more slowly[1] and become fragile and longitudinally ridged. Nails split, chip, and break; nail cosmetics are popular because they can improve the condition and appearance of the nails if used wisely. However, pain and disability may result from allergic reactions to or injudicious use of nail cosmetics and grooming tools. Examining the cosmetics used for manicures and nail care aids us in giving our patients practical advice.

NAIL ENAMEL REMOVERS

A first step in a manicure is the removal of nail enamel remaining on the nail plate from a prior application. Some people chip off old nail enamel with another fingernail; this habit damages the nail plate and, consequently, should be discouraged. Nail enamel removers are nitrocellulose solvents that can also remove lipids from the nail plate. Kechijian[2] maintained that these organic solvents dehydrate the nail plate and decrease corneocyte adhesion, contributing to brittleness. He observed that onychoschizia of the distal nail plate results from prolonged or frequent use of nail enamel removers. However, experiments producing lamellar separation of pieces of nail plate demonstrated that repeated wetting and drying of nails is a more important cause of onychoschizia.[3] A carefully performed manicure will last 1 to 2 weeks when defects are repaired with nail enamel and an extra layer of top coat is added periodically. Therefore, nail enamel removers need to be applied only weekly, minimizing any damage to the nail plate.

Solvents frequently used in nail enamel removers are acetone, ethyl acetate, butyl acetate, and methyl ethyl ketone (MEK).[4] Small amounts of lipid are added as a measure to counteract the drying effects of solvents. Nonsmearing nail enamel removers contain water-soluble solvents such as ethyl acetate to which a small amount of water has been added.

Although nail enamel removers are in contact with the skin a short time and rarely sensitize, these cosmetics contain chemicals that may cause dryness and irritation of the cuticle and surrounding nail folds.[5] If an allergic reaction is suspected, nail enamel removers should not be tested in a closed patch test. Ingredients may be tested in the following concentrations: 10 per cent acetone in olive oil; 10 per cent ethyl acetate in petrolatum; 25 per cent butyl acetate in olive oil[6]; plain MEK.

276

CUTTING AND FILING

The nails are shaped next in a manicure. Use a scissors or nail clipper to cut long, thick nails, clipping from one side to the other. If the clippers are placed across the nail, to span the entire nail, when they are snapped shut the nail tends to split. To finish shaping and smoothing the nail, a fine file should be used. Filing in a single direction rather than back and forth also prevents damage. Women should be counseled to carry a file in their purse to smooth small snags when they develop. Nails shaped with straight sides and gently rounded tops are stronger than pointed nails.

CUTICLE SHAPING AND GROOMING

The cuticle is softened by soaking the fingertips for several minutes in a dilute solution of detergent. The cuticle is an extension of the stratum corneum onto the nail plate. Cuticle removers contain alkaline materials, most commonly 2 to 5 per cent sodium or potassium hydroxide, in a liquid or cream vehicle to destroy keratin by attacking the disulfide bonds of cystine. The humectants glycerin and propylene glycol may be added to reduce irritation, decrease evaporation, and increase viscosity. Milder, less effective cuticle removers contain the inorganic salt trisodium phosphate or tetrasodium pyrophosphate. Organic bases such as triethanolamine have also been used in milder preparations.

Cuticle removers are applied to the base of the nail for several minutes. Then the softened cuticle is pushed back off the nail plate by rubbing with a wooden instrument called an orange stick or a similar tool. Manicurists may shape the remaining cuticle with a V-shaped sharp trimmer or nippers, which trims the cuticle. Hangnails are also trimmed back with sharp instruments during the manicure.

This manipulation of the cuticle may cause injury to the posterior nail fold. If caustic cuticle removers are left in place too long, irritation occurs. Between manicures, the cuticle should be pushed back gently after the hands are washed, when it is wet and soft. Inexperienced, rough handling of the cuticle may injure the matrix below it and was reported by Samman[7] to be a cause of leukonychia striata. Bauer and Baran[8] attributed transverse nail grooving to these practices. Carefully explaining to patients how the cuticle serves as a seal that prevents microorganisms and chemicals from invading the space below the posterior nail fold is important in winning their cooperation. Gentle care must be emphasized strongly; trauma with sharp instruments provides opportunities for infection. After visiting manicurists across the United States, Draelos observed that there were no consistent observations of disinfection techniques.[9] Regulations in the state of California require instruments to be washed clean in a detergent solution followed by a 10-minute soak in an Environmental Protection Agency–registered solution that is bactericidal, fungicidal, and virucidal. Advising patients to bring their own manicuring tools to salon appointments seems a wise precaution until they can be certain that the manicurist is practicing sound techniques of disinfection.

Cuticle removers and sodium or potassium hydroxide are irritants and should not be used for patch testing. Because almost all the reactions to these cosmetics are irritant type, ingredient patch testing is seldom, if ever, indicated.

Cuticle creams are not to be confused with cuticle removers. The creams are emollients to which quaternary ammonium compounds or urea is sometimes added to promote softening of the cuticle.[10] These creams are used not *during* a manicure but *between* manicures to maintain supple cuticle. Frequent, generous application of an emollient to the fingertips should discourage the formation of hangnails and improve brittle nails.

During a professional manicure, the hands are massaged with a lotion or cream, which is then removed from the nail plate with a dilute detergent solution.

BUFFING

Buffing nails is an alternative to wearing nail enamel. This technique is satisfactory only for people who have attractive nails and the necessary motivation to buff them regularly. Buffing powder, paste, or cream is applied to each nail, and a chamois-covered buffer is used to polish the nails until they shine. The abrasives used are fine powders of stannic oxide, talc, silica chalk, or kaolin.[10]

When this method is used persistently and gently, the results can be beautiful; however, rough buffing causes injury to the nail matrix and nail grooving.[11] After buffing, a white pencil may be used to color the undersurface of the unattached distal nail.

NAIL ENAMEL

Most women who manicure their nails choose to wear nail enamel. Nail enamel should be easy to apply, elastic, and glossy; it should dry quickly, adhere well, and resist chipping. The manufacture of nail enamel is highly specialized because of these performance standards and the hazards of fire and explosion during its production. For these reasons, most cosmetic firms purchase nail enamel from a small number of contract manufacturers, ensuring a certain uniformity in most of the products. Nail enamel is also called lacquer, varnish, and most commonly nail polish.

Nail polishes, including base coats and top coats, are of similar composition,[12] containing some or all of the following types of ingredients:

1. Film former, nitrocellulose, which forms a film that is hard and strong but does not adhere well and is inelastic

2. Resins, including toluene sulfonamide—formaldehyde resin (TSFR); alkyd, acrylate, polyamide, and vinyl resins[13]; and arylalkyl sulfonyl urethanes and toluene sulfonamide epoxy resin[14]; these improve adhesion and gloss

3. Plasticizers, including camphor; dibutyl, dioctyl, diphenyl phthalate; tricresyl or triphenylphosphate[12]; and glycerol tribenzoate[14]; these improve the flexibility of the enamel

4. Solvents and diluents, including ethyl, butyl, or isopropyl alcohol; butyl, ethyl, or amyl acetate; and toluene; these improve viscosity

5. Colorants,[15,16] for which organic colors must be approved by the Food and Drug Administration (FDA); cream enamels contain insoluble organic colors as well as titanium oxide or iron oxide; a few soluble organic dyes are used to tint colorless polishes; the nacreous pigments guanine, bismuth oxychloride, or mica are added to pearlized polishes

6. Suspending agent, stearalkonium hectorite, which prevents settling out of the pigments

Although nail solvents have been implicated in contributing to brittleness of nails, the frequency with which this may be a factor has not been established. Most women who manicure their nails regularly benefit from the protection polish can afford. Manufacturers can test the porosity of nail polishes and avoid producing occlusive enamels that could damage the nail by preventing the passage of water across the nail plate.

Colored nail polishes may cause yellow staining that is most prominent at the distal end of the nail. Samman[17] reproduced this phenomenon with dyes D&C red nos. 6, 7, and 34 and FD&C yellow no. 5 lake.

Reported allergic reactions to nail polish have usually been attributed to the TSFR. In a 1995 review of patch-testing results in 3549 patients conducted by the North American Contact Dermatitis Group[18] between 1992 and 1994, 1.9 per cent of the positive reactions were seen with TSFR. Eighty-five per cent of these were judged to be clinically relevant. Giorgini and associates[19] found reactions in 3.8 per cent of patients screened, and Tosti and associates[20] reported a rate of 6.6 per cent when only women who used nail polish were included. Allergic contact dermatitis to nail polish frequently affects the eyelids, sides of face, neck, or mouth and may spare the hands and fingers. The rash may appear anywhere on the body and even become generalized. Because of this sometimes confusing presentation, it is useful to include TSFR 10 per cent in petrolatum in screening patch tests for persons who wear nail polish. Tests with air-dried nail polish that the patient uses is another helpful screen. Liden and associates,[21] in their study of 18 TSFR-allergic patients diagnosed in an occupational dermatology clinic, demonstrated that this cause was seldom anticipated, and as a consequence patients had been on periods of sick leave (nine cases), stopped working with visual display units (two cases), and lost their jobs (two cases).

These reactions are attributed to the TSFR resin itself and not to the small amounts of free formaldehyde (0.15 per cent or less) present.[6] In the near future, we can anticipate that new allergens will be noted in cases of contact dermatitis relating to nail polish. Nail polishes are being reformulated because toluene was added to the list of chemicals for which California's Proposition 65 requires warning labels.[14,22] One large cosmetic manufacturer has already reformulated its nail polish so that it does not contain toluene or TSFR. From Finland, Kanerva and Associates[23] reported methyl acrylate as an allergen in a polish containing an acrylic resin.

NAIL "HARDENERS"

Physicians may be confused by the use of the term "nail hardener" for products that are only slightly modified nail enamels and are designated hardeners for marketing. Short nylon fibers are suspended in some polishes for added strength, and these enamels are called liquid wraps. None of these cosmetics contain added formaldehyde.

Hardeners with formaldehyde designed to be applied to the entire nail plate have been banned in the United States for more than 20 years. Severe reactions to these products reported in the 1960s included painful onycholysis and even hemorrhagic reactions about the lips in nail biters.[24–26] At present, hardeners sold in the United States may contain up to 5 per cent formaldehyde and are designed to be applied to the free edge of the nail while the surrounding skin is shielded. Norton[27] reported treating a wide variety of adverse reactions to these hardeners, including inflammatory and noninflammatory onycholysis, paronychia, chromonychia, temporary nail plate shedding, and painful pterygium inversum unguium as well as a dermatitis on distant skin and mucous membranes. These products are marketed by smaller companies, and their availability is variable.

MENDING KITS

Mending kits are convenient aids for women who wish to grow long nails. Splits in nails are bonded with cyanoacrylate glue. The repair is splinted by gluing on a patch of paper that has the consistency of heavy tissue paper. The glues used to saturate the papers are nail polishes with a high solid content. When using the mending kits at home, nonprofessionals often get the glue on their skin. In case of accidental bonding, the skin should not be separated by direct force. The surfaces should be soaked in warm, soapy water and rolled apart.

NAIL WRAPPING

When nail wrapping was first introduced, the techniques and material were the same as those used in nail repairing described previously. The skilled manicurist would wrap the end of the nail, using nail polish as a glue. Paper wrapping has been displaced by silk, linen, and fiber glass. The nail plate is often abraded or primed with methacrylic acid. The cloth is used to cover the entire nail plate and glued with cyanoacrylate. New layers are applied every 2 weeks. The materials are removed from the nail approximately every 2 months and fresh layers are applied. Patients sensitized to ethyl cyanoacrylate used to glue wraps may experience periungual dermatitis as well as eruptions on distant sites.[28]

PLASTIC NAILS

Artificial, preformed plastic nails are available in kits; even gold false nails are available to glue on. Plastic tips that are attached to the distal portion of the nail with cyanoacrylate glue have become popular. They are faster to use and require less skill than does nail sculpturing. Acrylics, gels, or wraps may be used to smooth and strengthen this form.

Burrows and Rycroft[29] reported an instructive case in which a woman had used a prosthetic nail for several years before becoming allergic to the p-tertiary butyl phenol formaldehyde resin adhesive and the tricresyl ethyl phthalate of the plastic nail itself. Neoprene has been used as an adhesive for plastic nails, also. Shelley and Shelley[30] reported a case of nail dystrophy and periungual dermatitis caused by an allergic reaction to cyanoacrylate glue used for false nails. Occupational exposure to cyanoacrylate among beauticians and manicurists is important.[31,32] In working up suspected cases of cyanoacrylate allergy, Jacobs and Rycroft[32] pointed out that cyanoacrylate glues may contain hydroquinone and contaminant acrylates, which may complicate a case.

NAIL SCULPTURE

Resins used in nail sculpture are made from mixing liquid acrylic monomers and powdered polymers. Then, using a template that surrounds the nail, the resins are molded into an attractive nail on the nail plate. The liquids may contain a stabilizer, such as hydroquinone, resorcinol, eugenol, thymol, or N,N-dimethyl-p-toluidine; plasticizers such as tricresyl or phthalate phosphate[33]; solvents; and dyes. The powdered polymer may have benzoyl peroxide added as an initiator. The nail plate is prepared by being painted with methacrylic acid primer[34] or by being abraded with a file. As the nail grows out, its base needs to be filled with applications of the resin. Despite the expense and time required for application, these sculptured nails are popular for women who have been unable to grow long nails and can have the appearance of extremely long nails that do not require enamel to look attractive. In addition, use of these resins allows the manicurist to make fanciful creations on the nails, painting airbrush decorations, or imbedding jewels. Unfortunately, trauma, irritant, and allergic reactions to these nails as well as infection may have painful and even long-lasting consequences for some users.

The first formulations of sculptured nails contained methyl methacrylate monomer; as early as 1957, Fisher and associates[35] reported severe allergic reactions to this monomer. Patients experienced painful paronychia, onychia, and nail distortion. Dermatitis on the face and fingers accompanied some local reactions. By 1974 the FDA had received so many complaints that methyl methacrylate was banned from these products. One case of permanent nail loss was reported,[36] and we have seen severe permanent distortion of psoriatic nails as a result of the Koebner phenomenon.

Despite reformulation using other methacrylate monomers, sensitization still occurs.[37,38] In addition, distressing, persistent paresthesias have been another consequence of nail sculpture.[39] In some instances, paresthesia may result in the absence of allergic sensitization. Many patients who experience inflammatory reactions to sculptured nails are never reported or patch tested because of the lack of information as to which monomers are being used in salon preparations. The chemistry of these acrylic resins is complex, there are common patterns of cross-reactions, and ingredient labeling of the products used exclusively in salons is done on a voluntary basis by the manufacturer. Koppula and associates[40] attempted to simplify this maze. After reviewing their data from patch-tested patients who used artificial nails and were patch tested with 33 acrylates, Koppula and coworkers proposed that the following five chemicals be used as screens: ethyl acrylate, 2-hydroxyethyl acrylate, ethylene glycol dimethacrylate, 5 ethyl cyanoacrylate, and triethylene glycol diacrylate. In their series of 11 patients, 0.1 per cent ethyl acrylate in petrolatum detected 91 per cent of the acrylate-allergic artificial-nail users. The 5 ethyl cyanoacrylate–sensitive patients had cross-reactions to other methacrylates. In September 1994, the Cosmetic Ingredient Review Expert Panel published a final report on ethyl methacrylate, a frequent ingredient used in nail sculpture, and declared it safe as used.[41] In Finland, Kanerva and associates, in their study of 23 acrylate-sensitive patients, reported that 6 patients were sensitive to ethyl methacrylate. They maintained that this chemical should be considered a significant allergen.[42]

Other similar systems are used to create artificial nails or artificial enhancements. For "porcelain" nails, a finely ground silica is added to the powder.[34] In gel systems, layers of resin are applied to the nail. These resins are usually hardened with light, either ultraviolet or lighting in the room. Ultraviolet-cured resins are combined with photochemically reactive substances that, on ultraviolet light exposure, form free radicals to initiate the polymerization.[43] Visible light systems are composed of urethane acrylate or urethane methacrylate.[44] Acute paronychia and paresthesia have been reported from the use of photo-bonded nails also.[45]

In the United States, the burgeoning number of nail salons is evidence of the popularity of all these artificial methods of decorating nails. Dermatologists must be prepared to recognize and treat the adverse reactions that occur.

In addition, the advisability of the use of nail adornment for health care workers has also been questioned. Protective latex gloves are more easily torn by long artificial nails. Chipped nail polish may harbor bacteria not removed by surgical scrubs,[46] and artificial nails appear to carry increased numbers of gram-negative bacteria.[47] This led the Association of Operating Room Nurses to recommend that nurses in restricted and semirestricted areas keep their nails unadorned.[48] Certainly, health care workers providing direct patient care need to avoid the use of cosmetics or cosmetic devices that cause rashes on their hands and fingers.

References

1. Orentreich N, Sharp NJ: Keratin replacement as an aging parameter. J Soc Cosmet Chem 18:537, 1967.
2. Kechijian P: Nail polish removers: Are they harmful? Semin Dermatol 10:26, 1991.
3. Wallis MS, Bowen WR, Guin JD: Pathogenesis of onychoschizia (lamellar dystrophy). J Am Acad Dermatol 24:44, 1991.
4. Dovaik WC: Nail lacquers and removers. In Balsam MS, Sagarin E (eds): Cosmetics: Science and Technol-

ogy, ed 2, vol 2. Wiley-Interscience, New York, 1972, pp 521–541.

5. Scher RK: Cosmetics and ancillary preparations for the care of nails—Composition, chemistry, and adverse reactions. J Am Acad Dermatol 6:523, 1982.

6. De Groot AC, Weyland JW, Nater JP: Unwanted Effects of Cosmetics and Drugs Used in Dermatology, ed 3. Elsevier, New York, 1994.

7. Samman PD: The Nails in Disease, ed 4. William Heinemann, London, 1986.

8. Bauer E, Baran R: Cosmetics: The care and adornment of the nail. In Baran R, Dawber RPR (ed): Diseases of the Nail and Their Management, ed 2. Blackwell, Boston, 1994, pp 285–296.

9. Draelos ZD: The potential risks of manicures and pedicures. Cos Derm 6:13, 1993.

10. Wilkinson JB, Moore RJ (eds): Harry's Cosmeticology. Chemical Publishing, New York, 1982.

11. Braun JB: Grooving of nails due to P. Shine: A new manicure kit. Cutis 19:323, 1977.

12. Schlossman ML: Modern nail enamel technology. J Soc Cosmet Chem 31:29, 1980.

13. Schlossman ML: Nail-enamel resins. Cosmet Tech 1:53, 1979.

14. Schlossman ML, Wimmer E: Advances in nail enamel technology. J Soc Cosmet Chem 43:331, 1992.

15. Schlossman ML: Nail polish colorants. Cosmet Toiletries 95:31, 1980.

16. Fotiu E: Modern formulations of coloring agents: Face, lips and nails. In Frost P, Horwitz SN (eds): Principles of Cosmetics for the Dermatologist. CV Mosby, St. Louis, 1982, pp 147–151.

17. Samman PD: Nail disorders caused by external influences. J Soc Cosmet Chem 28:351, 1977.

18. Marks JG, Belsito DV, Dedeo VA, et al: North American Contact Dermatitis Group standard tray patch test results (1992 to 1994). Am J Contact Dermatitis 6:160, 1995.

19. Giorgini S, Brusi C, Francalanci S, et al: Prevention of allergic contact dermatitis from nail varnishes and hardeners. Contact Dermatitis 31:325, 1994.

20. Tosti A, Guerra L, Vincenzi C, et al: Contact sensitization caused by toluene sulfonamide-formaldehyde resin in women who use nail cosmetics. Am J Contact Dermatitis 4:150, 1993.

21. Liden C, Berg M, Farm G, Wrangsjo K: Nail varnish allergy with far-reaching consequences. Br J Dermatol 128:57, 1993.

22. Nail polish. Consumer Reports 60:104, 1995.

23. Kanerva L, Lauerma A, Jolanki R, Estlander T: Prevention of nail lacquer dermatitis by substituting toluene sulfonamide formaldehyde resin? Methyl acrylate—A new sensitizer in nail lacquer. Allergologie 18:470, 1995.

24. March CH: Allergic contact dermatitis to a new formula to strengthen nails. Arch Dermatol 93:720, 1966.

25. Lazar P: Reaction to nail hardeners. Arch Dermatol 94:446, 1966.

26. Huldin DH: Hemorrhages of the lips secondary to nail hardeners. Cutis 4:709, 1968.

27. Norton L: Common and uncommon reactions to formaldehyde-containing nail hardeners. Semin Dermatol 10:29, 1991.

28. Bellsito DV: Contact dermatitis due to ethyl-cyanoacrylate containing glue. Contact Dermatitis 17:234, 1987.

29. Burrows D, Rycroft RJG: Contact dermatitis for PTBP resin and tricresyl ethylphthalate in a plastic nail adhesive. Contact Dermatitis 7:336, 1981.

30. Shelley ED, Shelley WB: Nail dystrophy and periungual dermatitis due to cyanoacrylate glue sensitivity (letter). J Am Acad Dermatol 19:574, 1988.

31. Tomb RR, Lepoittevin JP, Durepaire F, Grosshans E: Ectopic contact dermatitis from ethyl cyanoacrylate instant adhesives. Contact Dermatitis 28:206, 1993.

32. Jacobs MC, Rycroft RJG: Allergic contact dermatitis from cyanoacrylate? Contact Dermatitis 33:71, 1995.

33. Foussereau J, Benezra C, Maibach HI: Occupational Contact Dermatitis: Clinical and Chemical Aspects. Munksgaard, Copenhagen, 1982.

34. Artificial Fingernail Products: A Guide to Chemical Exposures in the Nail Salon. Hazard Evaluation System and Information Service, Berkeley, CA 1989.

35. Fisher AA, Franks A, Glick H: Allergic sensitization of the skin and nails to acrylic plastic nails. J Allergy 28:84, 1957.

36. Fisher AA: Permanent loss of fingernails due to allergic reaction to an acrylic nail preparation: A sixteen-year follow-up study. Cutis 43:404, 1989.

37. Marks JG, Bishop ME, Willis WF: Allergic contact dermatitis to sculptured nails. Arch Dermatol 115:100, 1979.

38. Fitzgerald DA, English JSC: Widespread contact dermatitis from sculptured nails. Contact Dermatitis 30:118, 1994.

39. Fisher AA, Baran RL: Adverse reactions to acrylate sculptured nails with particular reference to prolonged paresthesia. Am J Contact Dermatitis 2:38, 1991.

40. Koppula SV, Fellman JH, Storrs FJ: Screening allergens for acrylate dermatitis associated with artificial nails. Am J Contact Dermatitis 6:78, 1995.

41. Cosmetic Ingredient Review Expert Panel: Final Report of Safety Assessment of Ethyl Methacrylate. Cosmetic, Toiletry, and Fragrance Association, Washington, DC, 1994.

42. Kanerva L, Estlander T, Jolalnki R, Tarvainen K: Statistics on allergic patch test reactions caused by acrylate compounds, including data on ethyl methacrylate. Am J Contact Dermatitis 6:75, 1995.

43. Bjorkner B: Sensitizing Capacity of Ultraviolet Curable Acrylic Compounds. Department of Occupational Dermatology, Lund Sweden, 1984.

44. Baran R: Cosmetics for abnormal and pathological nails. In Baran R, Maibach HI (eds): Cosmetic Dermatology. Martin Dunitz, London, 1994, pp 169–180.

45. Fisher AA: Adverse nail reactions and paresthesia from "photobonded acrylate 'sculptured' nails." Cutis 45:293, 1990.

46. Wynd CA, Samstag DE, Lapp AM: Bacterial carriage on the fingernails of OR nurses. AORN J 60:796, 1994.

47. Pottinger J, Burns S, Manske C: Bacterial carriage by artificial versus natural nails. Am J Infect Control 17:340, 1989.

48. Association of Operating Room Nurses: Recommended Practices for Surgical Attire. In ARON standards and Recommended Practices for Perioperative Nursing. Denver, Association of Operating Room Nurses, 1991.

CHAPTER 17

Occupational Disease

David G. Kern

Medicine, like jurisprudence, should make a contribution to the well-being of workers and see to it that, so far as possible, they should exercise their callings without harm. So I for my part have done what I could and have not thought it unbecoming to make my way into the lowliest workshops and study the mysteries of the mechanic arts.

Bernardini Ramazzini 1700

NAILS AND WORK

During early human evolution, nails served as weapons, climbing aids, and eating tools. More recently, our nails have become less useful and more decorative. Because nails are continuously visible and growing, necessity and culture demand that our nails be groomed and decorated.

At odds with the integrity of our nails is the workplace, which may pose many threats to both nails and periungual tissues. The goal of this chapter is to provide a framework within which physicians can explore these threats. Attention is not addressed to the nail's function as a tool. Three decades ago, Francesco Ronchese wrote that "nails . . . are to man from important to essential in earning a living."[1] This remains true even today for some workers in the less industrially advanced nations of the world. In the United States, however, with the

growth of automation and the deskilling and fragmentation of the craft trades, our nails are no longer critical to our work.

AN APPROACH TO OCCUPATIONAL NAIL DISEASE

When as physicians we suspect a causal relationship between a patient's work and illness, some very exciting opportunities are created. As armchair sleuths, we may investigate the plausibility of our suspicions using the known facts. If this information is insufficient for forming a sound conclusion, we may then have to leave our armchair for a tour of the workplace. We can there assess firsthand the character of the specific work setting and the potential for hazardous working conditions. If we do find an occupationally related condition, changes in the employee's interaction with the workplace in concert with specific medical treatment may allow us the satisfaction of witnessing a reversible illness and a permanent cure. Given the fact that an individual's illness may represent the tip of an iceberg, there is also the potential for significant public health advocacy. Together with colleagues from other disciplines, we may investigate whether the patient's coworkers have been similarly affected or are currently at risk. If we find this to be the case, then with our colleagues' help, a solution can be crafted and recommended for implementation. These interventions offer the hope of limiting illness, Workers' Compensation premiums, and financial losses while simultaneously improving the quality of life of employees and increasing overall productivity. Finally, if the illness is not reversible and adversely affects the ability of the worker to earn a living, then there is some consolation in our being able to help our patients secure rehabilitative and job retraining services and, when appropriate, Workers' Compensation and Social Security disability benefits. Given the socioeconomic system of the United States, where social welfare programs are minimal in comparison with those of most other industrialized nations, the importance of these rehabilitation and disability compensation systems cannot be overemphasized.[2]

When we see a patient with nail disease suggestive of occupational origin, all of the preceding applies. In addition, the diagnosis of occupational nail disease should alert us to the possibility of more serious systemic illness. The same insult that produces a nail condition may, with time, lead to more serious bodily injury or systemic illness. If we can intervene when only the nail disease is present, then more serious consequences may be prevented.

REACTION PATTERNS IN OCCUPATIONAL NAIL DISEASE

Borrowing from traditional classifications of occupational skin disease, we can categorize the cause of most work-related nail disease as being of mechanical, chemical, physical, or biologic origin.[3] Although mechanical trauma is the most common, dermatologists will infrequently see patients with these conditions, because their cause is usually obvious. Chemical exposures, in contrast, are probably responsible for most evaluations of work-related nail disease.

Just as there are a limited number of causes of occupational nail disease, there are also a limited number of reaction patterns. These include nail discoloration, separation of the nail plate from the nail bed, configurational changes such as spooning and clubbing, and nail plate textural irregularities resulting from paronychia, other insults to the nail matrix, and direct trauma to the nail plate.

Chromonychia

Because a chapter in this book is devoted to chromonychia and because work-related nail pigmentation has been addressed elsewhere,[4] only a few observations are made here.

1. Pigment limited to the nail plate is responsible for most abnormally colored nails in the occupational setting. Pigment so limited will persist when the nail bed is blanched by depressing the nail plate and when a flashlight held in apposition to the underside of the nail's free edge is shone up through the plate.[5] Although nail plate pigmentation is typically due to topical staining, systemic conditions must be considered as well. Topical staining can be assumed if pigment can be removed by scraping or with acetone.[6]

2. Systemic absorption of a chemical through the skin or lungs may occasionally lead to pigmentary nail changes. If the color disappears on nail bed blanching, then the pigment is clearly in the blood. If blanching does not obliterate the pigment but the flashlight does, then the pigment is probably deposited in the nail bed. An example of the former is the purplish-blue pigment of methemoglobinemia, and an example of the latter is the blue nail of generalized argyria found in silver refinery workers.[7]

3. Nail pigmentation following systemic absorption symmetrically involves all digits and only rarely produces pigment changes limited to the nail unit. In generalized argyria, for example, the skin is diffusely pigmented a slate gray color. An exception, however, is methemoglobinemia that occasionally manifests as a lilac discoloration of only the fingertips and nail beds. In the workplace, such a limited lilac discoloration may occur in an otherwise asymptomatic worker following exposure to aromatic amines or aromatic nitrocompounds such as the nitrobenzenes, nitrotoluenes, anilines, phenylhydrazines, nitrophenols, naphthylamines, nitrophenyls, paraphenylenediamine, acetanilide, dinitro-*o*-cresol, and benzidine. These chemicals are found in the manufacture of dyestuffs, pigments, and explosives as well as in the chemical, textile, rubber, dyeing, and paper industries.[8] The substances are rather distinctive in that they are readily absorbed through the skin. Within the body, they lead to the oxidation of hemoglobin to methemoglobin ($Fe^{++} \rightarrow Fe^{+++}$). When roughly 10 to 15 per cent of one's hemoglobin has been oxidized to pro-

duce 1.5 g of methemoglobin per 100 mL of blood, the purplish-blue color appears, initially limited to the lips, nose, ears, and finger tips.[9,10] Methemoglobin cannot reversibly bind with oxygen and hence is ineffectual in delivering oxygen to the tissues. Furthermore, these nonfunctioning heme units increase the oxygen affinity of their neighboring unaffected units in the same hemoglobin tetramer. Consequently, there is an even further decrease in overall oxygen delivery to the tissues. Nevertheless, when cyanosis first develops, 85 to 90 per cent of one's hemoglobin is still in the normal ferrous state (Fe^{++}), and patients are generally asymptomatic. This is in marked contrast to the more common cyanosis of hypoxemia from cardiac or respiratory disease. For this type of cyanosis to be apparent, roughly 30 to 40 per cent of one's hemoglobin or, more specifically, 5 g of hemoglobin per 100 mL of blood must be deoxygenated.[9] This typically occurs only with a life-threatening hemoglobin-oxygen saturation (65 per cent) and is associated with obvious symptoms or signs of cardiorespiratory disease.

A concerned company nurse once called about four asymptomatic workers who were experiencing recurrent episodes of purplish-blue discoloration of their fingertips and nails while at work. The color would leave momentarily when the nail beds were blanched and would disappear within 16 hours of leaving work. Only methemoglobinemia could account for these findings. Another pigmented hemoglobin moiety, sulfhemoglobin, could explain the asymptomatic fingertips and nail discoloration observed. Cyanosis from sulfhemoglobinemia may occur when only 3 to 7 percent of one's hemoglobin is sulfurated.[11] However, in contrast to methemoglobinemia, the disappearance of this cyanosis is very slow because sulfhemoglobin only leaves the blood with the red blood cells, which have a normal life span of 120 days.[9]

4. Nonblanching transverse white bands of the nail plate (Mees' lines) have been said to occur in occupational arsenic[12,13] and thallium[13] poisoning. Although Mees' lines have occurred following grossly symptomatic, usually life-threatening illnesses as a result of the

oral ingestion of these toxins,[14–16] the author can find no report of their occurrence in work-related arsenic[17] and thallium[18,19] poisonings.*

This is because Mees' lines, presumably, are due to acute rather than chronic toxic exposures. They are not an indicator of any particular toxin and probably represent a response of the nail matrix to any one of a number of fairly acute local or systemic insults. For example, 7 weeks following an episode of near-fatal carbon monoxide poisoning, complicated by renal failure and hemolytic anemia, a patient acquired Mees' lines.[20] Local trauma leading to Mees' lines may be either of mechanical or chemical origin. Although there is a single case report of such lines (leukonychia striae) developing in a keypunch operator,[21] the usual causative workplace mechanical trauma is accidental and of great intensity. These same transverse white bands have occurred in herbicide sprayers as a result of the local matrix toxicity of paraquat,[22,23] diquat,[23] and dinitro-o-cresol.[24] Clearly, this nail condition has little diagnostic or prognostic significance. It does, however, allow an estimate of when some prior illness or local injury occurred.

Distal Onycholysis

Distal onycholysis refers to a separation of the nail plate from the nail bed (except in psoriasis) in a retrograde fashion. The fact that the separation begins distally indicates that this onycholysis is not a disease of the nail matrix. Rather, it is a reaction pattern common to any one of a number of local insults that take advantage of the leverage and access afforded by the nail's distal free end. Occupational onycholysis may develop as a consequence of mechanical, chemical, and biologic hazards.

Mechanical Onycholysis

Obviously, a sufficient mechanical force can acutely elevate the distal end of the nail plate. What is less obvious is that repetitive minor trauma can also lead to onycholysis. This was seen in a chicken-processing plant where a young worker had been using three of his bare fingers to remove 2800 chicken crops each hour over the prior 5 weeks.*[25]

---

*Dermatologists will find it interesting that the rodenticide thallium was used medically as late as the 1950s and most commonly as a depilatory in the treatment of tinea of the scalp. Of 3648 children treated with the standard 8 mg/kg single dose of thallium acetate, there were 216 poisonings and 6 deaths.[18]

---

*The reader will be pleased to learn that the chickens he or she eats are inspected much more slowly, at a rate of 1200 per hour.

More recently, onycholysis has been described in workers repeatedly lifting plastic bags filled with heavy loads.[26] Foreign bodies, such as hair fragments, that wedge themselves up under the nail plate can also result in onycholysis. Yet a review of the published case reports of hair-induced nail disorders concluded that such disorders occur only in the context of an underlying abnormality of the periungual tissue or nail matrix.[27]

Chemical Onycholysis

Allergic Dermatitis. A vast array of chemicals in the workplace may act as sensitizers and lead to onycholysis through involvement of the subungual and periungual tissues. Aware that methyl methacrylate monomer was a potent sensitizer, Fisher and colleagues correctly predicted that the use of this material in sculptured artificial fingernails would lead to allergic reactions. Among those affected were demonstrators of the nail products.[28] The reactions consisted of erythematous or eczematous eruptions of the fingertips, paronychia, and varying degrees of onycholysis. Although the Food and Drug Administration subsequently banned the use of nail preparations containing this material, other methacrylate monomers quickly took its place, and cross-reactions have been reported.[29] Methacrylate monomers now used in dentistry, orthopedics, ultraviolet-cured printing ink manufacture, and a host of other settings continue to produce contact dermatitis of the hands.[30–32] Nevertheless, it appears that nail changes are rare except when the chemical material has been directly and repeatedly applied to the nail.

Skin contact with methacrylate monomers should be avoided. This is easier said than done. Vinyl and latex gloves offer little protection.[30,31] Some have claimed that such gloves are more dangerous than using bare hands, because the rapidly penetrating monomer is occluded between the skin and the glove.[32] Butyl rubber gloves have permitted previously sensitized workers to continue handling methyl methacrylate monomer liquids.[31] Dental technicians apparently have not found it feasible to wear gloves while shaping the methacrylate dental prosthesis.[32] It has been suggested that methacrylate orthopedic bone cement should be mechanically mixed and applied with a spatula while the surgeon wears four pairs of gloves (two cotton gloves sandwiched between two surgical gloves). Following application of the cement, the surgeon should discard the outer three gloves.[33]

Although nail hardeners containing more than 1 to 2 per cent formaldehyde are no longer allowed in the United States, previous use of such products led to sensitization and onycholysis. At times there were accompanying periungual changes,[34,35] but at other times there were not.[36] Although nail dystrophies may occur following occupational exposure to formaldehyde,[37,38] reviews of the cutaneous effects of formaldehyde in the workplace suggest that this does not occur very often.[39]

These examples and others[40] demonstrate that onycholysis may occur as a manifestation of occupational allergic contact dermatitis. However, the relative paucity of these examples suggests that the nail bed is fairly well protected from allergens. We may, however, expect to see onycholysis when the mechanical aspects of work increase a sensitizer's access to the area beneath the nail's distal end. "Tulip finger" illustrates this point: Workers who manually peel daughter bulbs from remnants of the parent tulip bulb develop a debilitating dermatitis of the fingertips[41,42] and onycholysis.[13]

Irritant Dermatitis. Among the first reports of occupational onycholysis was the study of a ketchup bottling plant in 1931.[43] After labels were pasted onto the finished product, the ketchup bottles were thrown into a tub of lukewarm water. A number of women then used sponges to remove the excess paste from the bottles. No soap or other chemicals were used. Within 48 hours of beginning this work, which kept their hands almost continuously immersed, several of the women experienced progressive onycholysis. None of the other employees, including the pasters and the bottlers, had any problem. Observation revealed that the women were picking at resistant specks of paste with their nails. The authors concluded that it was the prolonged immersion in water plus the repetitive mechanical trauma that was responsible for the onycholysis. Twenty years earlier, this same type of careful observation led to a description of onycholysis in washerwomen, whose nails were repeatedly traumatized by water, soap, and friction while rubbing clothes over washboards and while wringing clothes by hand.[43] During the same era, sugar onychia was described in confectioners and bakers. Following 2 months of hand-stuffing jams and jellies into pastries, a woman experienced proximal and distal onycholysis, paronychia, yellow nails, and subungual debris. No fungal mycelia or spores were found.[44]

More recently, irritant-induced onycholysis has been reported in a lifeguard after several weeks of work. Each day, she was required to add a solution of 16 per cent sodium hypochlorite to the pool.[45] A woman laundering clothes in an enzyme detergent of unknown identity for an hour a day for 1 month was also claimed to suffer irritant onycholysis. Patch testing to 1 and 2 per cent solutions of the detergent were nonreactive.[46]

Separation of the distal nail plate from its underlying bed may occur following a single exposure to highly destructive toxins. An example is the onycholysis reported in a worker cleaning gold electrode contacts with a mixture of potassium cyanide and *m*-nitrobenezene sulfonic acid.[47] The most dramatic example is hydrofluoric acid, which may reach the subungual area through a pinhole in a worker's rubber glove.[48]

In 1771, Priestly and Scheele mixed sulfuric acid with the fluorine-containing rock fluorspar and produced a vapor that corroded the flask. This power to attack silica paved the way for hydrofluoric acid's use in foundries to remove sand from castings, in glassworks for etching and frosting glass, in the pottery trades for spot removal, and in the graphite industry for removing silica-containing impurities.[49] This acid is also used in the production of organic and inorganic fluorine compounds, in metal pickling, as a catalyst in petroleum production, for the etching of silicon products in semiconductor manufacture, and as a rust and spot remover.

The incredibly destructive power of hydrofluoric acid depends not on its strength as an acid but on its extremely penetrating fluoride ion. Consequently, it may wreak havoc under a discolored but otherwise benign-appearing skin surface. Contact with acid concentrations lower than 50 per cent may go unnoticed for hours before intense pain begins.

For the past 40 years there has been a safe and effective antidote for the treatment of hydrofluoric acid skin burns.[50] The treatment relies on the precipitation of fluoride ions and, consequently, on the cessation of their destructive advance. With as much speed as possible, the affected area is doused with water and then covered with either a 2.5 per cent calcium gluconate gel (made by mixing a 4-ounce tube of K-Y Jelly with four 10-mL vials of 10 per cent calcium gluconate),[51] an ointment containing magnesium oxide or magnesium sulfate, or iced solutions of either magnesium sulfate or high-molecular-weight quarternary ammonium compounds.[52,53] An experimental animal study of the comparative efficacy of these topical treatments led to the conclusion that calcium gluconate jelly was the only effective therapy.[54] Burns caused by 20 per cent or stronger hydrofluoric acid solution must be urgently evaluated by a physician. The involved tissues should be injected with 5 to 10 per cent calcium gluconate through a 25- to 30-gauge needle.[50,51] Efforts should be made to limit the dose to 0.5 mL/cm^2 to avoid tissue destruction from local pressure.[49,55,56] Local anesthesia should not be used, if possible, as the disappearance of pain indicates the adequacy of the treatment. Although calcium gluconate injection of the wound area has long been considered the definitive therapy of hydrofluoric acid skin burns, Browne has claimed that the topical application of calcium gluconate ointment is just as effective in reducing the extent of injury.[57]

When hydrofluoric acid penetrates under the free end of the nail plate, treatment is more difficult. Most recommendations call for splitting or removing the nail plate and injecting the nail bed with calcium gluconate.[49,52,56,58,59] In this situation, it is recognized that local or regional block anesthesia will be administered before the nail plate is removed. More recently, intra-arterial calcium gluconate (one 10-mL vial of 10 per cent calcium gluconate in 50 mL of 5 per cent dextrose in water [D$_5$W] infused over 4 hours, repeated twice as necessary) has been recommended in an effort to spare the nail plate.[60–62]

Although pinhole-sized burns produce sheer agony, they do not pose a systemic threat. Being splashed with hydrofluoric acid, however, is a medical emergency. Several years ago, there was a published case report of a worker who died following a 100 per cent hydrofluoric acid burn that involved only 2.5 per cent of his skin surface.[63] In spite of massive intravenous and burn area injections of calcium gluconate, the patient's serum calcium could not be raised above 3.1 mg/100 mL (normal 8.8 to 10.3). The only difference between this patient and the survivor of a similar accident reported[64] 7 years earlier was a 2-hour delay before subcutaneous and intravenous calcium gluconate was administered. Although emergency medical treatment is essential, it may not be sufficient to correct life-threatening hypocalcemia. Buckingham described intractable hypocalcemia and ventricular fibrillation in a petrochemical worker suffering a 5 per cent body surface area burn from anhydrous hydrofluoric acid.[65] Surgical excision of the entire burn area was credited with saving the worker's life when large doses of intravenous and subcutaneous calcium proved ineffective.

Three months following publication of the just-described case fatality, the author was asked to investigate yet another death, that of a young worker who suffered a 10 per cent body burn from 70 per cent hydrofluoric acid. Review of the records revealed that none of the treating physicians had been aware of the particular toxicity of hydrofluoric acid. Even more tragically, hydrofluoric acid was found to be unnecessary at the workplace in question.

A worker who suffers onycholysis secondary to a pinhole-sized burn from hydrofluoric acid will benefit from treatment. However, perhaps more importantly, steps should be taken to prevent more serious subsequent injuries. Industrial hygienists from state and federal agencies or from the private sector can help an employer determine the need for this toxic material as well as the appropriate engineering controls and personal protective equipment necessary for its safe handling.

Biologic Onycholysis

The most common microbial infection leading to onycholysis is dermatophytosis. Although host predisposition is generally offered in explanation for why some experience this condition, it is clear that environmental factors are extremely important. In hot climates, closed shoes increase sweating and maceration, ideal conditions for the development of dermatophytosis. During World War II, 80 per cent of the soldiers in the South Pacific experienced tinea pedis.[66] Once in the toes' web spaces, *Trichophyton rubrum* and *Trichophyton mentagrophytes* may spread to the toenails and fingernails, where they may produce onycholysis. It has been noted that when onycholysis occurs, one may suspect the coexistence of yeast.[67]

Workers required to wear heavy boots or gloves for long periods of time, workers using a factory's communal foot bath, and workers with frequent hand immersion in water all are more susceptible to dermatophyte infections. Although zoophilic dermatophytoses are more common in veterinarians, farmers, butchers, abattoir workers, and zoo keepers, it is unclear how often those infections lead to nail involvement.

Forty years ago, Peck and Schwartz explored the sticky issue of assigning causality to dermatophyte infections among the work force.[68] Their thoughts are still very relevant today. Adams has discussed the difficulty of determining whether a *T. rubrum* infection of the hand can be considered work related. He noted that an occupational origin may be presumed when the affected hand was just previously involved in mildly traumatic work and claimed that most compensation boards will accept the causal or contributory relationship.[69]

Configurational Changes of the Nail Unit

Koilonychia

Koilonychia (spoon nail) has been described in car mechanics,[70] cabinet makers (Fig. 17–1),[71] mushroom growers repeatedly lifting heavy plastic bags,[26] homemakers, glassworkers, chimney sweeps, ricksha pullers (toes),[72] a coil winder,[73] and a pin threader.[74] The affected nails have typically been those most involved in some repetitive minor mechanical trauma and those most exposed to oils, solvents, acids, and alkali. The condition is painless and poses no hardship.

Clubbing

Clubbing of the digits is anatomically explained as an overabundance of vascular connective tissue. Why clubbing develops and why there is an increased amount of blood flow through these digits have remained mysteries for the past 2500 years.[75] We typically see clubbing in patients with cyanotic congen-

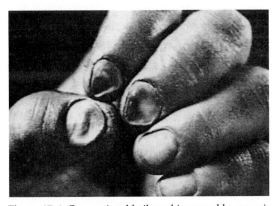

Figure 17–1. Occupational koilonychia caused by organic solvents. From Ancona-Alayon A: Occupational koilonychia from organic solvents. Contact Dermatitis 1:367, 1975. Used with permission.

ital heart disease, liver disease, pulmonary disease, and lung cancer. In the workplace, clubbing may develop in those with the pneumoconiotic lung diseases, which follow exposure to such materials as asbestos, talc, beryllium, and silica. In these disease processes, clubbing is not an early indicator of disease. Nevertheless, when clubbing is observed, further investigation is warranted. It should be easy to distinguish pathologic clubbing from the two forms of hereditary clubbing. True hereditary clubbing appears shortly after birth, whereas the incomplete form of pachydermoperiostosis develops around the time of puberty and progresses through the end of adolescence.[75] Neither of these conditions, then, would be developing at the same time as would clubbing secondary to a pneumoconiosis. This distinction is helpful only if the worker or the worker's family or physician can tell us when the clubbing first appeared. Adding additional difficulty is that until recently[76,77] there has been no qualitative or quantitative definitional scale to characterize this condition of painless uniform swelling of the soft tissues of the terminal phalanx.

The author saw an insulator who for a number of years was moderately short of breath but who was still working on asbestos removal projects. He had marked clubbing of all 20 of his digits (Fig. 17–2A). His work history, pulmonary function testing, and chest x-ray films (Fig. 17-2B) were diagnostic of severe asbestosis. This diagnosis, which should have been made years before, had important ramifications for his future health, his work, and his financial status.

Other work-related causes of clubbing are apparently rare. One of the early studies of vinyl chloride polymerization exposure described 31 workers with occupational acro-osteolysis, 8 of whom had clubbing as well.[78] Under unusual circumstances, clubbing also may occur as a result of repetitive trauma. Over a 13-year period, clubbing developed in a young man who exercised his fingers by ramming them into a bowl of raw rice 4 to 6 hours per day.[79]

Nail Plate Textural Irregularities From Paronychia, Other Insults to the Nail Matrix, and Direct Nail Plate Trauma

Paronychia

Stone and Mullins have described chronic paronychia as a paraungual inflammation of insidious onset and persistence.[80] The process

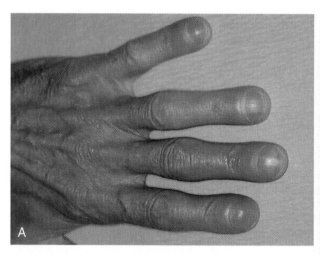

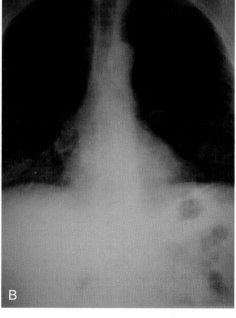

Figure 17–2. Manifestations of asbestosis in an insulator. *A,* Digital clubbing. *B,* Chest x-ray film.

typically starts at the lateral nail fold, which becomes swollen, mildly scaly, possibly pruritic, and eventually separated from the lateral nail margin. With time, the whole process moves proximally to involve the lateral aspect of the posterior nail fold. There, the cuticle separates from the nail plate and permits a pocket to form under the proximal fold. Periodically, acute inflammation with tenderness develops in this pocket. As a consequence of the inflammation, there is often an irregularity in nail growth manifesting as a wavy nail plate. Although *Candida albicans* can usually be cultured from this lesion, its role in the condition remains controversial.

It is fairly clear that certain working conditions predispose to or foster the development of chronic paronychia.[81] Schwartz and colleagues[82] have listed three dozen occupations associated with this condition. Common features of these occupations include prolonged immersion of the hands in water, alkali, solvents, oils, or soaps and conditions conducive to maceration.

Bakers are at risk from flour, baking powder, sugar, and fruit fillings; battery makers from sulfuric acid; building trades workers from cement, solvents, and trauma; and etchers from acids and chromates. Foreign bodies such as hair may be contributory,[83] as may crystals of oxalic acid and thorns. A number of biologic agents may cause paronychia. Herpes simplex infections of the fingertip are not uncommon in dental and medical personnel. Tuberculous paronychia has been described in pathologists, nurses, and laboratory technicians.[84,85] Fever, regional lymphadenopathy, and a minimally symptomatic paronychia are suggestive of this condition, which may be diagnosed by biopsy or aspiration. Erysipeloid (*Erysipelothrix insidiosa*) mainly occurs as an occupational disease from the handling of fish, poultry, and other animal carcasses. Obviously, many of the indolent microbial diseases that are characterized by skin invasion may present as chronic paronychia.

The general treatment of chronic paronychia requires avoidance of moisture, irritants, maceration, and trauma. This may be difficult in the workplace, because prolonged glove wearing may lead to even further maceration. Although this condition commonly persists for years, further investigation is warranted when the patient's occupation suggests the opportunity for invasion by an inert or microbial foreign body.

Other Matrix Insults

Many of the mechanical, biologic, and chemical agents discussed in this chapter can also produce textural irregularities of the nail plate. If an insult to the matrix is transitory and localized, pitting of the nail may occur. If the insult is transitory but not localized, then a transverse depression in the nail (Beau's line) may appear.[86–88] Physical forces in the form of microwave radiation have also been held responsible for the development of Beau's lines in two snack bar employees who were working with an allegedly malfunctioning microwave oven.[89] Prolonged continuous insults to the nail matrix may lead to thin, brittle, irregularly surfaced nails. At times it may be difficult to determine whether the insult was to the matrix or to the nail plate. However, the history of the condition's evolution should provide an answer to this question.

Onychorrhexis and Onychoschizia

Onychorrhexis and onychoschizia clearly are common problems in the workplace. Isolated and repetitive mechanical trauma account for most occupational nail splitting and breakage.[88] One cross-sectional study concluded that wet working conditions increase nail brittleness (and onychorrhexis and onychoschizia) in women but not in men.[90]

Hemorrhage Below the Nail

In the workplace, subungual hematomas and splinter hemorrhages frequently occur as a result of mechanical trauma.[91] This trauma may at times be so subtle as to go unnoticed. Pan washers wearing rubber gloves[92] and those who wear tight-fitting boots[93] have acquired subungual hematomas. To evacuate these hematomas and produce instant relief, trephining through the nail with a red-hot paper clip was "introduced" 30 years ago.[94] In the years since, others have recommended using an electric drill or twirling a venipuncture needle back and forth over the nail plate. The author's experience and patients' testimony[95] suggest that a heavy-gauge paper clip may be hard to beat for ease, efficacy, and acceptability. A disposable, hand-held, high-temperature cautery device has been promoted as the optimal tool with which to evacuate a subungual hematoma.[96] The physician should be certain that the discoloration thought to be due to the blood is not from melanin deposition. Ungual melanoma must always enter into the differential diagnosis, and if there is any doubt whatever, a biopsy is mandatory. Interestingly, some have proposed that trauma may predispose to subungual melanoma.[97]

SOURCES OF INFORMATION AND STRATEGIES IN THEIR USE

If both the occupational origin and the specific cause of a patient's nail condition are not readily apparent, then we require more information. The operational model depicted in Figure 17–3 can help organize our approach to the collection of this information.

Although we may find ourselves preoccupied with identifying "the exposure," we must be equally diligent in our evaluation of the other relevant factors. That is, the discovery of a nail-toxic chemical in the workplace cannot alone justify the presumption that the chemical is responsible for our patient's disorder. Rather, we need to determine whether the properties of the chemical together with the nature of our patient's actual exposure warrant the presumption. In making this determination, we must also consider any predisposing host factors or additional external influences that might make such a nail disease more likely to occur.

An orthopedic nurse had been mixing bone cement for a number of years. In the past, she had experienced a painful contact dermatitis of her fingertips from the cement despite her regular use of two pairs of latex gloves. The eruption and painful paresthesias disappeared after she had been out of work for 2 months. She subsequently resumed mixing the cement but wore butyl rubber gloves rather than latex because she learned they would protect her from the responsible sensitizer, a methyl methacrylate monomer liquid.[31] Now imagine that periodically the butyl rubber gloves were not available. She would then resort to latex gloves without difficulty. On one such day, however, after several days of prolonged hand immersion in water, she experienced pain and erythema of her periungual skin hours after mixing bone cement. We can assume that two important factors operate here. First, the patient was predisposed to an allergic reaction as a result of her earlier sensitization. Second, the prolonged immersion of her hands in water was a potentiating external influence.

With an organized approach, then, we should start our search for information with the patient.

The Patient and Beyond

In 1713, Bernadino Ramazzini, the father of occupational medicine, counseled that "when a doctor visits a working class home . . . he should take time for his examination, and to the questions recommended by Hippocrates, he should ask one more—what is your occupation?"[98] He further instructed us to inquire into the nature of our patients' work to determine the potential for toxic or hazardous exposures. Our patients can educate us through descriptions of their day-to-day workplace activities; with their help, we can estimate the potential for and extent of cutaneous and systemic exposure to various materials and conditions.

Our interview with the patient should provide us with information on the following:

1. The type of business, the services rendered, and the products manufactured
2. Work practices, including setup, at the beginning of the day and cleanup at the end of the day

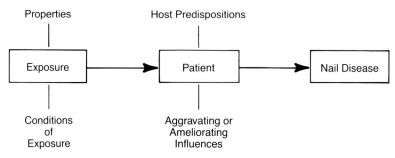

Figure 17–3. Host-exposure interactions in the development of nail disease.

3. Contact with dusts, fumes, vapors, gases, chemicals, radiation, vibration, and temperature extremes

4. The names or types of chemicals, cleaning materials, and metals and the frequency and extent of exposure to them

5. Personal protective equipment used, such as respirators, gloves, barrier creams, hand cleaners, and the rest room soap

6. Engineering controls, such as local exhaust ventilation, enclosures, and "no-touch" processes

7. Chronology of the nail condition with respect to the onset of work, task reassignment, periods away from work, accidents, and changes in materials, production processes, engineering processes, and personal protective equipment use

8. The presence of work-related cutaneous and mucosal irritation as well as respiratory, neurologic, and constitutional symptoms

9. The presence of similar nail disease in coworkers and their common conditions of exposure

10. Hobbies with potential chemical or metal exposures

11. Prior skin and nail disease and history of asthma, atopic dermatitis, and allergic rhinitis

12. Chronology of past jobs

Although one could spend hours eliciting answers to all these questions, 5 to 10 minutes of directed inquiry is often sufficient. Even if a definitive etiologic agent is not identified, we will probably have a fair idea as to whether or not the nail condition is work related. If at this point we still require further information, it will be of three types:

1. The actual names of the suspect chemicals or biologic materials in the workplace. Rarely, we will need to learn the characteristics of suspect physical or mechanical forces such as the vibratory frequency of a hand-held pneumatic tool.

2. The properties of these materials with regard to their inherent toxicity and paths of absorption, distribution, metabolism, and excretion.

3. The nature of the workplace exposure conditions. This information is needed to assess the opportunity for the required contact between a suspect workplace material and our patient.

There are a number of available sources of this information.

Identification of Chemical Names

Sometimes our patients will know only the brand names of the chemical materials they use at work, and other times they will not even know that. In both of these situations, the following information sources generally prove helpful.

Material Safety Data Sheet

The Material Safety Data Sheet (MSDS) is a brief form that lists the ingredients of brand name chemical products, the properties of these ingredients, the potential hazards of exposure, and handling precautions (Fig. 17–4). These forms are completed by the product's manufacturer and provided with the product to its commercial users. Although standard forms from the Occupational Safety and Health Administration (OSHA) are typically used, there are no strict quality or accuracy requirements. MSDSs are, however, an important starting point.

Right-To-Know Laws

Prior to 1984, approximately two dozen states and municipalities passed legislation requiring employers to maintain files of MSDSs for all toxic materials in use in the workplace.[99] Although each of these laws is somewhat different, they all require that copies of MSDSs be provided by employers to employees requesting them. Furthermore, nearly all of these statutes have sections that grant treating physicians this same right. To determine whether or not a right-to-know law is in force in your community, call your municipal government, State Department of Health, and State Department of Labor.

After a decade of frustrated action and inaction, OSHA promulgated a federal Hazard Communication Standard in 1984 that was subsequently extended to all employment sectors.[100] Despite the OSHA Standards' clear pre-emption provision, local statutes generally remain in force unless they have been legally challenged. If only a small number of MSDSs are required, and the brand names are known, it may be simpler to access this information on the Internet. The Vermont Safety Information on the Internet (http://hazard.com) currently lists more than 100,000 MSDSs.

MATERIAL SAFETY DATA SHEET

S–210
31:9203

Material Safety Data Sheet

May be used to comply with
OSHA's Hazard Communication Standard,
29 CFR 1910.1200. Standard must be
consulted for specific requirements.

U.S. Department of Labor

Occupational Safety and Health Administration
(Non-Mandatory Form)
Form Approved
OMB No. 1218-0072

IDENTITY *(As Used on Label and List)*

Note: *Blank spaces are not permitted. If any item is not applicable, or no information is available, the space must be marked to indicate that.*

Section I

Manufacturer's Name	Emergency Telephone Number
Address *(Number, Street, City, State, and ZIP Code)*	Telephone Number for Information
	Date Prepared
	Signature of Preparer *(optional)*

Section II — Hazardous Ingredients/Identity Information

Hazardous Components (Specific Chemical Identity; Common Name(s))	OSHA PEL	ACGIH TLV	Other Limits Recommended	% *(optional)*

Section III — Physical/Chemical Characteristics

Boiling Point	Specific Gravity (H_2O = 1)	
Vapor Pressure (mm Hg.)	Melting Point	
Vapor Density (AIR = 1)	Evaporation Rate (Butyl Acetate = 1)	

Solubility in Water

Appearance and Odor

Section IV — Fire and Explosion Hazard Data

Flash Point (Method Used)	Flammable Limits	LEL	UEL

Extinguishing Media

Special Fire Fighting Procedures

Unusual Fire and Explosion Hazards

Figure 17–4. Material Safety Data Sheet.

31:9204 REFERENCE FILE

Section V — Reactivity Data

Stability	Unstable		Conditions to Avoid
	Stable		

Incompatibility (*Materials to Avoid*)

Hazardous Decomposition or Byproducts

Hazardous Polymerization	May Occur		Conditions to Avoid
	Will Not Occur		

Section VI — Health Hazard Data

Route(s) of Entry: Inhalation? Skin? Ingestion?

Health Hazards *(Acute and Chronic)*

Carcinogenicity: NTP? IARC Monographs? OSHA Regulated?

Signs and Symptoms of Exposure

Medical Conditions
Generally Aggravated by Exposure

Emergency and First Aid Procedures

Section VII — Precautions for Safe Handling and Use

Steps to Be Taken in Case Material Is Released or Spilled

Waste Disposal Method

Precautions to Be Taken in Handling and Storing

Other Precautions

Section VIII — Control Measures

Respiratory Protection *(Specify Type)*

Ventilation	Local Exhaust	Special
	Mechanical *(General)*	Other

Protective Gloves	Eye Protection

Other Protective Clothing or Equipment

Work/Hygienic Practices

☆ USGPO 1986-491-529/45775

Figure 17–4. *Continued*

The Clinical Toxicology of Commercial Products[101]

This frequently updated book edited by Gleason, Gosselin, and Hodge lists the ingredients of about 20,000 trade name products and is readily available in nearly every medical library. In the absence of MSDSs, this volume can provide important information if correct trade names are known.

Poison Centers

City, state, or regional poison control centers can be reached from any telephone in the United States. Although most of us turn to such centers for help with the management of ingested toxins, we rarely think to call them for help with our evaluations of workplace exposures. This is another valuable resource, particularly when we know only a brand name.

National Institute for Occupational Safety and Health (NIOSH)

NIOSH was created by the Occupational Safety and Health Act of 1970. The institute has federal responsibility for training and research needs in occupational health and advises OSHA on the establishment of federal occupational exposure standards. Among its services, NIOSH maintains a large listing of trade name substances and their ingredients. One can gain access to this listing by calling 1-800-356-4674.

Occasionally, we'll reach a dead end and not even learn the trade name of a suspect material. Should this happen, we can turn to three excellent reference works that provide descriptions of various jobs and processes as well as the kinds of chemicals that would be used.[102–104] One of these books, *Occupational Skin Disease*,[102] is especially helpful in its detailed account of the specific irritant and sensitizing chemicals expected at various job sites.

Determining a Chemical's Toxicity and Other Properties

Once the chemicals contained in a suspect material are known, there are a number of options available to determine their toxicity, their routes of absorption, and other such informa-

tion. Reference librarians at the medical society, the university, or the hospital can be of great assistance in this area. Three especially helpful resources are listed next.

NIOSH Registry of Toxic Effects of Chemical Substances (RTECS)[105]

This quarterly updated work is a listing of nearly 100,000 toxins. In addition to printed form, the RTECS is also available on CD-ROM (see later discussion) and as a National Library of Medicine real-time interactive computer data base. For each of the entries, irritancy data are provided.

Patty's Industrial Hygiene and Toxicology[106]

This is a standard in the field of occupational health. Its recently updated volumes on toxicology provide exhaustive reviews of the properties of a multitude of toxins.

NIOSH Technical Information Clearinghouse (NIOSHTIC)

NIOSHTIC is a computerized bibliographic data base, maintained by the National Institute for Occupational Safety and Health (NIOSH), that contains more than 150,000 citations to workplace safety and health literature. Each NIOSHTIC citation includes a descriptive abstract of the reference as well as pertinent bibliographic information to permit the reference's retrieval from public or university libraries.

The data base is available commercially online from DIALOG Information Services, Inc. (1-800-334-2564) and Orbit Search Service (1-800-955-0906). It is also available in compact disc–read only memory (CD-ROM) format as "OSH-ROM" from SilverPlatter Information (1-800-343-0064) and as "CCINFOdisc" from the Canadian Centre for Occupational Health and Safety (250 Main Street East, Hamilton, Ontario, Canada L8N 1H6). For physicians without ready access to computerized literature retrieval systems, NIOSH might perform free searches (513-533-8328).

Workplace Exposure Conditions

If we detect a workplace chemical capable of producing our patient's nail disease, we still have to determine whether there was sufficient opportunity for contact at work. To determine this, if not clear from the patient's account, we can refer to the three works[102–104] previously cited for descriptions of various jobs and processes. We can also speak with industrial hygienists in our state's Department of Health or Department of Labor and in OSHA area and regional offices. Finally, we may wish to visit the patient's workplace.

THE PLANT VISIT

The visit may be prompted by a number of reasons. You may wish to observe your patient's working conditions to assess the work relatedness of his or her nail disorder, the specific cause of the disorder, and the appropriateness of various potential interventions. You may be asked by a plant's management, insurer, or union leadership to evaluate a clustering of a specific nail condition or to formulate a preventive program of nail health. Whatever the reason, the opportunity will enhance your appreciation of the material conditions and the dynamics of the workplace. You will also become more comfortable and capable and will derive greater satisfaction in your subsequent evaluation of patients with suspected work-related disease.

Preparations

In planning a visit, you should take care of the following matters:

1. Contact the plant's management and request permission for a tour. Explain your reasons for the visit in as constructive and positive a manner as possible.
2. Establish a date and time that will coincide with normal plant operations. Request that a knowledgeable guide be available to assist you. This would ideally be an industrial hygienist or, in decreasing order of preference, the production supervisor, the safety officer, the plant engineer, or the manager. The size of the facility will determine the availability of these personnel.
3. Notify any union representatives of your intended visit. Employee cooperation both at the time of your tour as well as with your subsequent recommendations will be influenced by perceptions of your integrity and concern for workers' health.

4. Review the work processes and conditions of exposure which you expect to witness.

At the Plant

Once at the facility, you should keep a detailed written log and proceed as follows:

1. Establish background information on:
   a. Names and positions of contacts and guides
   b. Number of employees, their demographics, and shifts
   c. Products manufactured or services provided
   d. Plant history
   e. Union representation and history
   f. Health and safety facilities, services, and personnel
   g. Medical services, programs, and personnel
   h. Workers' Compensation insurer and health benefit programs
2. Review with medical personnel, if available, the health experience of the workplace with particular reference to skin and nail disease.
3. Tour the plant, having first established any ground rules for your questioning of employees on the line. Beginning at the point of entry for raw materials, you should proceed in a logical fashion and end with the finished product. When applicable, you should spend additional time at your patient's work stations and observe all of his or her tasks and conditions of exposure. Those tasks that cannot be performed at the time can be simulated by your patient.
4. Inspect the plant's nonproduction areas such as the locker rooms, washstands, lavatories, and cafeteria.
5. In each area, assess the adequacy of engineering controls, personal protective equipment, work practices, and general sanitation.
6. Having thanked your hosts, leave the plant and legibly record your overall impressions of the potential hazards and suitable methods of control. When appropriate, go back to your reference works and consult with specialists in occupational health.

Your plant visit need not be as detailed as that just described. The purpose of your visit should determine what is reasonable. In the context of occupational nail disease, you will mainly be assessing the opportunity for repetitive mechanical trauma; immersion in or prolonged contact with alkali, acids, and other irritants; excessive confinement of hands and feet; and contact, however subtle, with sensitizing materials. You will simultaneously be evaluating the adequacy of existing controls and the need for additional or alternative controls.

TREATMENT AND PREVENTION OF OCCUPATIONAL NAIL DISEASE

There is actually nothing special about the treatment of occupational nail disease. What is special, however, is that we can afford to be extremely optimistic in our prognostication. A responsible etiologic agent can usually be identified and appropriate interventions made. It is clear that onycholysis resulting from repetitive trauma can be treated much more successfully than can onycholysis caused by psoriasis. Our treatment strategy, then, is one of prevention, both primary and secondary.

Pre-Employment Evaluation

The inclination to identify and exclude job applicants who are at high risk for the development of work-related skin or nail disease is tempting. Such an approach, however, comes into conflict with laws and principles of antidiscrimination. According to federal statute, a worker cannot be excluded from consideration simply because he or she is at significantly greater risk for experiencing or aggravating a medical condition when compared with other individuals. That is, a job applicant with psoriasis whose only hand involvement is nail pitting cannot be excluded from work as a dishwasher on the basis of a 10 per cent risk of onycholysis. Even though this risk may be 100 times greater than that of nonpsoriatic applicants, the fact remains that the probability of onycholysis developing cannot be considered excessive or inevitable. If the risk were 50 per cent, then we could recommend exclusion, but only if the risk could not be reduced through reasonable managerial efforts. Consequently, the author's contractual agreement with all employers includes the following statement:

Our health personnel will participate in pre-employment, preplacement, return-to-work, and job transfer examinations only if we are satisfied that such activities will not inherently discriminate by race, religion, national origin, age, sex, or handicap, medical or otherwise, as mandated by Title VII of the 1964 Civil Rights Act, the Age Discrimination in Employment Act of 1967 and 1975, and the American with Disabilities Act of 1990.[107] More specifically, we will find an employee or candidate not suitable for a given job only if: a) there is excessive risk that the worker will cause injury to him or herself or to other workers as a consequence of performing that job, b) this excessive risk cannot be alleviated by a reasonable accommodation by the employer, c) the excessive risk can be predicted in a manner that considers only the necessary tasks of the job, d) the test or factor used to predict the excessive risk is applied to all workers seeking a similar job, and e) the test or factor has reasonable accuracy.

Pre-employment and other similar examinations will only be performed after a job applicant has been informed that he or she will be hired pending successful completion of the health examination. The results of these examinations will be provided to the individuals so examined. The personnel department will receive a recommendation that excludes medical diagnoses.

These considerations in no way prevent the author from discussing a risk estimate with the job applicant. If he or she decides that a 10 per cent risk of onycholysis is unacceptable, that is a personal decision.

In a discussion of dermatologic risk assessment, Cohen[108] pointed out that at present our science of predicting risk is based on rather tenuous underpinnings. He concluded that the major determinant of predisposition to occupational skin disease is probably the working environment. From a practical viewpoint, Shmunes[109] suggested that certain dermatoses may in fact carry the predictive power required by law. Taking his lead, the author would concur and suggest that in the context of nail disease we carefully consider applicants with the job-host predisposition relationships listed in Table 17–1. The list is neither exhaustive nor meant to justify an applicant's exclusion. Rather, the individual applicant must be considered in the context of both the specific job requirements and reasonable accommodations by the employer.[110,111] For example, a worker with severe tinea pedis and onychomycosis need not be excluded from work requiring the use of heavy boots if every hour or two the boots could be removed and the feet cleaned, dried, and dusted.

Prevention in the Workplace

Whether you wish to minimize the risk to one of your patients with nail disease or are

Table 17–1. JOB-HOST PREDISPOSITION RELATIONSHIPS PREDICTIVE OF NAIL DISEASE

Predisposition	Working Conditions
Chronic paronychia	Wet or requiring skin occlusion
Onychomycosis	Wet or requiring skin occlusion
Onycholysis	Wet or repetitive trauma
Long nails	Repetitive trauma
Contact dermatitis	Opportunity for contact with an agent to which the applicant has been previously sensitized

asked to design a preventive program for workers subject to nail toxic conditions, it will be useful to consider the following questions:

1. Product substitution: Is there an irritant or sensitizing chemical that may be replaced by a safer alternative? An industrial hygienist can help answer this question.

2. Engineering controls: Can machinery that spares the nails be used? Examples include machine guards on foot presses, a dolly to carry heavy plastic bags, and a "no-touch" system for aromatic amino and nitro-compounds that penetrate all glove materials.

3. Administrative practices: Can job assignments and breaks be arranged so as to minimize uninterrupted periods of hand and foot immersion and occlusion?

4. Work practices: Have workers been provided with sufficient time and training to perform their work in the safest way possible? For example, bottle washers should be taught not to pick at things with their nails.

5. Personal protective equipment: Are there gloves of the proper size and are frequent changes available? Are gloves constructed of materials that can be expected to prevent penetration by the chemicals being handled? Are cotton liners available? Are solvent-free, minimally irritating, hypoallergenic skin cleaners available?

6. Education: Do the employees understand the risks of their work and the purpose of the required work practices, controls, and personal protective equipment?

Occupational Skin Disease[102] contains a wealth of information on personal protective equipment and product substitution, and *Recognition of Health Hazards in Industry*[103] contains much information on engineering controls and work practices. Under the entry "Safety Equipment and Clothing" in the yellow pages of your local telephone directory, you will find sources of information, brochures, and samples of personal protective equipment.

DISABILITY COMPENSATION

A book on nail disease is hardly the place for a lengthy dissertation on disability compensation. However, because skin disease accounts for half of all reported cases of occupational disease in the United States and because most physicians dread involvement in Workers' Compensation cases, the following points are germane:

1. The central tenet of the Workers' Compensation system is that workers disabled by circumstances arising out of and in the course of employment should be compensated for lost earning power.

2. It is important to recognize that in the United States the Workers' Compensation system did not evolve as a component of a social welfare state. At the turn of this century, an increasing number of successful lawsuits were being brought by injured workers against their employers. In response, the National Association of Manufacturers and the National Civic Federation, whose members included large corporations, began to lobby for state Workers' Compensation laws. All 50 states eventually had such laws, which substituted a limited, no-fault disability insurance program for the right to sue one's employer for a work-related injury.[112] Employers preferred the predictable cost of insurance premiums to the unpredictable risk of a court-ordered, financially catastrophic award.

3. The Workers' Compensation system in the United States, in contrast to that of most other industrialized nations, involves its participants in an adversarial contest. Unfortunately, the intensity of this needless battle is further heightened by the knowledge that an injured worker may have no other source of income.

The most striking difference in benefits between the eight programs and the United States is the availability abroad of significant and relatively generous alternatives to and supplements of workers' compensation benefits. These programs are particularly significant to persons whose disabilities are not work connected, and so are especially important in cases of disease. Benefits are always more generous when the disablement is due to an occupational disease (except in Holland); however, the next best alternative is often only slightly less substantial when the illness is not occupational in origin. The availability of alternatives must make it less difficult for a compensation administrator to rule against a claimant and a worker or a survivor to accept such a decision. Many decisions need never be made because some of these alternatives to workers' compensation provide the initial temporary support to workers without regard to the arising-out-of-and-in-the-course-of test. In many instances before benefits expire the person has been fully restored to his previous position and the issue of source of the condition is never raised.[2]

4. Physicians are obligated to inform their patients when an illness has been caused or aggravated by work. This is especially important when an illness has led to a loss of work time. It should be recognized that there may be no one other than the physician who is in a position to so inform the worker.

5. Physicians should be aware that in assessing the work relatedness of a patient's illness the standard of proof required under Workers' Compensation law is that the illness must be more likely than not to have been caused, contributed to, or aggravated by work. This is far different from the "beyond a shadow of a doubt" standard required in criminal law and far different from the scientific standard with which physicians are more familiar.

6. Physicians should also recognize that, in general, predisposing host factors are irrelevant in the determination of work relatedness. That is, the employer "takes the worker as (s)he is." This does not preclude secondary injury funds and apportionment schemes by which states attempt a more equitable allocation of costs.

7. The following practical suggestions should have immediate relevance to physicians who are providing written or verbal testimony before the Workers' Compensation system.

   a. Letters written in support of the work relatedness of a patient's medical condition should note the specific diagnosis; the causative, contributing, or aggravating factors; the degree of impairment; specific activity limitations; the expected duration of these limitations; the restrictions necessary to minimize further aggravation of the condition; the recommended therapy; and the degree of physician certainty as to the work relatedness of the condition. The phrase "possibly due to" is of no use in supporting a claim of work relatedness, whereas the phrase "probably due to," meaning more likely than not, is sufficient.

   b. The more precisely written such letters are, the less likely will be the need to provide further testimony in person or by deposition before the Workers' Compensation board.

   c. Some states offer physicians the option of giving testimony by formal deposition in their own medical offices rather than having to appear before the Workers' Compensation commission. Physicians are not always apprised of this option by the attorneys involved in the case.

   d. Some physicians have come to refuse all requests to serve as an expert witness for their patients because, in the past, they failed to receive promised witness fees from an attorney. Rather than penalizing all of their patients, such physicians could require advance payment from the requesting attorney.

   e. Each state Workers' Compensation system has its own idiosyncrasies. Some of these peculiarities can be found in the annually updated *Analysis of Workers' Compensation Laws*.[113] More practical assistance, however, may be available from individual Workers' Compensation commissions and from state bar associations.

References

1. Ronchese F: Occupational nails. Cutis 5:164, 1969.
2. Barth PS, Hunt HA: Workers' Compensation and Work-Related Illnesses and Diseases. MIT Press, Cambridge, MA, 1980, pp 146, 255–257.
3. Tucker SB, Key MM: Occupational skin disease. *In* Rom WN (ed): Environmental and Occupational Medicine. Little Brown, Boston, 1983.
4. Baran RL: Occupational nail disorders. *In* Adams RM (ed): Occupational Skin Disease. WB Saunders, Philadelphia, 1990, pp 160–171.
5. Daniel CR III, Osment LS: Nail pigmentation abnormalities. Cutis 25:595, 1980.
6. Harris AO, Rosen T: Nail discoloration due to mahogany. Cutis 43:55, 1989.
7. Bleehen SS, Gould DJ, Harrington CI, et al: Occupational argyria: Light and electron microscopic studies and x-ray microanalysis. Br J Dermatol 104:19, 1981.
8. Benya TJ, Cornish HH: Aromatic nitro and amino compounds. *In* Clayton GD, Clayton FE (eds): Patty's Industrial Hygiene and Toxicology, vol 2B. Wiley, New York, 1994, pp 947–1085.
9. Schmitter CR: Sulfhemoglobin and methemoglobin—Uncommon causes of cyanosis. Anesthesiology 43:586, 1975.

10. Harris JC, Rumack BH, Peterson RG, et al: Methemoglobinemia resulting from absorption of nitrates. JAMA 242:2869, 1979.

11. Park CM, Nagel RL: Sulfhemoglobinemia. N Engl J Med 310:1579, 1984.

12. Schwartz L, Tulipan L, Birmingham DJ: Occupational Diseases of the Skin. Lea & Febiger, Philadelphia, 1957.

13. Baran RL: Occupational nail disorders. In Adams RM (ed): Occupational Skin Disease. Grune & Stratton, New York, 1983, pp 99–109.

14. Welter A, Michaux M, Blondeel A: Lignes de Mees dans un cas d'intoxication aigue a l'arsenic. Dermatologica 165:482, 1982.

15. Aldrich CJ: Leuconychia striata arsenicalis transversus. Am J Med Sci 127:702, 1904.

16. Mees RA: The nails with arsenical polyneuritis. JAMA 72:1337, 1919.

17. Proceedings of the International Conference on Environmental Arsenic. Environ Health Perspect 19:1, 1977.

18. Munch JC: Human thallotoxicosis. JAMA 102:1929, 1934.

19. Richeson EM: Industrial thallium intoxication. Ind Med Surg 27:607, 1958.

20. Leavel UW, Farley CH, McIntyre JS: Cutaneous changes in a patient with carbon monoxide poisoning. Arch Dermatol 99:429, 1969.

21. Honda M, Hattori S, Koyama L, et al: Leukonychia striae. Arch Dermatol 112:1147, 1976.

22. Hearn CED, Keir W: Nail damage in spray operators exposed to paraquat. Br J Ind Med 28:399, 1971.

23. Samman PD, Johnston ENM: Nail damage associated with handling of paraquat and diquat. BMJ 1:818, 1969.

24. Baran RL: Nail damage caused by weed killers and insecticides. Arch Dermatol 110:467, 1974.

25. Ronchese F: Nail defect and occupational trauma. Arch Dermatol 85:404, 1962.

26. Schubert B, Minard JJ, Baran R, et al: Onychopathy of mushroom growers. Ann Dermatol Venereol 104:627, 1977.

27. DeBerker D, Dawber R, Wojnarowska F: Subungual hair implantation in hairdressers (letter). Br J Dermatol 130:400, 1994.

28. Fisher AA, Franks A, Glick H: Allergic sensitization of the skin and nails to acrylic plastic nails. J Allergy 28:84, 1957.

29. Fisher AA: Cross reactions between methyl methacrylate monomer and acrylic monomers presently used in acrylic nail preparations. Contact Dermatitis 6:345, 1980.

30. Mathias CGT, Caldwell TM, Maibach HI: Contact dermatitis and gastrointestinal symptoms from hydroxyethylmethacrylate. Br J Dermatol 100:447, 1979.

31. Kassis V, Vedel P, Darre E: Contact dermatitis to methylmethacrylate. Contact Dermatitis 11:26, 1984.

32. Seppalainen AM, Rajaniemi R: Local neurotoxicity of methylmethacrylate among dental technicians. Am J Ind Med 5:471, 1984.

33. Malten KE: Old and new, mainly occupational dermatological problems in the production and processing of plastics. In Maibach HI, Gellin GA (eds): Occupational and Industrial Dermatology. Year Book, Chicago, 1982.

34. Danto JL: Allergic contact dermatitis due to a formaldehyde fingernail hardener. Can Med Assoc J 98:652, 1968.

35. Lazar P: Reactions to nail hardeners. Arch Dermatol 94:446, 1966.

36. Mitchell JC: Non-inflammatory onycholysis from formaldehyde-containing nail hardener. Contact Dermatitis 7:173, 1981.

37. Chajes B: Formaldehyde, formalin. In Occupation and Health Encyclopedia of Hygiene, Pathology and Social Welfare. International Labour Office, Geneva, 1930.

38. Fisher AA: Contact dermatitis in medical and surgical personnel. In Maibach HI, Gellin GA (eds): Occupational and Industrial Dermatology. Year Book, Chicago, 1982.

39. NIOSH: Occupational Exposure to Formaldehyde. DHEW (NIOSH) Publication No. 77-126. U.S. Government Printing Office, Washington, DC, 1976.

40. Goh CL: Allergic contact dermatitis and onycholysis from hydroxylamine sulphate in colour developer. Contact Dermatitis 22:109, 1990.

41. Hjorth N, Wilkinson DS: Tulip fingers, hyacinth itch and lily rash. Br J Dermatol 80:696, 1968.

42. Verspyck Mijnssen GAW: Pathogenesis and causative agent of tulip finger. Br J Dermatol 81:737, 1969.

43. Templeton HJ: Onycholysis: An industrial dermatosis. JAMA 97:1950, 1931.

44. Cummer CL: Onychia due to handling sugar. Arch Dermatol Syphilol 41:142, 1940.

45. Coskey RJ: Onycholysis from sodium hypochlorite. Arch Dermatol 109:96, 1974.

46. Hodgson G, Mayon-White RT: Acute onychia and onycholysis due to an enzyme detergent. BMJ 7:352, 1971.

47. Budden MG, Wilkinson DS: Skin and nail lesions from gold potassium cyanide. Contact Dermatitis 4:172, 1978.

48. Baran R: Acute onycholysis from rust-removing agents. Arch Dermatol 116:382, 1980.

49. Dale RH: Treatment of hydrofluoric acid burns. BMJ 1:728, 1951.

50. Jones AT: The treatment of hydrofluoric acid burns. J Ind Hyg Toxicol 21:205, 1939.

51. Trevino MA, Herrman GH, Sprout WL: Treatment of severe hydrofluoric acid exposures. J Occup Med 25:861, 1983.

52. Shewmake SW, Anderson BG: Hydrofluoric acid burns. Arch Dermatol 115:593, 1979.

53. Reinhardt CG, Hume WG, Linch AL, et al: Hydrofluoric acid burn treatment. Am Ind Hyg Assoc J 27:166, 1966.

54. Bracken WM, Cuppage F, McLaury RL, et al: Comparative effectiveness of topical treatments for hydrofluoric acid burns. J Occup Med 27:733, 1985.

55. Dibbell DG, Iverson RE, Jones W, et al: Hydrofluoric acid burns of the hand. J Bone Joint Surg Am 52:931, 1970.

56. Iverson RE, Laub DR, Madison MS: Hydrofluoric acid burns. Plast Reconstr Surg 48:107, 1971.

57. Browne TD: Treatment of hydrofluoric acid burns. J Soc Occup Med 24:80, 1974.

58. Blunt CP: Treatment of hydrofluoric acid skin burns by injection with calcium gluconate. Ind Med Surgery 38:869, 1964.

59. National Institutes of Health: Hydrofluoric acid burns. Ind Med Surg 12:624, 1943.

60. Vance MV, Curry SC, Kunkel DB, et al: Digital hydrofluoric acid burns: Treatment with intraarterial calcium infusion. Ann Emerg Med 15:890, 1986.

61. Edelman PA: Hydrofluoric acid. In Rippe J (ed): Intensive Care Medicine. Little, Brown, Boston, 1991, pp 1286–1290.

62. Mistry DG, Wainwright DJ: Hydrofluoric acid burns. Am Fam Physician 45:1748, 1992.

63. Tepperman PB: Fatality due to acute systemic fluoride poisoning following a hydrofluoric acid skin burn. J Occup Med 22:691, 1980.

64. Burke WJ, Hoegg UR, Phillips RE: Systemic fluoride poisoning resulting from a fluoride skin burn. J Occup Med 15:39, 1973.

65. Buckingham FM: Surgery: A radical approach to severe hydrofluoric acid burns. J Occup Med 30:873, 1988.

66. Ganor S, Sagher F: Mycoses. In Parmeggiani L (ed): Encyclopedia of Occupational Health and Safety. International Labour Office, Geneva, 1983.

67. Norton LA: Nail disorders. J Am Acad Dermatol 2:451, 1980.

68. Peck SM, Schwartz L: Is dermatophytosis a significant occupational health problem. Am J Public Health 35:621, 1945.

69. Adams RM: Physical and biological causes of occupational skin disease. In Adams RM (ed): Occupational Skin Disease. Grune & Stratton, New York, 1983.

70. Dawber R: Occupational koilonychia. Clin Exp Dermatol 2:115, 1977.

71. Ancona-Alayon A: Occupational koilonychia from organic solvents. Contact Dermatitis 1:367, 1975.

72. Bentley-Phillips B, Bayles MAH: Occupational koilonychia of the toe nails. Br J Dermatol 85:140, 1971.

73. Smith SJ, Yoder FW, Knox DW: Occupational koilonychia. Arch Dermatol 116:861, 1980.

74. Pedersen NB: Persistent occupational koilonychia. Contact Dermatitis 8:134, 1982.

75. Shneerson JM: Digital clubbing and hypertrophic osteoarthropathy: The underlying mechanisms. Br J Dis Chest 75:113, 1981.

76. Bentley D, Cline J: Estimation of clubbing by analysis of shadowgraph. BMJ 3:43, 1970.

77. Bentley B, Moore A, Shwachman H: Finger clubbing: A quantitative survey by analysis of the shadowgraph. Lancet 2:164, 1976.

78. Wilson RH, McCormick WE, Tatum CF, et al: Occupational acroosteolysis. JAMA 201:577, 1967.

79. Craven SA: Clubbing of the digits of probable rare traumatic etiology. Practitioner 217:261, 1976.

80. Stone OJ, Mullins JF: Incidence of chronic paronychia. JAMA 186:71, 1963.

81. London L, Joubert G, Manjra SI, et al: Dermatoses—An occupational hazard in the canning industry. S Afr Med J 81:606, 1992.

82. Schwartz L, Tulipan L, Peck SM: Occupational Diseases of the Skin. Lea & Febiger, Philadelphia, 1947, pp 695–698.

83. Stone OJ: Chronic paronychia in which hair was a foreign body. Int J Dermatol 14:661, 1975.

84. Goette DK, Jacobson KW, Doty RD: Primary inoculation tuberculosis of the skin. Arch Dermatol 114:567, 1978.

85. O'Donnell TF Jr, Jurgenson PF, Weyerich NF: An occupational hazard—Tuberculous paronychia. Arch Surg 103:757, 1971.

86. DeBerker D: What do Beau's lines mean? Int J Dermatol 33:545, 1994.

87. Ward DJ, Hudson I, Jeffs JV: Beau's lines following hand trauma. J Hand Surg [Br] 13:411, 1988.

88. Sutton RL: Diseases of the skin. CV Mosby, St. Louis, 1956, pp 1348–1352, 1362–1365.

89. Brodkin RH, Bleiberg J: Cutaneous microwave injury. Acta Derm Venereol 53:50, 1973.

90. Lubach D, Beckers P: Wet working conditions increase brittleness of nails but do not cause it. Dermatol 185:120, 1992.

91. Scher RK: Occupational nail disorders. Dermatol Clin 6:30, 1988.

92. Long PI Jr: Subungual hemorrhage in pan washers. JAMA 168:1226, 1958.

93. Nail hemorrhages. Lancet 2:1351, 1978.

94. Willcock RD: Evacuation of subungual hematoma. BMJ 2:883, 1982.

95. Stewart PJ: Blood under the nail. Lancet 1:518, 1982.

96. O'Toole EA, Stephens R, Young MM, et al: Subungual melanoma: A relation to injury? J Am Acad Dermatol 33:525, 1995.

97. Palamarchuk HJ, Kerzner M: An improved approach to evacuation of subungual hematoma. J Am Podiatr Med Assoc 79:566, 1989.

98. Hunter D: The Diseases of Occupations. Little, Brown, Boston, 1955, pp 29–33.

99. Himmelstein JS, Frumkin H: The right to know about toxic exposures: Implications for physicians. N Engl J Med 312:687, 1985.

100. Hazard Communication Standard 29 CFR 1910 1200, 1984.

101. Gleason MN, Gosselin RE, Hodge HC, et al: Clinical Toxicology of Commercial Products. Williams & Wilkins, Baltimore, 1984.

102. Adams RM: Occupational Skin Disease. WB Saunders, Philadelphia, 1990.

103. Burgess WA: Recognition of Health Hazards in Industry: Review of Materials and Processes. Wiley, New York, 1995.

104. Encyclopedia of Occupational Health and Safety, vols I and II. International Labour Organization, Washington, DC, 1991.

105. Registry of Toxic Effects of Chemical Substances. DHEW (NIOSH) Pub. No. 79-100. U.S. Government Printing Office, Washington, DC, 1979.

106. Clayton GD, Clayton FE: Patty's Industrial Hygiene and Toxicology, vols 2A–E. Wiley, New York, 1993–1994.

107. The American With Disabilities Act: Impact, Enforcement, and Compliance. Bureau of National Affairs, Washington, DC, 1990.

108. Cohen SR: Risk factors in occupational skin disease. In Maibach HI, Gellin GA (eds): Occupational and Industrial Dermatology. Year Book, Chicago, 1982.

109. Shmunes E: Work preplacement. In Maibach HI, Gellin GA (eds): Occupational and Industrial Dermatology. Year Book, Chicago, 1982.

110. Hogan JC, Bernacki EJ: Developing job-related preplacement medical examinations. J Occup Med 23:469, 1981.

111. Lerner S: Editorial response. J Occup Med 23:475, 1981.

112. Ashford NA: Crisis in the Workplace. MIT Press, Cambridge, MA, 1976.

113. Chamber of Commerce of the United States. 1996 Analysis of Workers' Compensation Laws. Washington, DC, Chamber of Commerce, 1996.

CHAPTER 18

Podiatric Approach to Onychomycosis

Warren S. Joseph

Since the beginnings of the profession of podiatric medicine, toenail pathology has been of primary importance. In 1970 Krausz, reporting on nearly 30 years experience and almost 11,000 patients, found that 61 per cent of patients' presenting complaint was for nail pathology.[1] Early podiatrists, then known as chiropodists, were fairly limited in their scope of practice. Emphasis was placed on the treatment of hyperkeratotic lesions and dystrophic or ingrown nails. Treatment of these conditions was primarily local, including debridement and accommodative padding. Surgical therapy, including the use of local anesthetics, and systemic medical therapy were outside the scope of practice of these early pioneers. As the profession evolved and became more sophisticated, so did many of the approaches to different lower extremity pathologies. Surgical therapies were more commonly used. The pharmacopeia for podiatric physicians increased dramatically. With the scientific training and knowledge now on par with the rest of the medical community, old traditions still die hard. The roots of the profession continue to be taught to this day. Local, hands-on mechanical therapy is still a mainstay for the treatment of nails and keratotic lesions. However, with the development and release of safer, more effective oral antifungal agents, there is renewed interest and excitement in the exploration of new therapies for onychomycosis.

The causes and pathophysiology of onychomycosis are covered elsewhere in this book. The purpose of this chapter is to illustrate the way in which podiatric physicians approach the diagnosis and therapy of onychomycosis (Table 18–1).

PODIATRY VERSUS DERMATOLOGY

The two specialty groups most interested in the treatment of onychomycosis are podiatry and dermatology. Although the condition is seen by many general-family practitioners, there seems to be only minimal interest in the importance of this condition to the vast majority in these specialties. Much of the literature published on the topic of systemic therapy for onychomycosis has appeared in the dermatologic and mycologic literature. However, most of the work on the local, surgical, and cosmetic aspects of treatment has been performed by podiatrists.

Podiatry may, in fact, see more patients presenting with onychomycosis than does the dermatology community. Sheer numbers alone could account for this dichotomy. The American Podiatric Medical Association quotes 13,000 actively practicing podiatrists. This

Table 18–1. **A PODIATRIC APPROACH**

Podiatry vs. dermatology
Patient demographics
Historic issues
Debridement therapies
Surgical therapies
Medical therapies

Table 18–3. **MEDICARE GUIDELINES TO COVER ONYCHOMYCOSIS**

Clinical evidence of mycosis
Marked limitation of ambulation
Pain or secondary infection caused by the thickening
Debridement of mycotic nails is covered if there is a
    systemic condition that would pose a hazard if
    treatment was administered by a nonprofessional

compares with 6875 fellows and members of the American Academy of Dermatology (as of August 1995). According to the National Center for Health Statistics' National Health Interview Survey, the prevalence of toenail problems in the United States was 46 per 1000 people. Of those patients complaining of toenail problems who sought professional care, 70 per cent presented to a podiatrist.[2]

PATIENT DEMOGRAPHICS AND CONCERNS

The greatest difference between the two specialties and their respective approaches to onychomycosis can be traced to patient populations. Podiatrists have traditionally concentrated their efforts toward nail complaints in the older population. These patients generally complain of pain as a sequela of their thickened, dystrophic toenails. They are not as concerned about the cosmetic nature of the problem or some of the psychosocial stigmas that have been applied to this disease in younger patients. Furthermore, these patients may have significant underlying conditions and risk factors (Table 18–2), including peripheral vascular disease and diabetes mellitus, that make this frequently benign condition life and limb threatening. For this reason, the Health Care Financing Association has recognized toenail onychomycosis as a condition that may require professional care among the Medicare population. To be covered under Medicare, patients with onychomycosis must meet strict evidential criteria to prove the significance of the disease. Although regulations

Table 18–2. **GERIATRIC RISK FACTORS**

Diabetes
Vascular disease
Degenerative arthritis
Loss of visual acuity
Immune deficiencies
Polypharmacy
Chronic disease

may differ somewhat among states, the criteria established by Pennsylvania Blue Shield, the Medicare carrier for a number of eastern states, are paraphrased in Tables 18–3 and 18–4.

Despite having to satisfy these strict criteria for coverage of onychomycosis, podiatrists provided more than 8.8 million qualified services to Medicare patients in 1993. Of these patients, 70 per cent were 75 years of age or older, and a full 29 per cent were 85 years of age or older. These numbers give a feel for the size of the potential for serious sequelae of this condition in this population.

DIABETES MELLITUS AND ONYCHOMYCOSIS

By far the most significant risk factor for severe complications in patients with onychomycosis is diabetes mellitus. The skin of the diabetic patient is similar to geriatric skin. Loss of pliability secondary to increased collagen cross-linking may predispose the tissue to ulceration. Patients with diabetes frequently present with the triad of neuropathy, angiopathy, and immunopathy. Of these, the former is the most significant. Neuropathy may present as sensory, motor, or autonomic. Because of the sensory neuropathy, the patient may be unaware of the thickness or length of the toenail until the nail has damaged adjacent skin, potentiating a deep infection (Fig. 18–1). Furthermore, the patient with diabetic neuropathy tends to wear shoes that are too tight. Be-

Table 18–4. **SYSTEMIC CONDITIONS FOR WHICH ONYCHOMYCOSIS CARE IS COVERED**

Arteriosclerosis obliterans
Buerger's disease
Thrombophlebitis
Peripheral neuropathy secondary to
    Malnutrition
    Cancer
    Diabetes
    Multiple sclerosis

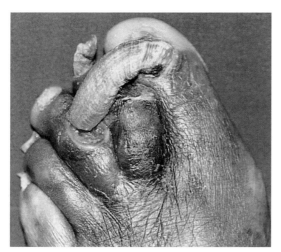

Figure 18–1. Ulceration of the third toe caused by an elongated mycotic toenail in a patient with diabetic peripheral neuropathy.

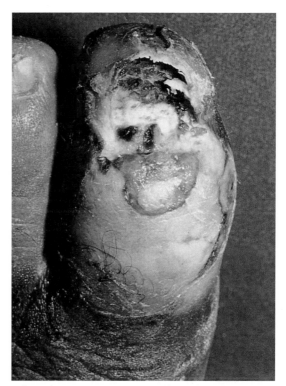

Figure 18–2. Neuropathic ulceration of the hallux toenail bed caused by pressure from the thickened mycotic toenail.

cause the patient has lost the ability to feel the presence of the shoe on the foot, he or she will try on shoes until they are tight enough to give the expected sensation. Combining a thickened, dystrophic, mycotic nail with a neuropathic nail bed placed into a shoe a few sizes too small potentially leads to subungual ulcerations of the nail bed (Fig. 18–2). Given the minimal amount of tissue present between the nail bed and the distal phalanx, osteomyelitis is a frequent result.

Even plantar ulcerations of the hallux may be traced to the combination of a neuropathic foot, a thickened nail, and a tight shoe. Excessive pressure from the shoe onto the top of the toe may cause increased plantar pressure, leading to ulceration (Fig. 18–3).

Another risk factor found in patients with and without diabetes is peripheral vascular disease. With poor perfusion to the digits, ulcerations and wounds heal with difficulty. If the patient attempts self-care and accidentally causes a laceration, this may progress to secondary infection, frank ischemia, and gangrene. Ischemia of the toes may also confuse the diagnosis of pain secondary to onychomycosis. Patients will relate a chief complaint of a painful toenail when in fact the cause of their discomfort is ischemic rest pain.

HISTORIC ISSUES

As mentioned, podiatric medicine has focused on diseases of the toenail since the be-

ginnings of the profession. Although this history lends a rich tradition to the local and surgical approaches that the specialty brings to therapy of nail conditions, in the area of systemic therapy for onychomycosis the profes-

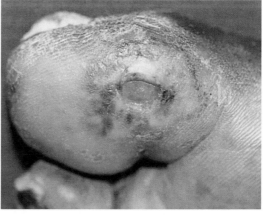

Figure 18–3. Plantar malperforans ulceration in a patient with diabetic neuropathy. Excessive dorsal shoe pressure on the thickened toenail may increase pressure on the plantar aspect of the toe, predisposing the patient to this type of ulcer.

sion has only more recently become actively involved. Reasons for this may include the following:

1. The importance of the disease. Although known to be a major potential problem in the patients with the risk factors described previously, is the disease important for otherwise healthy patients? The toenails looked unsightly, but is this only a cosmetic situation? Through the quality-of-life work originally performed by Lubeck and colleagues[3] and more recently by Drake, Scher (unpublished data), and others, it is now documented that a great number of these patients suffered with pain, missed days of work, and were subject to social castigation. In their article, Lubeck and coworkers concluded that "persons with onychomycosis also had significantly poorer ratings for mental health, social functioning, health concerns, physical appearance and functional limitations associated with activities involving standing on one's feet." Before these studies, this was mostly anecdotal knowledge.

2. Impossibility of a cure. Even if this disease was thought to be a true issue for the patient, there was little effective therapy. Although it could perhaps be controlled with local nail care and topical medication, results were less than spectacular. Patient dissatisfaction was high, as was physician frustration. All podiatrists have either heard a patient say or have muttered to themselves, "If only you (I) could find a cure for this, you'd (I'd) make a fortune!"

3. Distrust of griseofulvin. Even if systemic therapy was contemplated, what choices were there? Closely related to Point 2 is the concern instilled in podiatrists that griseofulvin is a dangerous, ineffective drug. Before the introduction of the newer antifungals, only griseofulvin was approved by the Food and Drug Administration (FDA). There is a pervasive feeling throughout much of the podiatric profession that hepatic and leukocyte toxicities of this agent, combined with a less than stellar success rate, render the only previously available choice as moot.

For these reasons, podiatric medicine has relied on its roots of local mechanical, chemical, and surgical therapy for the treatment of onychomycosis. Only recently with the introductions of terbinafine, itraconazole, and fluconazole is systemic therapy being used and a new paradigm being developed.

DEBRIDEMENT THERAPY

The mainstay of the podiatric approach to onychomycosis is the physical debridement of the dystrophic nail through manual, electric, and chemical means. The goal of this debridement therapy is to reduce the length and thickness of the nail significantly. Although not a cure for the condition, an aggressive debridement can render the patient pain free, reduce the risk for pressure-related sequelae, and make the nail more aesthetically pleasing. Removing the hypertrophied nail plate also facilitates the use of topical antifungals on the nail bed. Furthermore, the treatment is noninvasive and, therefore, safe for all patients, including those with advanced peripheral vascular disease and diabetes.

Manual debridement is performed using a hand-held nail nipper specifically designed for this task (Fig. 18–4). The nail is reduced from distal to proximal with angulation added to thin the nail as it is being shortened (Fig. 18–5A,B).

In many cases, after manual debridement, an electric drill with a rotary bur is used to reduce the thickened toenail further (Fig. 18–6).

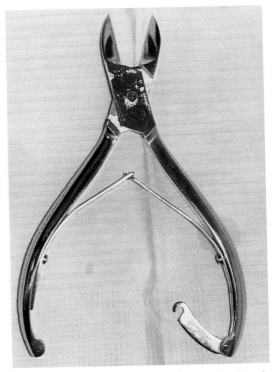

Figure 18–4. Curved jaw nail nipper designed for debridement of thickened mycotic toenails.

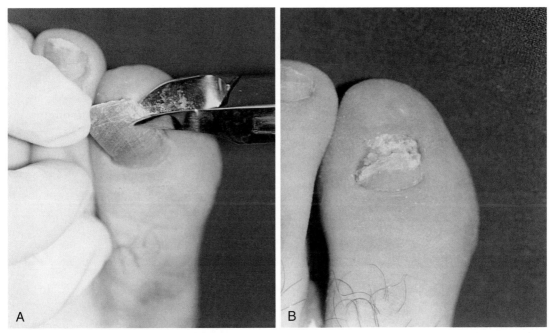

Figure 18–5. *A,* Proper use of the nipper to reduce the length and thickness of the mycotic nail. *B,* End result of a proper debridement. Note both the marked shortening and thinning of the nail plate.

This allows for closer reduction than would have been possible with the hand instrument alone. It also has the secondary benefit of smoothing any rough edges. This prevents the potential for irritation to an adjacent toe (Fig. 18–7*A, B*).

The greatest drawback to the use of the electric bur is the production of nail dust. To solve this problem, many different types of dust extraction devices have been marketed to the profession. These units range from small, inexpensive, easily installed canister vacuums to central externally ducted vacuums to the newer water or alcohol spray systems. According to a 1993 study by Harvey,[4] the efficacy of these different types of units ranges from 24.6 to 91.6 per cent. The water spray units were found to be the most effective at capturing debris, however, these units have the disadvantage of creating a "sludge." According to detractors, this becomes a neatness problem in the office. For this reason, along

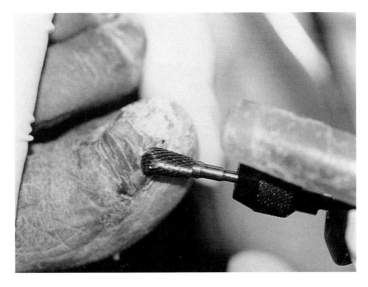

Figure 18–6. Electric rotary bur used to thin a thickened mycotic nail. The clear plastic hose attached to the hand piece is part of a dust extraction vacuum system.

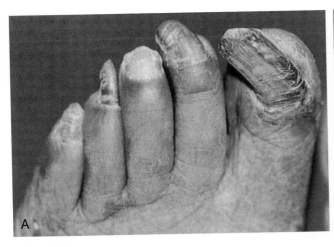
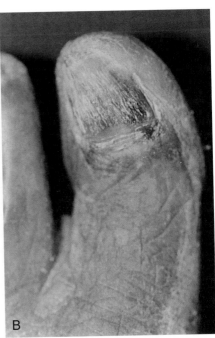

Figure 18–7. *A,* Markedly thickened and elongated mycotic hallux toenail. *B,* Marked shortening and thinning of the nail, which was possible with proper mechanical and electrical debridement technique.

with the relatively high cost of these units, they have not gained a significant foothold in the office setting. The conclusion drawn by Harvey was that the most important factors in the overall efficacy of the various units were (1) the distance of the vacuum nozzle to the nail, (2) the age of the collection bag, and (3) the power of the system.

Chemical debridement using 40 per cent urea is practiced to some extent in podiatric medicine. Overall, the technique is considered by many to be too time and labor intensive. In many cases, aggressive manual debridement obviates the need for the chemical therapy and can be performed in one visit. Some of the topical preparations frequently used in the profession such as Fungoid tincture and Gordochom contain agents to help soften the nail to facilitate regular debridement. Independent of the type of debridement performed, once the nail plate is removed topical antifungal therapy may be applied to the nail bed. Theoretically, this will provide activity against the organisms residing in the nail bed stratum corneum, allowing the new portion of nail to grow in more normally.

SURGICAL THERAPIES

In patients unresponsive to regular debridement therapy or those requesting a permanent cure, surgical removal of the nail and nail matrix has become a standard podiatric treatment. Contrary to the often-heard dermatologic axiom that "onychomycosis is a medical, not a surgical, disease," excellent results yielding patient satisfaction have been reported by podiatric surgeons. Concerns about loss of function after removal that may be relevant for fingernails seldom apply to toenails. The main function of the toenail is protection of the distal toe, and this duty has already been compromised by the deformity. In most cases, even the aesthetic result is quite acceptable. The remaining nail bed actually takes on the appearance of a more normal nail. It is not uncommon to see female patients apply nail polish to the bed and treat it as though a nail was present. Indications for surgical intervention include, but are not limited to, those found in Table 18–5. Entire chapters of textbooks have been written on the podiatric surgical approach to the toenail. There are multiple variations of similar approaches, all with advocates claiming superiority. Basically, partial or total

Table 18–5. **INDICATIONS FOR NAIL SURGERY**

Severely deformed nails
Painful nails unresponsive to conservative therapy
Failures with systemic oral antifungals
A desire for a reliable, permanent cure

Table 18–6. **ADVANTAGES AND DISADVANTAGES OF THE TWO COMMONLY USED MATRICECTOMY PROCEDURES**

Advantages	Disadvantages
Chemical	
Technically easy	Prolonged drainage
Relatively painless	Recurrences may be more frequent
Low infection rate	
Surgical	
Lower recurrence	More painful
Faster healing	More technically demanding
	Possibly higher infection rate

nail excisions can be broken down into two general classes: those performed with chemical matricectomy or those performed with surgical "cold steel" matricectomy. Both, again, have advocates and detractors. Advantages and disadvantages for each procedure are listed in Table 18–6. Other techniques such as carbon dioxide laser, radiotherapy, and electrocoagulation have been used to varying degrees and with varying success by some segments of the profession. The purpose of this section is not to present a primer on surgical procedures but rather to discusss briefly some of the techniques commonly practiced in podiatric surgery.

Anesthesia

Most podiatrists favor a digital block for local anesthesia. This may differ from the common dermatology technique of local, periungual infiltration of the anesthetic agent. The digital block is performed near the base of the toe using a two-stick (medial and lateral) or a three-stick "H" technique (medial, lateral, plantar) (Fig. 18–8). This technique is advantageous in that the greater volume of soft tissue in the area allows for greater expansion as the agent is injected and, therefore, minimal discomfort. Adequate anesthesia can usually be accomplished with 2 to 3 mL of lidocaine in the hallux. For lesser toes, a single-stick "V" block can be used, initiated at the dorsal aspect of the base of the toe using less lidocaine.

Chemical Matricectomy

After digital block, a tourniquet is placed around the base of the hallux. Once the toenail is avulsed (Fig. 18–9), the proximal and lateral folds are inspected for any remaining nail spicule. Phenolic acid, 89 percent, is applied to the matrix and proximal nail bed (Fig. 18–10). The timing and number of applications vary with different surgeons, but generally three applications of 30 seconds each is sufficient. This is followed with a copious flush of either an alcohol solution (thus the common name phenol and alcohol, or P&A, technique) or normal saline. A sterile, nonadherent dressing is applied, and the patient is discharged. The first postoperative visit usually occurs at 1 week, and the patient may then be monitored weekly (Fig. 18–11). Because the phenol causes a chemical burn, there is usually some inflammation and drainage. Both gradually subside, with the

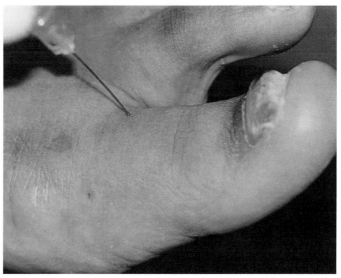

Figure 18–8. "Two-stick" technique performed at the base of the toe for proper preoperative anesthesia.

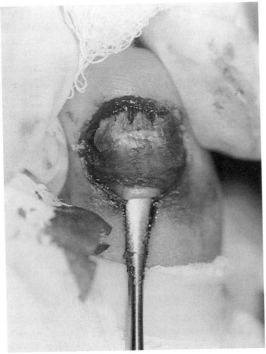

Figure 18–9. "Bottle cap" avulsion of the hallux nail by inserting a Freer periosteal elevator into the proximal nail fold and lifting distally.

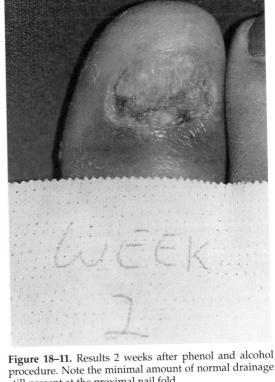

Figure 18–11. Results 2 weeks after phenol and alcohol procedure. Note the minimal amount of normal drainage still present at the proximal nail fold.

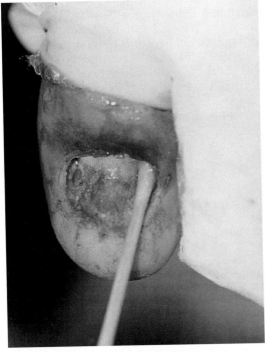

Figure 18–10. The use of a cotton-tipped applicator to apply the 89% phenolic acid in a phenol and alcohol procedure.

drainage lasting anywhere from 2 to 6 weeks or more. The patient should be made aware of the possibility for prolonged drainage to avoid untoward apprehension about infection. The end result is generally excellent (Fig. 18–12).

Although the phenol and alcohol procedure is by far the most common chemical matricectomy performed by podiatrists, variations do exist. The use of 10 per cent sodium hydroxide followed by a 5 per cent acetic acid flush was popularized in the early 1980s.[5] Proponents emphasized the lower recurrence rate with fewer postoperative complications, but the procedure has not achieved wide acceptance.[6]

Surgical Matricectomy

As mentioned, there are numerous variations on the approach to a surgical matricectomy. Whether the surgeon performs a proximal flap, performs an "acisional," or removes varying amounts of the nail bed is dependent on individual preference. Whichever method is chosen, the technique is performed under sterile conditions after avulsion of the nail plate. The matrix is identified and excised via

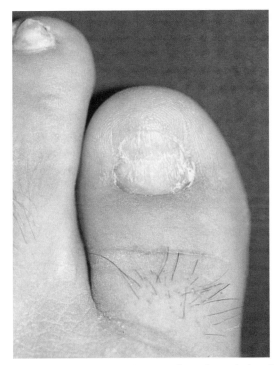

Figure 18–12. End result of a properly performed phenol and alcohol procedure. The result is usually aesthetically pleasing to the patient, and there is no possibility of pain from a thickened mycotic nail.

sharp dissection. The eponychium may then be sutured to the remaining nail bed. The wound is dressed with a sterile, nonadherent dressing. Frequently, a longer acting anesthetic agent is instilled into the base of the toe at the completion of the procedure. This is helpful in maintaining the patient's comfort through the immediate postoperative period.

MEDICAL THERAPIES

Although most podiatrists' experience with griseofulvin was not overly encouraging, the drug was helpful in a great number of patients. When used at a high enough dose for a long enough period of time, nails would clear. However, because of the previously discussed issues surrounding this drug's safety and efficacy, many podiatrists avoided the use of oral antifungal therapy. One limited survey of podiatric prescribing habits found that, before the introduction of the new drugs, the responding podiatrists averaged fewer than one prescription per week for oral antifungal med-

ications.[7] Instead, there was reliance on the use of topical therapy with or without nail avulsion. The same survey showed that this group of podiatrists was prescribing almost 10 topical antifungal prescriptions per week. Extrapolated out to the number of actively practicing podiatrists, this amounts to almost 130,000 antifungal prescriptions per week. Unfortunately, there is no way to determine from the survey how much of this topical usage was for onychomycosis versus tinea pedis.

Over the past few years, immense interest has been generated in the profession regarding the new oral antifungal drugs. Even before FDA approval of any of these agents for onychomycosis, podiatrists were monitoring the literature and, based on early study results, were beginning to experiment with the available compounds. Before the labeling of itraconazole for this indication, fluconazole was the most readily available and most widely used. The prescribing survey just discussed indicates this drug accounted for a majority of the usage up to the latest data of 1995. It should be pointed out that these data were probably collected before the release of itraconazole and, most certainly, before the availability of terbinafine in the United States. Despite the lack of federal approbation, it is interesting to note that podiatric usage of oral agents doubled in a 1-year period.

With the relabeling of itraconazole and the release of oral terbinafine, podiatric usage of these agents is bound to increase exponentially. Intensive marketing to the profession and the direct-to-consumer (DTC) campaigns initiated by these pharmaceutical houses are raising awareness of the disease and treatment options in the minds of both the professionals and the public. It is doubtful that there is a podiatrist in the United States who has not had a new patient enter the office waving a DTC advertisement for one of these products.

With each clinical exposure to the new drugs, podiatrists will become more and more comfortable with their safety profile, successes, and failures. Proper patient selection criteria will be determined. Mechanical, surgical, and topical therapy will continue to play an important role and may be useful in augmenting the new oral therapies. Only with time, clinical usage, and well-designed, large-scale postmarketing studies will any clearly superior treatment or combination of treatments be delineated.

References

1. Krausz CE: Nail survey (1942–1970). Br J Surg 35:117, 1970.
2. Greenberg L, Davis H: Foot problems in the US: The 1990 National Health Interview Survey. J Am Podiatr Med Assoc 83:475, 1993.
3. Lubeck DP, Patrick DL, McNulty P, et al: Quality of life of persons with onychomycosis. Quality Life Res 2:341, 1993.
4. Harvey CK: Comparison of the effectiveness of nail dust extractors. J Am Podiatr Med Assoc 83:669, 1993.
5. Travers GR, Ammon RG: The sodium hydroxide chemical matricectomy procedure. J Am Podiatr Assoc 70:476, 1980.
6. Greenwald L, Robbins HM: The chemical matricectomy. J Am Podiatr Assoc 71:388, 1981.
7. Donoghue SK: Keeping pace in the face of managed care. Podiatr Manage 14:44, 1996.

CHAPTER 19

Pedal Biomechanics and Toenail Disease

Justin Wernick and Richard C. Gibbs

Injuries to the nail plate are often the result of repeated microtrauma. This microtrauma may be secondary to faulty biomechanics during gait, eventually creating deformity of the digits and concomitant abnormal pressure on the nail plate. In order to understand the mechanism that may cause this injury, we must first understand normal biomechanics during gait.

NORMAL FUNCTION OF THE FOOT

The primary purpose of the foot is to perform specific dynamic functions at different phases of the gait cycle (Fig. 19–1). The total gait cycle is the time from heel contact of one foot until the next heel contact of that same foot. Initially, as the foot hits the ground, it is required to (1) react to terrain that is often uneven and (2) absorb shock by allowing increased knee flexion. The pedal mechanism allowing these movements occurs at the subtalar and midtarsal joints (Fig. 19–2) and is called pronation. Pronation is a complex motion that takes place at several joints of the foot, moving the sole plantarward and toward the midline of the body and lowering the arch.

Pronation (the contact phase of gait) occupies the first 27 per cent of the gait cycle and allows for "unlocking" of the foot. It is this un-locking mechanism that alters the structure of an otherwise rigid bony foot, creating a more flexible structure that is perfect for the purposes of adjusting to an uneven surface. Once the forefoot contacts the ground, the opposite limb then leaves the ground and swings past the planted limb. The planted foot then undergoes change in its architecture, moving from a flexible to a more rigid structure, thus providing stabilization for the total body as it swings over the support limb. This midstance phase occupies 40 per cent of the gait cycle.

Once the body weight has been stabilized over the support limb, the terminal event in the stance phase of the gait cycle, called propulsion, takes place. This action occupies the last 30 to 40 per cent of the cycle and is initiated when the opposite limb strikes the ground and the planted heel lifts from the surface, thrusting the body weight forward onto the forefoot. During this phase, the foot must be stable to balance the body solely on a small plantar area as it thrusts forward.

This propulsive phase allows transfer of the body weight from the support limb to the opposite limb, which is then in contact with the ground. This motion occurs mainly at the subtalar joint by supination. In supination, a complex motion involving several joints in the foot, the plantar surface of the foot moves dorsally and away from the midline, raising the arch.

311

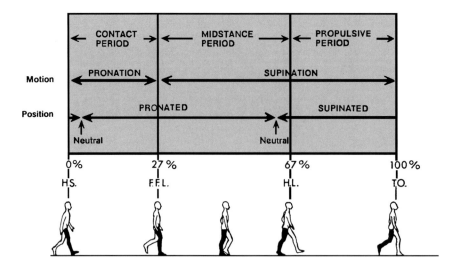

The foot is slightly supinated at the subtalar joint as heel strike initiates the stance phase of gait. During the contact period, the subtalar joint pronates. Momentarily after heel strike, the foot pronates to a neutral subtalar joint position and then continues into a pronated position. The foot reaches its maximum pronated position at the end of the contact period. Normally, the subtalar joint begins to supinate as the midstance period starts. The foot becomes less pronated during midstance, until the subtalar joint again reaches a neutral position late in the midstance period. Prior to heel lift, the foot should normally be slightly supinated. During the propulsive period, the subtalar joint continues to supinate, and the foot assumes its maximum supinated position shortly before toe off.

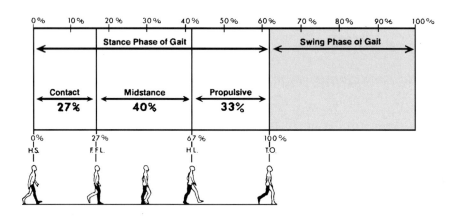

The stance phase of gait is divided into three periods. The contact period starts at heel strike (H.S.) and terminates with forefoot loading (F.F.L.). At the end of the contact period, all metatarsals are bearing weight. The midstance period is that period of stance in which the entire foot is making ground contact and is bearing the full weight of the body. The midstance period starts with forefoot loading and terminates with heel lift (H.L.). The propulsive period is initiated with heel lift and terminates with toe off (T.O.).

Figure 19–1. Gait cycle. From Root M, Weed J, Orion WD: Normal and Abnormal Function of the Foot—Clinical Biomechanics, vol 2. Clinical Biomechanics Corporation, Los Angeles, 1977. Used with permission.

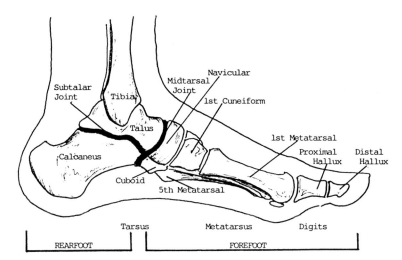

Figure 19–2. Diagram of foot showing anatomic parts important in locomotion.

The three phases (contact, midstance, and propulsion) that compose the stance or weight-bearing phase of gait occupy approximately 60 per cent of the total gait cycle and occur in approximately 0.6 second. The orderly transfer of body weight is essential for the normal propulsive sequence and for the efficient distribution of body weight from one area of the foot to the next.

ABNORMAL FUNCTION OF THE FOOT

The gait motions take place in a segmental and sequential manner, requiring specific time periods for each phase to occur. If these motions are interfered with, the foot is delayed in changing from its adaptive flexible structure to a more rigid one.[1] In that event, the supinatory phase, during which the foot is locked into a rigid propulsive lever, occurs much later in the cycle. As a result of this delay, the foot structure is still in a weakened and partially flexible state and is not prepared to accept the increase in the reactive force of the ground. This increased force reacts against the individual's body weight and eventually alters and deforms the osseous and muscular alignment, creating deformity.[2] Poorly fitting shoes can contribute to this deformity, because the ground strikes the shoe first, exaggerating the reactive force. Because these events occur in the final stage of propulsion, the digits bear most of the deforming forces. These deforming forces, inflicted thousands of times per day

over a period of time, traumatize the nail and nail tissue and cause damage and distortion.

Abnormal biomechanics of the limb resulting in abnormal timing mechanisms may be due to two major factors: congenital deformities and acquired deformities. Acquired deformities may be secondary to disease or abnormal development or to trauma, including that inflicted by shoes.

Congenital Deformities

Congenital deformities such as bowlegs (tibia vara) or flat feet (pes valgus) may directly alter function of the foot so that prolonged pronation occurs, increasing instability in the forefoot.

Acquired Deformities

Diseases such as poliomyelitis can cause talipes equinus, a deformity in which the foot is plantar flexed, forcing the patient to walk on the toes without touching the heel to the ground. The deformed foot resembles a horse's hoof. Limb length discrepancies resulting from diseases such as scoliosis may prematurely load the forefoot with the body weight, damaging the feet and nails. Specific disease processes such as arthritis, diabetes, or neuromuscular problems can also alter normal biomechanics, resulting in disturbances of the gait cycle.

Table 19–1. **BIOMECHANICALLY INDUCED ONYCHIAL DISEASES AND SUGGESTED THERAPY**

Biomechanical Abnormality	Resultant Onychodystrophy	Therapy
Common bunion (hallux valgus)—the hallux is shifted and rotated toward the second toe.	Hypertrophic nail—caused by abnormal pressure of the distal nail of the hallux against the shoe.	1. Periodic reduction and debridement of the nail plate. 2. Change to a shoe with a high toe box. 3. If severe hypertrophy, permanent removal of all or a portion of the nail plate.
	Onychocryptosis—caused by the lateral nail margin of the hallux being pushed against the second toe because of the abducted position of the hallux.	1. Surgical removal of the offending portion of the nail plate and perhaps destruction of a portion of the nail matrix.
	Subungual hematoma—caused by the shoe's pressure on the hallux nail, which overlaps the adjacent toe. Long-term pressure may eventually cause subungual exostosis. Hypertrophic nail usually accompanies or is subsequent to hematoma.	1. Relief of pressure from the hematoma by cutting back the nail periodically. 2. Surgical removal of the exostosis. 3. Change to a shoe with a high toe box. Note: All of these conditions generally improve with realignment of the hallux. Therefore, a comprehensive surgical procedure to realign the first metatarsal-hallucal mechanism or a functional orthotic device with or without the surgical procedure may be indicated.
Hallux rigidus—motion is lost in the first metatarsal phalangeal joint, resulting in excessive motion at the interphalangeal joint and a dorsiflexed position of the distal phalanx.	Hypertrophic nail plate and subungual hyperkeratosis—caused by the distal phalanx and nail plate contacting the dorsal and distal surface of the toe box, resulting in recurrent microtrauma. Subungual hematoma and exostosis.	1. Periodic reduction of the nail plate and subungual hyperkeratosis. 2. Permanent removal of the nail. 3. Surgical procedure to reestablish motion in the first metatarsal phalangeal joint and use of an orthotic device to maintain proper function.
Contracted toes (hammertoes)—the muscles that control the digits are shortened, resulting in a buckling of the toes.	Subungual hyperkeratosis and hypertrophic lesser nail plate caused by the distal phalanx applying direct pressure into the sole of the shoe.	1. Periodic reduction of the nail plate and subungual tissue. 2. Permanent removal of the offending nail plate. 3. Sometimes a shoe with a longer and higher toe box will help, as will use of softer lining material. 4. Surgical procedure to straighten the toe.
Overlapping and underlapping toes—severe dislocation of a toe, resulting in toes resting on top of or below one another.	Hypertrophic nail plate and subungual bleeding caused by pressure on the nail plate directly from the toe above or, in the case of an overlapping toe, pressure from the toe box of the shoe.	1. Periodic reduction of the nail plate and subungual hyperkeratosis. 2. Permanent removal of the nail. 3. Broad and deep toe box. 4. Surgical procedure to realign the digits.
Rotated toe—the fifth toe is rotated so that the individual walks on the lateral portion of the nail plate.	Onychoclavus—pressure from the shoe continues to traumatize the nail bed, resulting in hypertrophy and eventual cornification and heloma development; most often found in the nail groove itself. Note: Might be associated with hallux valgus deformity.	1. Periodic debridement of cornified tissue. 2. Change offending shoe if the problem persists. 3. Surgical removal of the lateral nail plate, nail groove, and osseous condyle of the underlying area. 4. Plastic surgery to derotate the fifth toe.

Table 19–1. **BIOMECHANICALLY INDUCED ONYCHIAL DISEASES AND SUGGESTED THERAPY**
(Continued)

Biomechanical Abnormality	Resultant Onychodystrophy	Therapy
Shoe-induced biomechanical abnormality—the shoe directly causes distorted growth of toenails.	Onychogryphosis—pressure from the shoe encourages abnormal growth of toenails, tennis toe, pincer toenails.	1. Periodic reduction of the nail plate and subungual hyperkeratosis. 2. Permanent removal of the nail. 3. Sometimes a shoe with longer and higher toe box will help, as will use of softer lining material.

Developmental problems such as inward or outward malpositions of the heel and forefoot can result in disruption of the pronation-supination sequence, leading to instability of the forefoot at propulsion. Deformities such as hallux valgus, hallux rigidus, under- and overlapping toes, and contracted digits can result.

Trauma to the extremities may result in asymmetric function, eventually increasing destructive forces on the leg or foot. A simple injury such as a sprained ankle or a fracture, for example, can initiate these problems.

Shoes can be a factor in distorting normal biomechanics. The height of the heel, the shape and design of the last, the construction of the shoe itself (particularly the toe box), and the material used can place excessive pressure on the nail and alter the mechanisms of the foot, resulting in injuries. These many factors and the resultant alterations in gait cause specific dystrophies of nails and skin. Table 19–1 outlines common congenital or acquired deformities and the nail dystrophies associated with them.

THERAPY

Biomechanical Therapy

The biomechanical factors that contribute to the faulty function of the foot should be assessed. Common assessment techniques include comprehensive static biomechanical examination, weight-bearing x-ray series, and visual gait analysis. Computerized gait analysis (electrodynogram) can contribute information to the decision-making process.

Once a proper assessment has been made, a functional orthotic device may be indicated (Fig. 19–3). A functional orthosis is a mechanical device made of various moldable materials and worn in a shoe to create more normal leg and foot motions. It captures the contour of the individual's foot in its anatomic neutral position, a position that is most efficient for a particular individual, and maintains this relationship. By effectively maintaining true osseous angular relationships, the orthosis permits more efficient locomotion by restoring normal anatomic relationships of bones.

The continual deforming forces that can create hallux valgus, hammertoes, and underlapping and overlapping toes can be eliminated or reduced with proper treatment. Continuing a particular treatment and having patients wear proper shoes and undergo physiotherapy can actually prevent or eliminate the pathologic process.

Minor Surgical Therapy

Minor surgery can sometimes reduce the signs and symptoms directly related to the nail condition. It may require the periodic reduction and debridement of the nail plate and subungual tissue. Total or partial removal of a nail plate may be necessary, either permanently or temporarily. These minor surgical techniques may use chemosurgery, electrosurgery, or a scalpel.

Major Surgical Therapy

The objective of podiatric surgical procedures is to realign the malpositioned digits, restoring proper function and position. By placing a digit and its associated metatarsal in proper alignment before propulsion, the recurrent deforming forces are neutralized. Nail dystrophies often respond once the concomitant pressure is relieved. The surgeon must

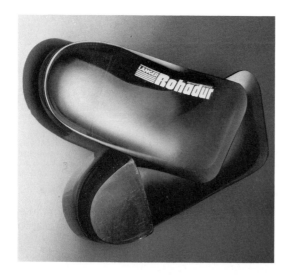

Figure 19–3. Orthotics seen from both sides.

judge whether a specific nail condition may require an extensive surgical procedure.

In conclusion, abnormal function of a foot in gait and its consequences can be the prime mechanism causing nail dystrophies. Recognizing underlying factors and implementing the proper treatment plan can be very effective in restoring normal nail tissue.

References

1. Wernick J, Langer S: A Practical Manual for a Basic Approach to Biomechanics. Langer Acrylic Laboratory, Deer Park, NY, 1972.
2. Root M, Weed J, Orien W: Normal and Abnormal Function of the Foot—Clinical Biomechanics, vol 2. Clinical Biomechanics Corporation, Los Angeles, 1977.

CHAPTER 20

Subungual Exostosis and Nail Disease and Radiologic Aspects

Harvey Lemont and Robert A. Christman

By far the most common osseous lesion associated with nail disease is the subungual exostosis. These poorly understood bony proliferations are found most notably in the hallux and rarely in the fingers[1-3] and lesser toes.[4,5] Although the lesion was described as early as 1847 by Dupuytren,[6] only a small number of cases have since been reported.[7-11] Discrepancies regarding the pathology and natural history of the subungual exostosis have appeared in the literature. Evison and Price[12] described the covering of the exostosis to be composed of fibrocartilage, whereas Landon and colleagues[13] reported it to be covered by either fibrous or hyaline cartilage. Although there have been numerous attempts to clarify the natural history of this lesion,[14-16] the cause remains an enigma.

We have found it convenient, based on the lesion's pathology, radiographic appearance, location, and age, to categorize subungual exostosis into genetic and acquired types (Table 20–1).

GENETIC SUBUNGUAL EXOSTOSIS (TYPE I)

Type I exostosis has a predilection to affect young females usually in their second and third decades of life, with the lesion almost always originating on the dorsomedial aspect of the distal phalanx. As a result of the gradual enlargement of a subungual exostosis, the nail bed and periungual tissue become compressed, resulting in increased periungual skin tension (Fig. 20–1). Paronychia and pyogenic granuloma often develop (Figs. 20–2 and 20–3). Nail plate elevation with accompanying subungual hemorrhage may be demonstrated histologically. In addition, small keratinized nail matrix inclusions are commonly implanted into the nail bed. These inclusions develop without a granular layer (Fig. 20–4). As a result of distal skin pressure, similar inclusions develop in the dermal hyponychium. These latter inclusions, in contrast, tend to form with a granular layer. Marked fibrosis is also noted in the dermal hyponychium (Fig. 20–5). Radiographic evaluation of patients with genetic subungual exostoses usually reveals a plateau or tabletop exostosis on lateral projection of the toe and increased circumscribed radiodensity at the medial aspect of the distal phalanx shaft on dorsoplantar view (Fig. 20–6). They may occasionally be dome or mushroom shaped (Figs. 20–7 and 20–8). Although less frequent, these lesions may appear on the lesser digits (Fig. 20–9) Histologically, this type of sub-

Text continued on page 322

Table 20–1. **COMPARISON OF GENETIC AND ACQUIRED SUBUNGUAL EXOSTOSIS**

Factor	Type I Genetic Subungual Exostosis	Type II Acquired Subungual Exostosis
Paronychia	Frequent	Usually absent
Nail bed hypertrophy	Medial aspect of nail bed	Entire nail bed
Nail shape	Elevation of nail plate medially	Incurvation of medial and lateral aspects of nail plate
Accentuation of interphalangeal skin crease	Absent	Present
Age	Second and third decades of life	Fourth through sixth decades of life
Location	Dorsomedial diaphysis	Distal dorsal and central ungual tuberosity
Histology	Hyaline or fibrous cartilage covering	No cartilage covering
Radiographic findings	Plateau or dome-shaped exostosis	Blunted or sharp protuberance

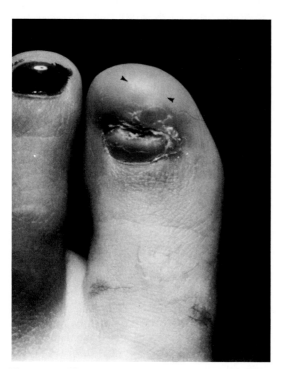

Figure 20–1. The growing genetic subungual exostosis has caused expansion and tightening of the periungual skin distally and medially (arrowheads).

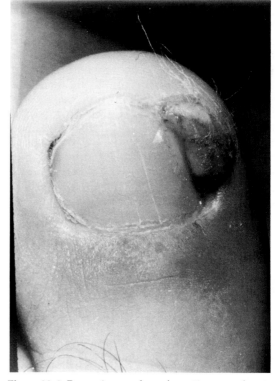

Figure 20–2. Pyogenic granuloma formation secondary to chronic irritation from a genetic subungual exostosis.

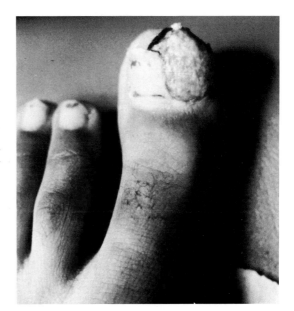

Figure 20–3. Advanced pyogenic granuloma formation resulting from long-standing pressure and low-grade infection.

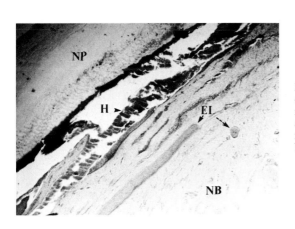

Figure 20–4. Note subungual nail plate hemorrhage secondary to nail plate elevation. Traumatic implantation of nail matrix into nail bed is also seen, lacking the presence of a granular layer. Note nail matrix inclusions in dermis. (NP, nail plate; EI, epidermal inclusions; H, hemorrhage; NB, nail bed.)

Figure 20–5. The genetic subungual exostosis exerts distal pressure on the hyponychium, promoting fibrosis and implantation of epidermis into dermis. Note keratinizing epidermal inclusion developing with the benefit of a granular layer, surrounded by fibrosis of the hyponychium. (HF, hyponychium fibrosis; GL, granular layer.)

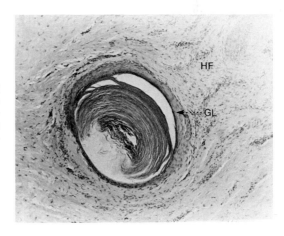

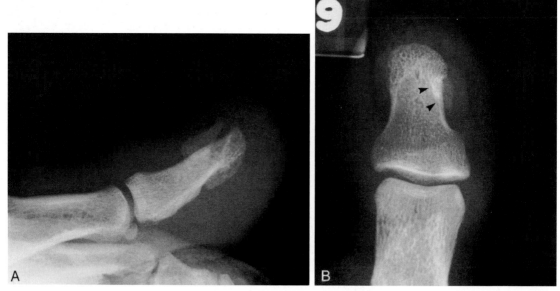

Figure 20–6. *A,* Tabletop genetic subungual exostosis, hallux lateral projection. Note its origin from the dorsal aspect of the distal shaft. *B,* Dorsoplantar projection. Arrowheads indicate the medial origin of the exostosis, extending medial to the shaft.

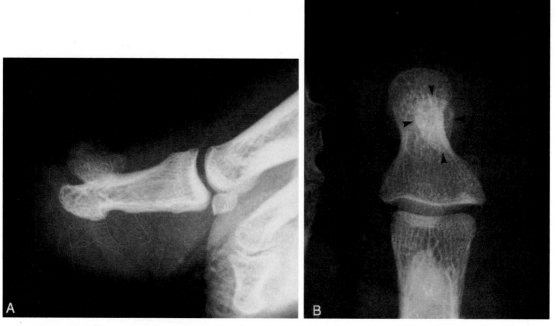

Figure 20–7. Dome-shaped genetic subungual exostosis. *A,* Lateral projection. *B,* Dorsoplantar projection.

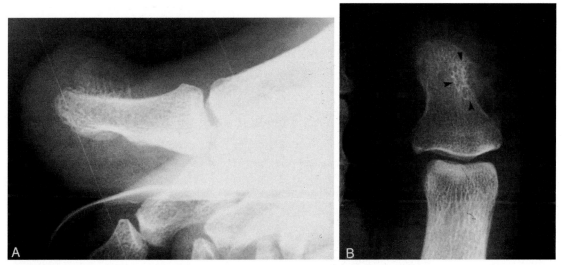

Figure 20–8. Dome-shaped genetic subungual exostosis. *A,* Lateral projection. *B,* Dorsoplantar projection.

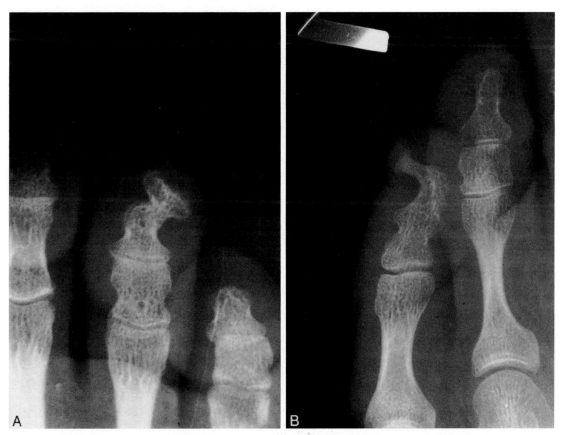

Figure 20–9. Genetic subungual exostoses, although more commonly affecting the hallux, can be located on the lesser digits. Note exostoses at distal phalanges of third *(A)* and fifth *(B)* digits.

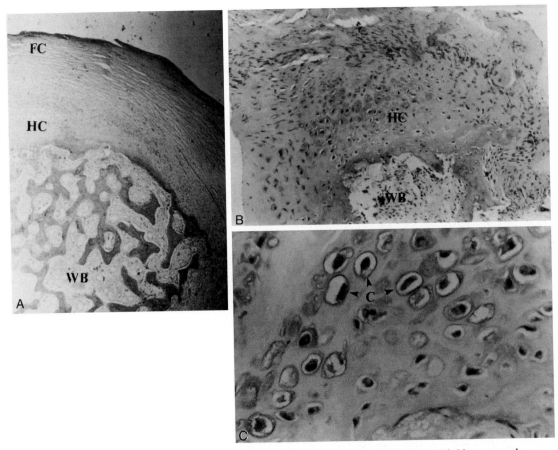

Figure 20–10. *A*, Histologic section of genetic subungual exostosis (hematoxylin and eosin, × 10). Note woven bone covered by hyaline cartilage capped by fibrous tissue. (WB, woven bone; HC, hyaline cartilage; FC, fibrous cap; C, chondrocyte.) *B*, Magnification of hyaline cartilage cap (hematoxylin and eosin, × 10). *C*, Note immature chondrocytes demonstrating large, plump nuclei, characteristic of immature hyaline cartilage (hematoxylin and eosin, × 10).

ungual exostosis demonstrates immature bone capped by hyaline or fibrocartilage (Fig. 20–10). This covering at times may be surrounded by a collarette of dense fibrous tissue.

ACQUIRED SUBUNGUAL EXOSTOSIS (TYPE II)

In contrast to genetic subungual exostosis, the acquired type usually is seen later in life, affecting females between the fourth and sixth decades. The lesion has a predilection for the distal, dorsal, and central aspects of the distal phalanx tuft. In our opinion, these exostoses develop as a result of an abnormal positional relationship between the first metatarsal and hallux, with secondary osteoarthritis or hallux limitus developing. This limited motion is subsequently compensated for at the interpha-

langeal joint, where excessive dorsiflexion occurs, subjecting the ungual tuberosity of the distal phalanx and its surrounding nail bed and plate to intermittent trauma. This sequence of events results in nail bed remodeling and osteoarthritic subungual spur formation (Fig. 20–11). Accentuation of the dorsal interphalangeal joint crease is a frequent skin marker of limited motion at the metatarsophalangeal joint, which may be associated with osteoarthritic subungual spur formation (Fig. 20–12). The nail plate in acquired subungual exostosis frequently appears as an inverted U, with nail bed hypertrophy being apparent (Fig. 20–13). Patients with these types of exostoses often complain of chronic ingrown toenails, with painful incurvation noted at both the medial and lateral margins of the nail plate. Microscopic evaluation of the spur reveals remodeling of the distal phalanx ungual tuberosity, with an extrusion of phalangeal

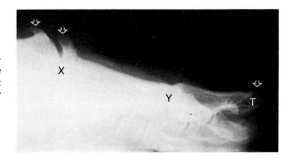

Figure 20–11. Limited motion at the first metatarsophalangeal joint (X) results in compensatory dorsiflexion at the interphalangeal joint (Y), subjecting the distal phalanx tuft (T) to intermittent trauma resulting in osteoarthritic spur formation (arrows).

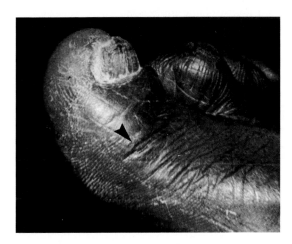

Figure 20–12. Accentuation of dorsal interphalangeal joint crease, a cutaneous marker of osteoarthritis at the first metatarsophalangeal joint. The accentuation of this crease also is commonly associated with acquired subungual exostosis.

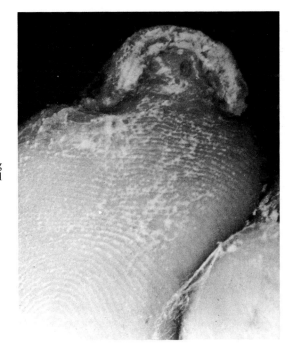

Figure 20–13. Acquired subungual exostosis demonstrating nail bed hypertrophy and characteristic inverted U-shaped appearance of nail.

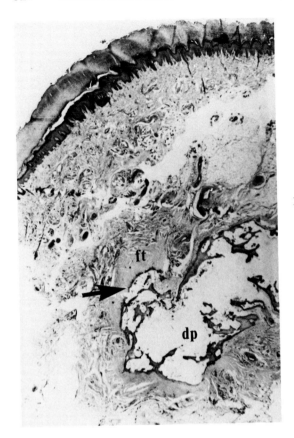

Figure 20–14. Histologic section of hallux distal phalanx (dp) demonstrating acquired subungual exostosis. The dorsal distal osteoarthritic exostosis (arrow) is surrounded by hyponychial fibrous tissue (ft).

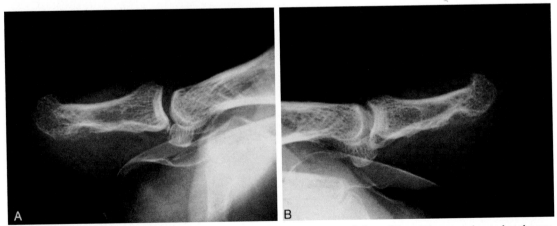

Figure 20–15. Variations of acquired subungual exostosis. Note blunt *(A)* and sharp *(B)* protuberances located at the central and distal ungual tufts of the distal phalanges.

bone noted distally, and dorsally. The spur is covered only with fibrous tissue. No cartilage is present in this type of exostosis (Fig. 20–14). Roentgenographic examination on lateral projection reveals a blunt or sharp protuberance at the distal and dorsal aspect of the distal phalanx (Fig. 20–15).

References

1. Matthewson MH: Subungual exostosis of the fingers. Are they really uncommon? B J Dermatol 98:187, 1978.
2. Bennett RG, Gammer S: Painful callus of the thumb due to phalangeal exostosis. Arch Dermatol 108:826, 1973.
3. Lowenthal K: Subungual exostosis on a forefinger. N Y State J Med 64:2691, 1964.
4. Chesler SM, Basler RSW: Subungual exostosis. J Am Podiatr Assoc 68:732, 1978.
5. Cohen HJ, Frank SB, Minkin W, et al: Subungual exostoses. Arch Dermatol 107:431, 1973.
6. Dupuytren G: On the injuries and diseases of the bones. Publications of the Sydenham Society, London, 20:408, 1847, cited by Zimmerman EH: Subungual exostosis. Cutis 19:185, 1977.
7. Bendl BJ: Subungual exostosis. Cutis 26:260, 1980.
8. Oliveira ADS, Picoto ADS, Verde SF, et al: Subungual exostosis: Treatment as an office procedure. J Dermatol Surg Oncol 6:555, 1980.
9. Brenner MA, Montgomery RM, Kalish SR: Subungual exostosis. Cutis 25:518, 1980.
10. Apfelberg DB, Druker D, Maser MR, et al: Subungual osteochondroma. Arch Dermatol 115:472, 1979.
11. Zimmerman EH: Subungual exostosis. Cutis 19:185, 1977.
12. Evison G, Price CHG: Subungual exostosis. B J Radiol 39:451, 1966.
13. Landon GC, Johnson KA, Dahlin DC: Subungual exostoses. J Bone Joint Surg Am 61:256, 1979.
14. Lewin P: The Foot and Ankle. Lea & Febiger, Philadelphia, 1947, p 270.
15. Williams WR: Subungual exostosis. Bristol Medico Chir J 22:17, 1904.
16. Kurtz AD: Subungual exostoses. Surg Gynecol Obstet 43:488, 1926.

CHAPTER 21

Surgery

Stuart J. Salasche

The purpose of gaining proficiency in nail unit surgery is to be able to perform appropriate diagnostic and therapeutic biopsies, definitively treat benign and malignant lesions, and restore anatomic and functional integrity in certain conditions such as ingrown toenail or posttraumatic split nails.

A thorough understanding of the anatomy and physiology of the nail unit is a prerequisite for performing safe and efficacious nail surgery.[1–3] The foundation skills of securing adequate local anesthesia, performing nail plate avulsions, and executing proper nail bed and matrix biopsies are then easy to learn. Most routine nail surgery involves these basic techniques.

It is helpful to have certain documentation before attempting nail surgery. Preoperative and serial postoperative photographs provide both educational and medicolegal documentation. Pictures should be taken from a close, consistent distance using the same background, lens, and lighting system. Each sequence of exposures should include an identifying shot with the patient's name and the date (Fig. 21–1). All digits look the same in a close-up picture once the nail plate and the pathology have been removed. Providing these data in the picture makes it possible to match up preoperative and follow-up pictures.[4] It is also prudent to obtain preoperative x-ray films or soft tissue xerograms when dealing with tumors of the distal digit. They will reveal the osteocartilaginous tumors (exostosis, enchondroma, or osteochondroma) and warn surgeons before they inadvertently expose or enter bony tissue (Fig. 21–2).

Finally, nail surgery requires special patient counseling. Patients should know beforehand that, despite the outpatient nature of the surgery, the effects may be long lasting. Even after a simple avulsion and biopsy, the nail will not be fully replaced for up to 6 to 12 months, and there is a risk of some permanent deformity. They must consider that even simple activities such as typing, bowling, sewing, and cooking may be compromised for a time. Likewise, toenail surgery will require that they wear a large open shoe or sandal to accommodate the bulky dressing. If the foot is numb or the dressing too bulky, driving may become dangerous, and other transportation arrangements must be made.

INSTRUMENTS

Specialized instruments make nail surgery safer and easier. Having a prepacked sterilized tray containing all the requisite instruments

326

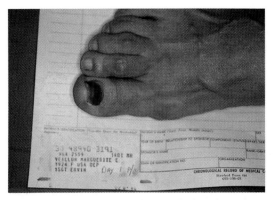

Figure 21–1. Postoperative photo with identifying data.

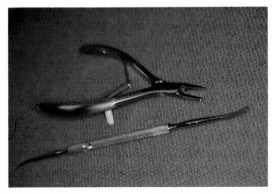

Figure 21–3. Septum elevator (bottom) and nail splitter (top).

avoids frustrating searches and delays once surgery has begun. Figures 21–3 through 21–8 illustrate these distinctive instruments.

Especially useful is the Freer septum elevator (Fig. 21–3).[5] This strong and beautiful instrument, whose graceful convex and concave surfaces closely match those of the nail plate and nail bed, is indispensable when performing both distal and proximal nail plate avulsions. It is also useful in defining the proximal nail groove (Fig. 21–4). Dental spatulas and hemostats have been used for the same purpose, although not as elegantly.[6]

Another unique instrument is the English nail splitter, which is as useful in partial nail avulsions as the septum elevator is in total avulsions (Figs. 21–3 and 21–5). The splitter has a standard scissors-like upper blade to cut through the nail plate. It also has a unique, wedge-shaped lower blade designed to sepa-

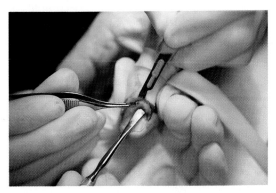

Figure 21–4. Septum elevator defines proximal nail groove and prevents cutting too deeply.

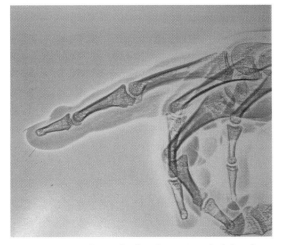

Figure 21–2. Radiograph showing no underlying bone disease related to proximal nail fold tumor.

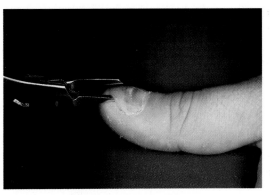

Figure 21–5. Nail splitter.

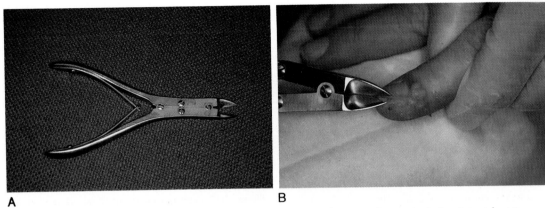

A   B

Figure 21–6. *A,* Double-action bone forceps. *B,* Nail plate is pared away to show extent of periungual wart.

rate the nail plate from the nail bed. Its smooth undersurface glides along the nail bed without causing trauma, while the anvil-like upper surface slides along under the nail plate, providing a platform for the cutting upper blade.[4]

Double-action bone forceps are excellent for trimming and paring the nail plate (Fig. 21–6). This instrument is especially useful for trimming back the nail plate beyond the free edge. This is particularly helpful when attempting to expose the extent of a periungual wart fully before treatment with any one of a number of modalities. The heavy-duty jawlike nail trimmer allows cutting of extremely thickened nails (Fig. 21–7).

For biopsy purposes, both standard and Beaver knife handles are useful. The smaller version of the regular no. 15 scalpel blade, no. 67 of the Beaver system, is helpful for small elliptical or crescentic biopsies. Likewise, the chisel-like no. 81 Beaver blade is an excellent nail splitter when dealing with thick, friable nails.

Single-pronged and double-pronged skin hooks are helpful in retracting the proximal nail fold when visualization of the matrix is required (Fig. 21–8). Small dermal curets are used for debriding subungual hyperkeratotic debris or exuberant granulation tissue. The tray is completed with 3/8-inch Penrose drains used for tourniquets and small mosquito hemostats to secure them.

DRESSINGS AND POSTOPERATIVE CARE

Like any surgical wound, postoperative nail unit wounds are subject to pain, bleeding, exudation, and possible infection. There are also some special considerations. The nail unit,

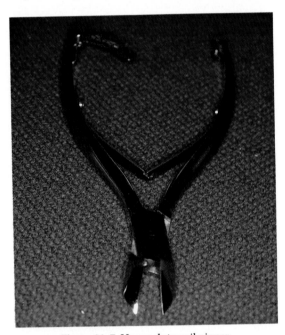

Figure 21–7. Heavy-duty nail nipper.

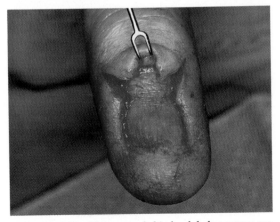

Figure 21–8. Double-pronged skin hook helps expose matrix.

when operated on, tends to throb spontaneously and is excruciatingly painful if traumatized. If the wound is improperly dressed, swelling may become dangerous. This section outlines general guidelines for postoperative care and dressings. Unique dressings, problems, and complications attendant to specific procedures are discussed later along with those procedures.

Patients are instructed to keep the hand or foot out of the dependent position and elevated as much as possible for 48 hours to reduce edema and pain. Pain can usually be controlled with combinations of oral acetaminophen and codeine or nonsteroidal antiinflammatory agents.

An ideal standard dressing should be nonocclusive, nonadherent, and absorbent enough to collect serosanguineous drainage without stimulating bleeding when the dressing is changed (Fig. 21–9). It should be bulky enough to absorb the shock of bumps and snug enough to assist hemostasis. Furthermore, it should be elastic enough to expand and accommodate any swelling. In this last regard, securing adhesive tape must not be placed completely around the digit because it may act as a constricting band if swelling occurs.

If hemostasis is difficult, it may be aided by the use of collagen matrix sponges (Instat, Helistat) (Fig. 21–10A). Similarly, strips of iodoform gauze may be packed under the nail folds to stop bleeding (Fig. 21–10B). A fine film of antibiotic ointment is applied to the wound bed. A square of Telfa, Release, or other nonadherent pad is placed directly on the wound (Fig. 21–10C). Although it usually stays in place by itself, it may be secured with strips of paper tape (Fig. 21–10D). The main body of

the dressing is fashioned by applying several overlapping layers of X-span tubing or Surgitube (Figs. 21–10E and 21–11). Paper tape is again used to secure the dressing. An orthopedic Reese or Zimmer boot will provide additional protection and immobilization (Fig. 21–12).

The dressing should be changed daily until exudation has stopped and pain abated. If the dressing is not changed frequently, the serosanguineous or seropurulent material may act as media for bacteria. During the initial week, open wounds may be compressed or soaked with dilute hydrogen peroxide before applying a fresh dressing. Sutured wounds need only be cleaned with a peroxide-soaked cotton swab and redressed. As healing progresses, a simple dressing of ointment, Telfa pad, and tape will suffice.

ANESTHESIA

For most people, nail surgery is an emotional experience. As with a visit to the dentist, patients are often more apprehensive about the needle stick than the actual procedure. It is best to have patients in a reclining position during the administration of anesthesia in the event a vasovagal episode occurs. It is also best to inform them when a needle stick is about to occur to avoid a dangerous reflex jerk. Use of a 30-gauge needle minimizes the pain, as does slow injection. The surgeon should allow 5 to 10 minutes for the full effect of the anesthesia.

Two basic techniques are used to achieve anesthesia of the nail unit, and each has its advocates and indications. These are the more distal "wing block" and the proximal digital nerve block. They may be used in combination to achieve excellent anesthesia.

The distal digital wing block is useful for procedures on the nail folds and matrix area, but should be supplemented with local injections at the fingertip if more distal procedures are planned.[1,4,7] The injection site is at a point about 3 mm proximal to the imaginary junction of the proximal nail fold and the lateral nail fold on each side (Fig. 21–13). By directing the needle first transversely and then distally, slow injection will distend and blanch both folds and anesthetize the terminal transverse and descending branches of the digital nerve. As the folds distend distally and medially from the focal injection point, a winglike appearance is noted (Fig. 21–13B). In practice it is

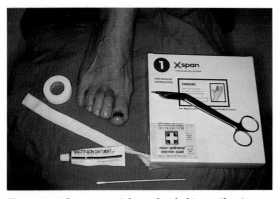

Figure 21–9. Some materials used to fashion nail unit standard dressing.

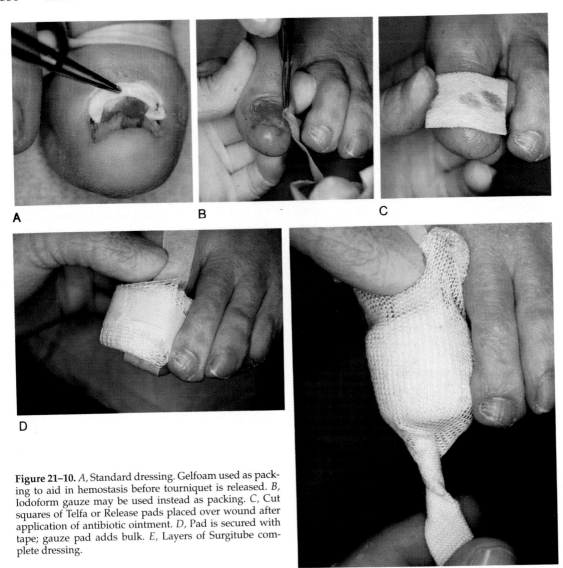

Figure 21–10. *A,* Standard dressing. Gelfoam used as packing to aid in hemostasis before tourniquet is released. *B,* Iodoform gauze may be used instead as packing. *C,* Cut squares of Telfa or Release pads placed over wound after application of antibiotic ointment. *D,* Pad is secured with tape; gauze pad adds bulk. *E,* Layers of Surgitube complete dressing.

often necessary to make intervening injections across the proximal nail fold to ensure complete anesthesia. Less than .5 mL of 1 or 2 per cent plain lidocaine is generally required at each site.

The digital nerve block is designed to anesthetize both the dorsal digital and the proper palmer sensory nerves.[8,9] The idea is to bathe the nerves with anesthetic fluid but not to enter directly into the nerve. This is best achieved by instilling 2 per cent plain lidocaine just under the dermis and allowing the fluid to diffuse down to the nerves. The use of vasoconstrictive agents such as epinephrine should be avoided to prevent prolonged vasospasm and vascular

compromise of the digit. The injection sites are on each side of the digit midway between the dorsal and ventral aspects. The exact site may vary in exact location from the web space to the middle proximal phalanx (Fig. 21–14*A*). Between 0.5 and 1.0 mL of anesthetic fluid, depending on the digit and the laxity of the skin, is introduced just under the dermis. The area will distend noticeably, but care should be taken not to forcibly pump in too much volume or tamponade of the venous flow may occur and compromise vascular integrity.[4,8] It will take several minutes for the anesthesia to diffuse around the nerves and achieve a block. Patience will be rewarded.

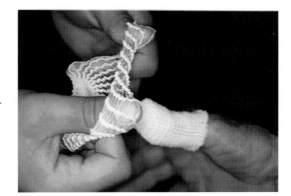

Figure 21–11. X-span also is used to secure dressing.

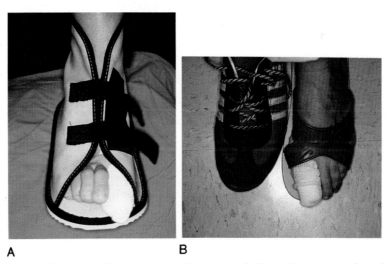

A   B

Figure 21–12. *A,* Special boot lends support and protection. *B,* Open shoe accommodates dressing.

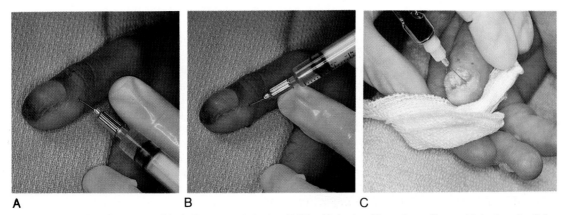

A   B   C

Figure 21–13. *A,* Distal or "wing" block. Transverse injection. *B,* Distal injection. Two wings off central injection site. *C,* Local injection.

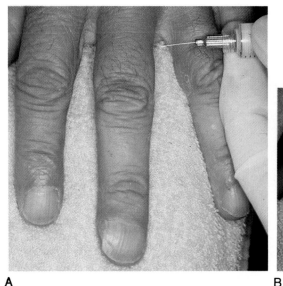
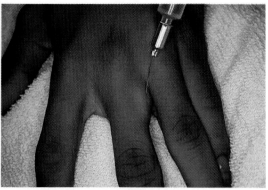

A   B

Figure 21–14. *A,* Digital block. *B,* Injection site nearer to web space.

Because plain lidocaine is a vasodilator and the use of epinephrine is usually not recommended for nail unit surgery, hemostasis is more problematic. Because most nail unit procedures are short, varying between 15 and 30 minutes, hemostasis can be achieved with a combination of lateral digital compression by the surgeon or surgical assistant and the use of tourniquet. Tourniquets can be fashioned from several materials, but one of the most useful is a sterile 3/8-inch Penrose drain secured by a straight hemostat at the base of the digit (Fig. 21–15). The tourniquet is applied only during those critical moments of a procedure that require a bloodless field such as incising a biopsy, placing sutures, or applying phenol. It is best to keep tourniquet use time to 10 minutes or less. Tourniquets create problems when they are small, thin, twisted, and constrictive like a rubber band or when they are left on too long.

Lidocaine 1 or 2 per cent is predictable and has an extraordinary safety record. Its only disadvantage is that it is a vasodilator. Mepivacaine (Carbocaine), which is not a vasodilator, may be used instead.[1] A combination of equal amounts of 0.5 per cent bupivacaine (Marcaine) and 1 per cent prilocaine (Citanest) is a longer acting alternative. If considerable postoperative pain is anticipated, a volume of 0.6 mL of 0.5 per cent bupivacaine with 0.4 mL of 4 mg/mL dexamethasone (Decadron) may be injected into the original wing block sites at the end of the procedure. The ensuing period of anesthesia lasts 8 to 12 hours.

NAIL PLATE AVULSION

Nail plate avulsion may be total or partial. Partial (segmental) avulsion usually refers to the technique of removing longitudinal lateral strips of nail plate in the treatment of ingrown toenails and is discussed later. Paring the nail plate refers to the transverse or longitudinal snipping of bits of nail to expose an area of nail bed more fully. This procedure may be used, for example, to reveal the full extent of a wart growing under the plate from the lateral nail fold (Fig. 21–6*B*). Total nail avulsion is the removal of an entire nail plate, and there are specific indications and techniques for accomplishing it.

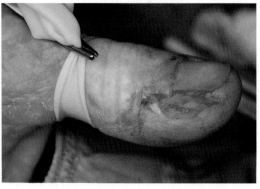

Figure 21–15. Placement of tourniquet.

The nail plate frequently obscures signs of nail bed or matrix pathology and hinders access to the lesion. One of the main indications for total removal of the plate is to allow clear visualization and exploration of the nail bed, nail matrix, and the proximal nail fold and lateral nail fold with their overhanging roofs and underlying grooves before obtaining a biopsy. The other main indication for avulsion is as a prelude to permanent surgical or chemical matricectomy.

There are two basic techniques for total nail avulsion: the usual distal approach and the somewhat more difficult proximal or anterior approach.[1-3,10-13] With either procedure, the object is to separate the plate as atraumatically as possible from its two foci of adherence: the nail bed and the proximal nail fold. With the distal approach, the Freer elevator, dental spatula, or blunt hemostat blade is introduced under the free edge of the nail plate and pushed proximally, forming a plane of cleavage between the bed and plate (Fig. 21–16). Considerable resistance is met until the matrix area is reached, when a characteristic "give" is

felt, indicating a much weaker attachment. Care must be taken not to push too far and shove the elevator into the proximal nail groove, causing injury. After the area over the matrix is reached, it has been recommended that the sides of the finger be held firmly and the elevator pulled or rocked from side to side until the lateral nail grooves are reached and the entire nail plate is separated from the bed. However, this is too traumatic to the nail bed, and it is preferable to reinsert the elevator in a side-by-side longitudinal fashion repeatedly until the entire bed is freed from the overlying plate. Next the elevator is inserted under the cuticle into the proximal nail groove in a similar manner, until all attachments are loosened. The nail plate is then secured with a hemostat and easily removed with a rolling motion.

The proximal approach (Fig. 21–17) is used when a cleavage plane at the distal free edge cannot be found or does not exist because of pathology caused by a disease process such as distal subungual onychomycosis.[1,11,12] The elevator is introduced under the cuticle into the proximal nail groove and then flipped around

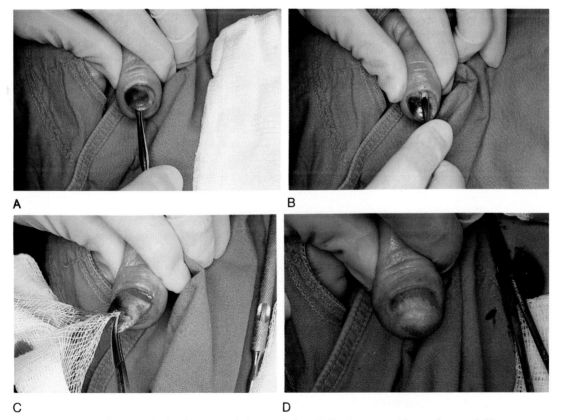

A   B

C   D

Figure 21–16. *A,* Distal approach: distal insertion below nail plate. *B,* Freeing up cuticle attachment. *C,* Hemostat to remove plate. *D,* Plate removed. Note digital compression to aid in hemostasis.

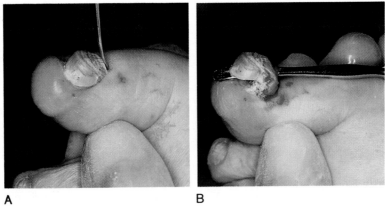

Figure 21–17. *A,* Distorted nail before proximal avulsion with elevator inserted under cuticle into proximal nail groove. *B,* Elevator rotated around proximal nail plate and advanced distally under free edge of plate.

the proximal edge of the plate into the natural cleavage plane between the plate and matrix. Note that the septum elevator is inserted "backward" so it conforms to the curve of the nail bed after it is turned and directed distally. The elevator is advanced until it emerges at the distal free edge. Successive insertions free the plate, which again can be removed by gentle traction with a hemostat.

NAIL MATRIX–PROXIMAL GROOVE EXPLORATION

Full exposure of the matrix and proximal nail fold is obtained by making two full-thickness tangential incisions laterally and proximally from a point where the lateral and proximal nail folds meet (Fig. 21–18).[2,14] The Freer elevator may be inserted into the proximal nail groove to act as a guide for these incisions and prevent the surgeon from cutting too deeply or proximally.[4] The flap is retracted with skin hooks or sutures to expose the matrix and proximal nail groove fully. At the completion of surgery, the flap is either sutured or fastened back into place with Steri-Strips.

NAIL UNIT BIOPSIES

Biopsies of the nail unit are often required to confirm or establish the diagnosis of a dermatosis or tumor. They are also necessary to explain a long-standing nail deformity or correctly diagnose what appears to be an unresponsive fungal infection. Most importantly, a biopsy may also be therapeutic for many of the tumors that arise on the nail unit.

Biopsy may be performed by punch through the nail plate, or the plate may be avulsed first,

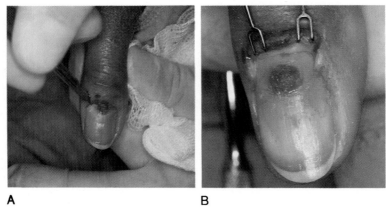

Figure 21–18. *A,* Incision to expose matrix area. *B,* Flap reflected with skin hooks to expose matrix.

with subsequent punch or excision. Combined biopsy of all nail unit components may be done by narrow central or lateral wedge excision. Because of these various biopsy techniques,[1–3,14–20] a certain amount of confusion has arisen about which approach is best. Because the nail is composed of distinct anatomic and physiologic units, it is best to discuss each separately. The nail matrix requires special surgical considerations that do not pertain to the nail bed, and vice versa. With only minor variations, biopsy of the paronychial tissue is similar to routine biopsies anywhere.

Frequent questions arise concerning nail unit biopsies. Is it necessary to remove the nail plate? Is a punch or excision better? Is it necessary to get representative tissue from all nail unit sites, including the nail fold, matrix, bed, and plate? The following guidelines should help in making a decision about the most appropriate type of biopsy:

1. Try to limit the biopsy to a single anatomic unit.

2. Biopsy only tissue that will help with the problem needing clarification.

3. Use the procedure with the most favorable risk-to-benefit ratio. Avoid scarring or deformity.

4. Take the smallest representative amount of tissue that will allow the pathologist to make a diagnosis.

5. If an option exists, biopsy nail bed tissue rather than nail matrix.

6. Use fusiform excisions when possible and suture them. These should be transverse in the matrix and longitudinal in the nail bed and less than 3 mm wide if possible.

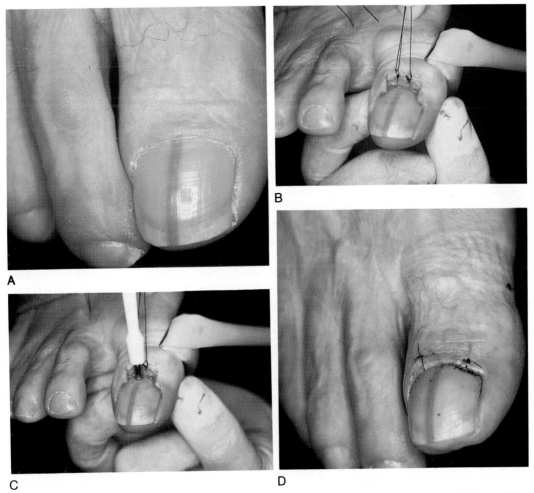

Figure 21–19. *A*, Pigmented longitudinal streak. *B*, Reflection of proximal nail fold to expose matrix. *C*, Three-millimeter punch biopsy of matrix. *D*, Lateral incisions sutured.

7. Incise the biopsy specimen all the way down to bone.

Using these guidelines, the original questions may be addressed. In most instances, it is preferable to think of the standard nail unit biopsy as one that includes total avulsion of the nail plate followed by either a fusiform excision or a punch biopsy small enough to allow primary closure. This includes biopsies of both the nail matrix and the nail bed. In general, this technique allows the surgeon clear visualization of the prospective operative site.

NAIL MATRIX BIOPSY

Indications for nail matrix biopsies include suspicious longitudinal pigmented streaks of nail plate, unexplained full-length nail plate deformities, or any tumor arising in the matrix area. After anesthesia is secured, the proximal nail fold is reflected to expose the entire matrix (Fig. 21–19). It is important to mark the proximal nail fold, if the nail plate is first avulsed, in line with the pigmented streak or suspected pathologic site to help identify it once the plate is removed. The two most important things to remember when obtaining a biopsy of the nail matrix are to orient the excision transversely and not to interfere with the configuration of the curvilinear distal border of the lunula. If possible, avoid the most proximal matrix, because its interruption might result in permanent defects of the surface plate. Whether sutured or not, narrow biopsies may be expected to result in a cosmetic nail plate (Fig. 21–20). Primary suturing is favorable, closure being secured with either a nonabsorbable material such as Prolene or absorbable suture material such as Vicryl. However, in some situations, such as with wider pigmented streaks or traumatically split nails, primary closure is difficult to affect because the nail matrix and bed are so bound down to the underlying periosteum. Undermining, by increasing movement of the wound edges, may be required to accomplish a primary closure. Undermining is best accomplished in the

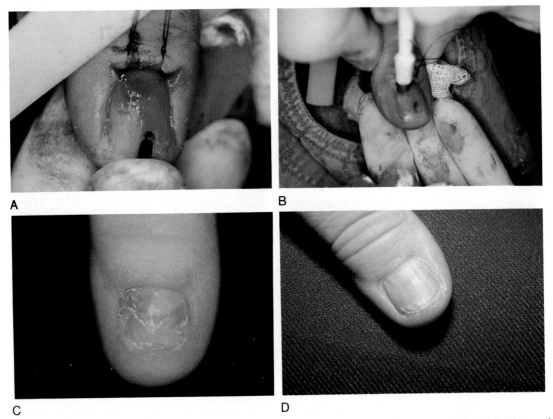

A

B

C

D

Figure 21–20. *A,* Glomus tumor of matrix. Note use of suture to retract proximal fold[4] (Courtesy of Cutis). *B,* Three-millimeter punch biopsy to encompass tumor left unsutured. *C,* Healing at 3 months. *D,* Healing at 6 months.

periosteal plane. More drastic mobilization may be attained by combining undermining with relaxing incisions in the lateral nail grooves. Two bipedicle flaps are created. The relaxing incisions do not require suturing.[21]

In any event, any biopsy of the nail matrix has the potential to result in permanent changes of the nail plate. There may be a depressed groove, a split nail, or a focal area of onycholysis. The patient must be thoroughly counseled before surgery of the indication for biopsy and possible sequelae (Fig. 21–21).

Nail Bed Biopsy

Indications for nail bed biopsy are similar to those for the nail matrix, as are the preoperative preparations. Fusiform excisions should be longitudinal if possible and limited to a width of about 3 mm (Fig. 21–22). The area to undergo biopsy should be outlined with surgical dye. It may be prudent to paint the entire epithelial surface of the specimen with a surgical mark to ensure it is properly oriented. The incision lines are cut perpendicular to the surface down to the periosteum. The base is re-

leased using a sharp tissue scissors. Care should be taken not to crush the specimen. This is best achieved by grasping the specimen lightly with delicate, toothed forceps. Undermining and suturing are recommended for best cosmetic results. Making sure that the biopsy material is oriented properly and not physically damaged will ensure the best opportunity for a correct histologic diagnosis.

The biopsy technique referred to as longitudinal resection is an en bloc removal of a wedge of tissue that includes nail fold, matrix, bed, and hyponychium and is a wonderful tool for defining disease processes of the nail unit. Recent clarification of the pathogenesis of diseases like psoriasis, lichen planus, Darier's disease, and alopecia areata have been possible only through obtaining such composite biopsies. However, this method is probably too extensive for routine biopsy by the clinician and is best left to the interested investigator who has a thoroughly informed patient. It is also an excellent therapeutic procedure for ablation of the lateral nail matrix in the treatment of an ingrown toenail or for treating tumors such as Bowen's disease or squamous cell carcinoma when they involve the area (Fig. 21–23).

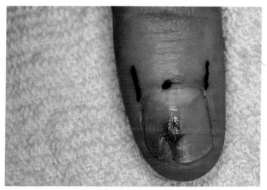

A

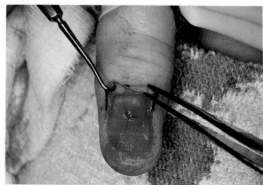

B

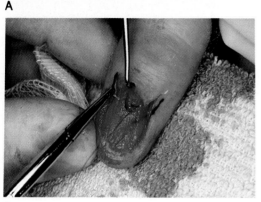

C

Figure 21–21. *A,* Split nail resulting from trauma of matrix. *B,* Proximal fold reflected to expose tear in matrix. *C,* Wound freshened and sutured.

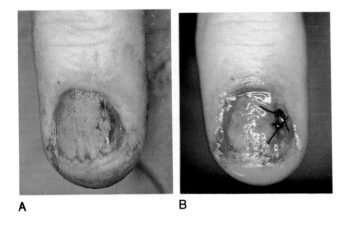

A   **B**

Figure 21–22. *A,* Longitudinal nail bed biopsy glomus tumor. From Salasche SJ, Peters V: Tips on nail surgery. Cutis 35:428, 1984. Used with permission. *B,* Sutured biopsy site.

PARONYCHIAL SURGERY

The paronychial region, which includes the proximal and lateral nail folds, is an anatomic site for which a systematized surgical approach has never been outlined.

Although not exhaustive, a catalogue of the most frequently occurring diseases of these tissues includes the following: infections such as acute and chronic paronychias, verruca vulgaris, deep fungi, and atypical mycobacteria; response to trauma, including foreign body granuloma, pyogenic granuloma, and keloid; and lesions unique to the area, such as focal mucinosis (myxoid cyst), acquired digital fibrokeratoma, and periungual fibroma associated with tuberous sclerosis.

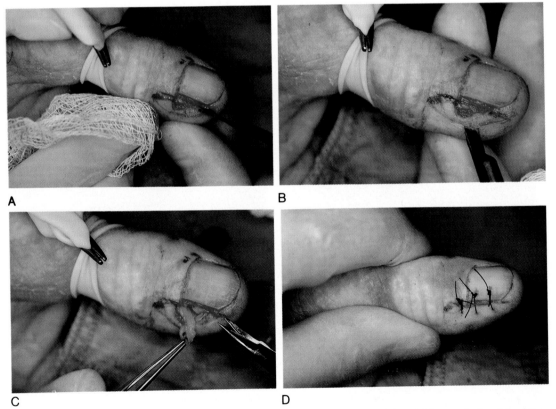

A   **B**

C   **D**

Figure 21–23. *A,* Lateral longitudinal resection vertical incision. *B,* Transverse incision. *C,* Removal of en bloc biopsy. *D,* Closure.

The requisite surgical skills at these sites include various biopsy techniques and the ability to perform an en bloc excision of the entire proximal nail fold.

Incisional Biopsy

When diagnostic tissue is required from the proximal or lateral nail fold, the procedure of choice is an incisional biopsy. This allows both acquisition of adequate tissue for histologic and other studies as well as the opportunity for primary closure with preservation of the normal nail fold anatomy.

On the proximal nail fold, a transverse incision that parallels the relaxed skin tension lines results in the easiest and most cosmetically acceptable closure (Fig. 21–24). Care should be taken to place the incision far enough beyond the distal interphalangeal joint to avoid cutting the tendon of the extensor digitorum communis, which inserts onto the proximal dorsal portion of the terminal phalanx. Likewise, avoid the distal free margin to prevent notched scarring. After a generous biopsy specimen is obtained, the lesion may be closed primarily without undermining. A relatively nonreactive suture material such as 4-0 or 5-0 Prolene may be used. The sutures are removed in about 7 days.

If required, the specimen may be divided and a portion processed routinely for hematoxylin and eosin sections and for special stains (periodic acid–Schiff, acid fast, Brown and Brenn). The remaining portion is submitted for tissue cultures to search for deep fungi or atypical mycobacteria. The specimen illustrated in Figure 21–24 grew *Mycobacterium marinum,* which responded to oral minocycline. Sporotrichosis or a foreign body granuloma would have a similar clinical appearance.

The most common indication for biopsy of the lateral nail fold is a hyperkeratotic plaque that is considered to be a wart or fungal infection and that persists or recurs despite seemingly adequate therapy. Under these circumstances, a high index of suspicion for Bowen's disease or squamous cell carcinoma is justified. Biopsies of the lateral nail fold are similar to those of the proximal nail fold, except the orientation should be longitudinal rather than transverse. However, the pathology frequently extends into the sulcus of the lateral nail groove or even under the nail plate and onto the nail bed. This requires paring back the nail plate for complete exposure and biopsy of the most suspicious area. Biopsies that involve the nail bed should be carried down to bone. Sutures may be placed from the skin of the lateral nail fold across to the nail bed and up through the adjoining nail plate.

En Bloc Excision of the Proximal Nail Fold

En bloc excision of the proximal nail fold, to include symmetric small portions of the lateral nail folds, is a useful procedure in the definitive treatment of selected conditions. The technique, which also includes healing by secondary intention, was originally described by Baran and Bureau[21] for the management of recalcitrant chronic paronychia. It has since been successfully adopted for treatment of stubborn myxoid cysts of the proximal nail fold,[23]

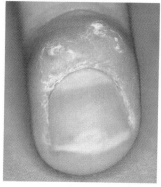 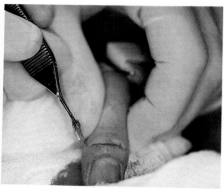

A B

Figure 21–24. *A,* Granulomatous swelling of proximal nail fold. *B,* Transverse proximal nail fold biopsy.

keloids (unpublished data), and collagen vascular disorders.[24]

Among the space-occupying lesions of the proximal nail fold, myxoid cyst is the most frequently encountered. In this location, these cysts appear as dome-shaped, translucent nodules that if large enough compress the nail matrix and cause various longitudinal nail plate dystrophies (e.g., grooves, ridges, or splits). Myxoid cysts over the distal interphalangeal joint as seen in patients with osteoarthritis are connected to the underlying joint space and are probably similar to synovial cysts.[22,25] These cysts are best definitively treated by those trained in hand surgery. Procedures include not only excising the cyst but also tracing the stalk back to the joint space and combining its excision with removal of the offending osteophytes.[26,27] Those cysts occurring on the proximal nail fold may not have such joint connection and may be due to overproduction of hyaluronic acid by focally deranged fibroblasts.[28] Puncture with a sterile needle yields a clear, viscous fluid. When conservative management, including intralesional corticosteroids or cryotherapy, fails, en bloc excision of the proximal nail fold to include the cyst has proved very successful.[23]

The digit is properly anesthetized, antiseptically prepared, and isolated, and a tourniquet fastened. The line of the intended incision is drawn with an appropriate surgical marker (Fig. 21–25). A Freer septum elevator is inserted into the proximal nail groove to define the proximal limit of this blind cul-de-sac and to act as a guide for the scalpel. Full-thickness excision is then carried out. By sliding the elevator along in concert with and below the advancing scalpel, the chance of inadvertently cutting too deeply into the nail matrix or the more proximal extensor tendon is avoided. The latter problem may also be avoided by beveling the blade to a less acute angle. This coincidently creates a gently sloped wound, which seems to heal more rapidly than the conventional vertical-edged wound.

Hemostasis is attained by judicious spot electrodesiccation of significant bleeders. Capillary bleeding is stemmed by pressing Gelfoam or Instat pads into the wound. A bulky dressing similar to that described in an earlier section is applied. Postoperative care consists of twice-daily cleansing with dilute hydrogen peroxide, application of an antibiotic ointment, and placement of a clean bulky dressing. A smaller dressing is used when healing is well under way and any tenderness has resolved.

Healing by second intention results in restoration of the proximal nail fold approximately 3 to 5 mm proximal to the original proximal nail fold. Rather than being deformed, the new configuration reveals more of the lunula and nail plate, giving the digit a slender, graceful appearance. The key elements contributing to the final cosmetic and functional outcome are full-thickness excision of the proximal nail fold to include symmetric small portions of the lateral nail fold and meticulous postoperative care consisting of daily dressing changes to keep the wound clean, moist, and covered. In most instances, exudation continues for 4 to 6 days postoperatively, with granulation tissue beginning in earnest at 7 to 10 days. By 6 weeks, a newly epithelialized proximal nail fold complete with a cuticle generally has regenerated. Full remodeling and maturation require several more weeks. Nail plate deformities on the fingers will grow out completely in about 6 months if there was no permanent matrix damage.

Acute flare-ups of chronic paronychia have a complicated pathogenesis. Repeated episodes lead to persistent edema, induration, and fibrosis of the proximal and lateral nail folds. This causes the nail folds to round up and retract away from the nail plate, thereby exposing the nail groove. This loss of an effective seal and the inability to form a cuticle leads to persistent retention of moisture within the groove with the subsequent overgrowth of bacteria (*Staphylococcus aureus* and *Pseudomonas aeruginosa*) and the cycle of recurrent acute infections.[1,22]

Excising the damaged nail folds as described previously results in restoration of the normal architecture and an effective seal (Fig. 21–26). If the patient will avoid water immersion, wear protective rubber gloves, and stop manipulating the cuticles, a good prospect for long-term remission exists.

Expansion of indications to include other space-occupying lesions has led to successful management of a keloid following trauma. Figure 21–27 depicts a keloid that developed 11 months before surgery in a 32-year-old black woman. The final size was reached 3 months after minor trauma and remained stable during the intervening time. A longitudinal depression developed, and it ultimately extended the length of the nail plate. Soft tissue xerograms failed to reveal a foreign body or origin from the underlying bone. Biopsy showed

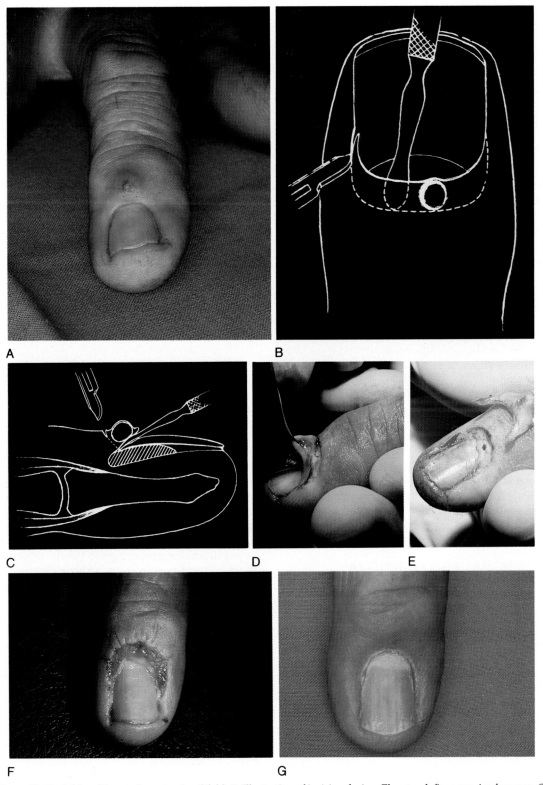

Figure 21–25. *A,* Myxoid cyst of proximal nail fold. *B,* Illustration of incision design. Elevator defines proximal groove. *C,* Beveled incision prevents cutting too deeply. *D,* Undersurface of myxoid cyst. *E,* Crescent-shaped full-thickness excision. *F,* One week postoperatively. *G,* One year postoperatively. From Salasche SJ: Myxoid cysts of the proximal nail fold: A surgical approach. J Dermatol Surg Oncol 10:35, 1984. Used with permission.

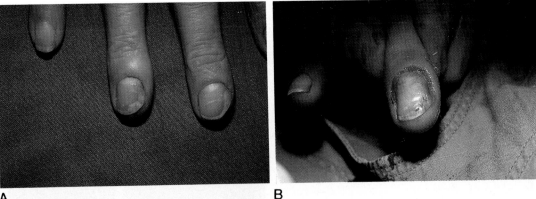

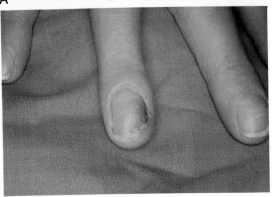

Figure 21–26. *A,* Chronic paronychia. *B,* Excision complete. *C,* Healing at 2 months.

large cords of dense collagen bundles in various directions and an absence of adnexal structures. Although postoperative intralesional corticosteroids had been considered as part of an overall plan, they were not required.

SUBUNGUAL AND PERIUNGUAL VERRUCA VULGARIS

Most warts have a finite life span, with two thirds resolving spontaneously within 2 years.[29] Likewise, most respond to relatively conservative measures such as cryotherapy.[30] Peri- and subungual verrucae, however, have special problems. In this location, they tend to be multiple and much more aggressive and destructive, often extending around and under the nail plate. Many patients find warts on the nail unit cosmetically unacceptable. Unfortunately, standard treatment modalities such as keratolytic agents, cantharidin, and liquid nitrogen are often unsuccessful and recurrences are frequent.[31,32]

When peri- and subungual warts have proved recalcitrant to therapy, surgical intervention with a technique of electrodesiccation and enucleation has proved efficacious.[32,33] After local anesthesia and removal of as much nail plate as necessary to visualize the wart fully, a two-step procedure is performed, aimed at separating the epidermal wart from its papillomatous moorings to the dermis (Fig. 21–28). The idea is to cause as little damage as possible to the latter to avoid scarring. The first stage (electrodesiccation) is designed to soften, destroy, and demarcate the wart tissue by "cooking" it with the current delivered by the ordinary monopolar terminal of the Birtcher Hyfrecutter. At the lowest possible current setting, the needle is applied either directly to the surface of small warts or intralesionally to larger, thicker warts. As the current passes through the wart tissue, it causes charring, dehydration, and retraction of the wart away from the dermis. Then in the second step, the peripheral plane of cleavage is found under the charred, shrunken wart and firmly swept away with a curet. After this enucleation stage, a white stringy or soupy material sometimes remains adherent to the base of the wound. This, too, may be lightly cauterized

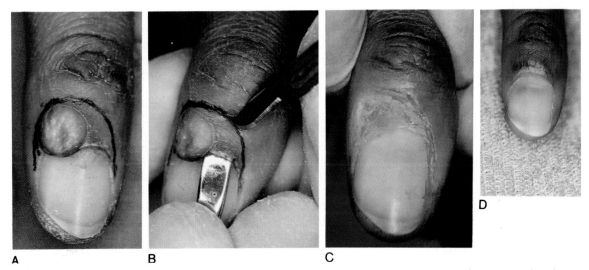

Figure 21–27. *A,* Keloid of proximal fold. *B,* Beveled excision. *C,* Postoperative view. *D,* Two months postoperative view.

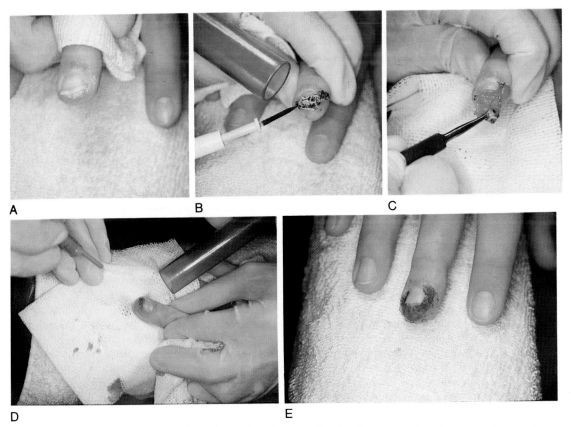

Figure 21–28. *A,* Periungual wart. *B,* Electrodesiccation of wart. *C,* Enucleation with curet. *D,* Laser vaporization of residual wart tissue. *E,* At completion of procedure.

and curetted. The brisk capillary bleeding resulting from interruption of the dermal papillomatosis is stemmed cautiously with further light electrodesiccation, 25 per cent aluminum chloride, or applications of Instat. Unless the electrodesiccation has been overzealous, healing by second intention without scarring is complete within 3 to 4 weeks to treat periungal warts.[34,35] An excellent cure rate may be expected.

A relatively recent advance has been the introduction of the use of the carbon dioxide laser to treat periungual warts.[34,35] The procedure is similar to that described previously except that the laser beam is used to vaporize the wart. In our practice, we initially char with the electrosurgical unit to debulk the major portion of the wart. Subsequently, the laser beam in the defocused mode eliminates any residual wart tissue (Fig. 21–28E).

PERMANENT MATRICECTOMY

Partial or total ablation procedures of the nail matrix are among the most useful techniques in the treatment of common nail unit disorders. The widest application of partial matricectomy is in the treatment of the ubiquitous ingrown toenail. Other indications include the pincer nail syndrome and the relatively common aging phenomenon of incurvature of the lateral nail plate.

Total ablation of the nail matrix is often indicated in extensive, symptomatic cases of onychomycosis, onychogryphosis, thickened nails, and other chronic painful or distorted nail conditions.

Although several scalpel surgery, laser surgery, and electrosurgical techniques are available for partial or total nail matrix ablation, they are generally complicated, are associated with considerable patient morbidity, and have unacceptable failure rates.[36–40] The simplest and most reliable and reproducible method is chemical matricectomy.[41,42] This phenol and alcohol technique uses the destructive protein-denaturing property of 88 per cent liquefied phenol. This effect is enhanced by a bloodless field, which is achieved by applying an "exsanguinating" tourniquet (Fig. 21–29). A 3/8-inch Penrose drain is placed at the end of the digit. Leaving an exposed end distally, the drain is wound firmly in successively overlapping loops in a proximal direction to a point proximal to the distal interphalangeal joint. The distal exposed end

is then unwound, again in a proximal direction. This effectively milks the blood from the digit. The final loop is firmly secured with a hemostat to function as a tourniquet.

Many causes have been ascribed to ingrown toenails, but the common denominator appears to be the soft tissue inflammatory response of the lateral nail fold. This is due either to sideways pressure of the nail plate secondary to tight-fitting shoes or to the irritating embedding of a spike of nail that is created from improperly trimmed toenails. The soft tissue responds as in a foreign body reaction, with edema, erythema, and tenderness. If the condition is allowed to progress, exudation, suppuration, and hypergranulation occur. In any event, even though the soft tissue of the lateral nail fold is overgrowing the nail plate, high cure rates are achieved only by removing the offending portion of the ingrowing plate.

The chemical-surgical approach consists of first achieving proper anesthesia, antiseptic preparation, and applying an exsanguinating tourniquet. Using an English nail splitter, a full-length, full-thickness split in the nail plate is created 2 to 3 mm from the affected lateral nail fold on the exposed nail plate (Fig. 21–30).[43]

The separated portion of the nail plate is grasped with a hemostat and rotated toward the remaining healthy nail plate. This effectively separates the buried nail plate from the lateral nail groove and prevents embedding a spicule of nail within the lateral nail fold, as may happen if the offending portion is rotated away from the main portion of the nail plate.

The matrix is then ablated by firmly pressing phenol-saturated cotton swabs directly onto it for 30 to 45 seconds. The phenol is diluted at the end of this time by flooding with isopropyl alcohol. The matrix is easily reached because the space formerly occupied by the nail plate remains widely patent. It is important to push aggressively into the lateral recesses of this space to bathe the lateral nail horn totally. Otherwise, a remnant of nail plate will reappear several months later.

Any significant granulation tissue is corrected by curetting it away with a 2- to 3-mm curet, followed by application of a silver nitrate stick to achieve hemostasis. The patent gap along the lateral nail groove and under the proximal nail fold is packed with iodoform gauze. If significant bleeding occurs, this same area may be packed with Instat or Gelfoam pads instead. A bulky dressing as described

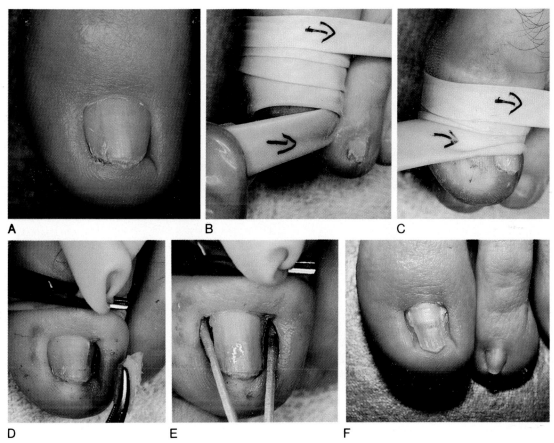

Figure 21–29. *A,* Bilateral incurved painful nails. *B,* "Exsanguinating" tourniquet winding in overlapping loops. *C,* Unwinding lower loop, also in proximal direction. *D,* Removal of lateral nail plate. *E,* Phenol application to lateral matrix. *F,* Healing, 3 months.

earlier is fashioned. Injecting 0.6 mL of 0.5 per cent bupivacaine and 0.4 mL dexamethasone at the original anesthesia site alleviates the patient's discomfort for 8 to 12 hours. A pain medication such as acetaminophen with codeine should nonetheless be given as well as instructions to keep the foot elevated. It is wise to advise the patient to bring appropriate footwear (sandals, slippers) to accommodate a bulky dressing.

Bilateral partial permanent matricectomies have been advocated for ingrown toenails and are useful in some cases of pincer nail or congenital bilateral ingrown toenail.[2] Even though the resulting nail plate is often very thin, the patient is delighted to be free of pain (see Fig. 21–29).

Soft tissue hypertrophy resolves spontaneously and usually does not require separate surgery. If necessary, however, wedge excisions, similar to lateral nail fold biopsies, will debulk the area.[1,44,45]

Partial matricectomies are also useful as adjunctive therapy. For example, Figure 21–31 demonstrates a myxoid cyst treated by en bloc excision of the proximal nail fold that had eroded into the matrix, causing a permanent split nail. Phenol destruction of the smaller segment of matrix eventuated in a cosmetically acceptable thin nail.

Total permanent matricectomies are performed in a similar manner. After avulsion of the nail, the phenol is applied to the entire matrix (i.e., the whole lunula), to the matrix under the proximal nail fold, and to both lateral nail horns. The grooves are again packed with iodoform gauze or collagen matrix pads, and a bulky dressing is applied. Daily cleansing with hydrogen peroxide, application of an antibiotic ointment, and dressing changes are identical to the procedure described earlier.

Indications for permanent matricectomies include recalcitrant onychomycosis in which the nail plate is thickened, discolored, fri-

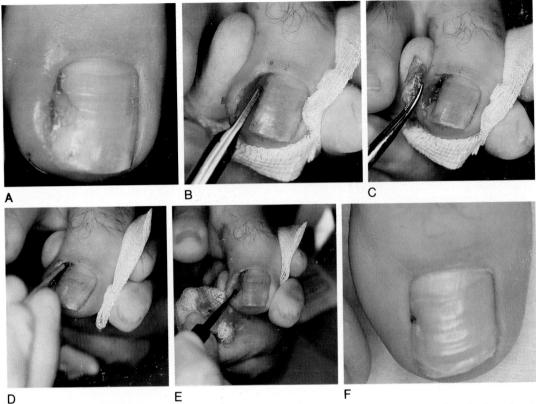

Figure 21–30. *A,* Ingrown toenail. *B,* Cut lateral nail plate. *C,* Remove lateral nail plate. *D,* Apply phenol to lateral matrix. *E,* Curet granulation tissue (Courtesy of Cutis). *F,* Result 6 months later.

able, and seemingly elevated by subungual debris. Painful onychogryphosis and ony-chauxis (thickened nails) are other indications (Fig. 21–32).

End-stage healing is attained when the nail folds fuse with the now thickened, leather-like nail bed. This acts as a pseudonail and serves to protect the digit as would a real nail plate. If lateral spicules of nail recur, these are easily treated by anesthetizing the digit and avulsing the remnant with a hemostat. Through the resultant tunnel, phenol is reapplied.

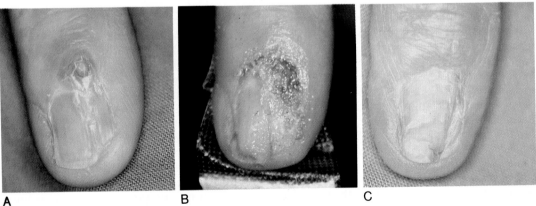

Figure 21–31. *A,* Myxoid cyst with destruction of matrix. *B,* En bloc excision of proximal nail fold, removal of lateral plate, and phenol application to lateral matrix. *C,* Result 6 months later.

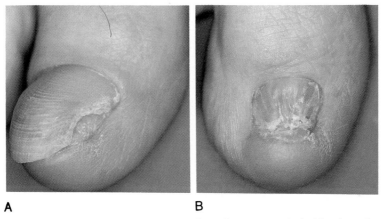

Figure 21–32. *A,* Thick, distorted, painful nail. *B,* View several months postoperatively. Note hyperkeratosis of nail bed.

MOHS' TECHNIQUE

As described in an earlier chapter, Bowen's disease and invasive squamous cell carcinoma of the nail unit, although capable of metastasizing, do so only rarely. If bony involvement has been ruled out by x-ray film, a tissue-sparing procedure rather than amputation is indicated. Mohs' technique, using either fresh or fixed tissue, has the advantage of frozen-section control of the surgical margins and enables the surgeon to trace out the subclinical tumor extensions and achieve high cure rates. This, coupled with the obvious tis-

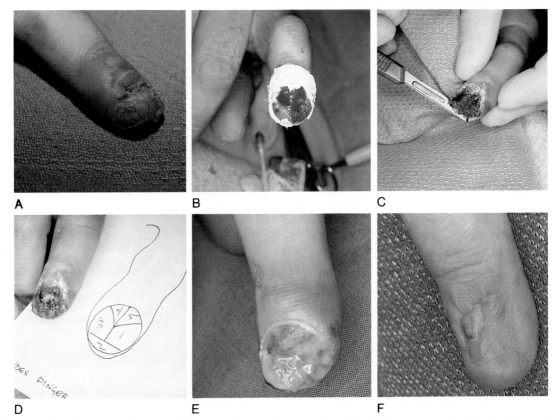

Figure 21–33. *A,* Preoperative Bowen's disease. *B,* Protective Lassar's paste. *C,* Excision of zinc chloride fixed tissue. *D,* Mapping tissue. *E,* Postoperative view. *F,* View several months postoperatively, secondary intention healing.

sue-sparing effect, makes it the treatment of choice for these relatively well-differentiated, nonaggressive, but potentially lethal tumors.

The fixed-tissue technique, which uses in situ fixation of the tissue with zinc chloride paste, is time consuming and uncomfortable for the patient. For the most part, it has been replaced by the fresh-tissue technique, which eliminates the use of paste.[46-48] However, in the nail bed region, where bleeding is a problem and paper-thin slices of tissue are often required, the fixed technique serves well (Fig. 21–33). The area is first debulked with a curet, and either bi- or trichloroacetic acid is applied to dekeratinize the skin and facilitate penetration of the paste. The surrounding area is protected by Lassar's paste, and the zinc chloride paste is applied in a thickness of about 1 mm. The area is covered with a dressing made from an eye patch and secured with paper tape. Twenty-four hours later, a thin saucerized excision is taken in a plane just above the level of the fixed tissue. This is cut into pieces of appropriate size for processing. A color-coded map is drawn to correspond to the sections. The tissue is inverted, and sections are cut, stained, and examined histologically for residual tumor. If tumor persists, the paste is reapplied and the procedure continued the next day until a tumor-free plane is achieved. The author now begins with the fresh-tissue approach and resorts to the fixed-tissue method if the tumor proves invasive.

Healing is by second intention. Daily wound care includes cleansing with hydrogen peroxide and application of an antibiotic ointment and a clean, dry dressing.

References

1. Baran R: Surgery of the nail. Dermatol Clin 2:271, 1984.
2. Siegle RJ, Swanson NA: Nail surgery: A review. J Dermatol Surg Oncol 8:659, 1982.
3. Scher RK: Nail Surgery. *In* Epstein E, Epstein E Jr (eds): Techniques in Skin Surgery. Lea & Febiger, Philadelphia, 1979, pp 164–170.
4. Salasche SJ, Peters V: Tips on nail surgery. Cutis 35:428, 1984.
5. Baran R: More on avulsion of the nail plates (letter). J Dermatol Surg Oncol 7:854, 1981.
6. Albom MJ: Surgical gems: Avulsion of a nail plate. J Dermatol Surg Oncol 3:34, 1977.
7. Scher RK: Punch biopsies of the nail: A simple valuable procedure. J Dermatol Surg Oncol 4:528, 1978.
8. Bennett RG: Fundamentals of Cutaneous Surgery. CV Mosby, St. Louis, MO, 1988, pp 218, 226–227.
9. Albom MJ: Digital block anesthesia. J Dermatol Surg 2:366, 1976.
10. Zaias N: The Nail in Health and Disease. Spectrum Publications, New York, 1980.
11. Scher RK: Surgical avulsion of nail plates by a proximal to distal technique. J Dermatol Surg Oncol 7:296, 1981.
12. Cordero FA: Ablacion ungueal: So uso en la onicomicosis. Dermatol Int 14:21, 1965.
13. Daniel CR III: Basic nail plate avulsion. J Dermatol Surg Oncol 18:685, 1992.
14. Scher RK: Biopsy of the matrix of the nail. J Dermatol Surg Oncol 6:19, 1980.
15. Zaias NJ: The longitudinal nail biopsy. J Invest Dermatol 49:406, 1967.
16. Bennett RG: Technique of biopsy of nails. J Dermatol Surg Oncol 2:325, 1976.
17. Scher RK: Longitudinal resection of nails for purposes of biopsy and treatment. J Dermatol Surg Oncol 6:805, 1980.
18. Stone OJ, Barr RJ, Horton RJ: Biopsy of the nail area. Cutis 21:257, 1979.
19. Baran R, Bureau H: Nail biopsy—Why, when, where, how? J Dermatol Surg Oncol 2:322, 1976.
20. Rich P: Nail biopsy: Indications and methods. J Dermatol Surg Oncol 18:673, 1992.
21. Ogo K: Split nails. Plast Reconstr Surg 86:1190, 1990.
22. Baran R, Bureau H: Surgical treatment of recalcitrant chronic paronychias of the fingers. J Dermatol Surg Oncol 7:106, 1981.
23. Salasche SJ: Myxoid cysts of the proximal nail fold: A surgical approach. J Dermatol Surg Oncol 10:35, 1984.
24. Scher RK, Tom DWK, Lally EV, et al: The clinical significance of periodic acid-Schiff positive deposits in cuticle-proximal nail fold biopsy specmens. Arch Dermatol 121:1406, 1985.
25. Newmeyer WI, Kilgore ES Jr, Graham WP: Mucus cysts: The dorsal interphalangeal joint ganglion. Plast Reconstr Surg 53:313, 1074.
26. Brown RE, Zook EG, Russell RC, et al: Fingernail deformities secondary to ganglions of the distal interphalangeal joint (mucous cysts). Plast Reconstr Surg 87:718, 1991.
27. Kasdan ML, Stallings SP, Leis VM, Wolens D: Outcome of surgically treated mucous cysts of the hand. J Hand Surg 19:504, 1994.
28. Johnson WC, Graham JH, Helwig EB: Cutaneous myxoid cysts: A clinicopathological and histochemical study. JAMA 191:15, 1965.
29. Massing AM, Epstein WL: Natural history of warts. Arch Dermatol 87:306, 1963.
30. Hall A: Advantages and limitations of liquid nitrogen in the therapy of skin lesions. Arch Dermatol 82:63, 1960.
31. Bunney MH, Nolan MW, Williams DA: An assessment of methods of treating viral warts by comparative treatment trials based on a standard design. J Dermatol 94:667, 1976.
32. Mahrle G, Alexander W: Surgical treatment of recalcitrant warts. J Dermatol Surg Oncol 9:445, 1983.
33. An YF: Intralesional electrodesiccation with a 30-gauge needle. J Dermatol Surg Oncol 3:520, 1977.
34. McBurney EI, Rosen DA: Carbon dioxide laser treatment of verrucae vulgaris. J Dermatol Surg Oncol 10:45, 1984.
35. Street ML, Roenigk RK: Recalcitrant periungual verrucae: The role of carbon dioxide laser vaporization. J Am Acad Dermatol 23:115, 1990.
36. Ceilley RI, Collison DW: Matricectomy. J Dermatol Surg Oncol 18:728, 1992.

37. Greig JD, Anderson JH, Ireland AJ, Anderson JR: The surgical treatment of ingrowing toenails. J Bone Joint Surg 73:131, 1991.
38. Van der Ham AC, Hackeng CAH, Yo TI: The treatment of ingrowing toenails: A randomized comparison of wedge excision and phenol cauterisation. J Bone Joint Surg 72:507, 1990.
39. Leshin B, Whitaker DC: Carbon dioxide laser matricectomy. J Dermatol Surg Oncol 14:608, 1988.
40. Hettinger DF, Valinsky MS, Nuccio G, Lim R: Nail matricectomies using radio wave technique. J Am Podiatr Med Assoc 81:317, 1991.
41. Siegle RJ, Harkness JJ, Swanson NA: The phenol alcohol technique for permanent matricectomy. Arch Dermatol 120:348, 1984.
42. Travers GR, Ammon RG: The sodium hydroxide matricectomy procedure. J Am Podiatr Assoc 70:476, 1980.
43. Gibbs RC: Treatment of uncomplicated ingrown toenails. J Dermatol Surg Oncol 4:438, 1978.
44. Orr CME, Photior S: Management of ingrowing toenails. Hosp Update 3:465, 1977.
45. Murray WR, Robb JE: Soft tissue resection for ingrowing toenails. J Dermatol Surg Oncol 7:157, 1981.
46. Tomsick R, Menn H: Chemosurgical excision of subungual squamous cell carcinoma. Hand 13:177, 1981.
47. Mohs FE: Chemosurgery in Cancer, Gangrene and Infections. Charles C Thomas, Springfield, IL, 1978, pp 131–152.
48. Albom MJ: Squamous cell carcinoma of the finger and nail bed: A review of the literature and treatment by Mohs surgical technique. J Dermatol Surg Oncol 1:43, 1975.

CHAPTER 22

Advanced Surgery

James H. Herndon, Steven R. Myers, and Edward Akelman

Surgical treatment of the nail unit has only recently received widespread attention. Textbooks on hand surgery have historically devoted only small segments to nail surgery, and dermatologists have not aggressively promoted work in this area.[1] Several modern clinicians, however, have pursued their interest in the techniques of nail surgery and have contributed significantly to our current understanding of the pathophysiology of nail diseases and their surgical treatment.

SURGICAL SET-UP

Preparation and draping of the extremity prior to surgery should be standardized for any procedure involving the hand (Fig. 22–1). Graft harvest sites should be prepared and draped appropriately before starting the operation. The instrument tray (Fig. 22–2) should include the basic tools for hand surgery, including a dental spatula or Freer septum elevator (Fig. 22–3), used to elevate the nail plate from the bed and matrix. When indicated, appropriate antibiotics are administered prior to exsanguination of the digit or extremity to ensure tissue exposure to the antibiotic during the procedure. Hemostasis is maintained by a tourniquet on either the finger or the proximal

arm; its placement is usually dictated by the predicted length of the procedure and type of anesthesia used. Caution should be exercised when using the finger tourniquet, because significant pressures can be generated, causing tissue necrosis. The use of surgical loupes in nail surgery is essential. Magnification (Fig. 22–4) in the range of 3.5 × is usually satisfactory.

ANESTHESIA

Anesthesia for surgery of the nail can be obtained through several routes. The dorsal sensory branches of the digital nerves can be anesthetized using 1 per cent lidocaine or 0.5 per cent mepivacaine (epinephrine is never used in the hand) inserted into the proximal and lateral nail folds with a 30-gauge needle.[2] This is contraindicated, however, in patients with a history of peripheral vascular disease.

The digital block is preferred to the nail fold block and is accomplished by injection of 2 to 3 mL of anesthetic 1.5 cm into the web spaces in the plane of the palm.[3] Intravenous regional (Bier block), wrist block, and axillary blocks are also useful, and general anesthesia is used for the patient who cannot remain stationary during a long surgical procedure.

350

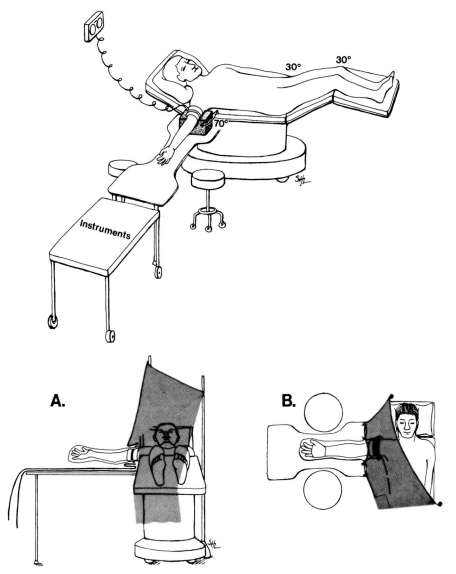

Figure 22–1. Draping of the patient for surgery of the hand. Two sheets are placed on the operating surface, and the upper one is carefully folded to form a cuff. A double-layer stockinette is rolled on the arm and carefully brought over the tourniquet. The vertical upper drape sheet is then clipped to the cuff on the table sheet, with the two clips adjacent to the arm, including the stockinette. The clips should *not* be placed through the patient's skin. From McCollister Evarts C (ed): Surgery of the Musculoskeletal System. Churchill Livingstone, New York, 1983. Used with permission.

TREATMENT OF ACUTE INJURIES

Subungual Hematoma

Subungual hematomas result from blunt injuries to the highly vascular nail bed. The contained bleeding often results in exquisite pain because of pressure on the periosteum. If 25 per cent or more of the nail is involved, to alleviate the pain, the hematoma should be decompressed with a needle, paper clip, or drill heated over an alcohol lamp.[4] Electrocautery units available in most emergency rooms can also painlessly release the hematoma. Large hematomas indicate significant nail bed injury. The nail bed should be explored and repaired accurately.

Complex Lacerations

Complex lacerations involve the proximal nail fold and germinal matrix and are associated with more serious posttraumatic compli-

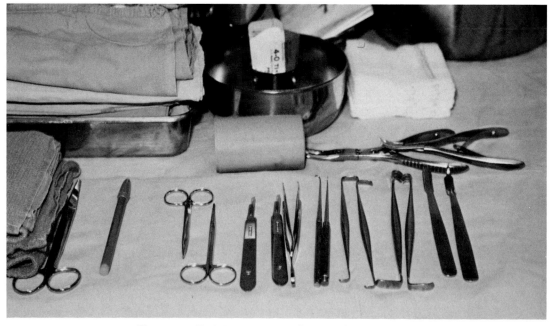

Figure 22–2. Basic instrument tray for general hand surgery.

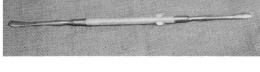

Figure 22–3. Freer septum elevator.

Figure 22–4. Surgical loupes allow examination of fine detail.

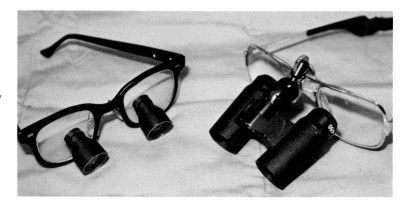

cations, including nail dystrophy, onycholysis, pterygium formation, and nail plate malalignment. In these injuries, the nail plate should always be removed for visualization of the matrix. This is accomplished by pushing the Freer elevator proximally until a characteristic "give" is felt and avulsing the nail plate with a hemostat. Anatomic restoration of the matrix

and proximal nail fold is then performed, using 5-0 or 6-0 absorbable suture for the matrix and 5-0 nylon for the nail fold. The postoperative dressing is especially important and takes into account three goals: to protect the nail bed during healing, to maintain the contour of the nail bed, and to prevent adherence of the proximal nail fold to the matrix. If the removed nail plate is large enough and can be sterilized by cleansing with an antibiotic solution, it can be replaced beneath the proximal nail fold to act as a stent.[5] An excellent alternative is a single layer of nonadherent petroleum jelly gauze or Xeroform, which can be replaced at each dressing change (Fig. 22–5).[6]

Simple Lacerations

Superficial lacerations into the nail plate without involvement of the matrix will heal as the nail grows. Jagged spikes that can catch on clothing should be trimmed flat.

Lacerations that extend into the nail matrix, however, require careful scrutiny and repair. The contour and appearance of the nail plate are largely dependent on the profile of the underlying matrix, and an irregularity in the matrix surface will lead to disfigurement of the nail plate. Anatomic restoration will prevent future deformity and dysfunction.[6]

Lacerations that involve the nail matrix must be fully visualized to achieve accurate repair. The overlying nail plate must be removed far enough proximally to allow placement of sutures in the lacerated matrix. A curved hemostat, Freer septum elevator, and dental spatula are suitable tools for sweeping under the nail plate to free it from its bed. A nail cutter or heavy scissors is then used to divide the nail proximal to the laceration.

After irrigating the wound, the area is carefully debrided, taking care not to excise viable tissue, which would make reapproximation more difficult. The matrix is then repaired us-

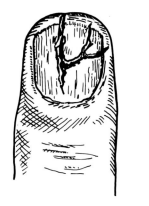
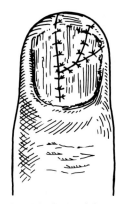

Figure 22–6. Stellate laceration of nail bed. Careful approximation of nail bed with fine absorbable sutures. From Kleinert H, et al: The deformed fingernail, a frequent result of failure to repair nail bed injuries. J Trauma 7:177, 1967. Used with permission.

ing interrupted simple sutures of 5-0 or 6-0 absorbable material (Fig. 22–6). A flat, even matrix will prevent ridge formation in the nail plate as it grows over the repaired area. A sterile dressing of petroleum jelly gauze or Xeroform with an overlying soft bulky dressing is then applied (Fig. 22–7). Circumferential tight wraps that would not allow for swelling should be avoided.

Avulsion and Crush Injuries

Injuries that result in tissue loss (avulsion) can frequently have an associated fracture of the distal phalanx of the digit.[31–33] Large gaps or poorly defined wound edges often make restoration of normal anatomy impossible.

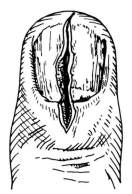
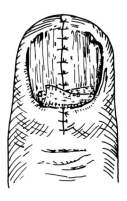

Figure 22–5. Laceration of nail bed, matrix, and skin fold. Careful approximation. Nonadherent gauze packed between matrix and skin fold. From Kleinert H, et al: The deformed fingernail, a frequent result of failure to repair nail bed injuries. J Trauma 7:177, 1967. Used with permission.

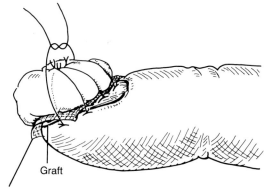

Graft

Nonadherent gauze

Figure 22–7. A dressing correctly applied to a nail matrix repair. From Kleinert H, et al: The deformed fingernail, a frequent result of failure to repair nail bed injuries. J Trauma 7:177, 1967. Used with permission.

Avulsions that involve the proximal nail fold can be treated by a split-thickness skin graft, local rotational pedicle flap, or cross-finger flap if skin loss is extensive (Fig. 22–8).

In distal phalanx crush injuries with associated nail bed injuries, the nail must be removed to enable full visual examination and thorough irrigation and debridement of small bony fragments. The nail matrix is repaired and dressed as previously described, and the prognosis is good. If the distal phalanx is not particularly comminuted, small Kirschner wires can be used to transfix the fragments, maintaining length and alignment. Failure to remove soft tissue and nail matrix from between the fracture fragments can lead to nonunion of the fracture. Pseudarthrosis of the distal phalanx, even with an intact nail apparatus, can make pinching painful and may require bone grafting to restore stability.[7]

When severe injury leads to inevitable deformity or loss of the nail unit and fingertip, the options for treatment must be considered with reference to the patient's goals and expectations. The patient whose self-image or livelihood requires restoration of normal cosmesis would choose a mode of treatment different from that chosen by the patient who wishes only to return to work as quickly as possible.

Injuries that devascularize or amputate the fingertip and a portion of the nail bed should be treated so that the bony phalanx has soft tissue coverage. Some length of the phalanx must frequently be sacrificed to allow flap advancement (Fig. 22–9),[8] split-thickness skin grafting, or healing secondarily.

Avulsion of a portion of the nail bed that leads to nonadherence of the nail plate or irregularity in the nail surface has successfully been treated with split-thickness nail matrix grafts taken from either the same nail bed or from the great toe.[9] Total loss or absence of the nail and matrix has been treated with free nail graft transfers, described by McCash in 1956.[10] He described three methods that can be chosen for the required amount of area (Figs. 22–10 and 22–11):

1. Partial nail graft: The central portion of the great toenail with nail plate, bed, and germinal matrix is transferred.

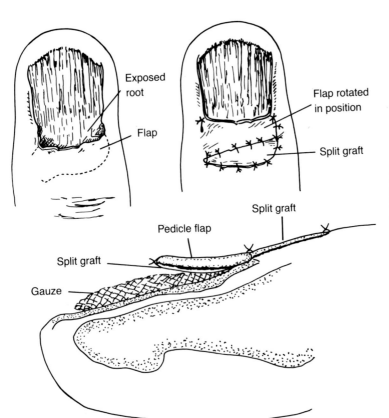

Exposed root

Flap

Flap rotated in position

Split graft

Split graft

Pedicle flap

Split graft

Gauze

Figure 22–8. Proximal nail fold avulsion treated with local rotational pedicle flap, with split-thickness skin grafting to defect left by flap. From Kleinert H, et al: The deformed fingernail, a frequent result of failure to repair nail bed injuries. J Trauma 7:177, 1967. Used with permission.

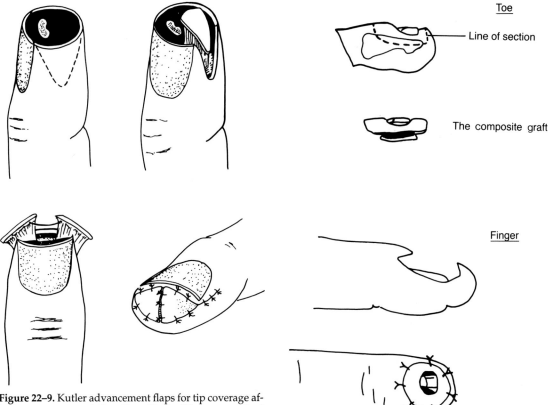

Figure 22–9. Kutler advancement flaps for tip coverage after transverse amputation. From Kutler W: A new method for finger tip amputation. JAMA 133:29, 1947. Used with permission.

Figure 22–10. Technique of composite nail graft. From Mc-Cash CR: Free nail grafting. Br J Plast Surg 8:19, 1956. Used with permission.

2. Complete nail graft: The entire nail plate, bed, and matrix are transferred.

3. Composite nail graft: The complete nail plate, matrix, bed, folds, and underlying periosteum of the distal phalanx are transferred as a unit.

A prosthetic nail has also been used after ablation of the nail matrix (see later) and creation of a pocket lined with a split-thickness skin graft folded on itself. An acrylic resin nail is then inserted and held in place with silicone adhesive.[11]

Nail deformity associated with traumatic bone loss can appear as a hooked nail deformity (Fig. 22–12). Ablation of the remaining germinal matrix with split-thickness skin grafting is usually definitive treatment. Verdan[4] described his method of elevating the nail bed, affixing a bone graft with small Kirschner wires, and applying a cross-finger flap for pulp coverage, creating an elongated distal phalanx (see Fig. 22–12). A similar procedure without the insertion of bone graft has also been used,

elevating the nail bed and providing support with soft tissue.[12] Shortening of the nail bed and matrix has also been reported.[13]

MATRICECTOMY

Permanent ablation of the matrix and nail plate has several indications: onychocryptosis (ingrown nail), pincer nail syndrome, onychomycosis, onychogryphosis (ram's horn deformity), onychauxis (thickened nail), split nails, and congenital nail dystrophies.[1,30]

Chemical matricectomy using liquefied phenol solution has been used with excellent results.[14] However, the use of chemical agents is contraindicated in patients with advanced vascular disease involving the digits. Travers and colleague[15] used a solution of 10 per cent sodium hydroxide to ablate the matrix.

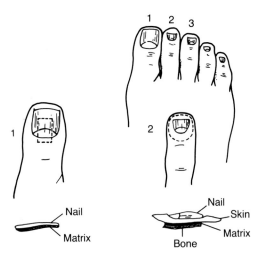

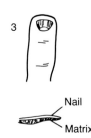

Nail
Matrix

Partial Nail Graft

Nail
Skin
Matrix
Bone

Composite Nail Graft

Nail
Matrix

Complete Nail Graft

Figure 22–11. Technique of composite nail graft. From McCash CR: Free nail grafting. Br J Plastic Surg 8:19, 1956. Used with permission.

The surgical treatment of onychocryptosis is aimed at removal of both the portion of the nail that is embedded beneath the lateral nail fold and the corresponding germinal matrix responsible for its production. If the ingrown nail is accompanied by local infection, the procedure may be staged by removing the offending strip of nail, curetting the inflammatory tissue, and providing antibiotics with local wound care. Later, when the lateral nail fold and bed are clear, the lateral germinal matrix is resected to prevent subsequent nail formation beneath the lateral nail fold. Excision of the central portion of the nail bed has been described by Suzuki and colleagues[17] for the treatment of the pincer nail syndrome. Baran[18] has supported total matricectomy for this unusual condition.

Total matricectomy, performed for the reasons previously mentioned, takes into account that the most proximal extent of the germinal matrix extends to the metaphyseal flares of the distal phalanx. To expose the entire germinal matrix, two oblique incisions are made from the junction of the lateral and proximal nail folds, extending proximally. The fold is then dissected carefully off the matrix, taking care to define the most lateral extent of the matrix. Next, under magnification, the distal nail bed, including the superficial periosteum, is elevated sharply with a no. 15 scalpel blade. The entire bed and matrix are elevated and removed totally.

Application of a split-thickness skin graft (Figs. 22–13 and 22–14) or free nail bed grafting (Fig. 22–15) is then possible, depending on

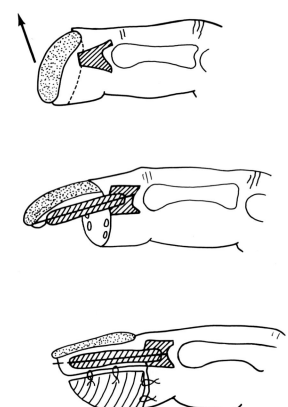

Figure 22–12. Lengthening of the terminal phalanx with a bone graft followed by cross-finger flaps (after Verdan). From Bureau R: Surgery of the hand. *In* McCollister Evarts C (ed): Surgery of the Musculoskeletal System. Churchill Livingstone, New York, 1983. Used with permission.

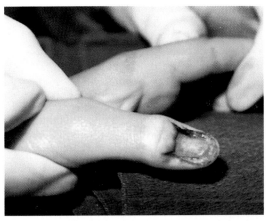

Figure 22–13. Total matricectomy in a 12-year-old patient.

the goals of treatment. Skin from the anterior thigh beneath the underwear line provides a graft of suitable color and leaves an inconspicuous scar.

TREATMENT OF PARONYCHIA

Acute Paronychia

Acute paronychia usually starts after minor trauma to the paronychium, with subsequent swelling, erythema, and pain. Conservative measures such as elevation, warm soaks, and antibiotics usually control an early infection. Once a localized area of pus is formed, a small incision parallel to the nail fold and directly over the abscess will relieve the pressure and allow for drainage. The tip of a small curved hemostat is used to break septations in the ab-

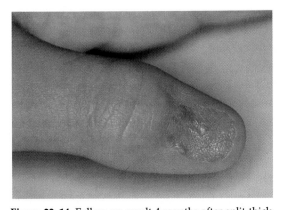

Figure 22–14. Follow-up result 4 months after split-thickness skin grafting after total matricectomy illustrated in Figure 22–13.

scess, if present. Removal of the lateral nail adjacent to the paronychia has been advocated by Bunnell.[19] However, this is necessary only when the infection tracks beneath the nail plate.

Chronic paronychia has been treated by excision and creation of an eponychial pouch,[20] but Baran and Bureau have found that simple crescentic excision of the involved nail fold will heal secondarily with dressing changes and local wound care in approximately 2 months.[21]

TREATMENT OF BENIGN TUMORS

Warts

Treatment of verruca vulgaris (warts) that involves the nail unit presents both cosmetic and functional problems. Several strains of weakly contagious human papillomavirus that produce the benign fibroepithelial tumors and are associated with squamous cell carcinomas have been identified.[22] Surgical removal of these rough, keratolytic growths is usually necessary after initial attempts to ablate the wart using keratolytic agents, cryotherapy, or liquid nitrogen have failed. The subungual wart can often be inaccessible to topical agents and can mimic the painful glomus tumor.

Cryosurgery is used to freeze and debride the wart, but special care must be used when treating the proximal nail bed because permanent damage to the underlying germinal matrix may occur. Electrodesiccation and enucleation are also advocated, using a low-voltage current to dehydrate the wart tissue, separating it from its attachments to the dermis. Debridement of the charred tissue can be performed using a small curet while preserving the underlying dermis and nail matrix. Bleeding can be brisk from neovascular ingrowth and is controlled with electrocautery or hemostatic topical agents.

Mucous Cysts

In patients with osteoarthritis involving the distal interphalangeal joints, small osteophyte formations (i.e., Heberden's nodes) at the joint margin may play an etiologic role in the formation of the mucous cyst, a small synovial fluid-filled cyst with a stalk arising from the synovium of the joint (Fig. 22–16). As the cyst

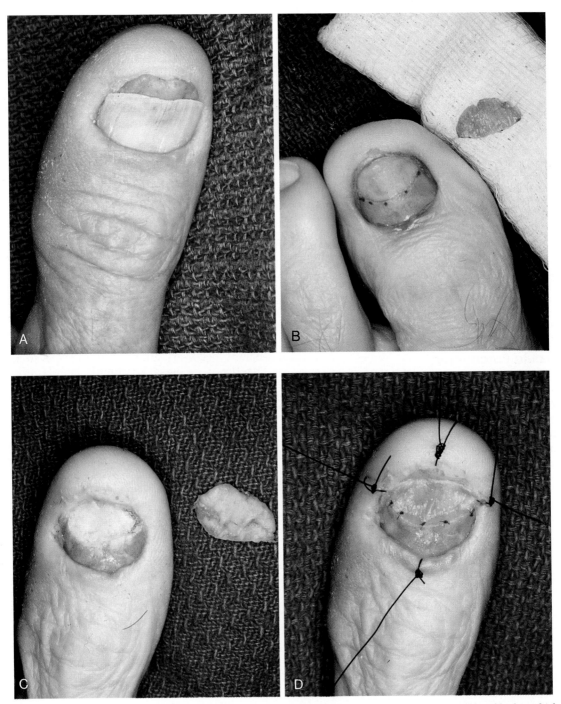

Figure 22–15. Free nail bed transfer from the great toe to the thumb. *A,* The posttraumatic scarred distal nail bed to which the nail does not adhere is seen. *B,* The toenail bed and the sterile matrix, which has been elevated as a split-thickness graft. *C,* The thumb and resected scarred matrix. *D,* Graft from toe sutures in place. Both nail beds show adherence as the nail grows over them.

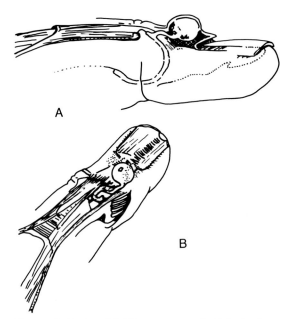

A

B

Figure 22–16. *A* and *B*, The mucous cyst originates from the distal interphalangeal joint, secondary to the osteoarthritic involvement in that joint from the extensor tendon passing to and fro over the marginal osteophytes arising from the head of the middle phalanx. From Eaton R, et al: Marginal osteophyte excision in treatment of mucous cysts. J Bone Joint Surg 55A:570, 1973. Used with permission.

enlarges, its thin, overlying dermal covering becomes tense, predisposing to rupture as a result of minor trauma or manicuring. Contamination of the joint may ensue, leading to septic arthritis. Another complication of the mucous cyst arises from direct pressure on the underlying germinal nail matrix. Chronic compression from the cyst leads to a furrowed nail with the longitudinal trough extending from the point of encroachment by the cyst. After meticulous dissection of the cyst and isolation of the stalk, removal of the adjacent osteophyte is thought to be the most important procedure in preventing recurrence of the cyst (Fig. 22–17).[23]

Pyogenic Granuloma

Pyogenic granuloma, a benign lesion consisting of granulation tissue, can occur after minor penetrating trauma where dermal and epidermal contents have been implanted into the subcutaneous tissues. The red papule may grow rapidly, and its surface can become eroded by pressure necrosis of the overlying skin. Total excision with a cautery or scalpel is indicated.

Glomus Tumor

First described by Barre and Masson,[24] the glomus tumor is a small hamartomatous tumor of the soft tissues. Seventy-five per cent occur in the hand, most commonly in the fingertips and particularly in the subungual area. They present as small blue or reddish-blue spots seen through the nail plate, usually less

Figure 22–17. *A* and *B*, Local rotational skin flap for coverage after excision of a mucous cyst and marginal osteophyte. From Haneke E, Baran R, Bureau H: Tumors of the nail apparatus and adjacent tissues. *In* Baran R, Dawber H (eds): Disease of the Nails. Blackwell Scientific Publications, Oxford, England, 1984. Used with permission.

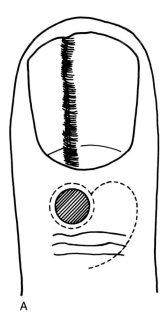
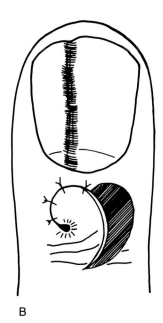

A   B

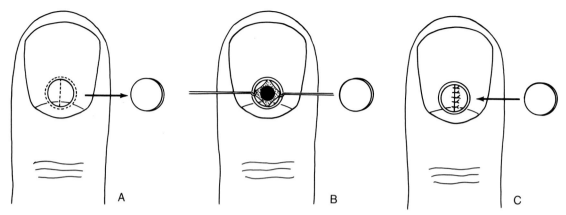

Figure 22–18. Glomus tumor: method of removal through a 6-mm hole in the nail plate. *A,* Circular 6-mm piece of nail plate removed. *B,* Removal of glomus tumor. *C,* Suture of defect and replacement of nail plate. From Haneke E, Baran R, Bureau H: Tumors of the nail apparatus and adjacent tissues. *In* Baran R, Dawber H (eds): Disease of the Nails. Blackwell Scientific Publications, Oxford, England, 1984. Used with permission.

than 1 cm in diameter. Clinical symptoms of intense, pulsating pain with compression or exposure to cold is the hallmark of the subungual glomus tumor. Treatment consists of total excision with preservation of the surrounding tissue. Small tumors may be excised through a punched-out hole in the nail plate, incising the nail bed and enucleating the lesion from its fibrous capsule (Fig. 22–18). Afferent arterioles, efferent venules, glomus cells, smooth muscle cells, and nerve fibers will be found on microscopic examination. Larger lesions require nail removal, incision and elevation of the matrix, tumor excision, and careful reapproximation of the matrix. As in posttrauma care, the nail bed should be held away from the skin fold using the nail or petroleum jelly gauze to prevent adherence.[6] Recurrence is unusual, and malignant degeneration has not been recognized (Fig. 22–19).[25]

Fibroadenoma

Many forms of fibroadenoma have been recognized in the periungual or subungual area. Although distinctly different in cause and clinical appearance, most are treated similarly, with local resection and reconstruction of the nail bed or skin grafting.

MALIGNANT TUMORS

Malignant tumors of the nail unit are unusual. In Smith and Koniuch's review of the literature, they found only 70 reported cases of

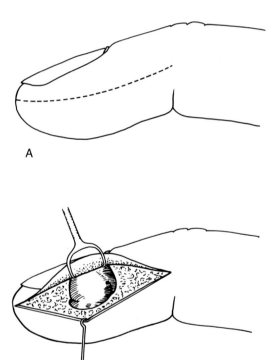

Figure 22–19. Site of incision *(A)* and removal *(B)* of a laterally placed glomus tumor. From Haneke E, Baran R, Bureau H: Tumors of the nail apparatus and adjacent tissues. *In* Baran R, Dawber H (eds): Disease of the Nails. Blackwell Scientific Publications, Oxford, England, 1984. Used with permission.

Table 22–1. DIFFERENTIAL DIAGNOSIS OF SUBUNGUAL SQUAMOUS CELL CARCINOMA AND BOWEN'S DISEASE

Malignant	Benign
Amelanotic melanoma	Common warts
Epithelioma cuniculatum	Keratoacanthoma
Basal cell carcinoma	Ingrowing nail
Radiodermatitis	Foreign body granuloma
Hemangioendothelioma	Chronic granulomatous inflammation
	Warty tuberculosis
	Pyogenic granuloma
	Subungual exostosis
	Subungual keratoma
	Paronychia

From Haneke E, Baran R, Bureau H: Tumors of the nail apparatus and adjacent tissues. *In* Baran R, Dawber H (eds): Disease of the Nails. Blackwell Scientific, Oxford, England 1984. Used with permission.

squamous cell carcinoma of the nail bed.[25] Bowen's disease, an intraepithelial carcinoma, is likewise an infrequent finding.[16] Subungual melanoma, which is usually presented to the physician because of its appearance, accounts for 0.7 to 3.6 per cent of all cutaneous malignant melanomas in the general population and 15 to 20 per cent in the black population.[26]

Table 22–2. CAUSES OF LONGITUDINAL NAIL PIGMENTATION

Addison's disease
Adrenalectomy for Cushing's disease
Bacterial infection
Drugs
Fungal infection
Hematoma, hemosiderosis
Idiopathic
Irradiation
Laugier-Hunziker's syndrome
Lentigo
Lichen planus
Malignant melanoma
Malnutrition
Melanotic hyperplasia (benign or atypical)
Metastatic melanoma
Nevocytic nevus
Peutz-Jeghers-Touraine syndrome
Photochemotherapy
Porphyria cutanea tarda
Pregnancy
Radiodermatitis
Splinter hemorrhages
Trauma
Vitamin B_{12} deficiency

Adapted from Haneke E, Baran R, Bureau H: Tumors of the nail apparatus and adjacent tissues. *In* Baran R, Dawber H (eds): Disease of the Nails. Blackwell Scientific, Oxford, England, 1984. Used with permission.

Diagnosis of a malignant lesion is usually confirmed after an incisional biopsy of a recalcitrant lesion that has been resistant to conservative therapy. Nonpigmented lesions can be mistaken for chronic infections, benign tumors, granuloma, or other benign lesions (Table 22–1). Subungual melanotic streaks likewise can be produced by several etiologic factors, most being benign or remote to the nail (Table 22–2).[29]

Recommendations for surgical management of malignant lesions of the nail bed are based on the experience of many workers with small series of cases. Basal cell and squamous cell carcinomas that have no bony involvement and can be excised with free margins will require skin graft coverage and continued observation for recurrence. If there is evidence of osseous involvement, however, amputation at the distal interphalangeal joint, or more proximally if necessary, is indicated. Subungual melanomas frequently mimic other malignant and benign conditions, thus leading to delays in diagnosis. Recommended treatment is metacarpal or metatarsal ray amputation, with or without regional node dissection.[27]

References

1. Bureau H, Baran R, Haneke E: Nail surgery and traumatic abnormalities. *In* Baran R, Dawber H (eds): Disease of the Nails. Blackwell Scientific Publications, Oxford, England, 1984.
2. Scher RK: Nail surgery. Clin Dermatol 5:135, 1987.
3. Burton R: Surgery of the hand. In McCollister Evarts C (ed): Surgery of the Musculoskeletal System, vol 2. Churchill-Livingstone, New York, 1983, p 61.
4. Verdan C: Plastic surgery and claw nail. *In* The Nail. Churchill Livingstone, New York, 1981, p 93.
5. Schiller C: Nail replacement in finger tip injuries. Plast Reconstr Surg 19:521, 1957.
6. Kleinert H, et al: The deformed fingernail: A frequent result of failure to repair nail bed injuries. J Trauma 7:177, 1967.
7. Itoh Y, et al: Treatment of pseudoarthrosis of the distal phalanx with the palmar midline approach. J Hand Surg 8:80, 1983.
8. Kutler W: A new method for finger tip amputation. JAMA 133:29, 1947.
9. Shepard GH: Treatment of nail bed avulsions with split thickness nail bed grafts. J Hand Surg 8:49, 1983.
10. McCash CR: Free nail grafting. Br J Plast Surg 8:19, 1956.
11. Bautista BN, Nery EB: Replacement of a malformed fingernail with acrylic resin material. Plast Reconstr Surg 55:234, 1975.
12. Atasoy E, et al: The "antenna" procedures for the "hook nail" deformity. J Hand Surg 8:55, 1983.
13. Dufourmental C: Problems Esthetiques dans la Reconstruction des Moignons Bouloureux. Monographie de Groupe de la Main. Les Mutilations de la Main. Expansion Scientifique, Paris, 1974, p 109.

14. Seigle R, et al: Phenol alcohol technique for permanent matricectomy. Arch Dermatol 120:348, 1984.
15. Travers GR, Ammon RG: The sodium hydroxide chemical matricetomy procedures. J Am Podiatr Assoc 70:476, 1980.
16. Strong MD: Bowen's disease in multiple nail beds—Case report. J Hand Surg 8:329, 1983.
17. Suzuki K, et al: Surgical treatment of pincer nail syndrome. Plast Reconstr Surg 63:570, 1979.
18. Baran R: Pincer and trumpet nails. Arch Dermatol 110:639, 1974.
19. Boyes JH: Pyogenic infections. In Bunnell's Surgery of the Hand, ed 4. JB Lippincott, Philadelphia, 1964, p 68.
20. Keyser J, Eaton R: Surgical cure of chronic paronychia by eponychial marsupialization. Plast Reconstr Surg 58:56, 1976.
21. Baran R, Bureau H: Surgical treatment of recalcitrant chronic paronychias of the fingers. J Dermatol Surg Oncol 7:106, 1981.
22. Moy RL, Eliezri YD, Nuovo GJ, et al: Human papilloma virus type 16 DNA in periungual squamous cell carcinomas. JAMA 261:2669, 1989.
23. Eaton R, et al: Marginal osteophyte excision in treatment of mucous cysts. J Bone Joint Surg 55A:570, 1973.
24. Barre JA, Masson PV: Anatomy—Clinical study of certain painful subungual tumors (tumors of the neuromyoarterial glomus of the extremities). Bull Soc Fr Dermatol Syphiligr 31:148, 1924.
25. Smith R, Koniuch M: Tumors of the hand. In McCollister Evarts C (eds): Surgery of the Musculoskeletal System. Churchill Livingstone, New York, 1983.
26. Tom D, Scher R: Melanonychia striata in longitudinem. Am J Dermatopathol 7:161, 1985.
27. Scher RK: Surgery of the nails. In Epstein E, Epstein E Jr (eds): Techniques in Skin Surgery. Lea & Febiger, Philadelphia, 1979.
28. Dawber R, Baran R: The nails and cosmetics. In Samman P, Fenton B (eds): The Nails in Disease, ed 4. Year Book, Chicago, 1986, pp 126–134.
29. Pack GT, Orpeza R: Subungual melanoma. Surg Gynecol Obstet 124:751, 1967.
30. White R, Noone R: Pachyonychia congenita (Jadassohn-Lewandowsky syndrome). Plast Reconstr Surg 59:855, 1977.
31. Zook EG: Injuries of the fingernail. In Green DP (ed): Green's Operative Hand Surgery. Churchill Livingstone, New York, 1982.
32. Zook EG: The perionychium. In Green DP (ed): Operative Hand Surgery, ed 2. Churchill Livingstone, New York, 1988.
33. Zook EG: Fingernail injuries. In Strickland J, Steichen J (eds): Difficult Problems in Hand Surgery. CV Mosby, St. Louis, MO, 1982.
34. Zook EG, et al: Anatomy and physiology of the paronychium: A review of the literature and anatomic study. J Hand Surg 5:528, 1980.
35. Zook EG, et al: A study of nail bed injuries: Causes, treatment, prognosis. J Hand Surg 9A:247, 1984.

Appendix 1
GLOSSARY

C. Ralph Daniel III

agnail[1] Hangnail; hard spicules at the edge of the nail.

anonychia Absence of nail plate or nail unit.

brachyonychia[2] Short nails.

chromonychia Color changes appearing in the nail unit.

clubbing Increase of the ungual-phalangeal angle greater than or equal to 180°; usually accompanied by fibrovascular hyperplasia of the more proximal nail unit (see Chapter 12).

defluvium unguium[1] Nail shedding starting at the base and extending forward; onychomadesis.

dolichonychia[2] Quotient between length and width of nail is greater than 1 ± 0.1; seen in Ehlers-Danlos syndrome and Marfan syndrome.

elkonyxis[3] Loss of nail substance (more than pitting); oval, 2 to 3 mm.

eponychium Most distal horny extension of the proximal nail fold–cuticle.

fragilitas unguium[1] Brittle nails.

hapalonychia[1] Soft nails.

heloma[4] Corn.

hyponychium Area of the nail unit distal to the nail bed having a granular layer (the only part of the nail unit normally having a granular layer).

koilonychia Spooning of the nail plate (see Chapter 12).

leukonychia Whitening of the nail plate (either apparent or real) (see Chapter 12).

lunula Half-moon; distal part (often visible) of the nail matrix.

macronychia Unusually large nail often wider than normal.

median nail dystrophy[1] Dystrophia mediana canaliformis; median canal or split in the nail plate, often idiopathic; usually thumbnails.

micronychia Small nail often shorter or narrower than normal.

nail apparatus Nail plate, nail folds, nail matrix, nail bed, hyponychium (nail plate and surrounding and underlying soft structures extending from the proximal nail matrix region distally).

nail bed Supporting structure of the nail plate extending from the nail matrix distally to the hyponychium.

nail field[5] Earliest anatomic sign of the nail, occurring at about 9 weeks of fetal development.

nail folds Two lateral, one proximal; outline and support the nail unit and guide the growth of the nail plate.

nail matrix Producer of the nail plate extending from under the proximal nail fold distally to the nail bed.

nail plate Horny, keratinized portion of the dorsal nail unit, usually extending from the proximal matrix region distally.

nail unit Same as nail apparatus.

onychalgia Nail unit pain.

onychia Inflammation somewhere in the nail unit.

onychoclavus[4] Subungual corn.

onychocryptosis[4] Ingrown nail.

onychogryphosis Ram's horn nail; hypertrophy of the nail plate, often hornlike, probably resulting from trauma. One side of nail seems to grow faster than the other, often curving the nail plate away from the site of trauma.

onychoheterotopia Abnormally placed nail on the digit as the result of displaced matrix material.

onycholysis Distal separation of the nail plate from underlying hyponychium and nail bed.

onychomadesis Proximal separation of the nail plate from the matrix–nail bed area.

onychomycosis Fungal infection of the nail unit.

onychophagia[1] Nail biting.

onychophosis[4] Localized or diffuse hyperkeratotic tissue of varying degree that develops on the lateral or proximal nail folds, in the space between the nail folds and the nail plate, or even subungually. Common in elderly patients in the first and fifth toes, and is due to repeated trauma.

onychoptosis Loss of the nail plate.

onychorrhexis Longitudinal striations of the nail plate, usually superficial.

onychoschizia Superficial splitting of the nail plate (layering), usually beginning distally.

onychotillomania Tearing, picking, destroying nails by some method.

pachyonychia Thickening of nail plate, often the entire plate.

panaritium[1] Abscess at the side or base of the nail (whitlow).

paronychia Inflammation or infection of the nail folds.

periungual Around the nail. One should *not* use paronychial as a synonym.

pincer (trumpet) nails Abnormally narrow, curved nails often caused by lateral pressure on the nail unit (as when shoes are too tight). Can occur idiopathically in fingernails.

platonychia[1] Increased nail curvature in the long axis.

polyonychia More than one nail on a digit.

pterygium Scarring of the proximal nail fold region involving the matrix.

pterygium inversus unguium Fusing (scarring) of the distal nail plate to the underlying hyponychium and nail bed.

tinea unguium Infection of the nail unit by a dermatophyte.

trachyonychia[2] Rough nails.

unguis incarnatus Ingrown nail.

usure des angles[1] Wearing away of nails usually from scratching.

References

1. Samman PD: The Nails in Disease, ed 2. Charles C Thomas, Springfield, IL, 1972.
2. Baran R: Diseases of the Nail and Their Management. Blackwell Scientific, Oxford, England, 1984.
3. DeNicola P: Nail Diseases in Internal Medicine. Charles C Thomas, Springfield, IL, 1974.
4. Cohen PR, Scher RK: Geriatric nail Disorders: Diagnosis and Treatment. J Am Acad Dermatol 26:521, 1992.
5. Zaias N: The Nail in Health and Disease. SP Medical and Scientific Books, New York, 1980.

Appendix 2

ONYCHOMYCOSIS

by Leanor D. Haley and C. Ralph Daniel III

1. Nail Micronizer: *Alas-Col Apparatus Company, Terre Haute, IN
2. 20 per cent potassium hydroxide (KOH)-glycerol solution

KOH	20 g
Glycerol	20 mL
Distilled water	80 mL

Dissolve KOH crystals in water; add glycerol. (Glycerol markedly prolongs shelf life of this reagent and also preserves KOH preparation for 2 or 3 days.)

10 per cent KOH is dimethyl sulfoxide (DMSO)

KOH	10 g
DMSO–water solvent	100 ml

(DMSO, 40 mL; distilled water, 60 mL; use a safety pipette when working with DMSO) 10 per cent KOH solution may be purchased in 50-mL aliquots from Remel Co., 12076 Santa Fe Drive, Lenexa, KS 66215; Cat. Number 21-230.
3. Periodic acid–Schiff (PAS) stain for nail scrapings

The PAS reaction is used to stain certain polysaccharides found in cell walls of fungi as well as some bacteria and tissue. The periodic acid is an oxidizing agent that breaks C-C bonds in polysaccharides where they occur as 1:2 glycol (HOHC-CHOH); these hydroxyl groups are converted to aldehyde groups (HOC-CHO). The basic fuchsin combines with these aldehyde groups in such a manner that it cannot be bleached out when treated with sodium metabisulfite.

A. Formulas for reagents

(1) Periodic acid

Periodic acid	5 g
Distilled water	100 mL

Place in a dark brown reagent bottle with a ground-glass stopper.

(2) Basic fuchsin solution

Basic fuchsin	0.1 g
Distilled water	95 mL
95 per cent ethyl alcohol	5 mL

Add the alcohol to the water and mix; carefully add the fuchsin to the mixture. Stir the solution with rotation of the container. The fuchsin very quickly goes into solution.

(3) Sodium metabisulfite solution ($Na_2S_2O_5$)

Sodium metabisulfite	1 g
1 N hydrochloride (HCl)	10 mL
Distilled water	190 mL

This is the bleaching agent; when freshly made, it usually requires approximately 3 minutes to bleach the fuchsin out of the material. As the solution ages, 5 minutes is adequate for bleaching. Seventy per cent, 85 per cent aqueous alcohol solutions; 95 per cent ethyl alcohol and absolute ethyl alcohol.

B. Technique for staining

Place fungal smear in absolute ethyl alcohol for 1 minute. Drain alcohol and

---

*Daniel CR, Elewski BE, Gupta AK: Surgical pearl: Nail Micronizer: J Am Acad Dermatol 34: 278, 1996.

immediately place slide in 5 per cent periodic acid for 5 minutes.

Wash in running water for 2 minutes.

Place in basic fuchsin for 2 minutes.

Wash 2 minutes in running water.

Immerse slide in sodium metabisulfite solution for 3 to 5 minutes.

Dehydrate by passing through 70 per cent, 85 per cent, 95 per cent, and absolute alcohol for 2-minute intervals.

Place in xylene for 2 minutes and mount with coverslip and Permount.

Do not allow slide to dry before mounting coverslip.

4. Sabouraud's dextrose agar with and without antibiotics can be obtained from BBL Microbiological Systems, P. O. Box 243, Cockeysville, MD 21030.

   Sabouraud's agar with antibiotics can be obtained in small rectangular bottles, and plain Sabouraud's agar in tubes can be obtained from Gibso Laboratories, P. O. Box 4385, 2801 Industrial Drive, Madison, WI. Sabouraud's agar with and without antibiotics can be obtained in tubes from Difco Laboratories, Detroit, MI.

5. Parafilm (4″ × 250″) can be obtained from American Can Co., Dexie/Marathon Div., Greenwich, CT 06830.

6. Lactophenol cotton blue is available in droppers from Remel Co. (see Item 2). One dropper is used for each lactophenol cotton blue preparation; 30 droppers in a carton. Cat. Number: 26-11-88.

7. Teasing needles are obtainable from any surgical or biologic supply house.

8. Cycloheximide is available as Actidione, from the Upjohn Co., Kalamazoo, MI.

INSTRUMENTS

1. English anvil nail splitter: Especially good for splitting nails as for ingrown nails.

2. Dual-action nail nipper: Excellent for practically painless trimming of onycholytic nails; expensive ($125 to $200).

3. Dental spatulas or nail elevators: 2 to 4 mm; helpful in obtaining subungual debris or elevating the nail from a subungual approach.

4. Mosquito hemostats: Applicable for small nail avulsion. Help loosen proximal nail fold from nail plate (keep teeth against nail plate) or loosening nail from nail bed.

5. Disposable punches (2-, 3-, and 4-mm) by Baker or by Accuderm, or Orentreich punches.

These should be available through your local medical supply house.

TREATMENT

Always be confident of your diagnosis before initiating therapy.

PSORIASIS

1. Keep the nails short.
2. Avoid trauma to the nails and aggressive cosmesis.
3. Avoid irritants (see irritant avoidance regimen under Chronic Paronychia).
4. Treat psoriasis elsewhere.
5. Intralesional triamcinolone acetonide, 2 to 4 mg/mL, injected with a 30-gauge needle into the area of the nail apparatus causing the clinical manifestation, every 3 to 4 weeks for 4 to 6 sessions.
6. Psoralen ultraviolet A, grenz ray, systemic retinoids, methotrexate topical 5-fluorouracil, cyclosporine, calcipotriene, high-potency fluorinated steroids, and so on have been used with varying degrees of success.
7. Side effects of the individual therapy should be taken into consideration when weighing risk and benefit.
8. Zinc pyrithione is being tested for nails at present.
9. See Chapter 11 for more details.

LICHEN PLANUS

1. See Items 1, 2, 3, and 5 under Psoriasis.
2. Consider systemic steroids for bullous lichen planus of the nail and for painful, active, nonbullous lichen planus in the matrix region to help prevent possible permanent scarring with subsequent permanent nail dystrophy or sometimes anonychia.
3. Griseofulvin and retinoids have been mentioned in the literature with varying results.
4. See Chapter 11 for more details.

PARONYCHIA

1. Acute
   A. Diminish predisposing factors such as trauma, irritants, overaggressive cosmesis, and so on.
   B. Gently incise and drain obvious abscesses.

C. Perform Gram's stain or culture purulent material, or both.

D. In milder cases initially begin erythromycin, 250 to 500 mg with food four times a day for 7 to 10 days. Polymyxin B sulfate–bacitracin zinc ointment or mupirocin ointment 2 per cent may be used. For more severe cases, begin on cephalexin, 250 to 500 mg with food four times a day for 7 to 14 days. These medications can be used until studies return or until the clinical situation dictates otherwise. Treat for 1 to 2 weeks.

E. Warm saline soaks three to four times a day may be used for an average of 5 to 7 days.

2. Chronic

A. See Item A under Acute Paronychia.

B. Treatment of bacterial component two to four times a day with a topical antibacterial solution as polymyxin B–bacitracin or ointments such as mupurocin 2 per cent or polymyxin B–bacitracin. Systemic erythromycin and cephalexin are warranted only occasionally.

C. Treatment of possible local yeast component with solutions of clotrimazole or sulconazole or broad-spectrum antifungal cream two to four times daily (apply before topical antibacterial agents if using at the same time). In more recalcitrant cases in which *Candida* species is strongly suspected as an exacerbating agent of the problem, systemic ketoconazole, itraconazole, or fluconazole can be instituted. The latter two may be given in pulse regimens. At the time of this printing, these drugs are not approved by the Food and Drug Administration (FDA) for this indication.

D. It is the firm belief of this author that contact irritants, trauma, and so on are the primary causes of most cases of chronic paronychia and onycholysis; therefore, a strict irritant-avoiding regimen is necessary.

E. Wear light cotton gloves under heavy-duty vinyl gloves for wet work. Heavy-duty vinyl gloves (Allerderm) are available at paint stores and pharmacies.

F. Wear the cotton and vinyl gloves when peeling or squeezing citrus fruits, handling tomatoes, and peeling potatoes or other raw food.

G. Avoid direct contact with paints, metal polish, paint thinner, turpentine, other solvents, and polish, and wear the cotton and vinyl gloves when using them.

H. Use lukewarm water and very little mild soap when washing hands; be sure to rinse the soap off and dry gently.

I. Protect hands from chapping and drying in windy or cold weather by wearing unlined leather gloves.

J. Push cuticles back as little as possible and do not use your fingernails, a metal file, or orange stick to do this. Cuticle removers are not good for people with paronychia or those predisposed to the development of paronychia.

K. If necessary, cuticles can be pushed back gently at the end of a shower or bath using a wet washcloth and the end of a finger.

L. Avoid nail cosmetics and artificial nails of all types while the disorder is healing. Frequent application and removal of nail cosmetics is harmful. Commercial cuticle treatments are often harmful.

M. See Chapter 10 for more details.

DERMATOPHYTE

1. Explain to the patient in advance that
   A. Therapy is slow.
   B. Therapy is not guaranteed.
   C. The problem may relapse.
   D. Therapy may be expensive.

2. Diminish heat, moisture, trauma, and other predisposing conditions.

3. Griseofulvin and ketoconazole are older drugs that are FDA approved for tinea unguium. In my experience, these drugs clear the nails about 20 to 30 per cent for toenails and about 60 per cent for fingernails. For an average-size adult, initially prescribe microsize griseofulvin, 500 mg twice daily with food. Dosage may be increased as warranted. Treat for an average of 6 months for fingernails and 12 months for toenails. Treat at least 1 month after the nails are clinically and mycologically clear.

4. I have found clearing rates of approximately 80 per cent or more for fingernails and 70 per cent or more for toenails for the drugs I have used in the following regimens:
   A. At present, intraconazole is FDA-approved for tinea of the toenails and a 2-month pulse regimen is used for fingernails. The earlier approved continuous therapy is 200 mg/day for 3 months. The author uses pulse therapy that is about one

half the price and seems to be more efficacious. For toenails, 200 mg is used twice daily for 1 week of the month for 3 months. The author uses two pulses for fingernails.

B. Lamisil is used at a dose of 250 mg/day for 3 months for toenails and 6 weeks for fingernails.

C. At present fluconazole is not FDA-approved for nails. The author has used 200 to 300 mg once a week for 4 to 6 months for fingernails and 10 to 12 months for toenails.

5. For all of these drugs, I discuss the possible side effects with the patient and I obtain baseline and periodic laboratory data (see Chapter 9 for more details).

ONYCHOLYSIS

1. The most important treatment consideration is finding, eliminating, and treating predisposing or causative factors.
2. Keep affected nails as short as possible.
3. See Items C to L under Chronic Paronychia.
4. Avoid nail cosmetics, artificial nails, and so on.
5. Keep in mind that the longer the onycholysis has persisted, the less likely it is that it will resolve.

BRITTLE NAILS

1. This condition is an enigma.
2. Explain the difficulty of therapy to the patient. Also explain to the patient that if the toenails are normal and the fingernails are brittle, usually external factors are of primary importance.
3. Divide the cases into hard and brittle and soft and brittle.
   A. Hard and brittle: too little moisture. At bedtime, soak the nails in water for about 5 to 10 minutes and then apply 10 per cent urea cream or 5 per cent lactic acid cream. Light cotton gloves may be worn to keep the agent on the nails. During the day, frequently apply a nongreasy cream to hands and nails. Use a humidifier in the house or workplace when the humidity is low. Avoid frequent wetting and then drying.
   B. Soft and brittle nails: Usually too much moisture. Wear cotton under vinyl gloves for wet work. Avoid contact with strong soaps and other irritants.

4. One packet of Knox gelatin in 6 ounces of water daily has been suggested by numerous dermatologists over the years. It has not been proven effective, but yet anecdotal testimonials are sometimes convincing.
5. Biotin, 300-μg tablets: try four to six tablets a day with food for 4 to 6 months. I have seen improvement in about one third to one half of my patients when using biotin.

GREEN NAIL (USUALLY *PSEUDOMONAS*, SOMETIMES *CANDIDA*)

1. Diminish predisposing conditions such as trauma, moisture, irritants, and incorrect cosmesis.
2. Treat onycholysis if present (see Onycholysis).
3. Keep afflicted nails as short as possible.
4. Apply no cosmetics to the nail until it has been normal for at least 1 month.
5. Twice daily, apply acetic acid (vinegar diluted with equal parts of water), gentamicin solution (Garamycin), or polymyxin B–bacitracin solution (Polysporin).

PERIUNGUAL AND SUBUNGUAL WARTS

1. Treat warts elsewhere on the body.
2. Have patient stop nail biting or finger sucking if applicable.
3. Gently debride the wart. For clinicians who are well versed in the use of liquid nitrogen, several freeze-thaw cycles should be attempted. Avoid neurovascular compromise and understand that the treatment is painful. Permanent nail dystrophy or neurovascular compromise may result from incorrect treatment.
4. Occlusion of the wart with adhesive tape (not too tight) for 7 to 9 days may be attempted.
5. Judicious use of cantharidin collodion (Cantharone) or salicylic acid solution (DuoFilm) may be helpful along with superficial debridement, taking care to avoid getting the solution on normal skin.
6. Subungual warts should be completely exposed by clipping back the nail.
7. X-ray films and biopsies should be taken to rule out malignancy in unusual or recalcitrant lesions.

8. Laser treatment has been sucessfully used.
9. Laser, intralesional bleomycin, or intralesional interferon may be helpful.
10. Discuss possible side effects and the fact that eventually warts usually resolve spontaneously.
11. See Chapter 15.

INGROWING TOENAILS

1. Always cut toenails straight across; do not round at the edges.
2. Do not tear or pull at the toenails.
3. Properly fitting shoes are essential. Avoid higher heels and narrow-toed shoes.
4. A wisp of cotton may be gently placed under an early ingrowing nail to help "guide" the nail outward. Place a teaspoon of salt in 1 quart of warm water. Soak the toe for 10 to 14 minutes three to four times a day for 5 to 7 days. For very early infection, try erythromycin, 250 to 500 mg with food four times a day for 7 days.
5. For more advanced cases, begin the soaks and cephalexin, 500 mg four times a day for 7 to 10 days. If the problem does not resolve promptly, once the swelling and infection have decreased, then excise the ingrowing portion of the nail using an English anvil nail splitter.
6. See Chapter 21 for more information.

Appendix 3

CONFIRMATORY TESTS USED IN IDENTIFYING SOME *TRICHOPHYTON* SPECIES

by Leanor D. Haley

CONFIRMATORY TESTS USED IN IDENTIFYING SOME *TRICHOPHYTON* SPECIES

Fungus	May Be Confused with	Confirmatory Test
T. mentagrophytes (granular)	*T. rubrum*	Kane's media (see Appendix 2), in vitro hair test (*T. rubrum* does not invade hair).
T. mentagrophytes (woolly)	White, woolly isolates of *T. tonsurans*	Growth of *T. tonsurans* is enhanced by thiamine.
T. rubrum	Some isolates of *T. mentagrophytes* and *T. tonsurans*	In vitro hair test; is not stimulated by thiamine.
T. tonsurans	Some isolates of *T. mentagrophytes* and *T. rubrum;* occasional isolate of *T. verrucosum*	Is enhanced by thiamine. *T. verrucosum* has an absolute requirement for thiamine and usually for inositol.
T. verrucosum	Some isolates of the white, woolly variety of *T. tonsurans;* occasional isolate of *T. schoenleinii* and *T. concentricum*	*T. schoenleinii, T. concentricum,* and *T. tonsurans* have no requirement for thiamine or inositol.

Appendix 4

COLONIAL MORPHOLOGY OF SOME DERMATOPHYTES

by Leanor D. Haley

COLONIAL MORPHOLOGY OF SOME DERMATOPHYTES

Fungus	Average Number of Days to Develop	Appearance of Colony
Trichophyton mentagrophytes (variety interdigitale)	6–10	*Flat, white woolly front, covers entire slant; back is colorless or a very light, nondiagnostic yellow*
Trichophyton mentagrophytes	4–10	*Flat or occasional shallow folds, granular or mixture of suede and granular; covers slant; usually white or a delicate buff or tan surface; rarely a reddish tinge may be seen on surface. Back of colony usually has a splotchy light brown to delicate reddish-brown color; often a band of reddish-brown color is noted at site where slant arises from the agar butt (this band of color is not noted on the back of colonies growing in Petri dishes). This type of colony is easy to confuse with some isolates of* T. rubrum.
Trichophyton rubrum (woolly)	7–12	*Flat, white woolly front, does not cover the entire agar surface. Back of colony has a red or pinkish red pigment; the entire back may be pigmented or only the center of the colony will have pigment. Occasionally, the pigment may form a ring on the edge of the colony back.*
Trichophyton rubrum (granular)	5–10	*Flat, granular surface, rarely with folds, a delicate pink or pinkish-red color may be present; occasional areas of white suede may be seen; colony rarely covers the entire slant. Back of colony is usually a deep red color. This type of colony may be mistaken for a young colony of the red variety of* T. tonsurans.
Trichophyton rubrum (yellow)	7–10	*Surface is beautiful yellow-orange suede to short woolly; usually the colony does not cover the entire agar surface. Back of colony is a deep yellow-orange suggestive of an old culture of* Microsporum canis. *These isolates may be confused with* M. ferrugineum *or* T. soudanense.
Trichophyton tonsurans	7–12	*Colony of either the red or yellow isolates is flat with deep radial folds; surface is a delicate suede that has been dusted with granules. The yellow isolates may be confused with* Epidermophyton floccosum; *the red isolates may be confused with some granular isolates of* T. rubrum. *The back of both of these isolates is deep brown. White isolates of* T. tonsurans *are short, woolly on the surface with occasional shallow folds. The back is light yellow to brownish.*
Trichophyton soudanense	7–12	*Surface is short woolly; usually a delicate light yellow pigment; does not cover entire agar slant. Back of colony is an apricot yellow.*
Microsporum ferrugineum	10–14	*Many isolates are flat, glabrous, and rust colored; occasional isolate may have a heaped center with suede. Back of colony is usually rust colored.*
Trichophyton megninii	10–14	*Surface is suede to short woolly with a delicate rose color; surface of the slant may be covered. Back of colony is a deep rose color.*
Trichophyton violaceum	10–14	*Surface is usually elevated with folds; it may be glabrous or a delicate suede; color is deep violet or purple. Growth is very restricted. Back of colony is deep purple.*
Trichophyton schoenleinii	14–18	*Surface is heaped with marked folding; usually glabrous; occasional isolate may have a suede periphery. Color is white. Back of the colony is colorless; as culture ages, the agar slant begins to pull from the sides of the tube and forms deep folds.*
Trichophyton concentricum	14–18	*Colony appears almost identical to that of* T. schoenleinii. *The surface may be a delicate honey color.*
Trichophyton verrucosum	8–14	*Surface may be very flat with little aerial mycelium or may be heaped and glabrous; an occasional isolate on primary isolation may be flat and short woolly. This fungus dies very quickly if Sabouraud's agar is not enriched by addition of thiamine. Color of surface is white to honey.*
Epidermophyton floccosum	8–14	*Surface is flat with marked folding; colony is granular with a gray-green-yellowish color. Back of the colony is usually a deep mahogany color.*

Appendix 5

THE POSSIBILITY OF HIV TRANSMISSION BY MANICURE

by Noreen Lemak and Madelein Duvic

The human immunodeficiency virus (HIV) is usually transmitted by sexual contact with infected semen or vaginal secretions, by contact with contaminated blood or blood products, or from an infected mother to the infant during pregnancy or the perinatal period.[1,2] An infected organ transplant also can transmit HIV.[3] Swimming pools, saunas, restaurants, social kissing, sneezing, or public water fountains or bathrooms are all unlikely sources of transmission.[4] Studies show that free infectious virus exists rarely in saliva or tears.[2]

Certain non–health care workers have the potential for exposure to small amounts of blood or body fluids. These workers include acupuncturists, tattoo artists, electrolysis specialists, ear piercers, and manicurists.[4] Thus far, the public has not been widely informed about the possibility of acquiring HIV from contaminated manicuring instruments. Minor bleeding is not unusual when a cuticle or a hangnail is clipped, and busy beauticians may be careless about sterilization of their tools between customers. It would be advisable for manicurists to wear gloves to protect themselves.

To be totally safe, clients should purchase their own manicuring instruments and take them to the beauty shop. Disposable instruments may be used once and discarded. In 1989, the Centers for Disease Control issued guidelines[5] for the prevention of transmission of HIV and the hepatitis B virus. Methods for sterilization of instruments include steam under pressure (autoclave), dry heat, or immersion in an Environmental Protection Agency–approved chemical sterilant for 6 to 10 hours or according to manufacturers' instructions. A 1:100 dilution of common household bleach (one-quarter cup of bleach per gallon of tap water) will disinfect surfaces such as metal, plastic, or wood but may require at least a 15- to 30-minute exposure time. There have been no documented cases of HIV transmission by a manicurist[6,7]; in such a case, the virus would be present in extremely low concentration.

Langerhans' cells colonize skin and mucosa and have been reported to be targets for the HIV virus.[8] Langerhans' cells are the primary cell type infected with HIV-1 within the epidermis of patients with acquired immunodeficiency syndrome (AIDS), and HIV-1 regulatory and structural genes are transcribed in these cells.[9] However, keratinocytes have also been shown to contain HIV viral transcripts.[10] Infected Langerhans' cells migrate to proximal lymph nodes, where they act as antigen-presenting cells through association with CD4+ (helper) lymphocytes. Data from 1994 show that Langerhans' cells play a key role in the pathogenesis of HIV infection, and they may be the vectors of infection for CD4+ T cells.[11] AIDS is now diagnosed when the number of T helper lymphocytes is less than $200/mm^3$ of blood if the patient is HIV seropositive, even if he or she has no opportunistic infections.[12] An HIV-positive patient may remain asymptomatic for many years.

In the hypothetical case of transmission of HIV by or to a manicurist, many months or years might pass before the client or beautician is diagnosed with HIV or AIDS, and it would be almost impossible to pinpoint the source. Hysteria and unreasonable fears should be discouraged, but precautions are necessary because transmission must be considered possible based on evidence of hepatitis B transmission by some non–health care workers.[6]

References

1. Brookmeyer R: Reconstruction and future trends of the AIDS epidemic in the United States. Science 253:37, 1991.
2. Levy JA: The transmission of HIV and factors influencing progression to AIDS. Am J Med 95:86, 1993.
3. McIntosh K: Transmissibility of HIV infection: What we know in 1993. J School Health 64:14, 1994.
4. Gershon RRM, Vlahov D, Nelson KE. The risk of transmission of HIV-1 through nonpercutaneous, non-sexual modes—A review. AIDS 4:645, 1990.
5. Centers for Disease Control: Guidelines for prevention of transmission of human immunodeficiency virus and hepatitis B virus to health-care and public-safety workers. Centers for Disease Control, Atlanta, 1989, p 29.
6. Backinger C: Personal service workers: A critical link in the AIDS education chain? AIDS Education Prevention 1:31, 1989.
7. Gershon RM, Vlahov D, Nelson KE: HIV infection risk to nonhealth-care workers. Am Ind Hyg Assoc J 51:A807, 1990.
8. Charbonnier AS, Mallet F, Fiers MM, et al: Detection of HIV-specific DNA sequences in epidermal Langerhans cells infected in vitro by means of a cell-free system. Arch Dermatol Res 287:36, 1994.
9. Henry M, Uthman A, Ballaun C, et al. Epidermal Langerhans cells of AIDS patients express HIV-1 regulatory and structural genes. J Invest Dermatol 103:593, 1994.
10. Mahoney S, Duvic M, Nickoloff BJ, et al: HIV transcripts identified in HIV related psoriasis and Kaposi's sarcoma lesions. J Clin Invest 88:174, 1991.
11. Schmitt D, Dezutter-Dambuyant C. Epidermal and mucosal dendritic cells and HIV1 infection. Pathol Res Pract 190:955, 1994.
12. Root-Bernstein R. Rethinking AIDS: The Tragic Cost of Premature Consensus. p 63. The Free Press, New York, 1993, p 63.

Appendix 6
TREATMENT

GENERAL FORM TO MODIFY FOR NAIL TREATMENT ACCORDING TO THE PATIENT

Your doctor has diagnosed a nail disorder, which he will discuss with you. At times, nail problems may be difficult to treat. Fingernails grow only about 0.1 mm to 0.15 mm a day, and toenails grow about one third that quickly. Therefore, it may take 3 to 6 months for your fingernails to completely regrow or about 9 to 18 months for a toenail to completely regrow. Different nails grow at different rates, and various factors affect nail growth. So it is important to be patient and expect no fast or miracle cures.

Please pay careful attention to the following items as well as other directions that Dr. Daniel has given you.

1. Keep your hands and feet cool and dry and away from moisture.

2. Wear sheer white cotton gloves underneath vinyl gloves when doing work around moisture or water or when preparing fresh food or using irritants such as strong soaps or cleaning fluids. Be sure the vinyl gloves stay dry inside, and change the cotton gloves frequently. If convenient, try to get someone else to help you with cleaning, washing, or work using irritating substances.

3. Call your doctor if a yeast infection, athlete's foot, "jock itch," or another fungal infection develops and have it promptly treated.

4. Do not pick at or push back your cuticles except as Dr. Daniel recommends.

5. Put _____ under and around your nails as Dr. Daniel will show you _____ times a day for_____ days.

6. Use only _____ to wash your hands or bathe with.

7. Do not clean far back under your nails because this may cause them to separate from the underlying nail bed.

8. Keep your nails cut back as short as possible without cutting or damaging the underlying nail bed.

9. Do not bite, pick, or tear at your nails.

10. Use nothing on your nails, such as nail cosmetics.

11. Do not use nail hardeners of any kind. Especially avoid formaldehyde or preparations with toluene-sulfonamide-formalin resin.

12. Do not wear shoes that are too tight or that have pointed toes.

13. Try not to bump or otherwise traumatize your nails.

Index

Note: Page numbers in *italics* refer to illustrations; those followed by t refer to tables.

ISBN 0-7216-7026-1

90071